A Study Guide for
GLAUCOMA

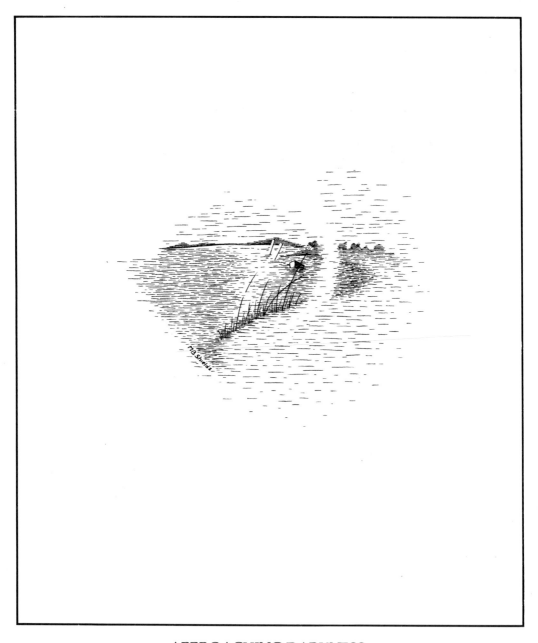

APPROACHING DARKNESS

Twilight along a Carolina shoreline
is superimposed on visual field defects of
glaucoma. Unlike the setting of the sun,
however, for the person who goes blind from
glaucoma, the dawn never comes.

A STUDY GUIDE FOR
GLAUCOMA

M. Bruce Shields, M. D.
Associate Professor of Ophthalmology
Duke University Medical Center
Durham, North Carolina

Drawings by:
Robert L. Blake, Sr.
Associate in Medical Art, Duke University
Durham, North Carolina

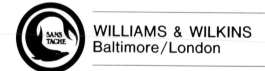

WILLIAMS & WILKINS
Baltimore/London

Library of Congress Cataloging in Publication Data

Shields, M. Bruce
    A study guide for glaucoma.
    Bibliography: p.
    Includes index.
    1. Glaucoma—Outlines, syllabi, etc. I. Title.
[DNLM: 1. Glaucoma. WW 290 S555s]
RE871.S447   617.7′41   81-13124
ISBN 0-683-07691-4   AACR2

Composed and printed at the
Waverly Press, Inc.
Mt. Royal and Guilford Aves.
Baltimore, MD 21202, U.S.A.

To
Sharon, Sarah, and John

PREFACE

The primary intent of this book is to provide an introduction to the subject of glaucoma, as well as a framework on which to expand the study of that discipline. The content of the text has been organized in modified outline form to facilitate its use as a study guide. Presentation of the material begins with the most fundamental aspects of glaucoma and builds on successive levels of knowledge. In keeping with the simplicity of the format, illustrations have been limited to schematic line drawings and are used only where they are felt to clarify material in the text.

A moderately extensive bibliography has also been included in the study guide, and it is hoped that this may serve at least two purposes. First, it provides the student with a reading list from which he can select material for more detailed study of specific subjects on glaucoma. In addition, it may be of value to the practitioner as a reference source to help him stay abreast of the current concepts regarding the diagnosis and management of the glaucomas. Along with the classic literature on glaucoma, an effort has been made to provide an up-to-date bibliography, insofar as this is possible for a field of medicine in which knowledge is expanding so rapidly.

A valid criticism of this study guide will be the confusion created by attempting to present more than one viewpoint on many issues. However, the complex nature of glaucoma is such that many questions remain unanswered, and the best one can do in these areas is to become familiar with the leading theories. With a few exceptions, an effort has been made to avoid imposing the author's bias into this text, but rather to present, as objectively as possible, the various schools of thought in areas where controversy exists.

It is in no way intended that this study guide should compete with the many excellent textbooks that are currently available on the various aspects of glaucoma. Rather, it is hoped that this book may supplement the others by filling what is felt to be a need for a study guide and limited reference source on glaucoma. During the course of initial study, or in refreshing oneself on this subject, both student and practitioner are urged to take full advantage of the wealth of outstanding textbooks on glaucoma, most of which are referenced throughout this study guide.

ACKNOWLEDGMENTS

I am deeply indebted to a large number of talented and thoughtful people who helped me in many ways during the preparation of this text. To each of these individuals I wish to express my most sincere gratitude.

The collection and organization of reference materials used in this study guide was started during my time with W. Morton Grant at the Massachusetts' Eye and Ear Infirmary. I am grateful to Dr. Grant for allowing access to his files and for the excellent teaching he and his staff provided.

The first several drafts of this book were prepared as outlines to accompany a series of lectures given to the residents at the Duke University Eye Center. The concept of developing this material into a study guide for publication was prompted by the kind words and encouragement of the Duke residents and senior staff. I am very indebted to all of these individuals, and especially to Robert Machemer, who urged me to embark on the project and was a strong source of support throughout its preparation.

The following experts kindly agreed to critically review preliminary drafts of certain chapters in this study guide (specific chapters noted in parentheses). Their helpful comments and suggestions were invaluable in preparing the final draft of each chapter.

A. Robert Bellows	Boston, Mass.	(30, 32, 33, 34)
Richard F. Brubaker	Rochester, Minn.	(2, 3)
David G. Campbell	Atlanta, Ga.	(12, 13, 17)
David L. Epstein	Boston, Mass.	(13, 14, 16)
Keith Green	Augusta, Ga.	(22, 27, 28, 29)
B. Thomas Hutchinson	Boston, Mass.	(30, 31, 32, 35)
Michael Kahn	Boston, Mass.	(13, 14, 16)
Gordon K. Klintworth	Durham, N. Car.	(10, 11, 12)
Marvin L. Kwitko	Montreal, Canada	(9, 10)
William E. Layden	Tampa, Fla.	(14, 18, 19)
Alan I. Mandell	Memphis, Tenn.	(26, 27, 28, 29)
Samuel D. McPherson, Jr.	Durham, N. Car.	(31, 33, 34, 35)
Arthur H. Neufeld	Boston, Mass.	(23, 24, 25, 26)
Charles D. Phelps	Iowa City, Iowa	(7, 15)
Irvin P. Pollack	Baltimore, Md.	(7, 8)
Harry A. Quigley	Baltimore, Md.	(4, 5)
Robert Ritch	New York, N. Y.	(20, 21, 22)
Richard J. Simmons	Boston, Mass.	(17, 18, 19)
George L. Spaeth	Philadelphia, Pa.	(4, 5)
E. Michael Van Buskirk	Portland, Ore.	(2, 3)
David S. Walton	Boston, Mass.	(9, 10, 11)

Martin Wand   Hartford, Conn.   (8, 15, 20, 21)
Myron Yanoff   Philadelphia, Pa.   (11, 12, 16)
Thom J. Zimmerman   New Orleans, La.   (23, 24, 25, 26)

I was extremely fortunate to receive the highly professional and conscientious assistance of the following individuals: Robert L. Blake, medical illustration; Margaret L. Hayes, manuscript typing; David L. Smith, library research, and Lori S. Fields and Pamela S. Weinert, secretarial assistance. I also wish to thank the publishers, Williams & Wilkins, and especially Barbara C. Tansill for her invaluable help.

CONTENTS

SECTION THREE: PHARMACOLOGY AND SURGERY FOR GLAUCOMA

Chapter 1

AN OVERVIEW OF GLAUCOMA

I. THE SIGNIFICANCE OF GLAUCOMA

Glaucoma is a leading cause of irreversible blindness in the United States. Based on an evaluation of government and commercial statistics, the prevalence of the disease was estimated to be approximately 1.4 million in this country in 1977.[1] Although the condition more commonly afflicts the elderly, it occurs in all segments of our society with significant health and economic consequences. The 1977 figures suggest that over $400 million was spent that year in direct treatment costs for glaucoma, and that another $1.9 billion was lost in productive work time.[1] Although these figures are undoubtedly limited by considerable sampling error, they provide an appreciation for the significance of glaucoma as a major public health problem.

II. A DEFINITION OF GLAUCOMA

A. A Group of Diseases

The most fundamental fact concerning glaucoma is that it is *not a single disease process.* Rather, it is a large group of disorders that are characterized by widely diverse clinical and histopathologic manifestations. This point is not commonly appreciated by the general public, or even by a portion of the medical community, which frequently leads to confusion. For example, a patient may have difficulty understanding why she has no symptoms with her glaucoma when a friend experienced sudden pain and redness with a disease of the same name. Again, a family physician may advise his patient not to use cold medications because the package insert cautions against it in patients with glaucoma, but fails to explain that this is only for certain types of glaucoma. In Section Two of this study guide, we will consider the many forms of glaucoma and the clinical and histopathologic features by which they are characterized.

B. The Common Denominators

If we were to attempt a definition that would encompass all the glaucomas, it might be "those situations in which *the intraocular pressure* is too high for the normal functioning of *the optic nerve head."* This definition, however, is a gross oversimplification of a highly complex and only partially understood discipline of medicine.

1

For example, we do not know what level of intraocular pressure will lead to glaucomatous damage in every case, nor do we fully understand the mechanism by which the optic atrophy occurs. We do know, however, that the damage to the optic nerve head is associated with progressive loss of *the visual field*, and it is this which, if untreated, can lead to total, irreversible blindness. It is these three common denominators (intraocular pressure, the optic nerve head, and the visual field) that provide the basis for our understanding of all forms of glaucoma. In Section One, these parameters will be discussed as they relate in general to the study of glaucoma.

III. THE PREVENTION OF BLINDNESS FROM GLAUCOMA

Once the blindness of glaucoma has occurred, there is no known treatment that will restore the lost vision. However, in nearly all cases, blindness from glaucoma is *preventable.* This prevention requires *early detection* and *proper treatment.* Detection depends on the ability to recognize the early clinical manifestations of the various glaucomas, while appropriate treatment requires an understanding of the pathogenetic mechanisms involved, as well as a detailed knowledge of the drugs and surgical procedures that are used to control the intraocular pressure. The clinical manifestations and the mechanisms of glaucoma are considered in Sections One and Two, while therapeutic modalities will be the subject of Section Three.

Reference

1. Roden, DR: The prevalence and cost of glaucoma. *In* Glaucoma Detection and Treatment. Proceedings of the First National Glaucoma Conference, Sponsored by the National Society to Prevent Blindness, Tarpon Springs, FL, 1980, p 20.

Section One

The Basic Features of Glaucoma

Chapter 2

AQUEOUS HUMOR DYNAMICS

AQUEOUS HUMOR DYNAMICS

The study of glaucoma deals primarily with the consequences of elevated intraocular pressure (IOP). A logical place to begin this study, therefore, is with the physiologic factors that control IOP, which are the dynamics of aqueous humor flow.

I. HOW AQUEOUS HUMOR DYNAMICS INFLUENCE INTRAOCULAR PRESSURE

To reduce a highly complex, and only partially understood, situation to its simplest form, IOP is a function of the rate at which aqueous humor enters the eye (inflow) and the rate at which it leaves the eye (outflow). When inflow equals outflow, a *steady state* exists, and the IOP remains constant.

Inflow is related to the rate of aqueous humor production, while outflow depends on the resistance to the flow of aqueous from the eye and the pressure in the episcleral veins. The control of IOP, therefore, is a function of: 1) production of aqueous humor; 2) resistance to aqueous humor outflow; 3) episcleral venous pressure.

The remainder of this chapter deals with these three parameters and their complex interrelationship with the IOP.

II. AN OVERVIEW OF THE ANATOMY

Aqueous humor is involved with virtually all portions of the eye, although the two main structures related to aqueous humor dynamics are the *ciliary body*, the site of aqueous production, and the *limbus*, the principal site of aqueous outflow. The step-wise construction of a schematic model, as shown in Fig. 2.1, illustrates the close relationship between these two structures and the surrounding anatomy. (The histology related to aqueous production and outflow is discussed later in this chapter, and the dimensions that are important in surgical procedures are considered in Section Three.)

1. *The limbus* is the transition zone between the cornea and the sclera. On the inner surface of the limbus is an indentation, the *scleral sulcus*, which has a sharp posterior margin, the *scleral spur*, and a sloping anterior wall that extends to the peripheral cornea (Fig. 2.1a).

2. A sieve-like structure, the *trabecular meshwork*, bridges the scleral sulcus and converts it into a tube, called *Schlemm's canal*. Where the meshwork inserts into the peripheral cornea, a ridge is created, known as *Schwalbe's line*. Schlemm's canal is connected by *intrascleral channels* to the episcleral veins (Fig. 2.1b).

The trabecular meshwork, Schlemm's canal, and the intrascleral channels comprise the main route of aqueous humor outflow.

3. *The ciliary body* attaches to the scleral spur and creates a potential space, the *supraciliary space*, between itself and the sclera.

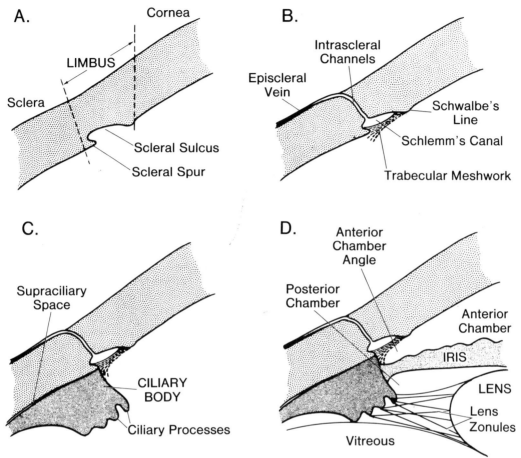

Figure 2.1. Step-wise construction of a schematic model depicts the relationship of structures involved in aqueous humor dynamics: **A:** Limbus; **B:** Main route of aqueous outflow; **C:** Ciliary body (site of aqueous production); **D:** Iris and lens.

On cross-section, the ciliary body has the shape of a right triangle, and the *ciliary processes* (the actual site of aqueous production) occupy the innermost and anteriormost portion of this structure, extending back for approximately 2 mm in the region called the *pars plicata* (or corona ciliaris). The posterior 4 mm of the ciliary body, the *pars plana* (or orbicularis ciliaris), has a flatter inner surface and joins the choroid at the ora serrata (Fig. 2.1c).

    4. *The iris* inserts into the anterior side of the ciliary body, leaving a variable width of the latter structure visible between the root of the iris and scleral spur. *The lens* is suspended from the ciliary body by zonules and separates the vitreous, posteriorly, from the aqueous, anteriorly. The iris separates the aqueous compartment into a posterior and an anterior chamber, and the angle formed by the iris and the cornea is called the anterior chamber angle (Fig. 2.1d).

    Thus, aqueous humor is produced by the ciliary processes and first enters the posterior chamber. It then passes forward, through the pupil, to the anterior chamber, where it leaves the eye by way of structures in the anterior chamber angle.

III. PRODUCTION OF AQUEOUS HUMOR

A. Histology of the Ciliary Body

The ciliary body is one of three portions of the uveal tract, or vascular layer of the eye. The other two structures in this system are the iris and choroid. The ciliary body measures 6 mm from the scleral spur to the ora serrata and is composed of 1) muscle, 2) vascular stroma, and 3) epithelium (Fig. 2.2):

1. *The ciliary muscle* consists of two main portions, the longitudinal and the circular fibers:

a. It is the *longitudinal fibers* which attach the ciliary body to the limbus at the *scleral spur.* The muscle then runs posteriorly to insert into the *suprachoroidal lamina* (fibers connecting choroid and sclera) as far back as the equator or beyond.

b. *The circular fibers* occupy the anterior and inner portion of the ciliary body and run parallel to the limbus.

c. A third portion of the ciliary muscle has been described as *radial fibers*, which connect the longitudinal and circular fibers.

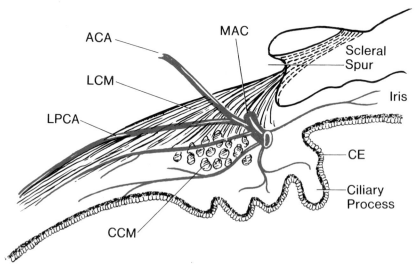

Figure 2.2. The ciliary body has three major components. (1) The ciliary muscle is primarily composed of longitudinal (**LCM**) and circular (**CCM**) fibers. (2) The vascular system is formed by branches of the anterior ciliary arteries (**ACA**) and long posterior ciliary arteries (**LPCA**). These vessels are shown forming the major arterial circle (**MAC**) in accordance with traditional teaching, although recent studies suggest that the major circle is supplied exclusively by the long posterior ciliary arteries.[1] (3). The ciliary epithelium (**CE**) is composed of an inner pigmented and an outer non-pigmented layer.

2. *The vascular stroma* of the ciliary body may be considered in two parts:

a. *The major arterial circle* lies in connective tissue stroma medial and anterior to the circular portion of the ciliary muscle. Traditional teaching holds that this vascular system is formed by anastomoses between the long posterior ciliary and the anterior ciliary arteries. However, scanning electron microscopic studies of plastic casts of human ocular microcirculation indicate that the major arterial circle is formed exclusively by paralimbal branches of the long posterior ciliary arteries.[1] The anterior ciliary arteries send branches to the iris and ciliary body, but the major arterial circle appears to be the main source of blood supply to both of these structures.

b. *The ciliary processes* consist of approximately 70 radial ridges composed of a capillary network and thin stroma covered by epithelium. Several precapillary arterioles from the major arterial circle supply each ciliary process. Sphincters have been noted in these arterioles just after they leave the major circle, and it has been suggested that they may influence aqueous humor production by regulating blood flow into the ciliary processes.[1] The precapillary arterioles break up into a plexus of interanastomosing capillaries within the ciliary processes and then drain predominantly into the pars plana veins.[1]

3. Two layers of *epithelium*, an outer *pigmented* and an inner *nonpigmented* layer, line the inner surface of the ciliary processes and the pars plana.

B. Ultrastructure of the Ciliary Processes

Each ciliary process is composed of *three basic components*; capillaries, stroma, and epithelia (Fig. 2.3):

1. The network of *capillaries* occupy the center of each process and are composed of[2]:

a. Very thin *endothelium* with fenestrae, or false "pores," which represent areas of absent cytoplasm with fusion of the plasma membranes, and which may be the site of increased permeability.

b. *A basement membrane* surrounding the endothelium.

c. *Mural cells*, or pericytes, within the basement membrane.

2. A very thin *stroma* surrounds the capillary network and separates it from the epithelial layers. The stroma is composed of[2]:

a. *Ground substance*, consisting of mucopolysaccharides, proteins, and solute of plasma (except those of large molecular size).

b. A very few collagen connective tissue fibrils.

c. Wandering cells of connective tissue and blood origin.

3. *Two layers of epithelium* surround the stroma, with the apical surfaces of the two cell layers in apposition to each other (Fig. 2.4)[2-5]:

a. *Pigmented epithelium* comprises the outer layer, adjacent to the stroma. These cells are low cuboidal and are characterized by numerous *melanin granules* in the cytoplasm and an atypical basement membrane on the stromal side.

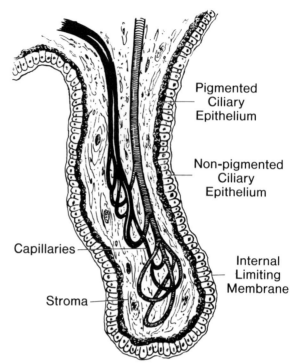

Pigmented
Ciliary
Epithelium

Non-pigmented
Ciliary
Epithelium

Capillaries

Internal
Limiting
Membrane

Stroma

Figure 2.3. A ciliary process is composed of three elements: (1) capillaries; (2) thin stroma; and (3) two layers of epithelium.

b. *Non-pigmented epithelium* makes up the inner layer, adjacent to the aqueous in the posterior chamber. The cells of this layer are columnar and have the following characteristics.

(1). The *basement membrane* is composed of fibrils in a glycoprotein. This membrane, which faces the aqueous, is also called the *internal limiting membrane* and fuses with the lens zonules.

(2). Numerous *mitochondria* are seen in the *cytoplasm*, along with poorly developed rough and smooth endoplasmic reticulum, and a scant amount of ribosomes. Rows of vesicles near the free surface, called "pinocytic vesicles," are seen only with osmium tetroxide fixation and are felt to represent artifactual tubules cut on end.[3]

(3). *The nucleus* has a nucleolus that appears to contain ribosomes.

(4). *The cell membrane* is 200 Å thick and is characterized by *infoldings* or interdigitations, especially surface infoldings on the free surface and lateral interdigitations, which are actually different cuts of the same structure. Na^+K^+-*activated ATPase* is located near the lateral interdigitations.

(5). A variety of *intercellular junctions* have been described which connect adjacent cells within each epithelial layer, as well as the apical surfaces of the two layers.[6] Tight junctions create a perme-

Posterior Chamber

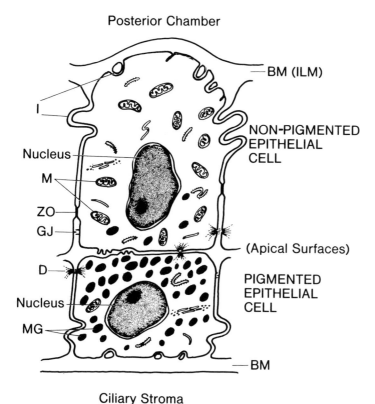

Ciliary Stroma

Figure 2.4. The two layers of ciliary epithelium are arranged with their apical surfaces in apposition to each other. Basement membrane (**BM**) lines the double cell layer and constitutes the internal limiting membrane (**ILM**) on the inner surface. The non-pigmented epithelium is characterized by mitochondria (**M**), zonula occludens (**ZO**), and lateral and surface interdigitations (**I**), while the pigmented epithelium contains numerous melanin granules (**MG**). Other intercellular junctions include desmosomes (**D**) and gap junctions (**GJ**).

ability barrier between the non-pigmented epithelial cells, which forms part of the *blood-aqueous barrier.* These tight junctions are said to be the "leaky" type, in contrast to the "non-leaky" type in the blood-retinal barrier, and may be the main diffusional pathways for water and ion flow.[7]

    c. Microvilli separate the two layers of epithelial cells. In addition, "ciliary channels" have been described as spaces between the two epithelial layers. They are felt to be related to the formation of aqueous humor, since they develop between the fourth and sixth months of gestation, corresponding to the start of aqueous production.[8]

C. Theories of Aqueous Humor Production

    1. Aqueous humor appears to be derived from *plasma* within the capillary network of the ciliary processes. To reach the posterior

chamber, therefore, the various constituents of aqueous must traverse the three tissue layers of the ciliary processes; *i.e.*, the capillary wall, stroma, and epithelia. The principal barrier to transport across these tissues is the *cell membrane* and related junctional complexes, and substances appear to pass through this structure by one of *three mechanisms*[9]:

a. *Diffusion*. Lipid-soluble substances are transported through the lipid portions of the membrane proportional to a concentration gradient across the membrane.

b. *Ultrafiltration*. Water and water-soluble substances (limited by size and charge) flow through theoretical "micropores" in the protein of the cell membrane in response to an osmotic gradient or hydrostatic pressure.

c. *Active transfer* (secretion). Water-soluble substances of larger size or greater charge are actively transported across the cell membrane. This mechanism is believed to be mediated by globular proteins in the membrane and requires the expenditure of energy.

2. All three transport mechanisms are probably involved in aqueous production, possibly in accordance with the following *simplified three-part scheme*:

a. Tracer studies suggest that most *plasma* substances pass easily from the capillaries of the ciliary processes, across the stroma, and between the pigmented epithelial cells before accumulating behind the tight junctions of the non-pigmented epithelium.[10, 11] This movement takes place primarily by *ultrafiltration*, and drugs that alter ciliary perfusion may exert their influence on intraocular pressure at this level.[12]

b. The tight junctions between the non-pigmented epithelial cells create part of the blood-aqueous barrier, and certain substances appear to be *actively transported* across this barrier into the posterior chamber, thereby establishing an osmotic gradient. Substances that are involved in active transport include:

(1). *Sodium*. There is a specific secretory pump for sodium,[13, 14] and approximately 70% of this electrolyte is actively transported into the posterior chamber,[15] while the remainder enters by passive ultrafiltration[9] or diffusion.[15] The active transport of sodium is ATPase-dependent,[16] but does not appear to be related to the concentration of sodium in the plasma.[17]

(2). *Chloride*. A much smaller percentage of the chloride ion is actively transported, and this appears to be dependent on the presence of sodium, as well as pH.[18, 19]

(3). *Potassium* is transported by secretion and diffusion.[20]

(4). *Ascorbic acid* is secreted against a large concentration gradient.[15]

(5). *Amino acids* are secreted by at least three carriers.[21]

(6). *Bicarbonate*. The rapid interconversion between bicarbonate and CO_2, which is catalyzed by *carbonic anhydrase*, makes it difficult to determine the relative proportions of these two substances.

However, bicarbonate formation has been shown to influence fluid transport through its effect on sodium,[22] possibly by regulating the pH for optimum active transport of sodium.[9]

c. *The osmotic gradient* across the ciliary epithelium, which results from the active transport of the above substances, leads to the movement of other plasma constituents by ultrafiltration and diffusion. There is evidence that *sodium* is the ion primarily responsible for the movement of water into the posterior chamber.[13, 23]

3. *The precise location* of aqueous humor production appears to be predominantly in the anterior portion of the pars plicata along the tips or crests of the ciliary processes, and the site of active transport is in the non-pigmented epithelial cells probably in the cell membrane of the lateral interdigitations. The following observations support this concept.

a. *The anterior portion of the pars plicata* has 1) increased basal and lateral interdigitations, mitochondria, and rough endoplasmic reticulum in the non-pigmented ciliary epithelium, 2) more numerous fenestrations in the capillary endothelium and 3) a thinner layer of ciliary stroma.[24]

b. When sodium fluorescein is administered systemically and the ciliary body is observed with a special gonioprism, fluorescein-stained aqueous is seen primarily at the *tips of the ciliary processes.*[25] In addition, an increase in cell organelles, fenestrations of capillary endothelium, and gap junctions between pigmented and non-pigmented epithelia has been observed at the *crests* of the ciliary processes.[26]

c. Evidence of active transport in the *non-pigmented epithelial cells*, especially in the cell membrane of the lateral interdigitations, comes from observations of the following in these areas:

(1). Abundant Na^+K^+-*activated ATPase.*

(2). Higher specific activity for glycolytic enzymes.[27]

(3). Preferential incorporation of labeled sulfate into macromolecules (primarily glycolipids and glycoproteins).[28, 29]

D. Rate of Aqueous Humor Production

1. **Values.** The rate at which aqueous humor is formed (inflow) is measured in microliters per minute. The actual volume in the human eye varies somewhat according to the measurement technique used. A figure of approximately 2.0 μl/min is generally quoted,[15] although fluorophotometric studies, which may provide the most reliable estimates, give a value of approximately *2.5 μl/min* in the undisturbed human eye.[30]

2. **Measurement techniques.** Tonography will be discussed in detail later in this chapter. The following is a brief overview of some of the more direct ways of estimating the rate of aqueous production:

a. *Fluorescein* techniques involve instillation of fluorescein into the anterior chamber by iontophoresis with subsequent measurement of either 1) the flow of unstained aqueous from the posterior to anterior chamber using *photogrammetric* methods[31] or 2) the change in concentration of fluorescein in the anterior chamber by *fluorophotometry.* [30, 32–35]

b. *Radioactive-labeled isotopes* have been used to measure inflow in animals by observing either 1) the *accumulation* of the isotope in the anterior chamber[36] or 2) *the decay rate* of the intracamerally injected isotope.[37]

c. *Perfusion* of eyes at a constant pressure can also be used to determine the inflow in animals.[38]

3. Many factors influence the rate of aqueous production, including the following:

a. *Intraocular pressure*

(1). *An elevation* of intraocular pressure is associated with a decline in aqueous production, which is referred to as *pseudofacility.* [39–45]

(2). *A decrease* in intraocular pressure may be associated with a transient increase in aqueous production.[43]

b. *Age.* Fluorophotometric studies agree with the traditional concept that aqueous production decreases with age,[30] although the degree of this change is less than previously thought.[46] The formation of aqueous humor is actually much more stable than the intraocular pressure or anterior chamber volume with respect to aging changes.[30]

c. *Inflammation* (uveitis) causes a *decrease* in inflow,[47, 48] possibly related to a disruption in ciliary epithelium.[49]

d. *Retinal detachment* is commonly associated with a reduction in the intraocular pressure. Whether this is due to a decrease in aqueous production, as has been suggested,[50] or an increase in aqueous outflow by an unconventional, posterior route, has yet to be determined.

e. Pharmacologic agents that reduce inflow are discussed in Section Three.

IV. FUNCTION AND COMPOSITION OF AQUEOUS HUMOR

A. Function[15, 21, 51]

In addition to its role in maintaining a proper intraocular pressure, aqueous humor has important metabolic requirements in providing substrates and removing metabolites from the avascular cornea and lens. For example, the cornea takes glucose and oxygen from the aqueous and releases lactic acid and a small amount of carbon dioxide into the aqueous.[15, 51] The lens also uses glucose and generates lactate and pyruvate.[15] In addition, it is reported that potassium and amino acids in the aqueous may be taken up by the lens, while sodium moves from the lens to the aqueous.[21] The metabolism of the vitreous and retina also appears to be associated with the aqueous humor in that substances such as amino acids and glucose pass into the vitreous from the aqueous.[15, 21]

B. Composition

From the above discussion, it may be seen that the composition of aqueous humor depends not only on the nature of its production, but also on the constant metabolic interchanges that occur throughout its intraocular course. However, close similarities in aqueous composition between the phakic and aphakic eye of the same individual suggest that lens metabolism has practically no influence on the composition of aqueous.[52] Diffusional exchange across the iris may be a more significant factor in the changing composition of the aqueous between the posterior and anterior chambers. Studies in rabbit eyes indicate that the total concentration of dissolved substances, pH, and osmotic pressure are the same in the posterior and anterior chambers, while the actual composition of the aqueous in the two chambers is different.[53] This difference appears to be related to active transport in the posterior chamber and passive transfer in the anterior chamber, where the iris vessels are permeable to anions and nonelectrolytes.[53]

The following statements describe only the general character of aqueous humor, expressed *relative to plasma*[51-57]:

1. Aqueous of both the anterior and posterior chamber is slightly *hypertonic* compared to plasma.

2. Aqueous is *acidic*, with a pH in the anterior chamber of 7.2.[55]

3. The two most striking characteristics of aqueous humor are:

a. A marked *excess* of *ascorbate*, which is fifteen times greater than that of arterial plasma.

b. A marked *deficit* of *protein* (0.02% in aqueous as compared to 7% in plasma). The albumin/globulin ratio is the same as plasma, although there is less gamma globulin. Human aqueous has been found to contain IgG, but no IgD, IgA, or IgM.[58] Protein and antibodies in the aqueous equilibrate with those in plasma to form a *plasmoid aqueous* under certain circumstances, including:

(1). *Uveitis.* Rabbit studies suggest the increased aqueous protein may come from proliferating blood vessels in the posterior chamber and vitreous and from disrupted, scarred ciliary epithelium.[49]

(2). *Paracentesis.* Following aspiration of aqueous, the newly formed fluid has a high protein content, which is suggested by monkey studies to result from[59, 60]:

(a). Blood reflux into Schlemm's canal with new gaps in the inner wall endothelial lining.

(b). Enlarged extracellular spaces in the ciliary epithelium of the anterior pars plicata.

4. The relative concentrations of free *amino acids* in the human aqueous varies, with aqueous/plasma concentrations ranging from 0.08 to 3.14; supporting the concept of active transport of amino acids.[61]

5. The concentrations of most other ions and nonelectrolytes are very close to those in the plasma, and conflicting statements in the literature primarily represent differences with regard to species and measurement techniques. In general, human aqueous has a slight excess of chloride and a deficiency of bicarbonate.[55, 56] However, several factors lead to rapid changes in aqueous bicarbonate levels,

and the concentrations measured may not accurately reflect the relative concentration of bicarbonate transported by the ciliary epithelia. Lactic acid is reported to be in relative excess in human aqueous[56]; however, this determination varies widely with the technique of measurement.[62] Glucose[56] and sodium[54] show a relative deficiency in the aqueous, although the later is based on rabbit studies.[54] The total CO_2 content in aqueous has considerable species variation, with a deficiency in man.[63]

V. AQUEOUS OUTFLOW

A. Histology of the Aqueous Outflow System

1. *Scleral Spur-roll.* The posterior wall of the scleral sulcus is formed by a group of fibers, the *scleral roll*, which run parallel to the limbus and project inward to form the *scleral spur* (Fig. 2.1).[64] The scleral spur-roll is composed of 75 to 80% collagen and 5% elastic tissue.[65] It has been suggested that this circular structure prevents the ciliary muscle from causing Schlemm's canal to collapse.[64]

2. *Schwalbe's line.* Just anterior to the apical portion of the trabecular meshwork is a smooth area, which varies in width from 50 μ to 150 μ and has been called *Zone S.*[66] The anterior border of this zone is represented by the transition from trabecular to corneal endothe-

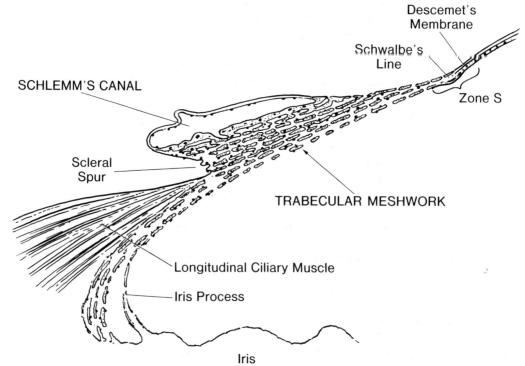

Figure 2.5. The trabecular meshwork extends from iris, ciliary body, and scleral spur to the sloping anterior wall of the scleral sulcus, converting the latter structure into Schlemm's canal.

lium and the thinning and termination of Descemet's membrane. The posterior border is demarcated by a discontinuous elevation, Schwalbe's line, that appears to be formed by the oblique insertion of uveal trabeculae into limbal stroma.[66]

3. *Trabecular meshwork* (Figs. 2.5 and 2.6). As previously discussed, the scleral sulcus is converted into a circular channel, Schlemm's canal, by the trabecular meshwork. This tissue consists of a connective tissue core surrounded by endothelium, and may be divided into *three portions.*[66, 67] (The ultrastructural details of these tissues will be considered later in this chapter.)

a. *The uveal meshwork*, the portion adjacent to the aqueous in the anterior chamber, is arranged in bands or rope-like trabeculae that extend from the iris root and ciliary body to the peripheral cornea. It is felt to be the oblique insertion of these trabecular bands into underlying limbal stroma that gives rise to the previously discussed Schwalbe's line.[66] The arrangement of the trabecular bands creates irregular openings that vary in size from 25 μ to 75 μ across.[67]

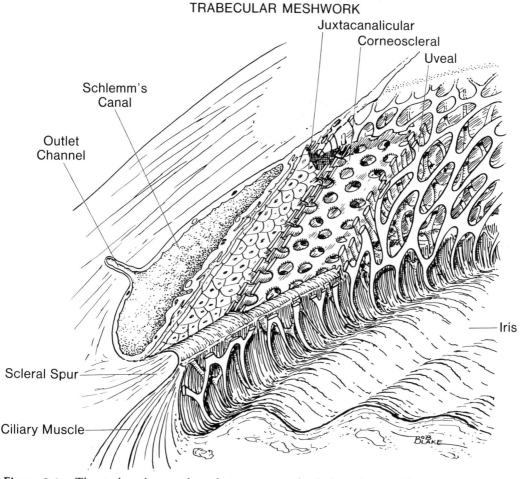

TRABECULAR MESHWORK

Figure 2.6. The trabecular meshwork is composed of three layers (shown in cut-away views): (1) uveal; (2) corneoscleral; and (3) juxtacanalicular.

b. *The corneoscleral meshwork* extends from the scleral spur to the lateral wall of the scleral sulcus and consists of sheets of trabeculae that are perforated by elliptical openings. These holes become progressively smaller as the trabecular sheets approach Schlemm's canal, with a range of 5 μ to 50 μ in diameter.[67]

c. *The juxtacanalicular tissue*[68] is the outermost portion of the meshwork (adjacent to Schlemm's canal) and consists of a layer of connective tissue lined on either side by endothelium. The outer endothelial layer comprises the inner wall of Schlemm's canal, while the inner layer is continuous with the remainder of the trabecular endothelium.

4. *Schlemm's canal* is an endothelial-lined channel averaging 190 to 370 μ in diameter.[69, 70] It may be a single channel, but occasionally branches into a plexus-like system.

5. *Intrascleral channels.* Schlemm's canal is connected to episcleral and conjunctival veins by a complex system of vessels (Fig. 2.7):

a. Intrascleral aqueous vessels, the *aqueous veins of Ascher,*[71] have been defined as originating at the outer wall of Schlemm's canal and terminating in episcleral and conjunctival veins in a laminated

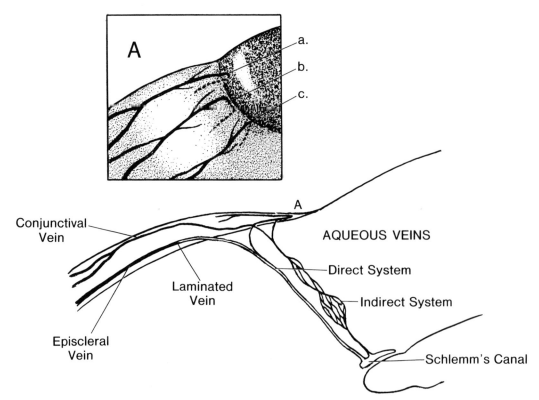

Figure 2.7. Intrascleral channels drain aqueous by direct and indirect (plexus) systems from Schlemm's canal to episcleral and conjunctival veins. Inset (A) shows three courses of anteriorly-directed veins: **a:** short course into cornea, **b:** short course parallel to limbus (most common pattern), and **c:** sharp loop at limbus.

junction, referred to as the "laminated vein of Goldmann."[72] However, others refer to the proximal portion of these vessels as "outflow channels"[70, 73] or "collector channels,"[69] since the structural pattern of the outer wall of Schlemm's canal extends into the first third of these channels.[73] The intrascleral vessels are divided into two systems:[69, 70, 73–75]

(1). A direct system. Large caliber vessels run a short intrascleral course and drain directly into the episcleral venous system.

(2). An indirect system. More numerous, finer channels form an intrascleral plexus before eventually draining into the episcleral venous system.

b. The intrascleral aqueous channels do not connect with vessels of the uveal system, except for occasional fine communications with the ciliary muscle.[74–76] There are no arterial communications,[74–76] although arteriovenous anastomotic vessels may occur in the anterior episcleral system.[74–77]

c. The aqueous vessels join the episcleral venous system by several routes[71]:

(1). Most aqueous vessels are directed posteriorly with the majority of these draining into episcleral veins, while a few cross the subconjunctival tissue and drain into conjunctival veins.

(2). Some aqueous vessels proceed anteriorly to the limbus, with most of these running a short course parallel to the limbus before turning posteriorly to conjunctival veins. Other vessels make a sharp loop to join conjunctival veins or rarely extend a short distance into the cornea before turning posteriorly.

6. The episcleral veins drain into the cavernous sinus via the anterior ciliary and superior ophthalmic veins, while the conjunctival veins drain into superior ophthalmic or facial veins via the palpebral and angular veins.[72]

7. Extracanalicular (uveoscleral) outflow pathways. The pathways described above are estimated to account for between 83[78] and 96%[79] of aqueous outflow in human eyes under normal circumstances. The other 5 to 15% of the aqueous leaves the eye by a system, or systems, that have been collectively called "uveoscleral,"[79–81] "uveo-vortex,"[82] "unconventional,"[83] or "secondary"[84] aqueous outflow pathways. The variety of names testifies to our incomplete understanding regarding this segment of the aqueous outflow system. Brubaker (personal communication) suggested the logical terms "canalicular" for the principal outflow pathway, involving Schlemm's canal, and "extracanalicular" for the other channels of aqueous outflow.

Although there is no universal agreement as to the anatomy of the extracanalicular outflow pathways, tracer studies in human[79] and animal[80–84] eyes suggest that the aqueous enters the stroma and vessels of the iris and ciliary body and then moves posteriorly, either in the suprachoroidal or choroidal vessels, to leave the eye through scleral pores surrounding long posterior ciliary arteries and nerves, or in vortex veins or vessels of optic nerve membranes.

B. Ultrastructure of Trabecular Meshwork and Schlemm's Canal

1. *Uveal* and *corneoscleral meshwork.* Although the gross structure of these two trabecular subunits differs, as previously discussed, their ultrastructure is the same. Each trabecular band or sheet is composed of *four concentric layers*[85]:

a. An inner *connective tissue core* is composed of typical collagen fibers, with the usual 640 Å periodicity.[85]

b. *"Elastic"* fibers are actually composed of otherwise typical collagen, arranged in a spiraling pattern with an apparent periodicity of 1,000 Å.[86, 87]

c. Between the spiraling collagen and the basement membrane of the endothelium is a broad zone composed of delicate filaments embedded in a ground substance.[86] This layer has been called a *glass membrane.*[85]

d. An *endothelial layer* provides a continuous covering over the trabeculae. The cells are larger, more irregular, and have less prominent borders than corneal endothelial cells.[66] Characteristics of trabecular endothelium include the following.

(1). *Phagocytic activity.* The cells have been shown to engulf and degrade foreign material,[88] or to engulf debri, detach from the trabecular core, and leave in Schlemm's canal.[89]

(2). *Microfilaments.* Two types of filaments have been found in the cytoplasm of human trabecular endothelium[91]:

(a). *6 nm filaments* are located primarily in the cell periphery, around the nucleus, and in cytoplasmic processes. These appear to be *actin filaments*[91] which are involved in 1) cell contraction and motility, 2) phagocytosis and pinocytosis, and 3) cell adhesion (the possible role in resistance to outflow will be discussed later in this chapter).

(b). *10 nm filaments* are more numerous in the cells and probably play a structural role.

(3). Preliminary reports show that the metabolism of trabecular meshwork tissue can be studied with biochemical techniques,[92] and that trabecular cells can be grown in tissue culture,[93] both of which may be useful approaches to further our understanding of this tissue in normal and disease states.

2. *Juxtacanalicular Tissue.* The portion of the trabecular meshwork adjacent to Schlemm's canal (and which actually makes up the inner wall of the canal) differs histologically from the other parts of the meshwork and has been given various names, depending on how one defines the anatomical limits of the tissue: "juxtacanalicular connective tissue,"[68] "pore tissue,"[67] and "endothelial meshwork."[94] In the broadest sense, this structure has *three layers*,[95] discussed here beginning with the innermost portion (Fig. 2.8).

a. A *trabecular endothelial layer* is continuous with the endothelium of the corneoscleral meshwork and might be considered as a part of this layer.

b. A central *connective tissue layer* of variable thickness is

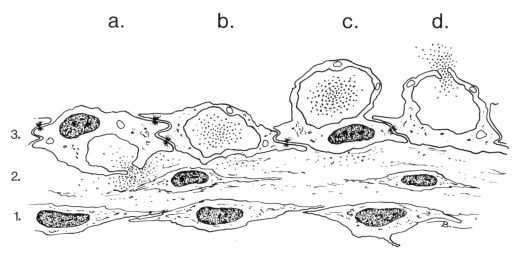

Figure 2.8. The juxtacanalicular portion of the trabecular meshwork, by the broadest definition, is composed of three layers: **1:** Trabecular endothelium, continuous with the corneoscleral meshwork; **2:** a central connective tissue layer; and **3:** the inner wall endothelium of Schlemm's canal. The theory of transcellular aqueous transport is depicted, in which a series of pores and giant vacuoles open on the connective tissue side (**a**), engulf aqueous (**b**), bulge into Schlemm's canal (**c**), and open to release aqueous into the canal (**d**).

unfenestrated and has several layers of parallel, spindle-shaped cells loosely arranged in a connective tissue ground substance.[68, 86, 95]

c. The *inner wall endothelium of Schlemm's canal* is also the outermost portion of the trabecular meshwork, *i.e.*, the last tissue that aqueous must traverse before entering the canal. This endothelial layer has significant morphological characteristics, which distinguish it from the rest of the endothelium in both the trabecular meshwork and in Schlemm's canal.

(1). The *surface is bumpy* due to protruding nuclei,[95] cyst-like vacuoles,[96] and finger-like projections[97] bulging into the canal. Johnstone[97] has shown that the finger-like projections are endothelial tubules with patent lumens, communicating between the anterior chamber and Schlemm's canal. Svedbergh,[98] however, interpreted them as protrusions with no significant openings. Further study will be needed to determine the significance of these structures.

(2). *Actin filaments*, as previously described in uveal and corneoscleral trabecular endothelium, are also present in the inner wall endothelium of Schlemm's canal.[91]

(3). *The intercellular spaces* are 150 to 200 Å wide and the adjacent cells are connected by a variety of intercellular junctions.[86, 95] It is not clear as to how tightly these junctions maintain the intercellular connections, although it has been shown that they will open to permit the passage of red blood cells.[95]

(4). The endothelial cells are anchored by cytoplasmic processes to underlying subendothelial cells and trabecular meshwork.[99]

(5). *Openings* in the endothelial cells have been described by many investigators. Considerable controversy has arisen as to the morphology and function of these structures. In general, the openings consist of *minute pores* and large, or *giant, vacuoles*. The reported sizes of the pores vary considerably, although most are in the range of 0.5 to 2.0 μ.[67, 69, 100-106] Tracer studies have shown that these pores communicate with the intertrabecular spaces and Schlemm's canal.[104, 105] The giant vacuoles in the endothelial cells were once felt to be postmortem artifacts,[107] but numerous studies have confirmed their existence and suggested that they are involved in aqueous outflow.[94, 108-112] It may be that the pores and vacuoles represent different parts of the same transcellular channels.[104] The possible significance of these structures in resistance to aqueous outflow will be discussed later in this chapter.

(6). Sonderman's "canals" are mentioned primarily for historical interest, and because the term may still be found in the literature. Although they were originally described as endothelial-lined channels communicating between the canal and intertrabecular spaces,[113] subsequent studies have variably interpreted them as tortuous communications wandering irregularly and obliquely through the meshwork,[114] deep grooves on cross-section,[94] slit-like spaces between cells,[115, 116] or artifacts.[67] It is unlikely that the structures, if they exist, have a significant role in aqueous outflow.

3. *The Outer Wall of Schlemm's Canal*

a. The *endothelium* of the outer wall is a single cell layer that is continuous with that of the inner wall.[86] The surface is smoother than that of the inner wall and has larger, less numerous cells[117] and no pores,[100, 101] but numerous, large *outlet channels*, as previously described.

b. Torus or lip-like thickenings have been observed around the openings of the outlet channels[70, 73] and septae have been noted to extend from these openings to the inner wall of Schlemm's canal, which presumably help to keep the canal open.[69, 70, 73]

c. The endothelium is separated from the collagenous bundles of the limbus by a basement membrane[86] and layers of fibrocytes and fibroblasts.[73]

C. Normal Resistance to Aqueous Outflow

1. *Trabecular meshwork and Schlemm's canal.* Grant[118, 119] demonstrated that a 360° incision in the trabecular meshwork of nonglaucomatous, enucleated human eyes eliminated 75% of the resistance to aqueous outflow. Whether this resistance is in the meshwork or is due to compression of Schlemm's canal is uncertain, but the following observations have been reported:

a. *Inner wall endothelium of Schlemm's canal.* Studies with tracer elements such as ferritin or thorotrast, suggest free flow through the trabecular spaces and juxtacanalicular connective tissue with heavy accumulation of the tracer on the inner surface of the inner wall endothelium of Schlemm's canal.[95, 104, 105, 110] This endothelial layer, therefore, appears to provide some degree of resistance to outflow, and the mechanism of transport across the layer is only partially understood:

(1). *Pores* and *giant vacuoles* in the inner wall endothelium of Schlemm's canal, as previously discussed, appear to be parts of a transcellular system for aqueous outflow, since tracer elements injected into the anterior chamber are seen in the vacuoles and pores.[95, 104, 105, 110, 120] The observation that the concentration of tracer material in the giant vacuoles is not always the same as in the juxtacanalicular connective tissue[95] suggests a dynamic system in which the vacuoles intermittently open and close to transport aqueous from the juxtacanalicular tissue to Schlemm's canal (Fig. 2.8).[110] Whether this transport is active or passive has been controversial.

(a). Indirect evidence for a *theory of active transport* has included the demonstration of enzymes[121] and electron microscopic structures[122] compatible with an active transport system in or near the endothelial layer.

(b). However, the bulk of evidence supports the *theory of passive (pressure-dependent) transport*, since the number and size of the vacuoles has been shown to increase with progressive elevation of the intraocular pressure.[123-126] Furthermore, this phenomenon is reversible in the enucleated eye,[124] and hypothermia has no effect on the development of the vacuoles in the enucleated eye[127] and only little effect on outflow in the eyes of living rabbits.[128]

It may be, therefore, that potential transcellular spaces exist in the inner wall endothelium of Schlemm's canal, which open as a system of vacuoles and pores, primarily in response to pressure, to transport aqueous from the juxtacanalicular connective tissue to Schlemm's canal (Fig. 2.8). The actual resistance to aqueous outflow provided by this system is unclear, although it has been calculated, based on the estimated size and total number of pores in the inner wall endothelium of Schlemm's canal, that resistance to outflow through the endothelial cells is a small fraction of the total resistance to outflow.[129]

(2). *Contractile microfilaments*, as previously described, occur in the inner wall endothelium of Schlemm's canal, as well as the endothelium lining the trabeculae. Perfusing monkey eyes with substances that are known to disrupt the microfilaments, such as cytochalasin B[130-132] or EDTA,[133, 134] significantly reduces the resistance to aqueous outflow, and histologic studies suggest that this is primarily due to an alteration in the trabecular meshwork or inner wall of Schlemm's canal.[131-134]

(3). *Fibrinolytic activity* has been demonstrated in the endothelium of Schlemm's canal,[135] but no evidence of coagulation factors has been found.[136] This suggests that a hemostatic balance, displaced towards fibrinolysis, protects this portion of the outflow system from occlusion by fibrin and platelets.[135, 136]

b. *Acid mucopolysaccharides* that are sensitive to hyaluronidase have been demonstrated in various portions of the trabecular meshwork.[137-139] In the polymerized form, mucopolysaccharides become hydrated, which may lead to increased resistance to outflow by closure of the trabecular spaces.[139] Enzymes that catabolize mucopolysaccharides have been demonstrated in the meshwork,[140] and these enzymes may be released by lysosomes to depolymerize the mucopolysaccharides, thereby minimizing this cause of resistance to outflow.[139, 140] In support of this theory, perfusion of eyes with hyaluronidase has been shown to increase outflow facility[119, 141] and increase the number of giant vacuoles.[142] In addition, prolonged perfusion of canine eyes caused a gradual increase in outflow facility, apparently due to a "washout" of a hyaluronidase-sensitive component of the barrier to aqueous outflow.[143, 144] However, perfusion studies with enucleated monkey eyes, using a trabeculotomy and hyaluronidase, suggest that resistance by mucopolysaccharides is only slightly related to the trabecular meshwork.[145]

c. *Resistance in Schlemm's Canal.* Once aqueous has entered Schlemm's canal, resistance to continued flow into the intrascleral outlet channels may depend on the spatial configuration of the canal.

(1). There is controversy as to whether the canal is normally entirely open and whether it allows *circumferential flow.* Perfusion studies in enucleated human adult eyes suggest that aqueous cannot flow more than 10° within the canal,[146] although there is less resistance to circumferential flow in infant eyes.[147] However, studies of segmental blood reflux into Schlemm's canal imply that the canal is normally entirely open and that there is circumferential flow.[148]

(2). *Elevation of intraocular pressure* is known to be associated with *increased resistance* to outflow,[149-151] which may be a result of *collapse* of *Schlemm's canal.*[152] Histologic studies of eyes perfused at different pressures suggest that compromise of the canal lumen with elevated intraocular pressure is due to distention of the trabecular meshwork,[153, 154] an increase in endothelial vacuoles,[123-126] and a ballooning of the inner wall endothelial cells into the canal.[99] Perfusion studies also suggest the resistance to aqueous outflow may normally depend in part on an intact, unyielding outer wall of Schlemm's canal, against which the intact inner wall is pressed by the intraocular pressure.[155] However, significant differences in the response to elevated perfusion pressure have been found among different mammalian eyes, and it has been suggested that factors other than, or in addition to, collapse of Schlemm's canal may be important regarding the influence of elevated intraocular pressure on resistance to outflow.[156]

(3). A *reduction in normal resistance* to outflow occurs with a *widening* of *Schlemm's canal.* Moses and Arnzen[157] have described the trabecular meshwork as a three-dimensional set of diagonally crossing collagenous fibers, which respond to a backward, inward displacement with a widening of Schlemm's canal. The effect of this form of traction on the meshwork has been demonstrated with deepening of the anterior chamber during perfusion studies when an iridectomy is not made,[118] posterior depression of the lens,[146, 158] or tension on the choroid.[159]

2. *Intrascleral Outflow Channels.* The remainder of the resistance to aqueous outflow appears to be within the intrascleral outflow channels. One monkey study has suggested the following distribution of resistance[160]:

    a. Trabecular meshwork: 60 to 65%

    b. Inner ⅓ to ½ of sclera: 25%

    c. Outer ½ to ⅔ of sclera: 15%

3. *Episcleral Venous Pressure.* The normal episcleral venous pressure is approximately 9 mmHg. Although this is not considered to be a part of resistance to outflow, it does contribute to the intraocular pressure. The precise interrelationship between episcleral venous pressure and aqueous humor dynamics is complex and only partially understood.

4. *Extracanalicular Outflow.* Unlike the canalicular (or conventional) outflow system, extracanalicular outflow has been reported to improve with an elevation of the intraocular pressure, presumably due to ultrafiltration of aqueous into uveal vessels.[80] It has also been shown that outflow by this route is reduced by miotics.[79] It should be noted that our understanding of the extracanalicular outflow system is based more on physiology than on anatomy, and further study is needed to correlate function and anatomy in this system.

VI. GONIOSCOPY

Gonioscopy is a clinical technique that is used to examine structures in the anterior chamber angle. Gonioscopic assessment is essential both for diagnosing the type of glaucoma and for planning the appropriate therapy, since the treatment for one type of glaucoma may be ineffective or contraindicated in another form. The subject is included in this chapter because of its relevance to the anatomy of aqueous humor dynamics. The present discussion, however, will be limited to technique and normal anatomic findings, while the alterations associated with the various forms of glaucoma will be considered in Section Two.

A. The Principle of Gonioscopy (Fig. 2.9)[161]

1. The *problem* is the *critical angle*

    a. When light passes from a medium with a greater index of refraction (n) to one of a lesser n, the angle of refraction (r) will be larger than the angle of incidence (i). When r equals 90°, i is said to have attained the critical angle. When i exceeds the critical angle, the light is reflected back into the first medium.

    b. The critical angle for the cornea-air interface is approximately 46°. Light rays coming from the anterior chamber angle exceed this critical angle and are, therefore, reflected back into the anterior chamber, preventing visualization of the angle.

2. The *solution* is to *eliminate the cornea* (optically).

Since the n of a contact lens approaches that of the cornea, there is minimal refraction at the interface of these two media, which eliminates the optical effect of the front corneal surface. Therefore,

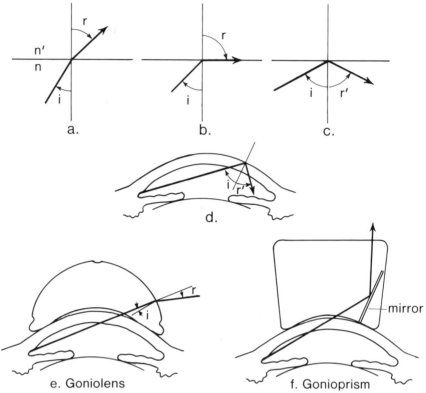

Figure 2.9. Principle of gonioscopy: **a:** Light ray is refracted when angle of incidence (**i**) at interface of two media with different indeces of refraction (**n** and **n'**) is less than the critical angle; **b:** Angle of refraction (**r**) is 90° when **i** equals the critical angle; and **c:** Light is reflected when **i** exceeds the critical angle. **d:** Light from anterior chamber angle exceeds the critical angle at the cornea-air interface and is reflected back into the eye; **e** and **f:** contact lenses have an index of refraction (**n**) similar to that of the cornea, allowing light to enter the lens and then be refracted (goniolens) or reflected (gonioprism) beyond the contact lens-air interface.

light rays from the anterior chamber angle enter the contact lens and are made to pass through the new contact lens-air interface by one of two basic designs[161-163]:

a. In *direct gonioscopy*, the anterior curve of the contact lens (goniolens) is such that the critical angle is not reached, and the light rays are refracted at the contact lens-air interface.

b. In *indirect gonioscopy*, the light rays are reflected by a mirror in the contact lens (gonioprism) and leave the lens at nearly a right angle to the contact lens-air interface.

B. Instruments and Techniques

1. *Historical background.*[162] In 1907, Trantas visualized the angle in an eye with keratoglobus by indenting the limbus and later coined the term, gonioscopy. Salsmann introduced the goniolens in 1914, and Koeppe improved it 5 years later by designing a steeper lens.

Troncoso also contributed to gonioscopy by developing the gonioscope for magnification and illumination of the angle. In 1938, Goldmann introduced the gonioprism, and Barkan established the use of gonioscopy in the management of glaucoma.

2. *Direct gonioscopy*

a. *Instruments*[164]

(1). The *Koeppe lens* is the prototype diagnostic goniolens and is available in different diameters and radii of posterior curvature. Additional types of goniolenses are listed in table one.

(2). A *gonioscope* provides 15 to 20× magnification. It may be hand-held or suspended from the ceiling with counterbalance.

(3). The *light source* is usually a separate hand-held unit, such as the Barkan focal illuminator, although it may be attached to the gonioscope.

b. *Technique.* Direct gonioscopy is performed with the patient in a supine position, preferably on a moveable diagnostic table. After applying a topical anesthetic, the goniolens is positioned on the cornea, using a bridge of balanced salt solution, a viscous preparation, or the patient's own tears.[165] The examiner usually holds the gonioscope in one hand and a light source in the other. Occasionally an assistant may be needed to move the goniolens to the desired position. Alternatively, a gonioscope with mounted light source may be used, which allows the examiner to control the goniolens with his other hand. In either case, the examiner scans the anterior chamber angle by shifting his position until all 360° have been studied.

Table 2.1
Contact Lenses for Gonioscopy

	Lens	Description/Use
I. Goniolenses (Direct Gonioscopy)	1. Koeppe	1. Prototype diagnostic goniolens
	2. Richardson-Shaffer	2. Small Koeppe lens for infants
	3. Barkan	3. Prototype surgical goniolens
	4. Siebeck	4. Tiny goniolens; floats on cornea
	5. Worst	5. Partial vacuum anchors lens to cornea
II. Gonioprisms (Indirect Gonioscopy)	1. Goldmann one-mirror	1. Prototype gonioprism
	2. Goldmann two-mirror	2. Both mirrors same as above
	3. Goldmann three-mirror	3. One mirror for gonioscopy; two for retina
	4. Zeiss four-mirror	4. All mirrors for gonioscopy; fluid bridge not required
	5. Allen-Thorpe	5. Four gonioscopy mirrors; requires fluid bridge between lens and cornea
	6. Worst Lo-Vac	6. Six mirrors; held to cornea by vacuum

3. Indirect Gonioscopy

a. *Instruments.* The gonioprism and a slit lamp are the only instruments needed for indirect gonioscopy. The *Goldmann one-mirror lens* is the prototype gonioprism. The mirror in this lens has a height of 12 mm and the posterior radius of curvature of the gonioprism is 8.15 mm. A large variety of additional gonioprisms are available and are listed in table one.

b. *Technique.* The cornea is anesthetized and, with the patient positioned at the slit lamp, the gonioprism is placed against the cornea with or without a fluid bridge, depending on the posterior radius of curvature of the instrument. The lens is then rotated to allow visualization of all 360° of the angle or the quadrants are studied with the four mirrors. Although visualization of the angle can be enhanced by manipulating the gonioprism, *e.g.*, asking the patient to look in the direction of the mirror being used, such maneuvers must be used with caution, since they can distort the appearance of the angle depth.[166] It has also been suggested that the Goldmann gonioprism can be used with a direct ophthalmoscope set at +10 or +20 when a slit lamp is not available.[167]

4. *Comparison of Direct and Indirect Gonioscopy.* There is no unanimity of opinion as to which basic method of gonioscopy is best. Advantages have been suggested for both approaches:

a. With *direct gonioscopy*, the height of the observer may be changed to look deeper into a narrow angle, while the gonioprism is limited in this regard by the height of the mirror. In addition, the goniolens may cause less distortion of the anterior chamber. Both features make it desirable when assessing the true depth of the anterior chamber angle.[168, 169]

b. In *indirect gonioscopy*, the slit lamp may provide better optics and lighting, which could be an advantage when looking for subtle details in the angle.[170] Furthermore, the method requires less additional instrumentation and space (assuming the slit lamp is already a part of the routine office examination) and is probably faster than direct gonioscopy. The latter is particularly true of the Ziess four-mirror lens, which is useful for rapid screening.

To minimize the two major disadvantages of gonioprisms, newer designs have included a posterior radius of curvature closer to that of the anterior corneal surface to reduce corneal distortion[166, 171] and taller mirrors to facilitate visualization of narrow angles.[166]

C. Normal Appearance of Adult Anterior Chamber Angle

1. Starting at the root of the iris and progressing anteriorly toward the cornea, the following structures can be identified by gonioscopy in a normal open adult angle (Fig. 2.10)[172]:

a. *The ciliary band* is that portion of the ciliary body which is visible in the anterior chamber as a result of the iris inserting into the ciliary body. The width of the band depends on the level of iris insertion, and tends to be wider in myopia and narrower in hyperopia. The color of the band is usually *gray* or *dark brown*.

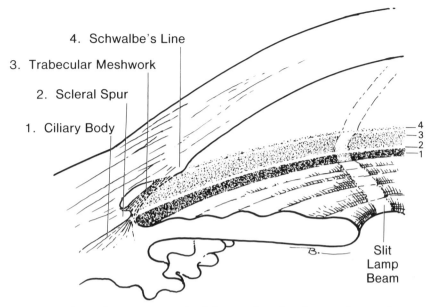

4. Schwalbe's Line

3. Trabecular Meshwork

2. Scleral Spur

1. Ciliary Body

Slit Lamp Beam

Figure 2.10. Normal appearance of adult anterior chamber angle, starting at the root of the iris and progressing anteriorly: **1:** Ciliary body band; **2:** Scleral spur; **3:** Trabecular meshwork (degree of pigmentation varies); and **4:** Schwalbe's line.

b. *The scleral spur* is the posterior portion of the scleral sulcus, which is attached to the ciliary body posteriorly and the corneoscleral meshwork anteriorly. It is usually seen as a *prominent white line* unless obscured by dense uveal meshwork or excessive pigment dispersion.

c. *The trabecular meshwork* is seen as a band just anterior to the scleral spur. It varies considerably in appearance, since it has no pigment at birth, but develops color with age from faint tan to dark brown, depending on the degree of pigment dispersion in the anterior chamber. The central one-third corresponds to the location of Schlemm's canal, where blood reflux may sometimes be seen as a red band.

d. *Schwalbe's line* marks the forward limit of the anterior chamber angle structures. It is a fine ridge just in front of the meshwork and is often identified by a small build-up of pigment, especially inferiorly.

2. *Blood vessels* are normally not seen in the angle, although loops from the major arterial circle may appear in front of the scleral spur and rarely over the meshwork. In addition, an anterior ciliary artery may occasionally be visible in the ciliary band of lightly pigmented eyes.

D. Recording Gonioscopic Findings

A variety of charts and classifications have been suggested for describing the observations made by gonioscopy. These will be discussed in Section Two, although descriptive words and drawings are probably the most useful technique. The drawings can be placed on a chart with concentric circles to represent the different parts of the anterior chamber angle, and the recorded data should include: 1) configuration of the angle, 2) degree of pigmentation, 3) presence of abnormal structures.

E. Cycloscopy[25, 45]

This technique is similar to gonioscopy, but allows visualization of ciliary processes under special circumstances, such as the presence of an iridectomy, wide iris retraction, aniridia, and some cases of aphakia in association with limbal indentation. The main value of the technique thus far has been in research studies of the ciliary processes, although it may hold promise for diagnostic and therapeutic purposes.

VII. TONOGRAPHY

Tonography is a clinical, non-invasive technique for estimating the facility of aqueous outflow. It has been extremely valuable in advancing our understanding of the mechanisms of glaucoma and the actions of antiglaucoma drugs, although its clinical usefulness in the detection and management of glaucoma remains a matter of controversy. Nevertheless, it is worth considering tonography in some detail, since an understanding of the involved physiology provides insight into the complex interplay of factors related to aqueous humor dynamics.

A. Historical Background

1. The mathematics
   a. *Poiseuille's law* (pronounced "pwah zoo' ez"). The 19th century French physician and physiologist, Poiseuille, pursued his interest in the circulation of blood by studying the flow of liquids in tubes of very small diameter.[173] This work led to the formulation of an equation that relates the velocity of flow (F) of fluid in a rigid tube to 1) the radius of the tube (r), 2) the pressure drop per length of tube ($P1-P2/1$), and 3) the coefficient of viscosity (n) of the fluid[174]:

$$F = \frac{\pi r^4}{8n} \cdot \frac{P1 - P2}{1}$$

b. In 1949, Goldmann sought to apply Poiseuille's law to aqueous outflow, suggesting that the rate of aqueous flow through the trabecular meshwork (F) is directly proportional to the intraocular pressure (Po) minus the episcleral venous pressure (Pv) and inversely proportional to the resistance to outflow (R)[175]:

$$F = \frac{Po - Pv}{R}$$

The equation implied that aqueous flow in living ocular tissue could be expressed in the same linear terms as that of fluid in rigid tubes, a belief that would subsequently be proven inaccurate. Nevertheless, it was modifications of Poiseuille's law that led to the mathematical foundation for tonography.

2. The technique[176]

a. At approximately the same time that Poiseuille was conducting his studies, Pagenstecher (1878) observed that massage of the eye lowered the intraocular pressure. In 1905, Schiøtz reported that repeated tonometry also lowered the pressure, although less so in eyes with glaucoma.

b. Polak-van Gelder, applying the above observations, described a technique in 1911 of repeated tonometer applications for 1 to 2 minutes to differentiate normal and glaucomatous eyes. Schoenberg modified this technique the following year by using a continuous application of the tonometer while reading the pressure fall on the scale of the instrument.

3. In 1950, Grant [177] introduced the modern concept of tonography by combining a modification of Poiseuille's law with electronic techniques of continuous intraocular pressure measurement.

B. Mathematical Basis

1. *Relationship of pressure to outflow*

a. As Goldmann[175] suggested, the rate of aqueous outflow (F), which is expressed in $\mu l/min$, is proportional to the intraocular pressure (Po), minus the episcleral venous pressure (Pv):

$$F \propto (Po - Pv)$$

b. Grant[177, 178] proposed that the factors which convert this proportionality to equality be expressed collectively as the *coefficient of outflow facility* (C), which is given in $\mu l/min/mmHg$:

$$F = C(Po - Pv)$$

The C-value is an expression of the degree to which a change in the intraocular pressure will cause a change in the rate of aqueous outflow, which is an indirect expression of the patency of the aqueous outflow system.

2. *Estimation of the C-value* [177]

a. Tonography is a means of estimating the C-value by raising the intraocular pressure with the weight of an indentation tonometer and observing the subsequent decay curve in the IOP. (This discussion presupposes an understanding of indentation tonometry, and the reader may wish to see the next chapter for an explanation of that technique.)

b. The weight of the tonometer plunger on the cornea raises the IOP from the baseline (Po) to a new, higher level (Pt). The elevated pressure causes an increased rate of aqueous outflow, leading to a change in the aqueous volume (ΔV), which is inferred from Friedenwald's tables relating volume change to Schiøtz scale readings.[179] Direct measurements of intraocular fluid volume change in enucleated eyes have supported Friedenwald's calculations.[180] Assuming for the moment that the elevated pressure does not alter other ocular parameters, the rate of volume decrease ($\Delta V/T$) equals the rate of outflow.

c. The standard tonographic technique is to measure the IOP for 4 minutes, *i.e.*, $T = 4$. The change in intraocular pressure during this time is computed as an arithmetical average of pressure increments for successive half-minute intervals (Ave. $Pt - Po$). The C-value is then derived from Grant's equation:

$$C = \frac{\Delta V}{T \text{ (Ave. } Pt - Po)}$$

d. Perfusion studies of enucleated human eyes have supported Grant's equation, although newer tables used in the formula have given C-values far higher than those generally accepted.[181] Sources of error in tonography include the following physiological and technical parameters.

3. *Other ocular parameters that influence tonography.* The tonographic calculation assumes that only the rate of aqueous outflow changes in response to a change in intraocular pressure. However, there are many other ocular parameters that respond to a pressure change, all of which can influence the tonographic result.

a. *Aqueous production decreases* with a rise in intraocular pressure, primarily due to an alteration in ultrafiltration.[182, 183] The subsequent intraocular pressure drop in response to reduced production of aqueous creates an impression of increased outflow and is called *pseudofacility*. This accounts for up to 20% of the total C-value.[182] Tonography measures the total C-value, without distinguishing between true facility and pseudofacility.

b. *Resistance to aqueous outflow increases* with an increase in the intraocular pressure, the physiologic basis of which was previously discussed. The tonographic result is that the C-value of an eye decreases with increasing intraocular pressure.[184] This phenomenon relates to the conventional, or canalicular, route of aqueous outflow. The influence of extracanalicular outflow on the tonographic result is not fully understood.

c. *Episcleral venous pressure rises* an average of 1.25 mmHg with the pressure elevation during tonography,[185] which is usually corrected for in the formula by adding 1.25 to *Po*.

d. *Ocular rigidity* is an expression of the "stretchability" of the eye in response to an increase in intraocular pressure and probably represents several characteristics of the eye. An average ocular rigidity of 0.0125 is used in calculating the tonographic C-value, although there is significant interpatient variation in this parameter, which leads to a potential source of error in tonography. For this reason it is useful to check the pressure by applanation tonometry before performing the tonography and to compare this with the *Po* obtained with the indentation tonometer, as a means of identifying any major discrepancy in ocular rigidity.[172]

e. *The expulsion of uveal blood* in response to elevated intraocular pressure probably influences tonography, although the actual effect is uncertain.[186]

C. Technique

The details of performing tonography are available in several excellent textbooks.[164, 172, 176] The purpose of the present discussion is to provide an overview of the technique.

1. *Basic steps.*

a. With the recorder running, the electronic tonometer is calibrated at scale readings of 0 and 7. The recording needle is then set at 0 for the subsequent readings.

b. The patient is in a supine position, fixing on a target overhead. After instilling a topical anesthetic on the cornea, the intraocular pressure is measured with two brief applications of the electronic tonometer.

c. The 4-minute pressure tracing is then made by gently applying the tonometer to the cornea and maintaining this position until a smooth tracing has been obtained for a full 4 minutes. A good tracing will have fine oscillations and a gentle downward slope. If the slope is steeper or irregular during the first few seconds, which is not uncommon, the study should be continued until a good 4-minute tracing has been obtained.

d. The slope of the tracing is then estimated by placing a free hand line through the middle of the oscillations. The scale readings are noted at the beginning and end of the 4-minute tracing.

e. Po is determined from the initial scale reading and a standard calibration table. Po and the change in scale readings over the four minutes (ΔR) are then used to obtain the C-value from special tonographic tables.

2. *Sources of error.*

a. Variations in *corneal curvature* from the assumed average of 7.8 mm may significantly influence the pressure measurements.[176]

b. *Moses effect.* The hole in the tonometer footplate must be slightly larger in electronic tonometers to prevent sticking. At low scale readings, the cornea may mold into the space between the plunger and hole, pushing the plunger up and leading to falsely high pressure readings.[187]

c. *Variations in line voltage* may produce an apparent drift in the intraocular pressure mesurements, which can be minimized with line voltage stabilizers and by avoiding magnetic fields.[176]

d. *Consensual pressure drop.* The intraocular pressure has been shown to drop approximately 1 mmHg in the fellow eye while tonography is being performed on the first eye. A neural etiology was once postulated for this phenomenon, but it was subsequently found to be secondary to the evaporation that results from keeping the eye open for fixation during the 4-minute test.[188] The problem can be eliminated by draping a plastic sheet over the fellow eye, while the first eye is being tested.[188]

e. *Patient relaxation effect*. During the first 15 to 20 seconds after the tonometer is placed on the cornea, the IOP will fall as the patient relaxes. Time should be allowed for this before starting the 4-minute tracing. Other patient-related factors, such as blinking, squeezing, or lack of fixation during the test, can also lead to a poor tonographic result.

f. *Operator error*, including improper cleaning, calibration, or positioning of the instrument, as well as improper calculation of the tracing, can also lead to inaccurate results.

D. Interpreting Tonographic Results

Despite the many potentials for error in tonography and the possibility that currently accepted values may be grossly inaccurate, it is nevertheless necessary to be familiar with the values that might be anticipated with current techniques.

1. In a study of 1379 eyes, Becker [189] reported the following values:
   a. *C-value*
      (1). The mean in 909 *normal* eyes was 0.28 μl/min/mmHg.
      (2). The prevalence of *low* C-values was:

C-Value	Normals (n = 909)	Glaucoma Patients (n = 250)	Family History of Glaucoma (n = 220)
<0.18	2.5%	65%	20%
<0.13	0.15%	43%	11%

   b. *Po/C ratio*
      (1). The mean of the *normal* population was 56.
      (2). The prevalence of *high* Po/C ratios was:

Po/C Ratio	Normals	Glaucoma Patients	Family History of Glaucoma
>100	2.5%	73%	21%
>138	0.15%	50%	14%

2. In a study of 7,577 eyes, the C-value was found to *decrease* with age, with an average of 0.2932 for ages 41 to 45 years, compared to 0.2518 in the 81- to 85-year-old group. There was no sex difference at any age level.[190]

3. When the C-value and Po do not seem to correlate, the following possibilities should be considered.[176]
   a. A *low C* with a *normal Po* may be due to:
      (1). a sticky tonometer
      (2). low ocular ridigity
      (3). hyposecretion
   b. A *high C* with *elevated Po* may be due to:
      (1). an artificially elevated Po
      (2). high ocular rigidity
      (3). high pseudofacility
      (4). elevated episcleral venous pressure
      (5). angle-closure glaucoma (the force of the tonometer may open the angle)

(6). the Moses effect
4. *The wave components* of a tonographic tracing include[191]:
    a. Fine oscillations, which reflect the *cardiac pulse.*
    b. Large waves, which reflect the *respiratory movement.*
    c. Still larger, irregular waves (Traube-Hering waves), which reflect periodic oscillations in the systemic blood pressure.
    d. Cardiac irregularities, *e.g.,* extrasystoli, bigeminy, etc., can also cause irregularities in the tonographic tracing.

E. The Clinical Value of Tonography

As previously noted, there is controversy regarding the value of tonography in the detection and management of glaucoma. The following are the main situations in which tonography is felt by some physicians to have clinical value:

1. As an *adjunct in diagnosing open-angle glaucoma*, tonography is suggested to have predictive value regarding the development of nerve damage in patients with elevated intraocular pressure,[192-194] although this has not been confirmed in all studies.[195] The *Po/C* ratio is generally felt to be the more sensitive parameter in this situation,[192-194] and a prior water-drinking test (discussed in Section Two under Open-Angle Glaucoma) has been suggested to further enhance the predictive value of tonography.[192] However, it has been stressed that abnormal tonometric and tonographic results do not make the diagnosis of glaucoma, but alert the ophthalmologist to follow the patient more closely.[196]

2. *A low C-value* was felt to correlate with a *wider diurnal fluctuation in intraocular pressure*, but a study of 388 eyes showed that a single tonometric reading correlated with the diurnal curve better than did the tonographic results.[197]

3. In *angle-closure glaucoma*, a 25 to 30% fall in the *C*-value may be used as adjunctive confirmation of a positive *provocative test*. In addition, once an acute attack is broken, a *C*-value of 0.10 or less suggests that a peripheral iridectomy alone may be insufficient.[176]

4. *Ocular inflammation*, as with surgery, trauma, disease, etc., may mask a compromised outflow system by temporarily reducing aqueous production, and tonography during this time can disclose the abnormal outflow.[176]

5. Additional suggested values for tonography include an adjunct in the diagnosis of *myasthenia gravis* by observing a rise in IOP of 2 to 5 mmHg in response to intravenous tensilon.[198]

6. Since both aqueous and blood are expelled from the eye in variable amounts during tonography, it may be that a future value of tonography lies in its ability to assess the posterior half of the eye, the portion directly related to visual loss, by measuring the *blood-ejection coefficient.* [186, 199]

References
1. Woodlief, NF: Initial observations on the ocular microcirculation in man. I. The anterior segment and extraocular muscles. Arch Ophthal 98:1268, 1980.

2. Smelser, GK: Electron microscopy of a typical epithelial cell and of the normal human ciliary process. Trans Am Acad Ophthal Otol 70:738, 1966.
3. Tormey, JM: The ciliary epithelium: an attempt to correlate structure and function. Trans Am Acad Ophthal Otol 70:755, 1966.
4. Holmberg, A: Ultrastructure of the ciliary epithelium. Arch Ophthal 62:935, 1959.
5. Holmberg, A: Differences in ultrastructure of normal human and rabbit ciliary epithelium. Arch Ophthal 62:952, 1959.
6. Raviola, G, Raviola, E: Intercellular junctions in the ciliary epithelium. Invest Ophthal Vis Sci 17:958, 1978.
7. Cunha-Vas, JG: The blood-ocular barriers. Invest Ophthal Vis Sci 17:1037, 1978.
8. Wulle, KG: Zelldifferenzierungen in Ciliarepithel wahrend der menschlichen Fetalentwicklung und ihre Bezichungen zur Kammerwasserbildung. Albrecht v Graefes Arch klin exp Ophthal 172:170, 1967.
9. Richardson, KT: Cellular response to drugs affecting aqueous dynamics. Arch Ophthal 89:65, 1973.
10. Uusitalo, R, Palkama, A, Stjernschantz, J: An electron microscopical study of the blood-aqueous barrier in the ciliary body and iris of the rabbit. Exp Eye Res 17:49, 1973.
11. Smith, RS, Rudt, LA: Ultrastructural studies of the blood-aqueous barrier. 2. The barrier to horseradish peroxidase in primates. Am J Ophthal 76:937, 1973.
12. Marci, FJ, Cevario, SJ: The formation and inhibition of aqueous humor production. Arch Ophthal 96:1664, 1978.
13. Becker, B: The effect of hypothermia on aqueous humor dynamics. III. Turnover of ascorbate and sodium. Am J Ophthal 51:1032, 1961.
14. Berggren, L: Effect of composition of medium and of metabolic inhibitors on secretion in vitro by the ciliary processes of the rabbit eye. Invest Ophthal 4:83, 1965.
15. Sears, ML: The aqueous. *In* Adler's Physiology of the Eye, 6th edition, Moses, RA, ed, CV Mosby Co, St Louis, 1975, p 232.
16. Bonting, SL, Becker, B: Studies on sodium-potassium activated adenosinetriphosphatase. XIV. Inhibition of enzyme activity and aqueous humor flow in the rabbit eye after intravitreal injection of ouabain. Invest Ophthal 3:523, 1964.
17. Cole, DF: Some effects of decreased plasma sodium concentration on the composition and tension of the aqueous humour. Br J Ophthal 43:268, 1959.
18. Holland, MG, Gipson, CC: Chloride ion transport in the isolated ciliary body. Invest Ophthal 9:20, 1970.
19. Holland, MG: Chloride ion transport in the isolated ciliary body. II. Ion substitution experiments. Invest Ophthal 9:30, 1970.
20. Bito, L, Davson, H: Steady-state concentrations of potassium in the ocular fluids. Exp Eye Res 3:283, 1964.
21. Reddy, VN: Dynamics of transport systems in the eye. Invest Ophthal Vis Sci 18:1000, 1979.
22. Maren, TH: The rates of movement of Na^+, Cl^-, and HCO^-_3 from plasma to posterior chamber: effect of acetazolamide and relation to the treatment of glaucoma. Invest Ophthal 15:356, 1976.
23. Cole, DF: Effects of some metabolic inhibitors upon the formation of the aqueous humour in rabbits. Br J Ophthal 44:739, 1960.
24. Hara, K, Lutjen-Drecoll, E, Prestele, H, Rohen, JW: Structural differences between regions of the ciliary body in primates. Invest Ophthal Vis Sci 16:912, 1977.
25. Mizuno, K, Asaoka, M: Cycloscopy and fluorescein cycloscopy. Invest Ophthal 15:561, 1976.
26. Ober, M, Rohen, JW: Regional differences in the fine structure of the ciliary epithelium related to accommodation. Invest Ophthal Vis Sci 18:655, 1979.
27. Russmann, W: Levels of glycolytic enzyme activity in the ciliary epithelium prepared from bovine eyes. Ophthal Res 2:205, 1971.

28. Feeney, L, Mixon, R: Localization of [35]sulfated macromolecules at the site of active transport in the ciliary processes. Invest Ophthal 13:882, 1974.
29. Feeney, L, Mixon, RN: Sulfate and galactose metabolism in differentiating ciliary body and iris epithelia: autoradiographic and ultrastructural studies. Invest Ophthal 14:364, 1975.
30. Brubaker, RF, Nagataki, S, Townsend, DJ, Burns, RR, Higgins, RG, Wentworth, W: The effect of age on aqueous humor formation in man. Ophthalmology (in press).
31. Holm, O: A photogrammetric method for estimation of the pupillary aqueous flow in the living human eye. I. Acta Ophthal 46:254, 1968.
32. Jones, RF, Maurice, DM: New methods of measuring the rate of aqueous flow in man with fluorescein. Exp Eye Res 5:208, 1966.
33. Bloom, JN, Levene, RZ, Thomas, G, Kimura, R: Fluorophotometry and the rate of aqueous flow in man. Arch Ophthal 94:435, 1976.
34. Coakes, RL, Brubaker, RF: Method of measuring aqueous humor flow and corneal endothelial permeability using a fluorophotometry nomogram. Invest Ophthal Vis Sci 18:288, 1979.
35. Brubaker, RF, Coakes, RL: Use of a xenon flash tube as the excitation source in a new slit-lamp fluorophotometer. Am J Ophthal 86:474, 1978.
36. Becker, B: The measurement of rate of aqueous flow with iodide. Invest Ophthal 1:52, 1962.
37. Macri, FJ, O'Rourke, J: Measurements of aqueous humor turnover rates using a gamma probe. Arch Ophthal 83:741, 1970.
38. Wickham, MG, Worthen, DM, Downing, D: A randomized technique of constant-pressure infusion. Invest Ophthal 15:1010, 1976.
39. Bárány, EH: A mathematical formulation of intraocular pressure as dependent on secretion, ultrafiltration, bulk outflow, and osmotic reabsorption of fluid. Invest Ophthal 2:584, 1963.
40. Brubaker, RF, Kupfer, C: Determination of pseudofacility in the eye of the rhesus monkey. Arch Ophthal 75:693, 1966.
41. Bill, A: Aspects on suppressability of aqueous humour formation. Doc Ophthal 26:73, 1969.
42. Brubaker, RF: The measurement of pseudofacility and true facility by constant pressure perfusion in the normal rhesus monkey eye. Invest Ophthal 9:42, 1970.
43. Leydhecker, VW, Rehak, S, Mathyl, J: Investigations on homeostasis: the effect of experimental changes of pressure on the production of aqueous humour in the living rabbit eye. Klin Monatsbl Augenheilkd 159:427, 1971.
44. Bill, A: Effects of longstanding stepwise increments in eye pressure on the rate of aqueous humour formation in a primate (cercopithecus ethiops). Exp Eye Res 12:184, 1971.
45. Mizuno, K, Asaoka, M, Muroi, S: Cycloscopy and fluorescein cycloscopy of the ciliary process. Am J Ophthal 84:487, 1977.
46. Becker, B: The decline in aqueous secretion and outflow facility with age. Am J Ophthal 46:731, 1958.
47. Auricchio, G: Der osmotische druck des kammerwassers im verlaufe einer anaphylaktischen uveitis beim kaninchen. Ophthalmologica 136:217, 1958.
48. Auricchio, G, Barany, E: Uber augendruckbestimmende Faktoren bei experimenteller Kaninchenuveitis. Ophthalmologica 136:249, 1958.
49. Howes, EL, Cruse, VK: The structural basis of altered vascular permeability following intraocular inflammation. Arch Ophthal 96:1668, 1978.
50. Dobbie, JG: A study of the intraocular fluid dynamics in retinal detachment. Arch Ophthal 69:53, 1963.
51. Cole, DF: Aqueous and ciliary body. In Biochemistry of the Eye, Graymore, CN, ed, Academic Press, London, New York, 1970, p 114.
52. de Berardinis, E, Tieri, O, Inglio, N, Polzella, A: The composition of the aqueous humour of man in aphakia. Acta Ophthal 44:64, 1966.
53. Kinsey, VE: Comparative chemistry of aqueous humor in posterior and anterior

chamber of rabbit eye. Its physiologic significance. Arch Ophthal 50:401, 1953.

54. Reddy, DVN: Chemical composition of normal aqueous humor. In Biochemistry of the Eye, Dardenna, MU, Nordmann, J, eds, Karger, Basel, New York, 1968, p 167.

55. Becker, B: Chemical composition of human aqueous humor. Effects of acetazoleamide. Arch Ophthal 57:793, 1957.

56. de Berardinis, E, Tieri, O, Polzella, A, Iuglio, N: The chemical composition of the human aqueous humour in normal and pathological conditions. Exp Eye Res 4:179, 1965.

57. Kinsey, VE, Reddy, DVN: Chemistry and dynamics of aqueous humor. In The Rabbit in Eye Research, Prince, JH, ed, Charles C Thomas, Springfield, Ill, 1964, p 218.

58. Sen, DK, Sarin, GS, Saha, K: Immunoglobulins in human aqueous humour. Br J Ophthal 61:216, 1977.

59. Okisaka, S.: Effects of paracentesis on the blood-aqueous barrier: a light and electron microscopic study on cynomolgus monkey. Invest Ophthal 15:824, 1976.

60. Bartels, SP, Pederson, JE, Gaasterland, DE, Armaly, MF: Sites of breakdown of the blood-aqueous barrier after paracentesis of the rhesus monkey eye. Invest Ophthal Vis Sci 18:1050, 1970.

61. Dickinson, JC, Durham, DC, Hamilton, PB: Ion exchange chromatography of free amino acids in aqueous fluid and lens of the human eye. Invest Ophthal 7:551, 1968.

62. de Berardinis, E, Tieri, O: Rapport entre les concentrations de l'acide lactique dans l'humeur aqueuse et dans le plasma. Ann d'Ocul 194:411, 1961.

63. Davson, H, Luck, CP: A comparative study of the total carbon dioxide in the ocular fluids, cerebrospinal fluid, and plasma of some mammalian species. J Physiol 132:454, 1956.

64. Moses, RA, Grodzki, WF Jr: The scleral spur and scleral roll. Invest Ophthal 16:925, 1977.

65. Moses, RA, Grodzki, WJ Jr, Starcher, BC, Galione, MJ: Elastin content of the scleral spur, trabecular mesh, and sclera. Invest Ophthal Vis Sci 17:817, 1978.

66. Spencer, WH, Alvarado, J, Hayes, TL: Scanning electron microscopy of human ocular tissues: trabecular meshwork. Invest Ophthal 7:651, 1968.

67. Flocks, M: The anatomy of the trabecular meshwork as seen in tangential section. Arch Ophthal 56:708, 1957.

68. Fine, BS: Observations on the drainage angle in man and rhesus monkey: a concept of the pathogenesis of chronic simple glaucoma. A light and electron microscopic study. Invest Ophthal 3:609, 1964.

69. Hoffmann, F, Dumitrescu, L: Schlemm's canal under the scanning electron microscope. Ophthal Res 2:37, 1971.

70. Rohen, JW, Rentsch, FJ: Morphology of Schlemm's canal and related vessels in the human eye. Albrecht v Graefes Arch Klin exp Ophthal 176:309, 1968.

71. Ascher, KW: The Aqueous Veins. Biomicroscopic Study of the Aqueous Humor Elimination. Charles C Thomas, Springfield, Ill, 1961.

72. Last, RJ: Wolff's Anatomy of the Eye and Orbit, 5th edition, WB Saunders Co, Philadelphia, 1961, p 49.

73. Rohen, JW, Rentsch, JF: Electromicroscopic studies on the structure of the outer wall of Schlemm's canal, its outflow channels and age changes. Albrecht v Graefes Arch klin exp Ophthal 177:1, 1969.

74. Jocson, VL, Sears, ML: Channels of aqueous outflow and related blood vessels. I. Macaca mulatta (rhesus). Arch Ophthal 80:104, 1968.

75. Jocson, VL, Sears, ML: Channels of aqueous outflow and related blood vessels. II. Cercopithecus ethiops (Ethiopian green or green velvet). Arch Ophthal 81:244, 1969.

76. Jocson, VL, Grant, WM: Interconnections of blood vessels and aqueous vessels in human eyes. Arch Ophthal 73:707, 1965.

77. Gaasterland, DE, Jocson, VL, Sears, ML: Channels of aqueous outlfow and

related blood vessels. III. Episcleral arteriovenous anastomoses in the rhesus monkey eye (*Macaca mulatta*). Arch Ophthal 84:770, 1970.

78. Jocson, VL, Sears, ML: Experimental aqueous perfusion in enucleated human eyes. Arch Ophthal 86:65, 1971.
79. Bill, A, Phillips, CI: Uveoscleral drainage of aqueous humour in human eyes. Exp Eye Res 12:275, 1971.
80. Pederson, JE, Gaasterland, DE, MacLellan, HM: Uveoscleral aqueous outflow in the rhesus monkey: importance of oveal reabsorption. Invest Ophthal Vis Sci 16:1008, 1977.
81. Inomata, H, Bill, A: Exit sites of uveoscleral flow of aqueous humor in cynomolgus monkey eyes. Exp Eye Res 25:113, 1977.
82. Sherman, SH, Green, K, Laties, AM: The fate of anterior chamber fluorescein in the monkey eye. I. The anterior chamber outflow pathways. Exp Eye Res 27:159, 1978.
83. Inomata, H, Bill, A, Smelser, GK: Unconventional routes of aqueous humor outflow in cynomolgus monkey (macaca irus). Am J Ophthal 73:893, 1972.
84. McMaster, PRB, Macri, FJ: Secondary aqueous humor outflow pathways in the rabbit, cata, and monkey. Arch Ophthal 79:297, 1968.
85. Ashton, N: The exit pathway of the aqueous. Trans Ophthal Soc U K 80:397, 1960.
86. Fine, BS: Structure of the trabecular meshwork and the canal of Schlemm. Trans Am Acad Ophthal Otol 70:777, 1966.
87. Iwamoto, T.: Light and electron microscopy of the presumed elastic components of the trabeculae and scleral spur of the human eye. Invest Ophthal 3:144, 1964.
88. Grierson, I, Chisholm, IA: Clearance of debris from the iris through the drainage angle of the rabbit's eye. Br J Ophthal 62:694, 1978.
89. Grierson, I, Lee, WR: Erythrocyte phagocytosis in the human trabecular meshwork. Br J Ophthal 57:400, 1973.
90. Grierson, I, Rahi, AHS: Microfilaments in the cells of the human trabecular meshwork. Br J Ophthal 63:3, 1979.
91. Gipson, IK, Anderson, Ra: Actin filaments in cells of human trabecular meshwork and Schlemm's canal. Invest Ophthal Vis Sci 18:547, 1979.
92. Anderson, PJ, Wang, J, Epstein, DL: Metabolism of calf trabecular (reticular) meshwork. Invest Ophthal Vis Sci 19:13, 1980.
93. Polansky, JR, Weinreb, RN, Baxter, JD, Alvarado, J: Human trabecular cells. I. Establishment in tissue culture and growth characteristics. Invest Ophthal Vis Sci 18:1043, 1979.
94. Speakman, JS: Drainage channels in the trabecular wall of Schlemm's canal. Br J Ophthal 44:513, 1960.
95. Feeney, L, Wissig, S: Outflow studies using an electron dense tracer. Trans Am Acad Ophthal Otol 70:791, 1966.
96. Anderson, DR: Scanning electron microscopy of primate trabecular meshwork. Am J Ophthal 71:90, 1971.
97. Johnstone, MA: Pressure-dependent changes in configuration of the endothelial tubules of Schlemm's canal. Am J Ophthal 78:630, 1974.
98. Svedbergh, B: Protrusions of the inner wall of Schlemm's canal. Am J Ophthal 82:875, 1976.
99. Johnstone, MA: Pressure-dependent changes in nuclei and the process origins of the endothelial cells lining Schlemm's canal. Invest Ophthal Vis Sci 18:44, 1979.
100. Segawa, K: Electron microscopic observations on the replicas of Schlemm's canal. Acta Soc Ophthal Jap 73:2013, 1969.
101. Segawa, K: Scanning electron microscopic studies on the iridocorneal angle tissue in normal human eyes. Acta Soc Ophthal Jap 76:659, 1972.
102. Holmberg, A: The fine structure of the inner wall of Schlemm's canal. Arch Ophthal 62:956, 1959.
103. Holmberg, A: Schlemm's canal and the trabecular meshwork. An electron microscopic study of the normal structure in man and monkey (cercopithecus

ethiops). Doc Ophthal 19:339, 1965.

104. Inomata, H, Bill, A, Smelser, GK: Aqueous humor pathways through the trabecular meshwork and into Schlem's canal in the cynomolgus monkey (*Macaca irus*). Am J Ophthal 73:760, 1972.

105. Segawa, K: Pores of the trabecular wall of Schlemm's canal ferritin perfusion in enucleated human eyes. Acta Soc Ophthal Jpn 74:1240, 1970.

106. Segawa, K: Pore structures of the endothelial cells of the aqueous outflow pathway: scanning electron microscopy. Jpn J Ophthal 17:133, 1973.

107. Reese, TS, Gaasterland, D: Postmortem formation of giant endothelial vacuoles in Schlemm's canal of the monkey. Am J Ophthal 76:896, 1973.

108. Tripathi, RC: Ultrastructure of Schlemm's canal in relation to aqueous outflow. Exp Eye Res 7:335, 1968.

109. Tripathi, RC: Ultrastructure of the trabecular wall of Schlemm's canal. Trans Ophthal Soc U K 89:449, 1969.

110. Tripathi, RC: Mechanism of the aqueous outflow across the trabecular wall of Schlemm's canal. Exp Eye Res 11:116, 1971.

111. Triphathi, RC: Ultrastructure of the exit pathway of the aqueous in lower mammals (a preliminary report on the "angular aqueous plexus"). Exp Eye Res 12:311, 1971.

112. Tripathi, RC: Aqueous outflow pathway in normal and glaucomatous eyes. Br J Ophthal 56:157, 1972.

113. Sondermann, R: Beitrag zur entwicklung und moorphologie des Schlemmschen kanals. Albrecht v Graefes Arch Klin Exp Ophthal 124:521, 1930.

114. Ashton, N, Brini, A, Smith, R: Anatomical studies of the trabecular meshwork of the normal human eye. Br J Ophthal 40:257, 1956.

115. Iwamoto, T: Light and electron microscopy of Sondermann's channels in the human trabecular meshwork. Albrecht v Graefes Arch klin Exp Ophthal 172:197, 1967.

116. Iwamoto, T: further observation on Sondermann's channels of the human trabecular meshwork. Albrecht v Graefes Arch Klin Exp Ophthal 172:213, 1967.

117. Lutjen-Drecoll, E, Rohen, JW: Uber die endotheliale auskleidung des Schlemmschen Kanals im silberimpragnationsbild. Albrecht v Graefes Arch klin Exp Ophthal 180:249, 1970.

118. Grant, WM: Further studies on facility of flow through the trabecular meshwork. Arch Ophthal 60:523, 1958.

119. Grant, WM: Experimental aqueous perfusion in enucleated human eyes. Arch Ophthal 69:783, 1963.

120. Tripathi, RC, Tripathi, BJ: The mechanism of aqueous outflow in lower mammals. Exp Eye Res 14:73, 1972.

121. Tarkkanen, A, Niemi, M: Enzyme histochemistry of the angle of the anterior chamber of the human eye. Acta Ophthal 45:93, 1967.

122. Vegge, T: Ultrastructure of normal human trabecular endothelium. Acta Ophthal 41:193, 1963.

123. Grierson, I, Lee, WR: Changes in the monkey outflow apparatus at graded levels of intraocular pressure: a qualitative analysis by light microscopy and scanning electron microscopy. Exp Eye Res 19:21, 1971.

124. Johnstone, MA, Grant, WM: Pressure-dependent changes in structure of the aqueous outflow system of human and monkey eyes. Am J Ophthal 75:365, 1973.

125. Grierson, I, Lee, WR: Pressure-induced changes in the ultrastructure of the endothelium lining Schlemm's canal. Am J Ophthal 80:863, 1975.

126. Kayes, J: Pressure gradient changes on the trabecular meshwork of monkeys. Am J Ophthal 79:549, 1975.

127. VanBuuskirk, EM, Grant, WM: Influence of temperature and the question of involvement of cellular metabolism in aqueous outflow. Am J Ophthal 77:565, 1974.

128. Pollack, IP, Becker, B, Constant, MA: The effect of hypothermia on aqueous humor dynamics. I. Intraocular pressure and outflow facility of the rabbit eye. Am J Ophthal 49:1126, 1960.

129. Bill, A, Svedbergh, B: Scanning electron microscopic studies of the trabecular meshwork and the canal of Schlemm—an attempt to localize the main resistance to outflow of aqueous humor in man. Acta Ophthal 50:295, 1972.

130. Kaufman, PL, Bárány, EH: Cytochalasin B reversibility increases outflow facility in the eye of the cynomolgus monkey. Invest Ophthal Vis Sci 16:47, 1977.

131. Svedbergh, B, Lütjen-Drecoll, E, Ober, M, Kaufman, PL: Cytochalasin B-induced structural changes in the anterior ocular segment of the cynomologus monkey. Invest Ophthal Vis Sci 17:718, 1978.

132. Johnstone, M, Tanner, D, Chau, B, Kopecky, K: Concentration-dependent morphologic effects of cytochalasin B in the aqueous outflow system. Invest Ophthal Vis Sci 19:835, 1980.

133. Kaufman, PL, Svedbergh, B, Lütjen-Drecoll, E: Medical trabeculocanalotomy in monkeys with cytochalasin B or EDTA. Ann Ophthal 11:795, 1979.

134. Bill, A, Lütjen-Drecoll, E, Svedbergh, B: Effects of intracameral Na_2EDTA and EGTA on aqueous outflow routes in the monkey eye. Invest Ophthal Vis Sci 19:492, 1980.

135. Pandolfi, M, Kwaan, HC: Fibrinolysis in the anterior segment of the eye. Arch Ophthal 77:99, 1967.

136. Pandolfi, M: Coagulation factor VIII localization in the aqueous outflow pathways. Arch Ophthal 94:656,, 1976.

137. Zimmerman, LE: Demonstration of hyaluronidase-sensitive acid mucopolysaccharide in trabecula and iris in routine paraffin sections of adult human eyes. A preliminary report. Am J Ophthal 441:1, 1957.

138. Berggren, L, Vrabec, F: Demonstration of a coating substance in the trabecular meshwork of the eye and its decrease after perfusion experiments with different kinds of hyaluronidase. Am J Ophthal 44:200, 1957.

139. Francois, J: The importance of the muucopolysaccharides in intraocular pressure regulation. Invest Ophthal 14:173, 1975.

140. Hayasaka, S, Sears, ML: Distribution of acid phosphatase, beta-glucuronidase, and lysosomal hyaluronidase in the anterior segment of the rabbit eye. Invest Ophthal 17:982, 1978.

141. Francois, J, Rabaey, M: Studies on outflow of aqueous humor. Trans. Ophthal Soc Australia 16:51, 1956.

142. Grierson, I, Lee, WR, Abraham, S: A light microscopic study of the effects of testiculaar hyaluronidase on the outflow system of a baboon (*Papio cynocephalus*). Invest Ophthal Vis Sci 18:356, 1979.

143. Van Buskirk, EM, Brett, J: The canine eye: in vitro dissolution of the barriers to aqueous outflow. Invest Ophthal Vis Sci 17:258, 1978.

144. Van Buskirk, EM, Brett, J: The canine eye: in vitro studies of the intraocular pressure and facility of aqueous outflow. Invest Ophthal Vis Sci 17:373, 1978.

145. Peterson, WS, Jocson, VL: Hyaluronidase effects of aqueous outflow resistance. Quantitative and localizing studies in the rhesus monkey eye. Am J Ophthal 77:573, 1974.

146. Van Buskirk, EM, Grant, WM: Lens depression and aqueous outflow in enucleated primate eyes. Am J Ophthal 76:632, 1973.

147. Van Buskirk, EM: Trabeculotomy in the immature, enucleated human eye. Invest Ophthal Vis Sci 16:63, 1977.

148. Moses, RA, Hoover, GS, Oostwouder, PH: Blood reflux in Schlemm's canal. I. Normal findings. Arch Ophthal 97:1307, 1979.

149. Ellingsen, BA, Grant, WM: The relationship of pressure and aqueous outflow in enucleated human eyes. Invest Ophthal 10:430, 1971.

150. Ellingsen, BA, Grant, WM: Influence of intraocular pressure and trabeculotomy on aqueous outflow in enucleated monkey eyes. Invest Ophthal 10:705, 1971.

151. Brubaker, RF: The effect of intraocular pressure on conventional outflow resistance in the enucleated human eye. Invest Ophthal 14:287, 1975.

152. Moses, RA: The effect of intraocular pressure on resistance to outflow. Surv Ophthal 22:88, 1977.

153. Grierson, I, Lee, WR: The fine structure of the trabecular meshwork at graded levels of intraocular pressure. 1. Pressure effects within the near-physiological

range (8–30 mmHg). Exp Eye Res 20:505, 1975.

154. Grierson, I, Lee, WR: The fine structure of the trabecular meshwork at graded levels of intraocular pressure. 2. Pressure outside the physiological range (0 and 50 mmHg). Exp Eye Res 20:523, 1975.

155. Ellingsen, BA, Grant, WM: Trabeculotomy and sinusotomy in enucleated human eyes. Invest Ophthal 11:21, 1972.

156. Hashimoto, JM, Epstein, DL: Influence of intraocular pressure on aqueous outflow facility in enucleated eyes of different mammals. Invest Ophthal Vis Sci 19:1483, 1980.

157. Moses, RA, Arnzen, RJ: The trabecular mesh: a mathematical analysis. Invest Ophthal Vis Sci 19:1490, 1980.

158. Van Buskirk, EM: Changes in the facility of aqueous outflow induced by lens depression and intraocular pressure in excised human eyes. Am J Ophthal 82:736, 1976.

159. Moses, RA, Grodzki, WJ Jr: Choroid tension and facility of aqueous outflow. Invest Ophthal Vis Sci 16:1062, 1977.

160. Peterson, WS, Jocson, VL, Sears ML: Resistance to aqueous outflow in the rhesus monkey eye. Am J Ophthal 72:445, 1971.

161. Rubin, ML: Optics for Clinicians, 2nd ed, Triad Scientific Publishing, Gainesville, Fla, 1974, p 56.

162. Becker, S: Clinical Gonioscopy—A Text and Stereoscopic Atlas. The CV Mosby Co, St Louis, 1972.

163. Kimura, R: Color Atlas of Gonioscopy. The Williams & Wilkins Co, Baltimore, 1974.

164. Kolker, AE, Hetherington, J Jr: Becker-Shaffer's Diagnosis and Therapy of the Glaucomas, 4th ed, The CV Mosby Co, 1976, St Louis, p 9.

165. Peczon, JD: Tears for gonioscopic fluid. Am J Ophthal 57:838, 1964.

166. Becker, SC: Unrecognized errors induced by present-day gonioprisms and a proposal for their elimination. Arch Ophthal 82:160, 1969.

167. Kingsley, B, Stanley, JA: Pocket gonioscopy. Ann Ophthal 10:1661, 1978.

168. Hetherington, J Jr: Koeppe Lens Gonioscopy. In Controversy in Ophthalmology, Brockhurst, FJ, Boruchoff, SA, Hutchinson, BT, Lessell, S, eds, WB Saunders Co, Philadephia, 1977, p 142.

169 Campbell, DG: A comparison of diagnostic techniques in angle-closure glaucoma. Am J Ophthal 88:197, 1979.

170. Schwartz, B: Slit Lamp Gonioscopy. In Controversy in Ophthalmology, Brockhurst, RJ, Boruchoff, SA, Hutchinson, BT, Lessell, S, eds, WB Saunders Co, Philadelphia, 1977, p 146.

171. Smith, RJH: An improved diagnostic contact lens. Br J Ophthal 63:482, 1979.

172. Chandler, PA, Grant, WM. Glaucoma, 2nd edition, Lea & Febiger, Philadelphia, 1979, pp 16–22, 30–56.

173. Bingham, EC: Biography of Dr. Jean Leonard Marie Poiseuille. Rheological Memoirs 1:VII, 1940.

174. Frank, NH: Introduction to Mechanics and Heat, 2nd edition, McGraw-Hill Book Co, Inc, New York, 1939, p 246.

175. Goldmann, H: Augendruck und glaukom. Die Kammerwasservenen und das Poiseuille sche Gesetz. Ophthalmologica 118:496, 1949.

176. Drews, RC: Manual of tonography. CV Mosby Co, St Louis, 1971.

177. Grant, WM: Tonographic method for measuring the facility and rate of aqueous flow in human eyes. Arch Ophthal 44:204, 1950.

178. Grant, WM: Clinical measurements of aqueous outflow. Arch Ophthal 46:113, 1951.

179. Friedenwald, JS: Some problems in the calibration of tonometers. Am J Ophthal 31:935, 1948.

180. Hetland-Eriksen, J, Odberg, T: Experimental tonography on enucleated human eyes. II. The loss of intraocular fluid caused by tonography. Invest Ophthal 14:944, 1975.

181. Hetland-Eriksen, J, Odberg, T: Experimental tonography on enucleated human

eyes. I. The validity of Grant's tonography formula. Invest Ophthal 14:199, 1975.

182. Kupfer, C, Sanderson, P: Determination of pseudofacility in the eye of man. Arch Ophthal 80:194, 1968.
183. Kupfer, C: Clinical significance of pseudofacility. Am J Ophthal 75:193, 1973.
184. Moses, RA: Constant pressure applanation tonography. III. The relationship of tonometric pressure to rate of loss of ocular volume. Arch Ophthal 77:181, 1967.
185. Linnér, E: Episcleral venous pressure during tonography. Acta XVII Cong Ophthal 3:1532, 1955.
186. Fisher, RF: Value of tonometry and tonography in the diagnosis of glaucoma. Br J Ophthal 56:200, 1972.
187. Moses, R: Tonometry-Effect of tonometer footplate hole on scale reading. Further studies. Arch Ophthal 61:373, 1959.
188. Grant, WM, English, FP: An explanation for so-called consensual pressure drop during tonography. Arch Ophthal 69:314, 1963.
189. Becker, B: Tonography in the diagnosis of simple (open angle) glaucoma. Trans Am Acad Ophthal Otol 65:156, 1961.
190. Johnson, LV: Tonographic survey. Am J Ophthal 61:680, 1966.
191. Haik, GM, Perez, LF, Reitman, HS, Massey, JY: Tonographic tracings in patients with cardiac rhythm disturbances. Am J Ophthal 70:929, 1970.
192. Becker, B, Christensen, RE: Water-drinking and tonography in the diagnosis of glaucoma. Arch Ophthal 56:321, 1956.
193. Roberts, W: Long-term handling of open-angle glaucoma: tonography and other prognostic aids. Ann Ophthal 9:557, 1977.
194. Portney, GL, Krohn, M: Tonography and projection perimetry. Relationship according to receiver operating characteristic curves. Arch Ophthal 95:1353, 1977.
195. Pohjanpelto, PEJ: Tonography and glaucomatous optic nerve damage. Acta Ophthal 52:817, 1974.
196. Podos, SM, Becker, B: Tonography-current thoughts. Am J Ophthal 75:733, 1973.
197. Phelps, CD, Woolson, RF, Kolker, AE, Becker, B: Diurnal variation in intraocular pressure. Am J Ophthal 77:367, 1974.
198. Wray, SH, Pavan-Langston, D: A reevaluation of edrophonium chloride (Tensilon) tonography in the diagnosis of myasthenia gravis with observations on some other defects of neuromuscular transmission. Neurology 21:586, 1971.
199. Spaeth, GL: Tonography and tonometry. In Clinical Ophthalmology, vol 3, chap 47, Duane, TD, ed, Harper & Row, Hagerstown, Md, 1976.

Chapter 3

THE INTRAOCULAR PRESSURE

THE INTRAOCULAR PRESSURE

I. WHAT IS NORMAL?

Within the context of a discussion on glaucoma, "normal" intraocular pressure (IOP) might be defined as that pressure which does not lead to glaucomatous damage of the optic nerve head. Unfortunately, such a definition cannot be expressed in precise numerical terms, since all eyes do not respond the same to given pressure levels. The best we can do is to describe the distribution of IOP in general populations and in groups of individuals with glaucomatous damage to establish *levels of risk* for glaucoma within different pressure ranges.

A. Distribution in General Populations

1. The most frequently cited population study is that by Leydhecker and associates[1] in which 10,000 persons with no known eye disease were tested with Schiøtz tonometers. They obtained a distribution of pressures that resembled a Gaussian curve, but was skewed toward the higher pressures, which they interpreted as two subpopulations: a large, "normal" group and a smaller group that was felt to represent previously unrecognized glaucoma (this included individuals with and without established glaucomatous optic nerve damage). The following data were reported for the "normal" group:

a. The *mean* IOP was 15.5 ± 2.57 mmHg.

b. Two standard deviations (±2 SD) above the mean was approximately 20.5 mmHg, which the authors interpreted as the upper limit of "normal," since 95% of the area under a Gaussian curve lies between the mean ± 2 SD. However, the latter principle does not apply when a frequency distribution is skewed, and the concept of "normal" IOP limits must be viewed as only a rough approximation.[2]

2. Subsequent IOP screening studies, using either indentation or applanation tonometry (these techniques are explained later in the chapter), have generally agreed with Leydecker's findings regarding pressure distribution in general populations, with small differences probably related to population selection and testing techniques (Table 3.1).[3-8] However, the division of IOP groups into normal and abnormal is not as simple as Leydecker and associates[1] originally suspected. Two reasons are: 1) many factors, in addition to glaucoma, influence the IOP, and 2) as previously noted, all eyes do not respond the same to given pressure levels. This leads to an overlapping of IOP distributions within non-glaucoma and glaucoma populations, which can only be illustrated theoretically (Fig. 3.1), since the precise boundaries of both groups are not known.[9] In this chapter, we will consider factors that influence IOP in the general population, while the significance of various pressure levels within specific types of glaucoma will be discussed in Section Two.

Table 3.1
Reported IOP Distributions in General Populations

Investigators	Number of Individuals	Ages (yr)	IOP (mmHg)	
			Mean	SD
A. Tested with Schiøtz Tonometers				
Leydhecker et al. ('58)[1]	10,000	10–69	15.5	2.57
Johnson ('66)[3]	7,577	>41	15.4	2.65
Segal & Skwierczyriska ('67)[4]	15,695	>30	15.3–15.9 (women) 15.0–15.2 (men)	
B. Tested with Applanation Tonometers				
Armaly ('65)[5]	2,316	20–79	15.91	3.14[a]
Perkins ('65)[6]	2,000	>40	15.2 14.9	2.5 (OD) 2.5 (OS)
Loewen et. al. ('76)[7]	4,661	9–89	17.18	3.78
Ruprecht et. al. ('78)[8]	8,899	5–94	16.25	3.45

[a] Computed from data reported according to sex and age groups.

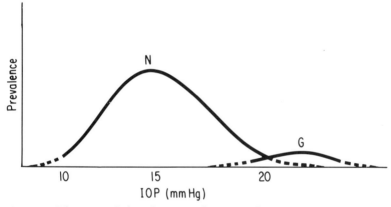

Figure 3.1. Theoretical distribution of intraocular pressures in non-glaucoma (**N**) and glaucoma (**G**) populations, showing overlap between the two groups (**dotted lines** represent uncertainty of extreme values in both populations).

B. Factors Influencing IOP

1. The following are factors (in addition to glaucoma) that influence the *long-term* IOP:

a. *Family history.* Relatives of patients with open-angle glaucoma tend to have higher IOP.[5]

b. *Age.* The IOP distribution is Gaussian in general populations between 20 and 40 years of age.[5] Thereafter, the curve begins to shift toward the higher pressures with advancing age,[5, 7, 8] which represents an increase in both the mean IOP and standard deviation.[5] This appears to be related to reduced facility of aqueous outflow,[10] despite a concomitant reduction in aqueous production.[10, 11] As noted in Chapter 2, the effect of age on aqueous humor formation in man is slight.[12]

c. *Sex.* IOP is equal between the sexes in ages 20 to 40 years. In older age groups, the previously noted increase in the *mean* IOP with age is greater in *females* and coincides with the onset of menopause, while the increase in the *standard deviation* of the IOP distribution is equal between the sexes.[5]

d. *Heredity* has been shown to influence the IOP,[13-15] possibly by a *polygenic, multifactorial* mode.[13, 14]

e. *Refractive error.* There is a positive correlation between axial length of the globe and the IOP,[16] so that *myopes* tend to have higher pressures.[16, 17] However, myopes also have a higher incidence of primary open-angle glaucoma, as will be discussed in Chapter 7, and it is hard to know whether the higher pressures in this group are a reflection of the early glaucoma cases or a truly higher IOP distribution throughout the myopic population.

f. *Race* may occasionally influence IOP distribution. For example, full-blood Indians in a New Mexican tribe were found to have a significantly lower mean IOP than a control population.[18] Furthermore, in a study of 7,638 blacks, using Schiøtz tonometry, only the standard deviation of IOP increased with age, while the mean remained constant, and there was no significant difference between the sexes.[19] However, the relationship between race and IOP is a question that requires considerably more study.

g. It has also been suggested, based on mathematical calculations, that the normal distribution of *"effective" pore diameters* in the aqueous outflow system could account for the skewed distribution of IOP.[20]

2. In addition to the aforementioned factors that have a long-term influence on IOP, the following are factors that have been reported to produce *transient fluctuations* in the pressure:

a. *Diurnal variation.* Like many biological parameters, the IOP is subject to cyclic fluctuations throughout the day.

(1). The mean *amplitude* of the daily fluctuation was 6.5 mmHg in one study of non-glaucomatous individuals.[21] An amplitude greater than 10 mmHg is generally considered to be pathologic,[21, 22] and glaucomatous eyes have been reported to exceed 30 mmHg of diurnal variation.[21]

(2). *The pattern* of the daily cycle has classically been described as having the peak IOP in the early morning hours.[23] However, subsequent studies have revealed many exceptions to this rule (if, indeed, it is the rule at all), with frequent peak pressures in the afternoon, as well as short-term fluctuations throughout the day.[21, 22, 24] This question needs further study.

(3). The *mechanism* of diurnal IOP variation is uncertain, but a relationship to *adrenocortical steroids* has been suggested, since the diurnal variation of plasma cortisol is reported by some investigators to parallel that of the IOP, peaking 3 to 4 hours before the latter.[25, 26] Furthermore, interruption of the normal daily corticosteroid cycle has been shown to alter the diurnal IOP curve.[25, 27] Serum osmolality was once thought to be correlated with the diurnal variation of IOP, but this has not been confirmed.[28] Results of tonographic studies are conflicting, with some showing an inverse relationship between IOP and outflow facility,[25] and others showing no relationship.[22]

b. *Postural variation.* Most studies show that the IOP *increases* when changing from the sitting to the *supine* position, with reported average pressure differences of 0.3 to 4.0 mmHg.[29-32] However, some investigators have been unable to confirm these findings in normal eyes.[33, 34] The postural influence on IOP is greater in eyes with glaucoma,[30, 32] or retinal vein obstruction,[34] and attempts have been made to use this phenomenon in the diagnosis of glaucoma.[35] The mechanism of pressure rise in the supine position has not been explained, but most likely relates to ocular hemodynamics.

c. *Exertional influences.* Exertion may lead to either a lowering or an elevation of the IOP, depending on the nature of the activity:

(1). *Prolonged exercise,* such as running or bicycling, has been reported to *lower* the IOP.[36-40] This reduction was found to average 24% of the baseline IOP in normal individuals[38] and 30% in open-angle glaucoma patients,[39] although reports vary. Theories of mechanism include increased serum osmolarity[38] and metabolic acidosis,[39] although most investigators agree that many factors are probably involved.

(2). *Straining,* as with valsalva[36] or electroshock therapy[41] has been reported to *elevate* the IOP. Mechanisms for this phenomenon likely include elevated episcleral venous pressure, especially with the valsalva manuever, and increased orbicularis tone. Blinking has been shown to raise the IOP 10 mmHg, while hard lid squeezing may raise it as high as 90 mmHg.[42] It has also been shown that repeated lid squeezing will lead to a slight reduction in IOP, although less so in glaucomatous eyes.[43] Reports differ as to whether decreased orbicularis tone, as with Bell's palsy or local facial nerve block, reduces IOP.[44, 45]

d. *Seasonal variation.* One study showed that the IOP tends to be higher in winter and lower in summer,[46] although this observation has yet to be confirmed.

e. The correlation between *blood pressure* and IOP is not clear. Although some studies have found no relationship,[47] others have shown a positive correlation after age 60 years.[48] The IOP is reported to rise and fall with corresponding transient fluctuations in blood pressure, as during cardiopulmonary bypass surgery,[49] and it may be that compensatory mechanisms effect the long-term correlation between these two parameters.

f. *Systemic hyperthermia* has been shown to cause an increased IOP of approximately 5 mmHg in rabbits.[50]

g. *Hormonal influences.* The possible correlation between diurnal IOP and plasma cortisol variations was previously discussed. In addition, preliminary evidence suggests that the IOP may *increase* in response to ACTH, glucocorticoids, and growth hormone, and *de-*

crease in response to progesterone, estrogen, chorionic gonadotropin and relaxin.[51] The IOP has also been reported to be higher in patients with hypothyroidism, and lower with hyperthyroidism.[52] However, the IOP does not appear to be influenced by gonadectomy in rabbits[53] or the menstrual cycle in humans.[54] Considerably more study is needed to clearly establish the relationship between hormonal disturbances and IOP.

h. *General anesthesia* is usually associated with a *reduction* in the IOP,[55, 56] although there are exceptions, such as with trichlorethylene[57] and ketamine,[58–60] which are reported to elevate the ocular pressure. There are two situations in which the ophthalmologist is particularly concerned about alterations in IOP during general anesthesia:

(1). In infants and children who are examined under anesthesia for suspicion of *congenital glaucoma*, the main concern is to avoid artificial reduction of IOP, which could mask a pathologic pressure elevation. Reported studies with halothane, the anesthetic agent most often used in this situation, are slightly inconsistent. Some investigators found that halothane anesthesia had no significant influence on IOP in children[61] or primates.[57] However, the mean IOP in infants without glaucoma under general anesthesia with halothane was found to be 9.56 ± 2.6 in one study[62] and 10.68 ± 6.0 mmHg in another series,[63] which is slightly lower than the reported 11.4 ± 2.4 mmHg in newborns without anesthesia.[64] *Hypnotics* that are used to produce unconsciousness, such as 4-hydroxybutyrate, are also reported to reduce the IOP,[65] and *barbiturates* and *tranquilizers* may, in some patients, cause a transient pressure reduction.[66]

(2). When operating on an *open eye*, as following penetrating injury or during intraocular surgery, the primary concern is to avoid sudden elevations of IOP that might lead to extrusion of ocular contents. *Depolarizing muscle relaxants*, such as succinylcholine[67] and suxamethonium,[68] cause a transient rise in IOP possibly due to a combination of extraocular muscle contraction and intraocular vasodilation. Pretreatment with non-depolarizing muscle relaxants, such as *d*-tubocurarine and gallamine, have not been proven to prevent IOP elevation during endotracheal intubation,[67, 68] although a newer agent, fazadinium, has been reported to be successful in this situation.[69]

It has also been noted that an elevated pCO_2[70–72] causes a rise in IOP, which is not blocked by pretreatment with acetazolamide,[72] and an increased concentration of oxygen is associated with an intraocular pressure reduction.[73]

i. Other *drugs* that have been studied for their effect on the intraocular pressure include the following (exclusive of antiglaucoma drugs, which will be discussed in Section Three):

(1). *Alcohol* has been shown to *lower* the IOP, although more so in patients with glaucoma.[74] This is not associated with a change in facility of aqueous outflow,[74] and it has been suggested that the mechanism may be a combination of suppressed circulating antidiuretic hormone, leading to a reduction of net water movement into the eye, and direct inhibition of aqueous secretion.[75]

(2). *Heroin*[76] and *marijuana* are also reported to *lower* the IOP. The latter will be discussed further in Section Three.

(3). *Tobacco* smoking may cause a transient *rise* in the IOP.[77] In one study, smoking one cigarette caused an increase in IOP of greater than 5 mmHg in 37% of open-angle glaucoma patients and 11% of non-glaucomatous individuals.[78]

(4). *Caffeine* may cause a slight, transient *rise* in IOP, although in the levels associated with customary coffee drinking this does not appear to cause a significant, sustained pressure elevation.[66]

(5). Other drugs that are reported to cause an *elevated* IOP include *LSD*[76] and *corticosteroids*. The latter will be discussed in Chapter 7 and 20.

(6). Systemic *vasodilators*, including glyceryl trinitrate (nitro-glycerine),[79, 80] pentaerythrityl tetranitrate,[79] isosorbide dinitrate,[80] be-cyclan,[80] nicotinic acid,[81] and cyclandelate,[81] are all reported to have no influence on IOP in normal or glaucomatous eyes with open angles. However, one study revealed that nitroglycerin, when administered by perfusion techniques, and isosorbide dinitrate lower the IOP in normal individuals as well as patients with open-angle or angle-closure glaucoma.[82]

(7). Systemic *anticholinergics*, such as atropine[83, 84] and pro-pantheline[85] have been found to have no influence on IOP in normal or glaucomatous eyes with open anterior chamber angles, especially with short-term therapy. However, topical cyclopentolate will elevate the IOP in some patients with open-angle glaucoma,[83, 86] and it has been suggested that these patients may also manifest a slight pressure rise in response to long-term administration of systemic anticholin-ergics.[84]

(8). *Anti-convulsants*, *e.g.*, diphenylhydantoin,[66] and *amphet-amines*, *e.g.*, dextro amphetamine,[66] have not been found to influence the IOP in normal or glaucomatous eyes with open anterior chamber angles.

(9). Drugs that may precipitate angle-closure attacks of glaucoma will be discussed in Chapter 8.

II. TONOMETERS AND TONOMETRY

A. Classification of Tonometers

All clinical tonometers measure the intraocular pressure by relating a *deformation* of the globe to the *force* responsible for the deformation. The two basic types of tonometers differ according to the *shape* of the deformation[87]:

1. *Indentation* (or impression) *tonometers*. The shape of the deformation with this type of tonometer is a *truncated cone* (Fig. 3.2a). The shape, however, is variable and unpredictable. In addition, these instruments displace a relatively large intraocular volume. As a result of these characteristics, conversion tables based on imperical data

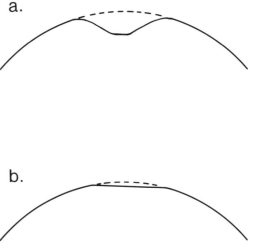

Figure 3.2. Corneal deformation created by **(a)** indentation tonometers (a truncated cone) and **(b)** applanation tonometers (simple flattening).

from in vitro and in vivo studies must be used to estimate the IOP. The prototype of this group is the *Schiøtz* tonometer.

2. *Applanation tonometers.* The shape of the deformation with these tonometers is a simple *flattening* (Fig. 3.2b) and, because the shape is constant, its relationship to the IOP can, in most cases, be derived from mathematical calculations. The applanation tonometers are further differentiated on the basis of the *variable* that is measured.

a. *Variable force.* This type of tonometer measures the force that is required to applanate (flatten) a standard area of the corneal surface. The prototype is the *Goldmann* applanation tonometer.

b. *Variable area.* Other applanation tonometers measure the area of cornea that is flattened by a known force (weight). The prototype in this group is the *Maklakov* tonometer. It should be noted at this point that the division between indentation and applanation tonometers does not correlate entirely with the grouping of instruments according to a relatively high or low volume displacement. In the case of Maklakov-type tonometers, the volume displacement is such that conversion tables are required.

3. A third type of tonometer measures the *time* required to deform the cornea in response to a standard force (a puff of air). This instrument is the *non-contact tonometer*.

We will first consider the descriptions and techniques of these various tonometers, and then compare their relative values and limitations.

B. Indentation Tonometry

1. *Description of Schiøtz tonometer* (Fig. 3.3).

a. The body of the tonometer has a *footplate*, which rests on the cornea.

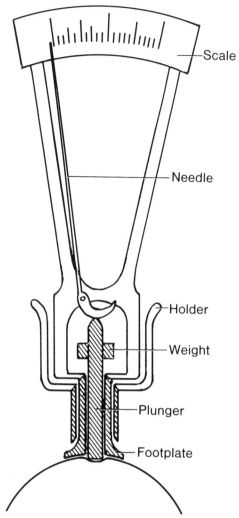

Figure 3.3. Cut-away view showing basic features of Schiøtz-type indentation tonometer.

  b. A *plunger* moves freely (except for the effect of friction)
within a shaft in the footplate, and the degree to which it indents the
cornea is indicated by the movement of a needle on a *scale*.
  c. A 5.5-g *weight* is permanently fixed to the plunger, which can
be increased to 7.5, 10, or 15 g by adding additional weights.
  2. *Basic Concept*.[88] When the plunger indents the cornea, the
baseline or resting pressure (P_0) is artificially raised to a new value
(P_t). Since the tonometer actually measures P_t, it is necessary to
estimate P_0 for each scale reading and weight.
  a. Schiøtz estimated P_0 by experiments in which a manometer
was attached to enucleated eyes by a cannula inserted through the
optic nerve. A stopcock was placed between the cannula and manom-

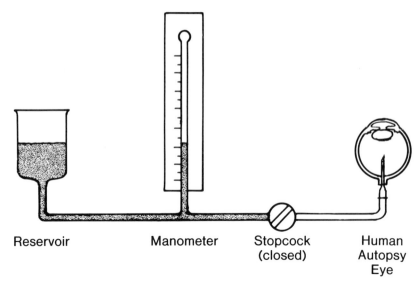

Reservoir   Manometer   Stopcock   Human
                          (closed)   Autopsy
                                       Eye

Figure 3.4. Apparatus used in manometric calibration of Schiøtz tonometer.

eter, and a reservoir was used to adjust the pressure in the eye (Fig. 3.4). He then made two sets of readings:

(1). In one set, *open manometer*, the stopcock was left open when the tonometer was placed on the cornea, which allowed correlation of P_t with the scale reading and weight.

(2). In the second set, *closed manometer*, the desired pressure was introduced in the eye and the stopcock was closed before placing the tonometer on the cornea, thereby allowing correlation of P_0 with the scale reading and weight. It was the data from this set of readings that were used to calibrate the tonometer.

b. The change in pressure from P_0 to P_t is an expression of the resistance an eye offers to the displacement of a volume of fluid (V_c). Friedenwald[88] developed an empirical formula for the linear relationship between the logarithm of the pressure and the volume change in a given eye. This formula has a single numerical constant, the *coefficient of ocular rigidity* (K), which is roughly an expression of the distensibility of the eye. He developed a *nomogram* for estimating K based on two tonometric readings with different weights,[88] and subsequent studies using applanation tonometry with different sized applanating areas confirmed his formulations.[89]

(1). Based on his formula and additional experiments, Friedenwald[90] calculated an average K of 0.0245 and used this to develop a set of conversion tables, referred to as the *1948 tables*.

(2). Friedenwald[91] later revised the average K to a value of 0.0215, on which he based a new set of tables that became known as the *1955 tables*.[92]

(3). Subsequent studies indicate that the 1948 tables agree more closely with measurements by Goldmann applanation tonometry.[93, 94]

3. Technique of Schiøtz tonometry

a. With the patient in a supine position and fixing on a target just overhead, the examiner separates the eyelids and gently rests the tonometer footplate on the anesthetized cornea in a position that allows free vertical movement of the plunger.

b. When the tonometer is properly positioned, the examiner will observe a fine movement of the indicator needle on the scale in response to the ocular pulsations. The *scale reading* should be taken as the average between the extremes of these excursions. It is customary to start with the fixed 5.5-g weight. However, if the scale reading is 4 or less, additional weight should be added to the plunger.

c. A *conversion table* is then used to derive the intraocular pressure in millimeters of Mercury (mmHg) from the scale reading and plunger weight. It is customary to record the scale reading, weight, IOP, and conversion table from which the pressure value was derived. For example, a scale reading of 7, using a 5.5-g weight, which corresponds to an IOP of 12 mmHg according to the 1955 conversion tables, would be written as 7/5.5 = 12 mmHg ('55).

4. Sources of error with indentation tonometry.

The accuracy of indentation tonometry depends on the assumption that all eyes respond the same to the external force of indentation, which is not the case. The following are some of the more common variables that introduce potential for error:

a. *Ocular rigidity.* Since conversion tables are based on an "average" coefficient of ocular rigidity (K), eyes that deviate significantly from this K value will give false IOP measurements. A *high* K will cause a falsely *high* IOP, while a *low* K will lead to a falsely *low* reading. There is some confusion in the literature as to how various conditions influence K:

(1). *Refractive errors* reportedly influence K, with the highest values in high hyperopes and the lowest in high myopes.[95] Another study, however, revealed an increased K with extreme myopia.[88]

(2). *Elevated IOP* is associated with a reduced K,[96] which may explain the lower K during water provocative testing.[95–97] However, in long-standing glaucoma, K has been found to be increased.[88]

(3). *Miotics*, especially strong cholinesterase inhibitors, are said to reduce K.[95] *Vasodilators* may also diminish K, while *vasoconstrictors* cause an increase.[88]

(4). *Surgery.* Ocular rigidity is reduced following retinal detachment surgery,[98, 99] or the intravitreal injection of a compressible gas,[100] leading to a falsely low IOP estimation with indentation tonometry. Keratoconus was once thought to be associated with an abnormally low K, but this may be an artifact due to the thin cornea, since it is not seen after keratoplasty for this disease.[101]

(5). *Age.* Reports vary widely regarding the correlation of K and advancing age.[88, 95, 102]

The technique for determining K is based on Friedenwald's[88] concept of *differential tonometry*, as previously discussed. Goldmann and Schmidt[103] suggested that it was more accurate to obtain the two readings with an applanation tonometer and a Schiøtz tonometer using a 10-g weight and to plot these readings on Friedenwald's nomogram. However, Chandler and Grant[104] have suggested that the estimation of ocular rigidity by any method is premature and of little value until more accurate calibrations are achieved.

b. *Blood volume alteration.* The variable expulsion of intraocular blood during indentation tonometry may also influence the IOP measurement.[105]

c. *Corneal influences.* Either a *steeper* or *thicker* cornea will cause a greater displacement of fluid during indentation tonometry, which leads to a falsely *high* IOP reading.[90]

d. The *Moses effect* on indentation tonometry was discussed under Tonography in chapter two.

5. *Electronic indentation tonometers.* Grant[106] combined the concept of Schiøtz tonometry with continuous electronic monitoring of the pressure for use in tonography, which was discussed in chapter two. Similar instruments were subsequently designed,[107, 108] and the importance of critical calibration of electronic tonometers has been emphasized.[109]

C. Applanation Tonometry with Variable Force

1. *Basic concept.* Goldmann[110] introduced a tonometer in 1954 based on a modification of the *Maklakov-Fick Law* (also referred to as the *Imbert-Fick Law*[111]):

a. The Imbert-Fick law states that an external force (w) against a sphere equals the pressure in the sphere (P_t) times the area flattened (applanated) by the external force (A) (Fig. 3.5):

$$W = P_t \times A$$

b. The validity of this law requires that the sphere is 1) perfectly spherical, 2) dry, 3) perfectly flexible, and 4) infinitely thin. The cornea fails to satisfy any of these requirements, since it is aspherical and wet, and neither perfectly flexible, nor infinitely thin. The moisture creates a surface tension (S), while the lack of flexibility requires a force to bend the cornea (B), which is independent of the internal pressure. In addition, since the cornea has a central thickness of approximately 0.55 mm, the outer area of flattening (A) is not the same as the inner area (A_1). It was, therefore, necessary to modify the Imbert-Fick Law in the following manner to account for these characteristics of the cornea (Fig. 3.6):

$$W + S = P_t A_1 + B$$

c. When $A_1 = 7.35$ mm^2, S balances B and $W = P_t$. This internal area of applanation is obtained when the diameter of the external area of applanation is 3.06 mm. The volume displacement produced by this amount of applanation is approximately 0.50 mm^3, so that P_t is very close to P_0, and ocular rigidity does not significantly influence the measurement.

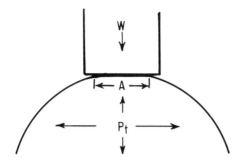

Figure 3.5.   The Imbert-Fick Law $(W = P_t \times A)$.

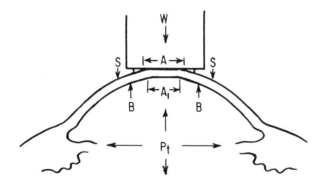

Figure 3.6.   Modification of Imbert-Fick Law for the cornea $(W + S = P_t \times A_1 + B)$.

2. Goldmann Applanation Tonometry

a. *Description of instrument.* The tonometer is mounted on a standard slit-lamp in such a way that the examiner's view is directed through the center of a *plastic biprism*, which is used to applanate the cornea. Two beam-splitting prisms within the applanating unit optically convert the circular area of corneal contact into semicircles. The prisms are adjusted so that the margins of the semicircles overlap when 3.06 mm of cornea is applanated. The biprism is attached by a rod to a housing, which contains a coil spring and series of levers that are used to adjust the force of the biprism against the cornea.[112]

b. *Technique* (Fig. 3.7).

(1). The tear film is stained with *sodium fluorescein,* and the cornea and biprism are illuminated with a *cobalt blue light* from the slit lamp. The resulting fluorescence of the stained tears facilitates visualization of the tear meniscus at the margin of contact between cornea and biprism. The staining may be accomplished by instilling

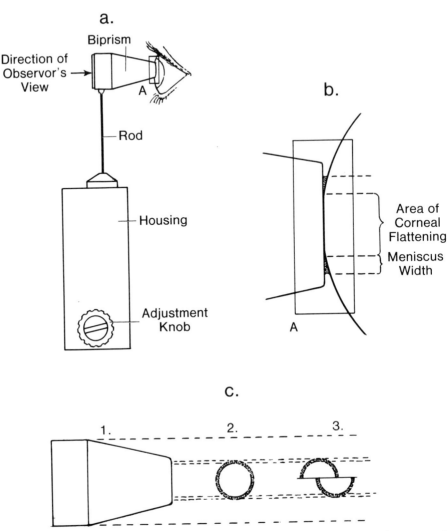

Figure 3.7. Goldmann-type applanation tonometry. **a:** Basic features of tonometer, shown in contact with patient's cornea. **b:** Enlargement (**A**) shows tear film meniscus created by contact of biprism and cornea. **c:** View through biprism (**1**) reveals circular meniscus (**2**), which is converted into semicircles (**3**) by prisms.

a drop of topical anesthetic and touching a fluorescein-impregnated paper strip to the tears in the lower cul-de-sac.[112] However, a 0.25% solution of sodium fluorescein has been shown to produce the optimum fluorescent semi-circles,[113] and commercial solutions are available in combination with topical anesthetics.[114] Studies have shown that the preservative in these commercial preparations imparts a satisfactory degree of resistance to bacterial contamination.[114-116] Some physicians have felt that Goldmann applanation tonometry could be performed without fluorescein, but this has been shown to give a significant underestimation of the IOP and is not recommended.[117]

(2). The *fluorescent semicircles* are viewed through the biprism, and the force against the cornea is adjusted until the *inner edges* overlap. As with the indentation tonometer, the influence of the ocular pulsations is seen when the instrument is properly positioned, and the excursions must be averaged to give the desired endpoint (Fig. 3.8a). The IOP is then read directly from a scale on the tonometer housing.

(3). It has been suggested that the biprism should be cleaned with water and cotton, since other agents may damage the methylmethacrylate or alter the accuracy of the instrument.[118]

c. *Sources of error.*

(1). The *meniscus width* may influence the reading slightly, with *wider* menisci causing falsely *higher* pressure estimates (Fig. 3.8b).[111]

(2). Improper *vertical alignment* (one semicircle larger than the other) will also lead to a falsely high IOP estimate (Fig. 3.8c).[112]

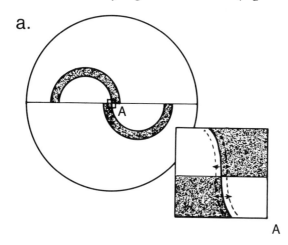

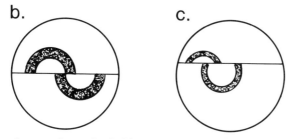

Figure 3.8. Semicircles of Goldmann-type applanation tonometry. **a**: Proper width and position. Enlargement (**A**) depicts excursions of semicircles caused by ocular pulsations. **b**: Semicircles are too wide. **c**: Improper vertical and horizontal alignment.

(3). *Corneal thickness* has been shown to influence the pressure estimate, with thin corneas producing falsely low readings.[119] A thick cornea causes a falsely high measurement if the thickness is due to increased collagen fibrils,[119, 120] whereas low readings occur if the thickness is due to edema.[119]

(4). *Corneal curvature* was also shown to influence IOP measurements, with an increase of approximately 1 mmHg for each 3 diopters of increase in corneal power.[121]

(5). Marked *corneal astigmatism* will produce an elliptical area of corneal contact. To minimize the error that this may induce, the biprism should be rotated until the dividing line between the prisms is 45° to the major axis of the ellipse.[112]

(6). An *irregular cornea* will also distort the semicircles and interfere with the accuracy of the IOP estimates.[112]

(7). *Prolonged contact* of the biprism with the cornea leads to corneal injury, as manifested by staining, which makes multiple readings unsatisfactory.[112] In addition, prolonged contact causes an apparent decrease in IOP over a period of minutes.[112] The latter phenomenon is less pronounced in eyes with carotid occlusive disease, suggesting that it may be related to intraocular blood.[122]

3. *Other Applanation Tonometers with Variable Force.*

a. *Hand-held Goldmann-type tonometers.*

(1). *Perkins applanation tonometer.* This instrument utilizes the same biprism as the Goldmann applanation tonometer. The light source is powered by a battery, and the force is varied manually. A counterbalance makes it possible to use the instrument in either the vertical or horizontal position.[123]

(2). *Draeger applanation tonometer.* This instrument is similar to the Perkins tonometer, but utilizes a different biprism and has an electric motor which varies the force.[124, 125]

(3). An inexpensive model has also been described in which a Goldmann biprism is mounted on a dynamometer and attached to a blue penlight.[126]

b. *Mackay-Marg tonometer* (Fig. 3.9).

(1). *Basic concept.* The force measured is that which is required to keep the flat plate of a plunger flush with a surrounding sleeve against the pressure of corneal deformation. The effect of corneal rigidity, *i.e.*, the force required to bend the cornea, is transferred to the sleeve, so the plate reads only the IOP.[127]

(2). *Description of instrument.* The plate has a diameter of 1.5 mm and is surrounded by a rubber sleeve. The force required to keep the plate flush with the sleeve is *electronically* monitored and recorded on a paper strip.[128]

(3). *Technique.* As the instrument tip momentarily touches the cornea, the *tracing* (representing the force required to keep the plate flush with the sleeve) rises until the applanated area reaches a diameter of 1.5 mm. At this point (the crest), the pressure against the plate represents the IOP plus the force required to bend the cornea.

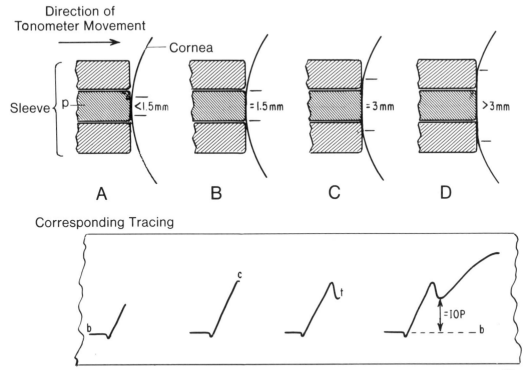

Figure 3.9. Mackay-Marg tonometry (modified from Marg, E, Mackay, RS, Oechsli, R[128]). A: As plate (p) contacts cornea, tracing begins to rise. B: Crest (c) is reached when diameter of contact equals that of plate surface (1.5 mm). C: With further corneal flattening, force of bending cornea is transferred to sleeve, and tracing falls to trough (t) when diameter of contact equals 3 mm. D: Still further corneal flattening leads to artificial elevation of intraocular pressure (IOP). Distance from baseline (b) of tracing to trough is read as the IOP.

The tracing then falls as the effect of corneal rigidity is transferred to the surrounding sleeve. When a corneal diameter of 3 mm is flattened (the initial trough), the plate is considered to be reading only the IOP. The tracing then rises due to artificial elevation of the IOP.[128]

    c. *Pneumatic "applanation" tonometer* (Fig. 3.10).

        (1). *Basic concept.* This is neither a true applanation tonometer, nor one which causes a very low volume displacement. However, the concept is similar to that of the Mackay-Marg tonometer in that a central sensing device measures the IOP, while the force required to bend the cornea is transferred to a surrounding structure. The sensor in this case is *air pressure*, rather than an electronically controlled plunger.[129, 130]

        (2). *Description of instrument.* At one end of a pencil-like holder is a sensing nozzle, which has an outer diameter of 0.25 inch and a central chamber of 2.0 mm. The nozzle is covered with a silastic diaphragm, and pressurized air in the central chamber exhausts at the face of the nozzle between the orifice of the central chamber and the diaphragm. The air pressure is dependent on the resistance to the

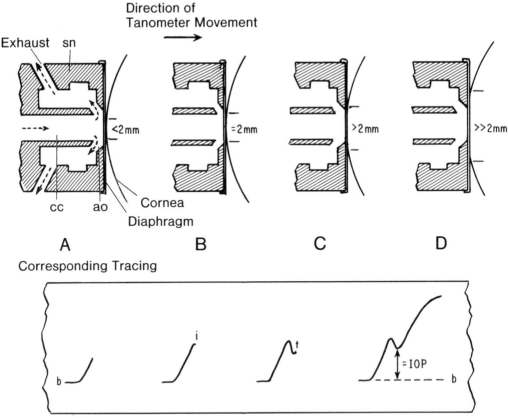

Figure 3.10. Pneumatic tonometry (modified from Durham, DG, Bigliano, RP, Masino, JA[129]). **A:** As sensing nozzle (**sn**) touches cornea, resistance to air flow (dotted lines) begins to increase at annular opening (**ao**), with corresponding rise in tracing. **B:** When diameter of corneal contact equals 2 mm, an initial inflection (**i**) is recorded. **C:** With further corneal flattening, force of bending cornea is transferred to face of sensor, and air pressure in central chamber (**cc**) measures IOP, represented by distance from baseline (**b**) to trough (**t**) of tracing. **D:** Further corneal compression by tonometer leads to artificial IOP rise.

exhaust, and a pneumatic-to-electronic transducer converts the air pressure to a recording on a paper strip.[129]

(3). *Technique.* As the sensing nozzle touches the cornea, the tracing rises as an increasing area of corneal surface comes in contact with the diaphragm. When the area of contact equals that of the central chamber, an initial inflection is recorded, which represents the IOP and the force required to bend the cornea. With further enlargement of the corneal contact, the bending force is transferred to the face of the nozzle and the tracing falls to a trough, which is interpreted as the actual IOP. Still further contact leads to artificial pressure elevation and a second inflection.[129] The instrument can be used for continuous IOP monitoring.

D. Applanation Tonometry with Variable Area

1. *Maklakov Tonometer.*

a. *Basic concept.* In 1885, Maklakov introduced a tonometer with which IOP is estimated by measuring the area of cornea that is flattened by a known weight.[131] It is still popular in Russia.

b. *Instrument and technique*. A dumbbell-shaped metal cylinder has flat *endplates* of polished glass on either end with diameters of 10 mm. A set of four such instruments are available, weighing 5, 7.5, 10 and 15 g, and a cross-action wire handle is supplied to support the instrument on the cornea. A layer of dye (a suspension of argyrol, glycerin, and water) is applied to either endplate and, with the patient in a supine position and the cornea anesthetized, the instrument is allowed to rest vertically on the cornea for 1 second. This produces a circular white imprint on the endplate, which corresponds to the area of cornea that was flattened. The diameter of the white area is measured with a transparent plastic measuring scale to 0.1 mm, and the IOP is read from a conversion table in the column corresponding to the weight used.[131, 132]

c. *Conversion tables*. Although the volume displacement with Maklakov-type applanation tonometry is less than with indentation tonometry, it is large enough that ocular rigidity must be considered in computing the IOP. Kalfa recognized this problem at approximately the same time that Friedenwald was applying the concept of ocular rigidity to Schiøtz tonometry. He too used different weights to estimate the average ocular rigidity of the eyeball, which he called an "elastometric rise."[133] New conversion tables have been developed which provide nomograms for the differential tonometry.[134]

d. *Other Maklakov-type tonometers* are listed in table two.

E. Non-Contact Tonometer

The *non-contact tonometer* (NCT) was introduced by Grolman[141] in 1972, and has the unique advantage over other tonometers of not touching the eye, other than with a *puff of air*. This instrument should not be confused with the pneumatic tonometer, which was previously discussed.

1. *Basic concept*. A puff of room air creates a constant force, which momentarily deforms the cornea. It is difficult to determine the exact nature of the corneal deformation, although it is postulated that the central cornea is flattened at the moment the pressure measurement

Table 3.2
Applanation Tonometers with Variable Area

Tonometer	Description/Use
1. Maklakov-Kalfa[131]	1. Prototype
2. Applanometer[135]	2. Ceramic endplates
3. Tonomat[136]	3. Disposable endplates
4. Halberg tonometer[137]	4. Transparent endplate for direct reading: multiple weights
5. Barraquer tonometer[138]	5. Plastic tonometer for use in operating room
6. Ocular Tension Indicator[139]	6. Utilizes Goldmann biprism and 2.1-g weight: for screening clinic (measures above or below 21 mmHg)
7. GlaucoTest[140]	7. Screening tonometer with multiple endplates for selecting different "cut-off" pressures

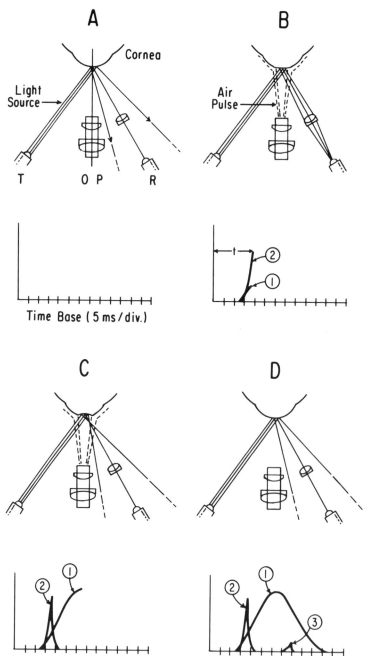

Figure 3.11. Non-contact tonometry (modified from Grolman, B[141]). **A**: Light source from transmitter (**T**) is reflected from undisturbed cornea toward receiver (**R**), while cornea is aligned by optical system (**O**). **B**: Air puff (**1**) from pneumatic system (**P**) deforms cornea, which increases the number of light rays (**2**) received and detected by **R**. Time (**t**) from internal reference point to moment of maximum light detection (which presumably corresponds to applanation of the cornea) is converted to IOP (based on calibrations with Goldmann applanation tonometer) and displayed on digital readout. **C**: Continued air pulse produces momentary concavity of cornea, causing sharp reduction in light rays received by R. **D**: As cornea returns to undisturbed state, a second moment of applanation causes another light peak (**3**). (Reprinted by permission from Shields, MB: Surv Ophthal 24:211, 1980.)

is made. The *time* from an internal reference point to the moment of presumed flattening is measured and converted to IOP based on prior comparisons with readings from Goldmann applanation tonometers.

2. *Description of instrument.* The NCT is mounted on a table and consists of three subsystems:[141, 142]

a. *An alignment system* allows the operator to optically align the patient's cornea in three dimensions (axial, vertical, and lateral).

b. An *opto-electronic applanation monitoring system* consists of 1) a transmitter, which directs a collimated beam of light at the corneal vertex, and 2) a receiver and detector, which accepts only parallel, coaxial rays reflected from the cornea.

c. A *pneumatic system* generates a puff of room air, which is directed against the cornea.

3. *Technique* (Fig. 3.11)[141–143]

a. The patient observes an internal target while the operator aligns the cornea by superimposing a reflection of the target from the patients cornea on a stationary ring. During this time, light from the transmitter is reflected from the undisturbed cornea, which allows only a small number of rays to enter the receiver.

b. When the cornea is properly aligned, the operator depresses a trigger which causes a puff of air to be directed against the cornea. At the moment that the central cornea is flattened, the greatest number of reflected light rays are received, which is recorded as the peak intensity of light detected. The time from an internal reference point to the moment of maximum light detection is converted to IOP and displayed on a digital readout.

c. The time interval for an average NCT measurement is 1 to 3 msec ($\frac{1}{500}$ of the cardiac cycle) and is random with respect to the phase of the cardiac cycle so that the ocular pulse becomes a significant variable, *i.e.*, cannot be averaged as with other tonometers. For this reason, it is recommended that a minimum of three readings within 3 mmHg be taken and averaged as the IOP.

F. Miscellaneous Tonometers

1. Attempts have been made to estimate the IOP by measuring the duration of contact of a spring driven hammer with the eye (impact tonometer),[144] or the frequency of a vibrating probe in contact with the cornea (Vibra-Tonometer).[145]

2. *Continuous IOP monitoring devices.* In the diagnosis and management of glaucoma, there is need for a tonometer that can continuously monitor the IOP for hours, days, or indefinitely without artificially altering the pressure. Preliminary laboratory studies have investigated the feasibility of remote IOP monitoring with *telemetric devices. Strain gauges* can be used to drive the monitor. The strain gauge can be placed in a contact lens to measure changes in the meridional angle of the corneo-scleral junction,[146] or it can be embedded in an encircling scleral band to measure the distention of the globe.[147] Another approach is to use a *scleral applanating device* attached to a passive radio telemetric pressure transducer.[148–150] Considerably more research is needed in this area.

G. Comparison of Tonometers

1. *Comparison with Goldmann tonometer in eyes with regular corneas.* The most precise method for evaluating the accuracy of a tonometer is to compare it with manometric measurements of the cannulated anterior chamber. While this technique is frequently used with animal and autopsy eyes, it has obvious limitations in large scale human studies. The alternative is to compare the tonometer in question against the instrument which previous studies have shown to be the most accurate. In eyes with regular corneas, the *Goldmann applanation tonometer* is generally accepted as the standard against which other tonometers must be compared. It should be noted, however, that even when two readings are taken on the same eye with Goldmann tonometers within a short time frame, using either one instrument and one examiner[151] or two instruments and two examiners,[152] at least 30% of the paired readings will differ by 2 and 3 mmHg or more, respectively. Therefore, an error of approximately 2 mmHg is assumed to be inherent in even the most accurate of pressure measurements.

a. *Schiøtz tonometer.* Studies consistently indicate that the Schiøtz tonometer reads *lower* than the Goldmann,[153-155] even when the postural influence on IOP is eliminated by performing both measurements in the supine position.[93, 156, 157] In one study, age was found to be the most important source of variation, with the greatest discrepancies occurring in the fifties and sixties.[158] The magnitude of disagreement between the two tonometers and the influence of ocular rigidity are such that the Schiøtz tonometer is felt to indicate only that the IOP is within a certain range,[93] and is of limited value even for screening purposes.[154, 155, 159] The Schiøtz tonometer is particularly unsuitable for situations in which ocular rigidity is known to be significantly altered, such as following retinal detachment surgery,[98, 99] or in eyes containing compressible gas.[100]

b. *Perkins applanation tonometer.* This instrument has compared favorably against the Goldmann tonometer.[160, 161] In one study, the difference between readings with the two instruments, expressed as the root mean square difference, was 1.4 mmHg.[160] This instrument is especially useful in infants and children and is accurate in the horizontal as well as the vertical position.

c. *Draeger applanation tonometer.* Comparative studies with Goldmann tonometry have given inconsistent results, with one showing satisfactory agreement,[161] while another found the Draeger instrument to be no better than a properly-used Schiøtz tonometer.[162] Because of its more complex design, the Draeger tonometer is more difficult to use than the Perkins, and patient acceptance tends to be worse.

d. *Mackay-Marg tonometer.* A highly significant correlation was found between IOP readings with the Mackay-Marg and Goldmann tonometers using topical anesthesia for both instruments, with the Mackay-Marg reading systematically *higher* and the Goldmann systematically *lower* than their mean results.[163] When the Mackay-Marg was used without anesthesia the mean IOP was approximately 2 mmHg higher than that obtained by the same instrument with anesthesia.[163] One study showed significant discrepancies between Mackay-Marg and Goldmann measurements when the former was used by a technician.[164] (See additional discussion under Tonometry on Irregular Corneas.)

e. *Pneumatic tonometer.* Comparative studies with one pneumatic tonometer, the *pneumatonograph*, showed close correlations with Goldmann tonometers,[165, 166] even when the pneumatic tonometer was operated by a technician.[155] However, the pneumatonograph read statistically *higher*,[165, 166] and one study of an early model revealed an unsatisfactory correlation.[167] In a laboratory analysis of the pneumatonograph, the investigators found several errors that resulted in compression of the scale readings and an overestimation of the IOP even in the physiologic range.[168] They concluded that the instrument was not suitable for tonography. (See additional discussion under Tonometry on Irregular Corneas.)

f. *Halberg applanation tonometer.* This instrument compared more favorably with the Goldmann tonometer than did the Schiøtz,[155, 169] although it compared less favorably than the pneumatonograph in one study.[155] It was felt to be easier to learn than Perkins hand-held tonometry,[170] although medical students in another study preferred and were more accurate with a Schiøtz tonometer.[171]

g. *GlaucoTest.* Evaluations of this tonometer suggest that it is a good screening instrument,[140] even when used by a technician.[155]

h. *Non-contact tonometer.* Comparisons against Goldmann applanation tonometers indicate that the NCT is reliable within the normal IOP range, although the reliability is reduced in the higher pressure ranges and is limited by an abnormal cornea or poor fixation.[141-143] Potential hazards with all contact tonometers include 1) abrasion of the cornea, 2) reactions to topical anesthetics, and 3) spread of infection, such as epidemic keratoconjunctivitis. The NCT eliminates all of these. In addition, the instrument can be used reliably by paramedical personnel and has particular value in mass screening and possibly in studies of topical antiglaucoma drugs.[143]

2. *Tonometry on irregular corneas.* The accuracy of Goldmann- and Maklakov-type applanation tonometers and the non-contact tonometer is limited in eyes with irregular corneas. In cases of scarred or edematous corneas, the *Mackay-Marg tonometer* is generally considered to be the most accurate.[172-174] However, the pneumatic tonometer has also been shown to be useful in eyes with diseased corneas,[174, 175] and one study, using cannulated eye-bank eyes with abnormal corneas, showed that the pneumatonograph gave more consistent and objective measurements than the Mackay-Marg.[176]

The Mackay-Marg was found to be more satisfactory than the pneumatonograph for measuring the IOP of canine eyes.[177] Investigators should be cautious of using the pneumatonograph in animals, since it has only been calibrated for human eyes. It has been claimed that both the Mackay-Marg[178] and pneumatonograph[175] can measure the IOP through soft contact lenses with sufficient accuracy to indicate significant pressure elevation. Applanation measurements are said to be effected by the power of the contact lenses with high water content, and correction tables have been developed to compensate for this.[179]

III. MASS SCREENING FOR GLAUCOMA

Early detection of glaucoma is essential in preventing loss of vision from this group of disorders. The absence of symptoms during the initial phases of the disease in the majority of cases requires that screening techniques be employed to identify patients with early glaucoma. For this reason, *mass IOP screening programs* have been established, although the efficacy of these efforts to detect glaucoma has yet to be proven. Some of the problem areas are the following:

A. The Screening Level

As noted in the outset of this chapter, there is an overlap of the IOP distributions between non-glaucoma and glaucoma populations, so that a simple "cut-off" pressure level between these two groups does not exist. Therefore, a screening level must be selected that is felt to provide the optimum balance between sensitivity and specificity[180, 181]:

1. *Sensitivity* is the ability to identify the screenees who truly have glaucoma, and is expressed as the percentage screening positive of the total number of confirmed cases, *i.e.*, a screening level with high sensitivity has few false negatives.

2. *Specificity* is the ability to give a negative finding when the screenee is truly free of glaucoma, and is expressed as the percentage screening negative of those who do not have the disease, *i.e.*, a screening level with high specificity has few false positives.

The optimum screening level is one that minimizes false negatives without significantly sacrificing specificity. This level is generally taken to be 21 mmHg, although factors which influence IOP distribution (see discussion earlier in this chapter), as well as those that increase the risk of glaucoma (see Chapter 7) may necessitate an adjustment of this level for certain populations.[180]

B. The Tonometer

The efficacy of a screening program is greatly influenced by the reliability of the tonometer used.[182] For example, the Schiøtz tonometer, as previously discussed, reads significantly lower than the Goldmann applanation tonometer, which increases the chance of missing patients who actually have glaucoma. Furthermore, the effect of ocular rigidity on Schiøtz tonometry makes it difficult to simply adjust the screening level for this instrument. The *Perkins applanation tonometer*, because of its accuracy and portability, is a useful instrument for mass screening,[160, 161] but it requires a highly skilled operator. The *non-contact tonometer* can be operated with considerable accuracy by paramedical personnel with minimal training and eliminates the risk of corneal abrasion, spread of infection, and reactions to topical anesthetics.[143] These advantages make the NCT particularly useful in mass screening programs, although the cost of the instrument remains a problem in many communities. Less expensive instruments that may have value in glaucoma screening include the Halberg applanation tonometer[170] and the GlaucoTest.[140, 155]

C. The Screening Site

In general, glaucoma detection programs are conducted in one of the three following settings[183]:

1. *Mass public screening clinics.* An essential criterion for success in any detection program is the percentage of positive screenees who follow through with an adequate medical examination. Mass clinics have been found to be the least efficient in this regard,[183] possibly because they are usually conducted on a periodic basis by volunteers, and lack adequate mechanisms of follow-up.

2. *Inhouse screening in industrial plants* was found to have the highest follow-up rate,[183] and appears to be an excellent screening setting for those in a position to take advantage of it.

3. *Public health departments*, as a part of *multiphasic screening*, offer the most logical setting for a community glaucoma detection program, since they are staffed by full-time professionals and provide a potential for long-term follow-up. A study in North Carolina has supported the feasibility of such a program, but also indicated the need for better methods of ensuring that positive screenees follow-up with an adequate medical examination.[183]

4. A fourth potential setting for glaucoma detection is in the office of the family physician, and the importance of educating the internist and general physician in this area has been stressed.[180]

D. The Legal Implications

A detailed appraisal of mass IOP screening for glaucoma concluded that it is legally permissible since the potential benefit, *i.e.*, detection of a sight-threatening disease, outweighs the potential hazards, such as rare ocular injury, the emotional trauma of a false positive test, and the risk of false-negative testing. It also concluded that full disclosure to the potential screenee of all possible hazards of the test was not required.[184]

E. Additional Tests

A major criticism against mass screening with tonometry alone is that false negatives and false positives are inevitable. This leads to a false sense of security among some individuals with glaucoma on the one hand, and the expense of detailed examinations for people without the disease on the other hand. This problem can be significantly reduced by adding one or more additional screening tests to tonometry; specifically, evaluation of the *optic nerve head* and visual field testing. A consideration of these two subjects constitutes the remainder of this section.

References

1. Leydhecker, W, Akiyama, K, Neumann, HG: Der intraokulare Druck gesunder menschlicher Augen. Klin Monatsbl Augenheilkd 133:662, 1958.
2. Colton, T, Ederer, F: The distribution of intraocular pressures in the general population. Surv Ophthal 25:123, 1980.
3. Johnson, LV: Tonographic Survey. Am J Ophthal 61:680, 1966.
4. Segal, P, Skwierczynska, J: Mass screening of adults for glaucoma. Ophthalmologica 153:336, 1967.
5. Armaly, MF: On the distribution of applanation pressure. I. Statistical features and the effect of age, sex, and family history of glaucoma. Arch Ophthal 73:11, 1965.
6. Perkins, ES: Glaucoma screening from a public health clinic. Br J Ophthal 1:417, 1965.
7. Loewen, U, Handrup, B, Redeker, A: Results of a glaucoma mass screening program. Klin Monatsbl Augenheilkd 169:754, 1976.
8. Ruprecht, KW, Wulle, KG, Christl, HL: Applanation tonometry within medical diagnostic "check-up" programs. Klin Monatsbl Augenheilkd 172:332, 1978.
9. Schwartz, B: Primary open-angle glaucoma. In Clinical Ophthalmology, Duane, TD, ed, vol 3, chap 52, Harper & Row, Hagerstown, Md, 1976.
10. Becker, B: The decline in aqueous secretion and outflow facility with age. Am J Ophthal 46:731, 1958.
11. Gartner, J: Aging changes of the ciliary epithelium border layers and their significance for intraocular pressure. Am J Ophthal 72:1079, 1971.
12. Brubaker, RF, Nagataki, S, Townsend, DJ, Burns, RR, Higgins, RG, Wentworth, W: The effect of age on aqueous humor formation in man. Ophthalmology 88:283, 1981.
13. Armaly, MF: The genetic determination of ocular pressure in the normal eye. Arch Ophthal 78:187, 1967.
14. Armaly, MF, Monstavicius, BF, Sayegh, RE: Ocular pressure and aqueous outflow facility in siblings. Arch Ophthal 80:354, 1968.
15. Levene, RZ, Workman, PL, Broder, SW, Hirschhorn, K: Heritability of ocular pressure in normal and suspect ranges. Arch Ophthal 84:730, 1970.
16. Tomlinson, A, Phillips, CI: Applanation tension and axial length of the eyeball. Br J Ophthal 54:548, 1970.
17. Deodati, F, Fontan, P, Mouledous, JM: La tension oculaire du grand myope. D'Ophthalmologie 34:77, 1974.
18. Kass, MA, Zimmerman, TJ, Alton, E, Lemon, L, Becker, B: Intraocular pressure and glaucoma in the Zuni Indians. Arch Ophthal 96:2212, 1978.
19. Kashgarian, M, Packer, H, Deutsch, AR, Deweese, MW, Lewis, PM: The frequency distribution of intraocular pressure by age and sex groups. JAMA 197:611, 1966.
20. Davanger, M, Holter, O: The statistical distribution of intraocular pressure in the population. Acta Ophthalmologica 43:314, 1965.
21. Kitazawa, Y, Horie, T: Diurnal variation of intraocular pressure in primary open-angle glaucoma. Am J Ophthal 79:557, 1975.
22. Newell, FW, Krill, AE: Diurnal tonography in normal and glaucomatous eyes. Trans Am Ophthal Soc 62:349, 1964.
23. Duke-Elder, S, Jay, B: Glaucoma and Hypotony. In System of Ophthalmology, Duke-Elder, S, ed, vol XI, Diseases of the Lens and Vitreous; Glaucoma and Hypotony, Henry Kimpton, London, 1969, p 456.
24. Henkind, P, Leitman, M, Weitzman, E: The diurnal curve in man: new observations. Invest Ophthal 12:705, 1973.
25. Boyd, TAS, McLeod, LE: Circadian rhythms of plasma corticoid levels, intraocular pressure and aqueous outflow facility in normal and glaucomatous eyes. Ann NY Acad Sci 117:597, 1964.

26. Weitzman, ED, Henkind, P, Leitman, M, Hellman, L: Correlative 24-hour relationships between intraocular pressure and plasma cortisol in normal subjects and patients with glaucoma. Br J Ophthal 59:566, 1975.
27. Kimura, R, Maekawa, N: Effect of orally administered hydrocortisone on the ocular tension in primary open-angle glaucoma subjects. Preliminary report. Acta Ophthalmologica 54:430, 1976.
28. Iverson, DG, Brown, DW: Diurnal variation of intraocular pressure and serum osmolality. Exp Eye Res 6:179, 1967.
29. Galin, MA, McIvor, JW, Magruder, GB: Influence of position on intraocular pressure. Am J Ophthal 55:720, 1963.
30. Anderson, DR, Grant, WM: The influence of position on intraocular pressure. Invest Ophthal 12:204, 1973.
31. Krieglstein, GK, Brethfeld, V, Collani, Ev: Comparative intraocular pressure measurements with position independent hand-applanation tonometers. Albrecht v Graefes Arch Klin Exp Ophthal 199:101, 1976.
32. Jain, MR, Marmion, VJ: Rapid pneumatic and Mackay-Marg applanation tonometry to evaluate the postural effect on intraocular pressure. Br J Ophthal 60:687, 1976.
33. Kindler-Loosli, C, Schmidt, T: Intraocular pressure after changing the patient's position. Albrecht v Graefes Arch Klin Exp Ophthal 194:17, 1975.
34. Williams, BI, Peart, WS: Effect of posture on the intraocular pressure of patients with retinal vein obstruction. Br J Ophthal 62:688, 1978.
35. Carenini, BB, Molfino, A: Postural tonographic test for the early diagnosis of glaucoma. Br J Ophthal 49:315, 1965.
36. Biro, I, Botar, Z: On the behaviour of intraocular tension in various sport activities. Klin Monatsbl Augenheilkd 140:23, 1962.
37. Lempert, P, Cooper, KH, Culver, JF, Tredici, TJ: The effect of exercise on intraocular pressure. Am J Ophthal 63:1673, 1967.
38. Stewart, RH, LeBlanc, R, Becker, B: Effects of exercise on aqueous dynamics. Am J Ophthal 69:245, 1970.
39. Kypke, W, Hermannspann, U: Glaucoma physical activity and sport. Klin Monatsbl Augenheilkd 164:321, 1974.
40. Shapiro, A, Shoenfeld, Y, Shapiro, Y: The effect of standardised submaximal work load on intraocular pressure. Br J Ophthal 62:679, 1978.
41. Epstein, HM, Fagman, W, Bruce, DL, Abram, A: Intraocular pressure changes during anesthesia for electroshock therapy. Anesthesia Analgesia 54:479, 1975.
42. Coleman, DJ, Trokel, S: Direct-recorded intraocular pressure variations in a human subject. Arch Ophthal 82:637, 1969.
43. Green, K, Luxenberg, MN: Consequences of eyelid squeezing on intraocular pressure. Am J Ophthal 88:1072, 1979.
44. Losada, F, Wolintz, AH: Bell's palsy: a new ophthalmologic sign. Ann Ophthal 5:1093, 1973.
45. Starrels, ME, Krupin, T, Burde, RM: Bell's palsy and intraocular pressure. Ann Ophthal 7:1067, 1975.
46. Blumenthal, M, Blumenthal, R, Peritz, E, Best, M: Seasonal variation in intraocular pressure. Am J Ophthal 69:608, 1970.
47. Leydhecker, W: The intraocular pressure: clinical aspects. Ann Ophthal 8:389, 1976.
48. Bulpitt, CJ, Hodes, C, Everitt, MG: Intraocular pressure and systemic blood pressure in the elderly. Br J Ophthal 59:717, 1975.
49. Levy, NS, Rawitscher, R: The effect of systemic hypotension during cardiopulmonary bypass on intraocular pressure and visual function in humans. Ann Ophthal 9:1547, 1977.
50. Krupin, T, Bass, J, Oestrich, C, Podos, SM, Becker, B: The effect of hyperthermia on aqueous humor dynamics in rabbits. Am J Ophthal 83:561, 1977.
51. Kass, MA, Sears, ML: Hormonal regulation of intraocular pressure. Surv Ophthal 22:153, 1977.
52. Aziz, MA: The relationship of I.O.P. to hormonal disturbance. Bull Ophthal Soc Egypt 60:303, 1967.

53. van den Pol, A, Maul, E, Sears, M: Unilateral gonadectomy does not alter contralateral intraocular pressure in rabbit eyes. Invest Ophthal Vis Sci 16:246, 1977.
54. Feldman, F, Bain, J, Matuk, AR: Daily assessment of ocular and hormonal variables throughout the menstrual cycle. Arch Ophthal 96:1835, 1978.
55. Duncalf, D: Anesthesia and intraocular pressure. Trans Am Acad Ophthal 79:562, 1975.
56. Adams, AP, Freedman, A, Henville, JD: Normocapnic anaesthesia for intraocular surgery. Br J Ophthal 63:204, 1979.
57. Schreuder, M, Linssen, GH: Intra-ocular pressure and anaesthesia. Direct measurements by needling the anterior chamber in the monkey. Anaesthesia 27:165, 1972.
58. Maddox, TS Jr, Kielar, RA: Comparison of the influence of ketamine and halothane anesthesia on intraocular tensions of nonglaucomatous children. J Ped Ophth 11:90, 1974.
59. Schutten, WH, Van Horn, DL: The effects of ketamine sedation and ketamine-pentobarbital anesthesia upon the intraocular pressure of the rabbit. Invest Ophthal Vis Sci 16:531, 1977.
60. Antal, M, Mucsi, G, Faludi, A: Ketamine anesthesia and intraocular pressure. Ann Ophthal 10:1281, 1978.
61. Ausinsch, B, Graves, SA, Munson, ES, Levy, NS: Intraocular pressures in children during isoflurane and halothane anesthesia. Anesthesiology 42:167, 1975.
62. Dominguez, A, Banos, MS, Alvarez, MG, Contra, GF, Quintela, FB: Intraocular pressure measurement in infants under general anesthesia. Am J Ophthal 78:110, 1974.
63. Grote, P: Augeninnendruckmessungen bei Kleinkindern ohne Glaukom in Halothanmaskennarkose. Ophthalmologica 171:202, 1975.
64. Radtke, ND, Cohan, BE: Intraocular pressure measurement in the newborn. Am J Ophthal 78:501, 1974.
65. Wyllie, AM, Beveridge, ME, Smith, I: Intraocular pressure during 4-hydroxy-butyrate narcosis. Br J Ophthal 56:436, 1972.
66. Peczon, JD, Grant, WM: Sedatives, stimulants, and intraocular pressure in glaucoma. Arch Ophthal 72:178, 1964.
67. Meyers, EF, Krupin, T, Johnson, M, Zink, H: Failure of nondepolarizing neuromuscular blockers to inhibit succinylcholine-induced increased intraocular pressure, a controlled study. Anesthesiology 48:149, 1978.
68. Bowen, DJ, McGrand, JC, Hamilton, AG: Intraocular pressures after suxamethonium and endotracheal intubation. Anaesthesia 33:518, 1978.
69. Couch, JA, Eltringham, RJ, Magauran, DM: The effect of thiopentone and fazadinium on intraocular pressure. Anaesthesia 34:586, 1979.
70. Samuel, JR, Beaugie, A: Effect of carbon dioxide on the intraocular pressure in man during general anaesthesia. Br J Ophthal 58:62, 1974.
71. Kielar, RA, Teraslinna, P, Kearney, JT, Barker, D: Effect of changes in pCO$_2$ on intraocular tension. Invest Ophthal Vis Sci 16:534, 1977.
72. Petounis, AD, Chondrell, S, Vadaluka-Sekioti, A: Effect of hypercapnea and hyperventilation on human intraocular pressure during general anaesthesia following acetazolamide administration. Br J Ophthal 64:422, 1980.
73. Gallin-Cohen, PF, Podos, SM, Yablonski, ME: Oxygen lowers intraocular pressure. Invest Ophthal Vis Sci 19:43, 1980.
74. Peczon, JD, Grant, WM: Glaucoma, alcohol, and intraocular pressure. Arch Ophthal 73:495, 1965.
75. Houle, RE, Grant, WM: Alcohol, vasopressin, and intraocular pressure. Invest Ophthal 6:145, 1967.
76. Green, K: Ocular effects of diacetyl morphine and lysergic acid diethylamide in rabbit. Invest Ophthal 14:325, 1975.
77. Shephard, RJ, Ponsford, E, Basu, PK, LaBarre, R: Effects of cigarette smoking on intraocular pressure and vision. Br J Ophthal 62:682, 1978.

78. Mehra, KS, Roy, PN, Khare, BB: Tobacco smoking and glaucoma. Ann Ophthal 8:462, 1976.
79. Whitworth, CG, Grant, WM: Use of nitrate and nitrite vasodilators by glaucomatous patients. Arch Ophthal 71:492, 1964.
80. Leydhecker, W, Waller, W, Krieglstein, G: The effect of vasodilators on the intraocular pressure. Klin Monatsbl Augenheilk 164:293, 1974.
81. Peczon, JD, Grant, WM, Lambert, BW: Systemic vasodilators, intraocular pressure, and chamber depth in glaucoma. Am J Ophthal 72:74, 1971.
82. Wizemann, AJS, Wizemann, V: Organic nitrate therapy in glaucoma. Am J Ophthal 90:106, 1980.
83. Lazenby, GW, Reed, JW, Grant, WM: Short-term tests of anticholinergic medication in open-angle glaucoma. Arch Ophthal 80:443, 1968.
84. Lazenby, GW, Reed, JW, Grant, WM: Anticholinergic medication in open-angle glaucoma. Arch Ophthal 84:719, 1970.
85. Hiatt, RL, Fuller, IB, Smith, L, Swartz, J, Risser, C: Systemically administered anticholinergic drugs and intraocular pressure. Arch Ophthal 84:735, 1970.
86. Valle, O: Effect of cyclopentolate on the aqueous dynamics in incipient or suspected open-angle glaucoma. Acta Ophthalmologica: XXI Meeting of Nordic Ophthalmologists 52, 1973.
87. Macri, FJ, Brubaker, RF: Methodology of eye pressure measurement. Biorheology 6:37, 1969.
88. Friedenwald, JS: Contribution to the theory and practice of tonometry. Am J Ophthal 20:985, 1937.
89. Moses, RA, Tarkkanen, A: Tonometry: The pressure-volume relationship in the intact human eye at low pressures. Am J Ophthal 47:557, 1959.
90. Friedenwald, JS: Some problems in the calibration of tonometers. Am J Ophthal 31:935, 1948.
91. Friedenwald, JS: Tonometer calibration: An attempt to remove discrepancies found in the 1954 calibration scale for Schiotz tonometers. Trans Am Acad Ophthal Otol 61:108, 1957.
92. Kronfeld, PC: Tonometer calibration empirical validation. The committee on standardization of tonometers. Trans Am Acad Ophthal Otol 61:123, 1957.
93. Anderson, DR, Grant, WM: Re-evaluation of the Schiotz tonometer calibration. Invest Ophthal 9:430, 1970.
94. Bayard, WL: Comparison of Goldmann applanation and Schiøtz tonometry using 1948 and 1955 conversion scales. Am J Ophthal 69:1007, 1970.
95. Drance, SM: The coefficient of scleral rigidity in normal and glaucomatous eyes. Arch Ophthal 63:668, 1960.
96. Draeger, VJ: Die Abhangigkeit des Rigiditatskoeffizienten von der Hohe des intraokularen Druckes. Ophthalmologica 140:55, 1960.
97. Vucicevic, ZM, Ralston, J: Influences of the volume and hydration changes on scleral rigidity. Ann Ophthal 4:715, 1972.
98. Pemberton, JW: Schiøtz-applanation disparity following retinal detachment surgery. Arch Ophthal 81:534, 1969.
99. Harbin, TS Jr, Laikam, SE, Lipsitt, K, Jarrett, WH II, Hagler, WS: Applanation-Schiøtz disparity after retinal detachment surgery utilizing cryopexy. Ophthalmology 86:1609, 1979.
100. Aronowitz, JD, Brubaker, RF: Effect of intraocular gas on intraocular pressure. Arch Ophthal 94:1191, 1976.
101. Foster, CS, Yamamoto, GK: Ocular rigidity in keratoconus. Am J Ophthal 86:802, 1978.
102. Draeger, J: Untersuchungen uber den rigiditatskoeffizienten. Doc Ophthal 13:431, 1959.
103. Goldmann, VH, Schmidt, T: Der rigiditatskoeffizient. (Friedenwald). Ophthalmologica 133:330, 1957.
104. Chandler, PA, Grant, WP: Glaucoma, 2nd ed., Lea & Febiger, Philadelphia, 1979, p 16.
105. Hetland-Eriksen, J: On tonometry. 2. Pressure recordings by Schiotz tonometry

on enucleated human eyes. Acta Ophthalmologica 44:12, 1966.

106. Grant, WM: Tonographic method for measuring the facility and rate of aqueous flow in human eyes. Arch Ophthal 44:204, 1950.
107. Francois, J, Moens, R, Moens, R: A new electronic tonometer. Br J Ophthal 36:694, 1952.
108. Horven, I: Dynamic tonometry. I. The dynamic tonometer. Acta Ophthalmologica 46:1213, 1968.
109. Horven, I: Electronic tonometer calibration. Acta Ophthalmologica 45:1083, 1967.
110. Goldmann, MH: Un nouveau tonometre a aplanation. Bull Soc Franc Ophthal 67:474, 1954.
111. Goldmann, VH, Schmidt, T: Uber applanationstonometrie. Ophthalmologica 134:221, 1957.
112. Moses, RA: The Goldmann applanation tonometer. Am J Ophthal 46:865, 1958.
113. Grant, WM: Fluorescein for applanation tonometry. More convenient and uniform application. Am J Ophthal 55:1252, 1963.
114. Quickert, MH: A fluorescein-anesthetic solution for applanation tonometry. Arch Ophthal 77:734, 1967.
115. Stewart, HL: Prolonged antibacterial activity of a fluorescein-anesthetic solution. Arch Ophthal 88:385, 1972.
116. Holtz, SJ: Clinical study of the safety of a fluorescein-anesthetic solution. Ann Ophthal 7:1101, 1975.
117. Roper, DL: Applanation tonometry with and without fluorescein. Am J Ophthal 90:668, 1980.
118. Corboy, JM, Borchardt, KA: Mechanical sterilization of the applanation tonometer. 1. Bacterial study. Am J Ophthal 71:889, 1971.
119. Ehlers, N, Bramsen, T, Sperling, S: Applanation tonometry and central corneal thickness. Acta Ophthalmologica 53:34, 1975.
120. Johnson, M, Kass, MA, Moses, RA, Grodzki, WJ: Increased corneal thickness simulating elevated intraocular pressure. Arch Ophthal 96:664, 1978.
121. Mark, HH: Corneal curvature in applanation tonometry. Am J Ophthal 76:223, 1973.
122. Bynke, H, Wilke, K: Repeated applanation tonometry in carotid occlusive disease. Acta Ophthalmologica 52:125, 1974.
123. Perkins, ES: Hand-held applanation tonometer. Br J Ophthal 49:591, 1965.
124. Draeger, J: Simple hand applanation tonometer for use on the seated as well as on the supine patient. Am J Ophthal 62:1208, 1966.
125. Draeger, J: Principle and clinical application of a portable applanation tonometer. Invest Ophthal 6:132, 1967.
126. Yablonski, ME: A new portable applanation tonometer. Am J Ophthal 80:547, 1975.
127. Mackay, RS, Marg, E: Fast, automatic, electronic tonometers based on an exact theory. Acta Ophthalmologica 37:495, 1959.
128. Marg, E, Mackay, RS, Oechsli, R: Trough height, pressure and flattening in tonometry. Vision Res 1:379, 1962.
129. Durham, DG, Bigliano, RP, Masino, JA: Pneumatic applanation tonometer. Trans Am Acad Ophthal Otol 69:1029, 1965.
130. Langham, ME, McCarthy, E: A rapid pneumatic applanation tonometer. Comparative findings and evaluation. Arch Ophthal 79:389, 1968.
131. Posner, A: An evaluation of the Maklakov applanation tonometer. EENT Monthly 41:377, 1962.
132. Posner, A: Practical problems in the use of the Maklakov tonometer. EENT Monthly 42:82, 1963.
133. Friedenwald, JS: Contribution to the theory and practice of tonometry. II. An analysis of the work of Professor S. Kalfa with the applanation tonometer. Am J Ophthal 22:375, 1939.
134. Schmidt, TFA: Calibration of the Maklakoff tonometer. Am J Ophthal 77:740, 1974.

135. Posner, A: A new portable applanation tonometer. EENT Monthly 43:88, 1964.
136. Posner, A, Inglima, R: The tonomat applanation tonometer. EENT Monthly 46:996, 1967.
137. Halberg, GP: Hand applanation tonometer. Trans Am Acad Ophthal Otol 72:112, 1968.
138. Barraquer, JI: New applanation tonometer for operating room. Ophthalmologica 153:225, 1967.
139. Jensen, JB: An ocular tension indicator of the applanation type. Acta Ophthalmologica 45:546, 1967.
140. Kaiden, JS, Zimmerman, TJ, Worthen, DM: An evaluation of the GlaucoTest screening tonometer. Arch Ophthal 92:195, 1974.
141. Grolman, B: A new tonometer system. Am J Optom Arch Am Acad Optom 49:646, 1972.
142. Forbes, M, Pico, G, Grolman, B: A noncontact applanation tonometer description and clinical evaluation. Arch Ophthal 91:134, 1974.
143. Shields, MB: The non-contact tonometer. Its value and limitations. Surv Ophthal 24:211, 1980.
144. Dekking, HM, Coster, HD: Dynamic tonometry. Ophthalmologica 154:59, 1967.
145. Roth, W, Blake, DG: Vibration tonometry—principles of the vibra-tonometer. J Am Optom Assoc 34:971, 1963.
146. Greene, ME, Gilman, BG: Intraocular pressure measurement with instrumented contact lenses. Invest Ophthal 13:299, 1974.
147. Wolbarsht, ML, Wortman, J, Schwartz, B, Cook, D: A scleral buckle pressure gauge for continuous monitoring of intraocular pressure. Int Ophthal 3:11, 1980.
148. Cooper, RL, Beale, D: Radio telemetry of intraocular pressure *in vitro*. Invest Ophthal Vis Sci 16:168, 1977.
149. Cooper, RL, Beale, DG, Constable, IJ: Passive radiotelemetry of intraocular pressure *in vivo*: calibration and validation of continual scleral guard-ring applanation transensors in the dog and rabbit. Invest Ophthal Vis Sci 18:930, 1979.
150. Cooper, RL, Beale, DG, Constable, IJ, Grose, GC: Continual monitoring of intraocular pressure: effect of central venous pressure, respiration, and eye movements on continual recordings of intraocular pressure in the rabbit, dog, and man. Br J Ophthal 63:799, 1979.
151. Moses, RA, Liu, CH: Repeated applanation tonometry. Am J Ophthal 66:89, 1968.
152. Phelps, CD, Phelps, GK: Measurement of intraocular pressure: a study of its reproducibility. Albrecht v Graefes Arch Klin Exp Ophthal 198:39, 1976.
153. Smith, JL, et al: The incidence of Schiøtz-applanation disparity. Cooperative study. Arch Ophthal 77:305, 1967.
154. Bengtsson, B: Comparison of Schiøtz and Goldmann tonometry in a population. Acta Ophthalmologica 50:445, 1972.
155. Krieglstein, GK: Screening tonometry by technicians. Albrecht v Graefes Arch Klin Exp Ophthal 194:221, 1975.
156. Armaly, MF, Salamoun, SG: Schiotz and applanation tonometry. Arch Ophthal 70:603, 1963.
157. Schwartz, JT, Dell'osso, GG: Comparison of Goldmann and Schiotz tonometry in a community. Arch Ophthal 75:788, 1966.
158. Bengtsson, B: Some factors affecting the relationship between Schiotz and Goldmann readings in a population. Acta Ophthalmologica 51:798, 1973.
159. Stepanik, J: Why is the Schiotz tonometer not suitable for measuring intraocular pressure? Klin Monatsbl Augenheilk 176:61, 1980.
160. Dunn, JS, Brubaker, RF: Perkins applanation tonometer clinical and laboratory evaluation. Arch Ophthal 89:149, 1973.
161. Krieglstein, GK, Waller, WK: Goldmann applanation versus hand-applanation and Schiotz indentation tonometry. Albrecht v Graefes Arch Klin Exp Ophthal 194:11, 1975.

162. Finlay, RD: Experience with the Draeger applanation tonometer. Trans Ophth Soc UK 90:887, 1970.
163. Moses, RA, Marg, E, Oechsli, R: Evaluation of the basic validity and clinical usefulness of the Mackay-Marg tonometer. Invest Ophthal 1:78, 1962.
164. Petersen, WC, Schlegel, WA: Mackay-Marg tonometry by technicians. Am J Ophthal 76:933, 1973.
165. Quigley, HA, Langham, ME: Comparative intraocular pressure measurements with the pneumatonograph and Goldmann tonometer. Am J Ophthal 80:266, 1975.
166. Jain, MR, Marmion, VJ: A clinical evaluation of the applanation pneumatonograph. Br J Ophthal 60:107, 1976.
167. Wuthrich, UW: Postural change and intraocular pressure in glaucomatous eyes. Br J Ophthal 60:111, 1976.
168. Moses, RA, Grodzki, WJ Jr: The pneumatonograph. A laboratory study. Arch Ophthal 97:547, 1979.
169. Francois, J, Vancea, P, Vanderkerckhove, R: Halberg tonometer. An evaluation. Arch Ophthal 86:376, 1971.
170. Zimmerman, TJ, Worthen, DM: A comparison of two-hand applanation tonometers. Arch Ophthal 88:421, 1972.
171. Kaiden, JS, Zimmerman, TJ, Worthen, DM: Hand-held tonometers. An evaluation by medical students. Arch Ophthal 89:110, 1973.
172. Kaufman, HE, Wind, CA, Waltman, SR: Validity of Mackay-Marg electronic applanation tonometer in patients with scarred irregular corneas. Am J Ophthal 69:1003, 1970.
173. McMillan, F, Forster, RK: Comparison of MacKay-Marg, Goldmann and Perkins tonometers in abnormal corneas. Arch Ophthal 93:420, 1975.
174. West, CE, Capella, JA, Kaufman, HE: Measurement of intraocular pressure with a pneumatic applanation tonometer. Am J Ophthal 74:505, 1972.
175. Krieglstein, GK, Waller, WK, Reimers, H, Langham, ME: Intraocular pressure measurements on soft contact lenses. Albrecht v Graefes Arch Klin Exp Ophthal 199:223, 1976.
176. Richter, RC, Stark, WJ, Cowan, C, Pollack, IP: Tonometry on eyes with abnormal corneas. Glaucoma 2:508, 1980.
177. Gelatt, KN, Peiffer, RL Jr, Gum, GG, Gwin, RM, Erickson, JL: Evaluation of applanation tonometers for the dog eye. Invest Ophthal Vis Sci 16:963, 1977.
178. Meyer, RF, Stanifer, RM, Bobb, KC: Mackay-Marg tonometry over therapeutic soft contact lenses. Am J Ophthal 86:19, 1978.
179. Draeger, J: Applanation tonometry on contact lenses with high water content: problems, results, correction factors. Klin Monatsbl Augenheilk 176:38, 1980.
180. Pollack, IP: The challenge of glaucoma screening. Surv Ophthal 13:4, 1968.
181. Packer, H, Deutsch, AR, Deweese, MW, Kashgarian, M, Lewis, PM: Efficiency of screening tests for glaucoma. JAMA 192:693, 1965.
182. Schwartz, JT: Vagary in tonometric screening. Am J Ophthal 64:50, 1967.
183. McPherson, SD Jr: The challenge and responsibilities of a community approach to glaucoma control. The Sightsaving Rev 50:15, 1980.
184. Franklin, MA: Medical mass screening programs: a legal appraisal. Cornell Law Qtly 47:205, 1962.

Chapter 4

THE OPTIC NERVE HEAD

THE OPTIC NERVE HEAD

The primary consequence of elevated intraocular pressure in an eye with glaucoma is progressive atrophy of the optic nerve head. Since it is this pathologic alteration which leads to the irreversible loss of vision, an understanding of glaucomatous optic atrophy is essential in the diagnosis and management of glaucoma.

I. ANATOMY AND HISTOLOGY

A. Terminology

The term, "optic nerve head," is generally preferred over "optic disc," since the latter suggests a flat structure without depth. Within the context of a discussion on glaucoma, the optic nerve head is the distal portion of the optic nerve that is directly susceptible to elevated intraocular pressure. In this sense, the optic nerve head is defined as extending from the retinal surface to the myelinated portion of the optic nerve that begins just outside the sclera. However, the term, "disc," is frequently used when referring to the portion of the optic nerve head that is clinically visible by ophthalmoscopy.

B. General Description[1,2]

The optic nerve head is composed of the *axons* of approximately 1.2 million neurons, which originate in the ganglion cell layer of the retina and converge upon the nerve head from all points in the fundus (the pattern of the retinal nerve fiber layer is discussed in Chapter 5). On the surface of the nerve head, the neurons bend acutely to leave the globe through a fenestrated scleral canal, the *lamina cribrosa*. Within the nerve head, the axons are grouped into approximately 1,000 fasicles, or bundles, and are supported by *astrogliocytes*. The intraocular portion of the nerve head has an average diameter of 1.5 mm, although this is reported to vary from 1.18 to 1.75 mm.[3] The cross-section of the nerve expands to approximately 3 mm just behind the sclera, where the neurons acquire a *myelin* sheath. The optic nerve head is also the site of entry and exit of the *retinal vessels*. This vascular system supplies some branches to the optic nerve head, although the predominant blood supply for the nerve head comes from the *ciliary circulation*.

C. Divisions of the Optic Nerve Head

The nerve head may be arbitrarily divided into the following four portions from anterior to posterior (Fig. 4.1)[4]:

1. *Surface nerve fiber layer.* The innermost portion of the optic nerve head is composed predominantly of *neurons*. In the Rhesus monkey, this layer is 94% neurons and 5% astrocytes.[5] The axonal bundles acquire progressively more interaxonal glial tissue within the

Optic Nerve Head

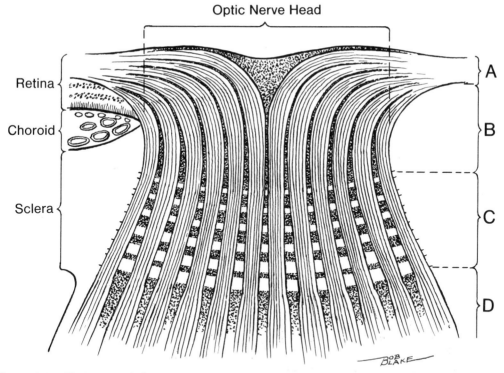

Figure 4.1. Divisions of the optic nerve head. **A:** Surface nerve fiber layer. **B:** Prelaminar region. **C:** Lamina cribrosa region. **D:** Retrolaminar region.

intraocular portion of the nerve head as this structure is followed posteriorly.[5]

2. *Prelaminar region*[4] (also called the anterior portion of the lamina cribrosa[6]). The predominant structures at this level are neurons and astrocytes, with a significant increase in the quantity of *astroglial tissue*.

3. *Lamina cribrosa region.* This portion contains fenestrated sheets of scleral *connective tissue* and occasional elastic fibers. Astrocytes separate the sheets and line the fenestrae,[6] and the fasicles of neurons leave the eye through these openings.

4. *Retrolaminar region.* This area is characterized by a decrease in astrocytes and the acquisition of *myelin* that is supplied by *oligodendrocytes*. The axonal bundles are surrounded by connective tissue septae.

The posterior extent of the retrolaminar region is not clearly defined. An India ink study of monkey eyes showed non-filling for 3 to 4 mm behind the lamina cribrosa, when the intraocular pressure was elevated.[7] However, a similar study with unlabeled microspheres showed an increased flow in the retrolaminar region close to the lamina even when the intraocular pressure was elevated high enough to stop retinal flow.[8]

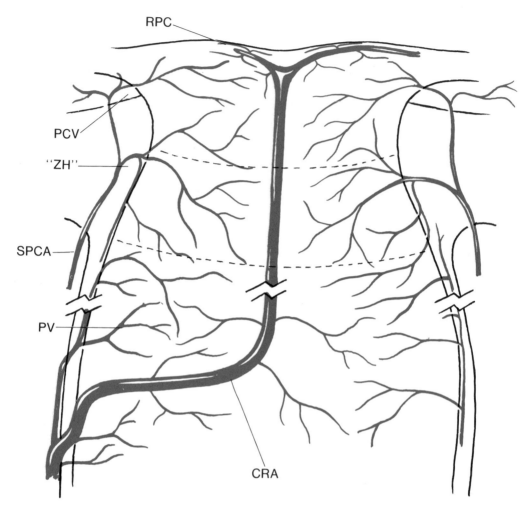

Figure 4.2. Vascular supply of the optic nerve head: central retinal artery (**CRA**); radial peripapillary capillaries (**RPC**); pial vessels (**PV**); short posterior ciliary arteries (**SPCA**); peripapillary choroidal vessels (**PCV**); "circle" of Zinn-Haller ("**ZH**").

D. Vasculature

1. The four divisions of the optic nerve head, as described above, correlate roughly with a four-part *vascular supply* (Fig. 4.2):

a. The *surface nerve fiber layer* is mainly supplied by *retinal* arterioles, which anastomose with vessels of the prelaminar region[9] and are continuous with the peripapillary retinal and long radial peripapillary capillaries.[4] One or more of the ciliary-derived vessels from the prelaminar region may occasionally enlarge to form *cilio-retinal arteries.*[4]

b. The *prelaminar region* is supplied by precapillaries and capillaries of *ciliary* origin. There is lack of agreement as to whether these vessels are derived primarily from the peripapillary choroidal system,[4] or from separate branches of the short posterior ciliary arteries.[9, 10]

    c. The *lamina cribrosa region* is also supplied by *ciliary* vessels, which come directly from short posterior ciliary arteries to form a dense plexus in the lamina.[4, 9] These arteries also provide an incomplete and inconsistent vascular system around the lamina, called the "circle" of Zinn-Haller.[4, 9]

    d. The *retrolaminar region* is supplied by both the *ciliary* and *retinal* circulations, with the former coming from recurrent pial vessels. The central retinal artery provides centripetal branches from the pial system and frequently, but not always, gives off centrifugal vessels.[11] A "central optic nerve artery" was described as a branch of the ophthalmic artery, supplying the axial portion of the optic nerve.[12] This has not been confirmed in subsequent studies, but may represent a rare variant of the normal anatomy.[11]

A continuity between small vessels from the retrolaminar region to the retinal surface has been observed,[9] and the optic nerve head microvasculature is said to represent an integral part of the retina-optic nerve vascular system.[10]

2. The *capillaries* of the optic nerve head, although derived from both the retinal and ciliary circulations, resemble more closely the features of retinal capillaries than the choriocapillaris. These characteristics include 1) tight junctions, 2) abundant pericytes, and 3) non-fenestrated endothelium.[10] They do not leak fluorescein and may represent a *nerve-blood barrier*, supporting the concept of the retina-nerve vasculature as a continuous system with the central nervous system.[9, 10] The capillaries become fewer behind the lamina, especially along the margins of the larger vessels.[13]

3. The *venous return* in the optic nerve head is primarily by the central retinal vein, although some enters the choroidal system, thereby establishing another communication between the retina and choroid.[4] Occasionally, these communications are enlarged as retino-ciliary veins, which drain from the retina to the choroidal circulation, or cilio-optic veins, draining from the choroid to the central retinal vein.[14]

E. Glial Support

1. *Astrocytes* provide a continuous layer between the neurons and blood vessels in the optic nerve head.[15] In the Rhesus monkey, astrocytes occupy 5% of the nerve fiber layer, as previously noted, but increase to 23% of the laminar region, and then decrease to 11% in the retrolaminar area.[5] The astrocytes are joined by "gap junctions," which resemble tight junctions, but have minute gaps between the outer membrane leaflets.[16]

2. The astroglial tissue also provides a covering for portions of the optic nerve head (Fig. 4.3):

    a. *The internal limiting membrane of Elschnig* separates the nerve head from the vitreous and is continuous with the internal

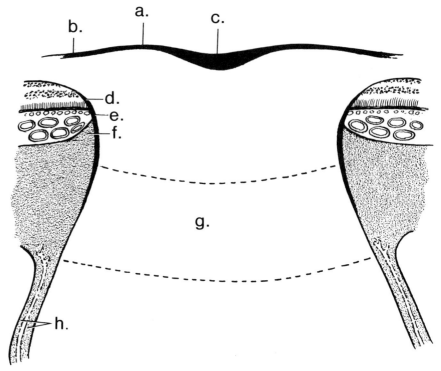

Figure 4.3. Supportive structures of the optic nerve head: internal limiting membrane of Elschnig (**a**), continuous with internal limiting membrane of the retina (**b**); central meniscus of Kuhnt (**c**); intermediary tissue of Kuhnt (**d**); border tissue of Jacoby (**e**); border tissue of Elschnig (**f**); lamina cribrosa (**g**); meningeal sheaths (**h**).

limiting membrane of the retina.[15, 17, 18] When the central portion of the internal limiting membrane is thickened, it is referred to as the *central meniscus of Kuhnt*.[18]

b. The *intermediary tissue of Kuhnt* separates the nerve from the retina, while the *border tissue of Jacoby* separates the nerve from the choroid.[6, 18]

F. Collagen Support

In addition to forming the lamina cribrosa in the optic nerve head, a rim of connective tissue, the *border tissue of Elschnig*, occasionally extends between the choroid and optic nerve tissues, especially temporally.[18] Posterior to the globe, the optic nerve is surrounded by *meningeal sheaths* (pia, arachnoid, and dura), which consist of connective tissue lined by meningothelial cells, or mesothelium.[19] Vascularized connective tissue extends from the undersurface of the pia mater to form longitudinal septae, which partially separate the axonal bundles in the intraorbital portion of the optic nerve.[18]

G. Influence of Age

At birth, the optic nerve is small and nearly unmyelinated.[20] In addition, the connective tissue of the lamina cribrosa is incompletely developed, which may account for the greater susceptibility of the infant nerve head to cupping, as well as its potential for reversible cupping.[21] With increasing age, there is a progressive loss of axons and a corresponding increase in the cross-sectional area occupied by the leptomeninges and fibrous septae.[20]

II. THE PATHOGENESIS OF GLAUCOMATOUS OPTIC ATROPHY

A. The Theories

The pathogenesis of glaucomatous optic atrophy has remained a matter of controversy since the mid-19th century when two concepts were introduced in the same year. In 1858, Müller[22] proposed that the elevated intraocular pressure led to direct compression and death of the neurons (the *mechanical theory*), while von Jaeger[23] suggested that a vascular abnormality was the underlying cause of the optic atrophy (the *vascular theory*). Initially, the mechanical theory received the greatest support.[24-26] In 1892, Schnabel[27] proposed another concept in the pathogenesis of glaucomatous optic atrophy, suggesting that atrophy of neural elements created empty spaces, which pulled the nerve head posteriorly (Schnabel's cavernous atrophy).

The mechanical concept held sway through the first quarter of this century until LaGrange and Beauvieux[28] popularized the vascular theory in 1925. In general, this belief held that glaucomatous optic atrophy was secondary to ischemia, whether the primary result of elevated intraocular pressure, or an unrelated vascular lesion.[29-31] In 1968, however, the role of *axoplasmic flow* in glaucomatous optic atrophy was introduced,[32] which revived support for the mechanical theory but did not exclude the possible influence of ischemia.

B. The Evidence

Continued investigation into the pathogenesis of glaucomatous optic atrophy has led to the following bodies of information:

1. *Histopathologic observations* of human eyes with glaucoma provide the most direct method of studying the alterations associated with glaucomatous optic atrophy, although they do not fully explain the mechanisms that caused the damage. One of the limiting factors has been that many of the specimens studied have represented advanced glaucomatous change, which led to possible misconceptions regarding the early pathogenic features. The recent studies of Quigley and co-workers,[33, 34] in which the histopathology of human eyes with varying stages of glaucoma were correlated with clinical records, appear to clarify many of these points.

a. It has been suggested that loss of *astroglial supportive tissue* may precede neuronal degeneration (astroglial hypothesis of disc cupping),[35] wl   was thought to explain the early and reversible cupping in infants.[36] However, subsequent studies indicate that glial cells not only are not selectively lost in early glaucoma, but that these are the only remaining cells after loss of axons in advanced cases.[33] Furthermore, as previously discussed, the incomplete development of the lamina cribrosa at birth may explain the unusual susceptibility to cupping in infants.[21]

b. It has also been suggested, based primarily on clinical observations, that loss of *small vessels* in the optic nerve head may accompany atrophy of axons.[37] In addition, one histologic study suggested a selective loss of retinal radial peripapillary capillaries in eyes with chronic glaucoma.[38] However, another study showed no correlation between atrophy of this vascular system and visual field loss.[39] Furthermore, the studies of Quigley and Green[33] revealed no major selective loss of optic nerve head capillaries in early cases of glaucoma.

c. Although backward bowing of the *lamina cribrosa* is a characteristic of late glaucomatous cupping,[33, 34, 40, 41] and may also occur early in the infant eye,[21] it does not occur in the early stages of adult glaucoma in a magnitude that is sufficient to explain the observed cupping.[33, 34] Nevertheless, the possibility of small posterior movements of the lamina, which could cause compression of the axons, still exists, and it has been suggested that the structure of the lamina cribrosa may be an important determinant in the susceptibility to damage from elevated intraocular pressure.[33, 34]

d. The cause of early cupping in glaucoma is an actual loss of *axonal tissue.*[33, 34, 42] The damage occurs at the level of the lamina cribrosa and first involves axonal bundles in the inferior and superior poles of the nerve head.[33, 34, 42] Experimental models of primate eyes exposed to chronic intraocular pressure elevation support these observations, and suggest that the damage is associated with a posterior and lateral displacement of the lamina cribrosa.[43]

2. *Fluorescein angiographic observations.* Although the preceding discussion of histopathology seems to preclude a possible vascular role in the pathogenesis of glaucomatous optic atrophy, it will be seen from the following fluorescein angiographic studies that alterations in the optic nerve head vasculature are associated with both the early and late stages of glaucomatous nerve head damage.

a. *The normal fluorescein pattern* of the optic nerve head is usually described as having *three phases*[4]:

(1). *An initial filling* or *preretinal arterial phase* is felt to represent filling of the prelaminar and lamina cribrosa regions by the posterior ciliary arteries. Fluorescein in the retrobulbar vessels may also contribute to this phase.[44]

(2). *The peak fluorescence* or *retinal arteriovenous phase* is primarily due to filling of the dense capillary plexus on the nerve head surface from retinal arterioles. With increasing age, there is a decrease in the filling time of both the retinal and choroidal circulations.[45, 46]

(3). *A late phase* consists of 10 to 15 minutes of delayed staining of the nerve head, which is probably due to fluorescein in the connective tissue of the lamina cribrosa. Tracer studies in monkeys suggest the leakage may come from the adjacent choroid.[47]

b. *The effect of artificially elevated intraocular pressure* on the fluorescein angiographic pattern has provided an understanding of the relative vulnerability of ocular vessels to elevated pressure in the normal and glaucomatous eye.

(1). There is a *general delay* in the entire ocular circulation in response to an elevation of the intraocular pressure.

(2). *The prelaminar portion of the nerve head* appears to be the most vulnerable of the ocular vascular systems to elevated pressure in monkeys.[4, 48]

(3). Studies regarding the vulnerability of the *peripapillary choroid* have provided inconsistent results. Fluorescein angiography of monkey eyes has revealed a marked susceptibility of this vascular system to elevated intraocular pressure,[4, 48, 49] and fluorescein studies of human eyes with glaucoma have shown similar delays in peripapillary choroidal filling.[48, 50-53] Other factors, such as increased diastolic blood pressure,[46] may also delay filling of peripapillary choroidal vessels in normal and glaucomatous eyes. Nevertheless, the delay appears to be sensitive to elevated intraocular pressure,[50] and it has been suggested that this vascular disturbance of the peripapillary choroid contributes to glaucomatous optic atrophy.[52]

Fluorescein angiographic studies of normal human eyes, however, have shown similar delayed or irregular choroidal filling at normal pressures,[54, 55] and the peripapillary choroidal capillaries of normal human eyes were relatively resistant to artificial pressure elevations.[56] Furthermore, a fluorescein study of patients with low-tension or chronic simple glaucoma provided no evidence that hypoperfusion of the peripapillary choroid contributed to optic nerve hypoperfusion.[57]

(4). A selective non-filling of the *retinal radial peripapillary capillaries* during India ink perfusion has been demonstrated in cats.[58] As previously discussed, histopathologic observations are conflicting with regard to alterations of this vascular system in glaucomatous eyes.[38, 39]

(5). Most studies of monkey[4, 48] and normal human eyes[59, 60] have found the choroidal circulation in general to be more vulnerable than that of the retina to elevated intraocular pressure, although one study found the two systems to fill at the same level of increased pressure.[61]

c. *Fluorescein angiographic studies of glaucomatous and nonglaucomatous eyes* have revealed two types of *filling defects* of the optic nerve head[62-64]:

(1). *Persisting hypoperfusion*[62, 63] or *absolute*[64] *filling defects* are more common in eyes with glaucoma,[62-64] especially low-tension glaucoma,[62, 63] and are said to correlate with visual field loss.[62-64] The characteristics of a filling defect include decreased blood flow, a smaller vascular bed, narrower vessels, and increased permeability of the vessels.[65] The filling defect may be *focal*, which is felt to reflect susceptible vasculature with or without elevated intraocular pressure and is the typical defect in low-tension glaucoma.[57] Focal defects occur primarily in the inferior and superior poles of the optic nerve head.[62-64, 66] In glaucomatous eyes, they are most often seen in the wall of the cup, while in normal eyes they occur more commonly, in the floor of the cup.[67] In other eyes, the defect is *diffuse*, which is felt to represent prolonged pressure elevation.[57]

Patients with elevated intraocular pressure, but normal optic nerve heads and visual fields (so-called "ocular hypertension") have more filling defects than the normal population, although fewer than in eyes with glaucoma.[64, 68] The only other condition reported to give absolute filling defects is sectorial ischemic optic neuropathy.[69] However, the nature of the defect in open-angle glaucoma is felt to be specific, and it has been suggested that fluorescein angiography of the optic nerve head may help to differentiate open-angle glaucoma from other conditions that have similar clinical changes in the optic disc.[69] A correlation between vascular changes of the optic nerve head and visual field loss in glaucoma has not been fully established. However, it has been reported that the development of new visual field defects is associated with changes in the optic nerve head circulation, as determined by fluorescein angiography.[70]

(2). *Transient hypoperfusion*[62, 63] or *relative (delayed)*[64] *filling defects* are seen in the normal population and do not correlate with optic nerve head or visual field changes.[62-64] However, it has been postulated that they may progress to absolute defects, which is felt to provide a sign of impending field loss.[64]

d. One study revealed *fluorescein leakage* of the optic nerve head associated with advanced glaucomatous optic atrophy in nine of 150 patients with primary open-angle glaucoma,[71] and *staining* of the nerve head was seen in 30% of glaucomatous eyes in one fluorescein study.[62, 63]

3. *Observations of axoplasmic flow* in animal models have provided insight into the ultrastructural changes that may be occurring in the human eye with glaucomatous optic atrophy.

a. *Axoplasmic flow* (or axonal transport) refers to the movement of materials (axoplasm) along the axon of a nerve (although the dendrite may also have transport) in a predictable, energy dependent manner.[72]

(1). This movement has been characterized as having fast and slow components,[72, 73] although numerous intermediate rates may also exist.[72] The *fast phase* moves approximately 410 mm/day in various species and may supply material to synaptic vesicles, the axolemma, and agranular endoplasmic reticulum of the axon, while the *slow phase* moves at 1 to 3 mm/day and is believed to subserve growth and maintenance of axons.[73]

(2). The flow of axoplasm may be *orthograde* (from retina to lateral geniculate body) or *retrograde* (lateral geniculate body to retina).[74]

b. An *experimental model* for studying axoplasmic flow has been developed in which *radioactive amino acids*, such as tritiated leucine, are injected into the vitreous of animals (usually monkeys). The amino acid is incorporated into the protein synthesis of retinal ganglion cells and then moves down the ganglion cell axon into the optic nerve, allowing histologic study of the movement of radioactively labeled protein.[75] In addition, the movement of certain unlabeled neuronal components, such as mitochondria, can be studied by electron microscopy under various conditions.[76] These models can be used to study factors that cause abnormal blockade of axoplasmic flow.

c. *Elevated intraocular pressure* causes obstruction of axoplasmic flow at the lamina cribrosa in monkey eyes,[74, 77-81] which involves both the fast[78, 81] and slow[78] phases as well as the orthograde and retrograde components.[74, 80] The height and duration of pressure elevation influences the onset, distribution, and degree of axoplasmic obstruction in the optic nerve head.[81-83] Two general mechanisms have been considered regarding the obstruction of axoplasmic flow in response to elevated intraocular pressure:

(1). The *mechanical theory* suggests that physical alterations in the optic nerve head, such as a misalignment of the fenestrae in the lamina cribrosa due to its backbowing, may lead to the axoplasmic obstruction.[32, 41, 80] In support of this hypothesis, it has been observed that elevated intraocular pressure leads to blockage of axonal transport despite an intact nerve head capillary circulation and an elevated arterial pO_2.[74, 84] Furthermore, obstruction of axoplasmic flow has also been reported in response to ocular hypotony,[78, 80, 85] leading some investigators to suggest that a pressure differential across the optic nerve head, whether due to a relative increase or decrease in intraocular pressure, causes mechanical changes with compression of the axonal bundles.[78, 80, 85, 86] However, elevated intracranial pressure in monkeys neither caused obstruction of rapid axoplasmic flow, nor prevented it in response to elevated intraocular pressure despite reduction in the pressure gradient across the lamina.[87] This suggests that more than a simple mechanical or hydrostatic mechanism may be involved with obstruction of axoplasmic flow in response to elevated intraocular pressure.[87]

(2). The *vascular theory* suggests that *ischemia* at least plays a role in the obstruction of axoplasmic flow in response to elevated intraocular pressure. Interruption of the short posterior ciliary arteries in monkeys has been reported to block both slow[88, 89] and fast[90] axoplasmic flow, although it did not cause glaucomatous cupping.[88, 89] It has also been noted in monkey eyes with elevated intraocular pressure that leakage from microvasculature of the nerve head was associated with blockade of axonal transport at the lamina cribrosa.[91] These observations suggest, but do not prove, a cause-and-effect relationship between ischemia and obstruction of axoplasmic flow in the optic nerve head of eyes with elevated intraocular pressure. Against a vascular mechanism for pressure-induced obstruction of axoplasmic flow was the observation that ligation of the right common carotid artery in monkeys, which reduced the estimated ophthalmic artery pressure by 10 to 20 mmHg below the left side, did not significantly affect the extent to which intraocular pressure elevation interrupted axonal transport.[92]

4. A study of *oxygen tension* in the monkey optic nerve head suggested that *autoregulation* compensates for changes in the perfusion pressure, and it was hypothesized that glaucomatous optic atrophy results from a breakdown in this homeostatic mechanism.[93]

5. *Electrophysiologic studies* have also contributed to our understanding of optic nerve disease in glaucoma. When the intraocular tension is artificially elevated in normal[94, 95] and glaucomatous[95] human eyes, a significant reduction in the amplitudes of electroretinogram components[94, 95] and visual evoked potentials[95] occurs only when the pressure approaches or exceeds the ophthalmic blood pressure. These findings appear to challenge the vascular theory of glaucomatous optic atrophy in chronic glaucoma, in which the intraocular pressure is often well below diastolic blood pressure,[94] but are consistent with an ischemic mechanism of optic nerve damage in acute glaucomas.[95]

6. *Studies of other ocular disorders* provide some indirect insight into the possible mechanism of glaucomatous optic atrophy. For example:

a. A histopathologic study of severe *peripapillary choroidal atrophy* revealed a normal optic nerve head, suggesting that the vascular supply of these two structures may be independent.[96]

b. Studies of *non-glaucomatous optic atrophy* have been used both to support and to refute an ischemic basis for glaucomatous optic atrophy. In patients with *anterior ischemic optic neuropathy*, cupping similar to that seen in glaucoma is frequently observed when the ischemia is due to giant cell arteritis, but in a significantly lower percentage of non-arteritic cases.[97, 98] These observations have led to the suggestion that glaucoma and anterior ischemic optic neuropathy have the same vasogenic basis of optic nerve damage, but differ according to the rate of change.[97] If this is true, the difference in visual field loss suggests that there is also a difference in the nature or distribution of the ischemia.[98] It has also been suggested that acute ischemic optic neuropathy may be one of several mechanisms of optic nerve disease in chronic glaucoma.[99]

In contrast to the above studies, a review of 170 eyes with non-glaucomatous optic atrophy of varied origin revealed a small, but significant increase in cupping.[100] However, the cups were morphologically different than those seen in glaucoma, which was suggested as evidence against a vascular etiology in glaucomatous cupping. Furthermore, a study of 18 patients with vasogenic shock and poor peripheral tissue perfusion revealed no evidence of glaucomatous optic nerve head or visual field change.[101]

c. *Optic atrophy* has been created in *animal models* by sectioning the optic nerve[102, 103] or disrupting the nerve fiber layer with retinal photocoagulation.[104] In either case, the atrophy was not associated with decreased vasculature of the nerve head,[102-104] and histologic findings suggested the pallor was due to proliferation[103] or reorganization[102, 104] of the glia, which obscured visualization of the vessels. These studies suggest that loss of axons from the optic nerve does not invariably lead to a secondary loss of vasculature in the nerve head. In other words, the vascular changes observed in glaucomatous optic atrophy are not readily explained as a secondary phenomenon.

d. *Cavernous atrophy* of the optic nerve, as originally described by Schnabel,[27] has been considered to be a form of glaucomatous optic atrophy due to severe elevations of intraocular pressure. However, this also occurs in patients with normal intraocular pressures, in which case it may represent an aging change associated with generalized arteriosclerosis.[105]

C. The conclusions

The present evidence suggests that obstruction to axoplasmic flow may be involved in the pathogenesis of glaucomatous optic atrophy. However, it is still not clear as to whether mechanical or vascular factors are primarily responsible for this obstruction, and whether other alterations are also important in the ultimate loss of axons. It may be that all of these factors are involved to some degree or, as Spaeth[62, 63] has suggested, that there is more than one mechanism of optic atrophy in eyes with glaucoma.

III. CLINICAL APPEARANCE OF GLAUCOMATOUS OPTIC ATROPHY

While investigators continue to study the pathophysiology of glaucomatous optic atrophy, the clinician has a responsibility to become thoroughly familiar with the morphology of this condition, since it provides the most reliable early evidence of damage in glaucoma.

A. Morphology of the Normal Optic Nerve Head

In order to recognize pathologic alternations of the optic nerve head, one must first be familiar with the wide range of normal variations.

1. *General features.* The ophthalmoscopic appearance of the optic nerve head is generally that of a vertical oval, although there is considerable variation in size and shape. One large study revealed a greater than 4-fold difference in the area of normal nerve heads.[106]

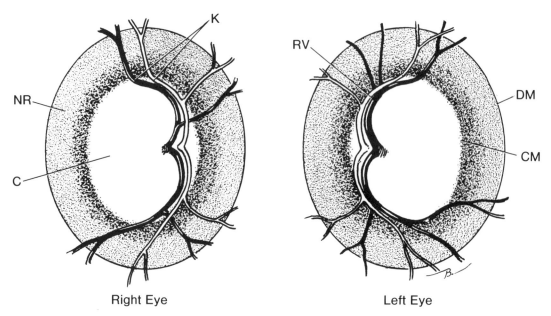

Right Eye   Left Eye

Figure 4.4. Normal optic nerve heads: neural rim (**NR**); disc margin (**DM**); cup margin (**CM**); cup (**C**); retinal vessels (**RV**): kinking of vessels at cup margin (**K**). Note that cups are symmetric between the two eyes and neural rims are even for 360°.

The central portion of the disc may contain a depression, the *cup*, and an area of *pallor*. While the area of cup and pallor are frequently the same, it is important to note that this is not always the case, especially in disease states,[107] and these two parameters should not be thought of as being synonymous. The tissue between the cup and disc margins is referred to as the *neural rim*. It represents the location of the axons and normally has an orange-red color, while the central pallor represents exposure of the underlying lamina cribrosa. *Retinal vessels* ride up the nasal wall of the cup, often kinking at the cup margin before crossing the neural rim to the retina (Fig. 4.4).

    2. *The physiologic cup* varies considerably in size and shape:

    a. The *size* of the optic nerve head cup, which is commonly described as the horizontal cup/disc ratio (C/D), is said to be determined in normal eyes by a ratio between 1) the width of the scleral canal and 2) the volume of glial supportive tissue.[3] Reports of C/D distribution within the general population differ, which is probably due to examination techniques. When the discs were studied by direct ophthalmoscopy, the distribution was found to be non-Gaussian with most eyes having a C/D of 0.0 to 0.3 and only 1 to 2% being 0.7 or greater.[108] However, when a stereoscopic view was utilized, which is probably more accurate, a Gaussian distribution was found with a mean C/D of 0.4 and approximately 5% with 0.7.[109] It is important to notice, however, that physiologic cups tend to be symmetrical,[108-111] with a C/D difference of greater than 0.2 between fellow eyes occurring in only 1% of the normal population.[108]

The following factors have been studied regarding their relationship to the size of physiologic cups:

(1). The size of a physiologic cup is frequently similar to that of parents and siblings,[108, 112] and is felt to be *genetically* determined on a polygenic, multi-factorial basis.[108] It is helpful, therefore, to examine other members of the family when attempting to distinguish between a large physiologic cup and glaucomatous cupping.

(2). In contrast to the above, the normal C/D does not appear to correlate with a family history of open-angle glaucoma.[108, 113] However, most studies show an increased frequency of larger C/D values among individuals with higher intraocular pressures,[109, 113, 114] abnormal tonographic outflow facilities,[113, 114] or highly positive pressure responses to topical corticosteroids.[115]

(3). *Age* has not been found to correlate with the size of the physiologic cup in most studies,[108, 112, 113, 116] although a slight, but significant, increase with age has been reported for both cup[109] and pallor.[117] It is important to note, however, that this enlargement, if it occurs, is gradual and should not be confused with the more rapid progression of glaucomatous cupping.

(4). Most studies have found no correlation with *sex*,[108, 109, 112] although one report described larger relative areas of pallor in white males than in white females.[117]

(5). *Refractive errors* in the mid-range do not appear to correlate with physiologic cup size.[109, 112] However, the depth of the physiologic cup, which usually correlates with the width of the cup,[114] tends to be shallower in myopic eyes.[118]

b. *The shape* of the physiologic cup is significantly correlated with the shape of the disc, which means that the margins of cup and disc tend to run parallel for the full 360°.[119] The *contour* of the bed of the cup, however, varies considerably. In 1899, Elschnig classified physiologic cups on the basis of configuration, and this has subsequently been supported by contour mapping[120, 121] (a technique discussed later in this chapter):

(1). Type I: Small cup with funnel-shaped walls.

(2). Type II: Temporal, cylindrical (steep-walled) cup.

(3). Type III: Central, trough-shaped cup.

(4). Type IV: Temporal or central cup with a well developed nasal wall, but a temporal wall that gradually slopes to disc margin. This is particularly common along the infero-temporal margin and can be confused with early glaucomatous cupping.[122]

(5). Type V: Developmental anomalies (discussed later in this chapter).

3. *The physiologic neural rim.* By tradition, more is said about the cup than the neural rim of both normal and glaucomatous nerve heads. However, it is actually alterations in the neural rim of an eye

with glaucoma that leads to changes in the cup as well as to loss of visual field. As previously noted, the margins of the cup and disc run parallel in normal eyes,[119] which results in an *even neural rim.* However, there are factors that can interfere with the interpretation of an even neural rim:

a. *A gray crescent in the optic nerve head* has been described, which typically is slate gray and located in the temporal or inferotemporal periphery of the neural rim. It is more common in black individuals and apparently represents a variation of the normal anatomy. However, mistaking the gray crescent for a peripapillary pigmented crescent could result in a physiologic neural rim being misinterpreted as pathologically thin in that area.[122, 123]

b. The *optic nerve head in a myopic eye* has several features that make interpretation difficult. As previously noted, the cup is shallower, which makes early glaucomatous deepening harder to recognize.[118] In addition, the *oblique insertion* of the optic nerve may create a temporal peripapillary crescent, that could be confused with a halo seen around some glaucomatous discs, and may lead to obstruction of the temporal neural rim from funduscopic view, suggesting pathologic thinning of this tissue.[118, 122]

4. In *summary*, normal optic nerve heads and their associated cups vary considerably in size and shape, but are characterized by *symmetry of the cups* between fellow eyes and an *evenness of the neural rim.* Most important from the standpoint of evaluating for glaucomatous cupping, however, is the observation that physiologic cups *do not change.*

B. Morphology of Glaucomatous Optic Atrophy

The disc changes of glaucoma are typically *progressive* and *asymmetric* and present in a variety of characteristic clinical patterns.

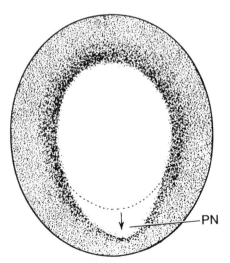

Figure 4.5.   Glaucomatous optic atrophy. Focal enlargement of cup inferotemporally (**arrow**) from original cup margin (**dotted line**), creating a polar notch (**PN**).

1. *Patterns of early glaucomatous cupping.* As bundles of axons are destroyed in the neural rim of an eye with glaucoma, the cup begins to enlarge in one of several patterns:

a. *Focal enlargement.* Selective loss of neural rim tissue in the *inferior* and *superior* poles of the optic nerve head due to glaucoma leads to enlargement of the cup in a vertical direction.[124-130] It is important to note that the concept of the "vertical cup" in glaucoma does not refer to the actual geometry of the cup, since many physiologic cups also have a vertically oval shape. Rather, it denotes the relationship between the shape of the cup and the disc. More specifically, thinning of the neural rim in an inferior or superior quadrant results in a cup that is "more oval" than the disc (Fig. 4.5).

The focal enlargement of the cup often begins as a small, discrete defect in the neural rim, usually in the inferior temporal quadrant, which has been referred to as "polar notching,"[127, 128] "focal notching,"[129] or "pit-like changes."[130] As the focal defect enlarges and deepens, it may develop a sharp nasal margin, often adjacent to a major retinal vessel, the "sharpened polar nasal edge."[127] When the local cupping reaches the disc margin (*i.e.*, no visible neural rim remains in that area), a "sharpened rim" may be produced.[127] If a retinal vessel crosses the sharpened rim, it will bend sharply at the edge of the disc, creating what has been termed "bayoneting at the disc edge"[127] (Fig. 4.6).

b. In contrast to focal enlargement, glaucomatous cups may also enlarge in *concentric* circles, which are sometimes horizontal, but are

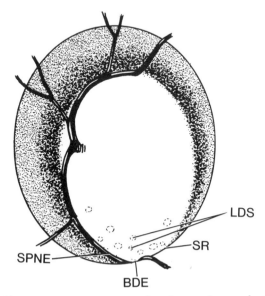

Figure 4.6. Glaucomatous optic atrophy. Loss of neural rim infero-temporally, creating a sharpened rim (**SR**) at the disc margin, a sharpened polar nasal edge (**SPNE**) along the cup margin, bayoneting at the disc edge (**BDE**), where the vessels cross the sharpened rim, and a laminar dot sign (**LDS**) due to exposure of fenestrae in lamina cribrosa.

more often directed infero-temporally or supero-temporally.[128] Since the loss of neural rim tissue usually begins temporally and then progresses circumferentially toward these poles, this has been called "temporal unfolding."[127, 128] In one study, this generalized expansion of the cup, with retention of its "round" appearance, was the most common form of early cupping in glaucoma.[131] Since it is difficult to distinguish this type of glaucomatous cup from a physiologic cup, it is important to compare the cup in the fellow eye for symmetry and to study serial photographs for evidence of *progressive change.*

 c. In some cases, the predominant pattern of early glaucomatous cupping is a *deepening* of the cup, which has been said to occur only when the lamina is not initially exposed.[132] This may produce the picture of "overpass cupping," in which vessels initially bridge the deepened cup and later collapse into it.[127, 128]

 d. *Pallor/cup discrepancy.* In the early stages of glaucomatous optic atrophy, the area of cupping may progress ahead of the area of pallor. This biphasic pattern differs from other causes of optic atrophy in which the area of pallor is typically larger than the cup.[107] A potential pit-fall in interpreting optic nerve head cupping is to look only at the area of pallor and miss the larger area of cupping. The latter can usually be recognized by observing kinking of vessels at the cup margin or by examining the disc with stereoscopic techniques. Although the pallor/cup discrepancy is typical and strongly suggestive of glaucomatous cupping, it has also been observed in physiologic optic nerve heads.[122]

Pallor/cup discrepancy may occur with diffuse or focal enlargement of the cup:

 (1). *"Saucerization"* refers to a pattern of early glaucomatous change in which diffuse, shallow cupping extends to the disc margins with retention of a central pale cup (Fig. 4.7).[133]

 (2). *"Focal saucerization"* is a more localized shallow, sloping cup usually in the inferior temporal quadrant.[128] The retention of normal disc color in the periphery of the cup has been called the "tinted hollow."[127] As the glaucomatous damage progresses, the color is replaced by a grayish hue, termed the "shadow sign," or by the sieve-like appearance of the lamina cribrosa, referred to as the "laminar dot sign" (Fig. 4.7).[127]

 2. *The neural rim.* Although the preceding discussion referred more often to the cup of the optic nerve head, it is re-emphasized that these changes actually reflect selective loss of neural rim tissue. An additional sign of glaucomatous damage to the neural rim has been called "thinning of the neural rim."[134] This finding is independent of changes in the cup and is seen as a crescentic shadow adjacent to the disc margin as the intense beam of a direct ophthalmoscope passes across the neural rim. The histologic explanation for this phenomenon is uncertain, but it is felt to be associated with early glaucomatous damage,[135] and should not be confused with the previously discussed gray crescent in the optic nerve head.[122, 123] Another

A

B

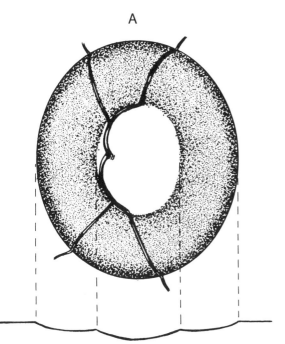
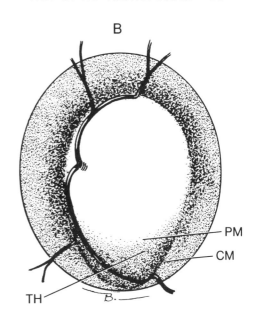

Figure 4.7. Glaucomatous optic atrophy. Pallor/cup discrepancy. **A:** Saucerization with corresponding cross-sectional view. **B:** Focal saucerization with tinted hollow (**TH**) between pallor margin (**PM**) and cup margin (**CM**). Note kinking of vessels in both cases.

sign of glaucomatous damage to the neural rim is thinning of the nerve fiber layer as it crosses the temporal margin of the disc.[136]

3. *Vascular changes in glaucomatous optic atrophy.*

a. It was once taught that *nasal displacement of the retinal vessels* on the optic nerve head was a sign of glaucomatous cupping. However, since these vessels enter and leave the eye along the nasal margin of the cup, their location on the disc is a function of cup size, whether physiologic or glaucomatous, and does not provide a useful diagnostic parameter.[114]

b. Another vessel sign that does appear to have diagnostic value has been called *"baring of the circumlinear vessel."*[137] In many normal optic nerve heads, one or two vessels may curve to outline a portion of the physiologic cup. With glaucomatous enlargement of the cup, and possibly some other forms of optic atrophy, the circumlinear vessel may be "bared" from the margin of the cup (Fig. 4.8).[137]

c. *Splinter hemorrhages*, usually near the margin of the optic nerve head (Fig. 4.8), may also be associated with early glaucomatous damage or may occur whenever the glaucoma is out of control.[138, 139] This finding is more prevalent in eyes with open-angle glaucoma than those with elevated intraocular pressure alone.[139] It is also associated with a higher incidence of field loss than eyes that have primary open-angle glaucoma or elevated intraocular pressure without hemorrhages.[138]

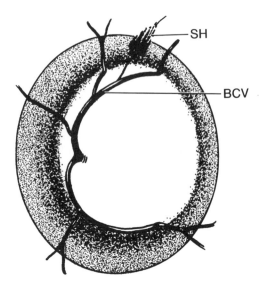

Figure 4.8. Glaucomatous optic atrophy. Vascular changes: splinter hemorrhage (**SH**) and baring of circumlinear vessel (**BCV**).

d. *Tortuosity of vessels* on the disc may be seen with advanced glaucomatous optic atrophy and in some cases with only moderate damage. It is believed to represent loops of collateral vessels in response to chronic central retinal vessel occlusion.[140] Veno-venous anastomoses associated with chronic branch retinal vessel occlusion, as well as the typical picture of acute central retinal vessel occlusion with massive flame hemorrhages, also occur with increased frequency in eyes with chronic glaucoma.[140]

e. *Bridging of vessels* on the disc, another useful diagnostic sign, was previously discussed in association with overpass cupping.

4. *Peripapillary changes associated with glaucomatous optic atrophy.*

a. *Nerve fiber bundle defects.* Striations in the retinal nerve fiber layer are normally seen as light reflexes, apparently due to the variable thickness of nerve fibers in this layer.[141] The loss of axonal bundles, which leads to the neural rim changes of glaucomatous optic atrophy, also produces visible defects in the retinal nerve fiber layer. These defects appear as dark stripes in the peripapillary area, paralleling the normal retinal striations,[142-144] and monkeys studies confirm that they are due to loss of axons.[145] This sign may have prognostic value, since it has been shown to correlate highly with visual field changes,[142-144] and may precede field loss.[142] However, the stripes are also seen in many neurological disorders.[146]

b. *Peripapillary depigmentation* is frequently associated with glaucomatous optic atrophy,[147] but is also seen with other conditions, such as myopia and aging changes. A distinction has been made between two forms of peripapillary depigmentation[148]:

(1). *Peripapillary halos* are defined as narrow, homogeneous light bands at the edge of the disc. The incidence of prominent halos is higher in glaucoma, although the average degree of halos is statistically the same as in nonglaucomatous eyes.

(2). *Peripapillary atrophy* is defined as an irregular, variably depigmented area peripheral to the halo and occurs with statistically greater frequency in glaucoma.

5. *Advanced glaucomatous cupping.* If the progressive changes of glaucomatous optic atrophy are not arrested by appropriate measures to reduce the intraocular pressure, the typical course is eventual loss of all neural rim tissue. The utlimate result is *total cupping,* which is seen clinically as a white disc with loss of all neural rim tissue and bending of all vessels at the margin of the disc. This has also been called "bean-pot cupping," because the cross section of a histologic specimen reveals extreme posterior displacement of the lamina cribrosa and undermining of the disc margin (Fig. 4.9).[128, 129]

6. One additional clinical sign that may be associated with glaucomatous optic atrophy is the *relative afferent pupillary defect* (Marcus-Gunn pupil), which is characteristic of unilateral or asymmetric optic nerve damage of any cause. This finding has been reported in

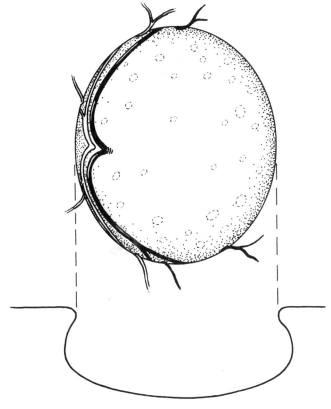

Figure 4.9. Advanced glaucomatous optic atrophy with total (or bean-pot) cupping with corresponding cross-sectional view.

patients with asymmetric glaucomatous cupping but normal kinetic visual fields.[149]

7. In *summary*, glaucomatous optic atrophy is characterized by *progressive*, asymmetric enlargement of the optic nerve head cup in a variety of characteristic patterns.

C. Differential Diagnosis of Glaucomatous Optic Atrophy

The following conditions may resemble glaucomatous cupping and lead to diagnostic confusion:

1. *Normal variations* in the size and shape of the physiologic cup and in the appearance of the neural rim, which may be confused with glaucomatous changes, were discussed previously under Morphology of the Normal Optic Nerve Head.

2. *Developmental anomalies* of the optic nerve head may lead to *colobomas*, which can simulate glaucomatous cupping.[150] In some cases, the diagnostic problem is compounded by associated field defects, which may resemble those of glaucoma but are not progressive.[151] Another congenital anomaly of the optic nerve head has been called the "morning glory syndrome," and is characterized by a funnel-shaped nerve head with white central tissue, elevated peripapillary pigment disturbance, and multiple radially oriented retinal vessels.[152] Yet another anomaly is the *congenital pit* of the optic nerve head, which is a localized, pale depression, usually near the temporal or inferotemporal margin of the disc. These may have associated visual disturbance due to macular or extramacular serous detachment.[153] Cases have also been reported in which congenital pits were noted to enlarge when observed for many years.[154]

3. *Non-glaucomatous causes of acquired cupping.* Studies have shown that ophthalmologists are not always able to distinguish between glaucomatous and non-glaucomatous optic atrophy on the basis of the optic disc appearance alone. Parameters that were found to be most useful in making this differentiation were pallor and obliteration of the neural rim.[156] Non-glaucomatous conditions that may cause acquired cupping include *anterior ischemic optic neuropathy*, as previously discussed, especially when the ischemia is due to arteritis.[97,98] A similar entity has been described in which infarction of the optic nerve head caused shallow cupping inferotemporally, associated with arcuate field defects.[157] This differed from glaucoma in that it was not progressive. Acquired cupping may also occur with compressive lesions of the optic nerve, such as an intracranial aneurysm, which was reported to cause cupping indistinguishable from that of early glaucoma.[158]

IV. RECORDING TECHNIQUES

Progressive cupping of the optic nerve head in a patient with glaucoma is the most reliable indicator that the intraocular pressure is not being adequately controlled. It is essential, therefore, to record the appearance of the nerve head in a way that will accurately reveal *subtle glaucomatous changes* over the course of follow-up evaluations. The following recording techniques have been used or evaluated for this purpose.

A. Techniques of Office Evaluation and Recording

Subjective estimates of cup dimensions have been shown to vary greatly, even among expert observers.[159-161] The complex and variable patterns of glaucomatous optic atrophy, as previously discussed, make simple descriptive statements, such as the horizontal cup/disc ratio, grossly inadequate. Attention to the vertical cup/disc ratio[162] or the amount of neural rim in the inferior and superior quadrants correlates more closely with field loss, but still fails to consider many of the glaucomatous changes in the nerve head and peripapillary area. The most useful office approach is to carefully study these structures with *stereoscopic techniques*, such as the Hruby lens attachment to the slit lamp, and to make detailed drawings that include the area of cupping and pallor in all quadrants, the position and kinking of major vessels, splinter hemorrhages, and peripapillary changes. However, no degree of attention to detail is sufficient to detect subtle changes in all cases, and the office evaluation should be considered only an adjunct to the indispensible use of photographic records.

B. Photographic Techniques

1. *Two-dimensional photos*, whether in color or black-and-white, have the advantages of simplicity and lower cost. In addition, the relative dimensions of the pallor and cup can be measured directly on the photograph.[122, 162] However, this technique is frequently limited by the inability to precisely determine the cup margins. Efforts have been made to enhance the contrast of structures in the optic nerve head and surrounding tissue by using appropriate monochromatic illumination[163, 164] or other special filters.[162, 165] The projection of fine, parallel lines onto the disc has also been used to improve recognition of the cup contours,[166] and techniques have been developed to electronically scan black-and-white disc photos to obtain an objective measure of the amount of optic disc pallor.[167, 168] A photo slit lamp and a fundus camera have been shown to be comparable for photographing the optic disc.[169]

2. A method that may be more reliable for recording disc cupping, as well as the other aspects of glaucomatous optic atrophy, is the use of *color stereophotographs.*[107, 124, 125] Stereophotographs can be obtained either by taking two photos in sequence on the same film with the use of a sliding carriage adapter (Allen separator),[170] or by taking simultaneous photos with a camera that utilizes the indirect ophthalmoscopic principle (Donaldson stereoscopic fundus camera),[171, 172] or a twin-prism separator.[173] These three techniques were compared for reproducibility, and the Donaldson camera was found to be superior.[174] A special viewer has also been developed in which two stereophotographs can be compared simultaneously.[175]

C. Newer Techniques

Even color stereophotographs are limited by the need for subjective evaluations and comparisons, and the following techniques have been studied in the search for more *objective, quantitative* ways to record and evaluate glaucomatous cupping:

1. *Index of cupping* involves charting the *circumference* of the cup and disc on tracings of nerve head photographs with a map measure and computing the ratio of these two values.[176]

2. *Photogrammetry* involves the mathematical determination of the *volume* and *contour* of the optic nerve head cup with stereoscopic photographs.[132, 177-180] With this technique, the *area/depth relationship* showed a high correlation in normal eyes, but no correlation in glaucomatous eyes, and was the most sensitive parameter in distinguishing glaucomatous from physiologic cupping.[181]

3. *Stereochronoscopy.* The stereoscopic principle has also been used to detect subtle changes in photographs of a disc taken at different times. If there has been any progression of the cupping, the disparity in the cup margins of the superimposed photographs will produce a stereoscopic effect.[180, 182]

4. *Colorimetric measurements* have also been studied in an effort to detect reduced or changing color intensity of the optic nerve head.[183-185]

5. *Ultrasonography* has been shown to detect glaucomatous cupping of 0.7 cup/disc ratio or greater, although systems with better resolution are needed to make this a useful method for examining the optic disc.[186]

6. *Fluorescein angiographic* studies of the optic nerve head were discussed earlier in this chapter and may one day have practical clinical application in the detection and management of glaucoma.

References

1. Last, RJ: Wolff's Anatomy of the Eye and Orbit, 5th ed, WB Saunders, Philadelphia, 1961, pp 408–410.
2. Hogan, MJ, Alvarado, JA, Weddell, JE: Histology of the Human Eye. An Atlas and Textbook, WB Saunders, Philadelphia, 1971, pp 523–606.
3. Kronfeld, PC: Normal variations of the optic disc as observed by conventional ophthalmoscopy and their anatomic correlations. Trans Am Acad Ophthal Otol 81:214, 1976.
4. Hayreh, SS: Anatomy and physiology of the optic nerve head. Trans Am Acad Ophthal Otol 78:240, 1974.
5. Minckler, DS, McLean, IW, Tso, MOM: Distribution of axonal and glial elements in the rhesus optic nerve head studied by electron microscopy. Am J Ophthal 82:179, 1976.
6. Anderson, DR: Ultrastructure of human and monkey lamina cribrosa and optic nerve head. Arch Ophthal 82:800, 1969.
7. Hamasaki, DI, Fujino, T: Effect of intraocular pressure on ocular vessles. Arch. Ophthal 78:369, 1967.
8. Geijer, C, Bill, A: Effects of raised intraocular pressure on retinal, prelaminar, laminar, and retrolaminar optic nerve blood flow in monkeys. Invest Ophthal Vis Sci 18:1030, 1979.

9. Liebermann, MF, Maumenee, AE, Green, WR: Histologic studies of the vasculature of the anterior optic nerve. Am J Ophthal 82:405, 1976.
10. Anderson, DR, Braverman, S: Reevaluation of the optic disk vasculature. Am J Ophthal 82:165, 1976.
11. Hayreh, SS: The central artery of the retina. Its role in the blood supply of the optic nerve. Br J Ophthal 47:651, 1963.
12. Francois, J, Neetens, A: Vascularization of the optic pathway. I. Lumina cribrosa and optic nerve. Br J Ophthal 38:472, 1954.
13. Goder, G: The capillaries of the optic nerve. Am J Ophthal 77:684, 1974.
14. Zaret, CR, Choromokos, EA, Meisler, DM: Cilio-optic vein associated with phakomatosis. Ophthalmology 87:330, 1980.
15. Anderson, DR, Hoyt, WF, Hogan, MJ: The fine structure of the astroglia in the human optic nerve and optic nerve head. Trans Am Ophthal Soc 65:275, 1967.
16. Quigley, HA: Gap junctions between optic nerve head astrocytes. Invest Ophthal Vis Sci 16:582, 1977.
17. Anderson, DR: Ultrastructure of the optic nerve head. Arch Ophthal 83:63, 1970.
18. Anderson, DR, Hoyt, WF: Ultrastructure of intraorbital portion of human and monkey optic nerve. Arch Ophthal 82:506, 1969.
19. Anderson, DR: Ultrastructure of meningeal sheaths. Normal human and monkey optic nerves. Arch Ophthal 82:659, 1969.
20. Dolman, CL, McCormick, AQ, Drance, SM: Aging of the optic nerve. Arch Ophthal 98:2053, 1980.
21. Quigley, HA: The pathogenesis of reversible cupping in congenital glaucoma. Am J Ophthal 84:358, 1977.
22. Müller, H: Anatomische Beitrage zur Ophthalmologie: Ueber Nervean-Veränderungen an der Eintrittsstelle des Schnerven. Arch Ophthal 4:1, 1858.
23. von Jaeger, E: Ueber Glaucom und seine Heilung durch Iridectomie. Z Ges der Aerzte zu Wien 14:465, 484, 1858.
24. Laker, C: Ein experimenteller Beitrag zur Lehre von der glaukomatösen Excavation. Klin Monatsbl Augenheilkd 24:187, 1886.
25. Schreiber, L: Ueber Degeneration der Netzhaut naut experimentellen und pathologisch-anatomischen Untersuchungen. Albrecht von Graefes Arch Ophthal 64:237, 1906.
26. Fuchs, E: Ueber die Lamina cribrosa. Albrecht von Graefes Arch Ophthal 91:435, 1916.
27. Schnabel, J: Das glaukomatose Sehnervenleiden. Archiv fur Augenheilkunde 24:18, 1892.
28. LaGrange, F, Beauvieux, J: Anatomie de l'excavation glaucomateuse. Arch Ophthal (Paris) 42:129, 1925.
29. Duke-Elder, S: Fundamental concepts in glaucoma. Arch Ophthal 42:538, 1949.
30. Gafner, VF, Goldmann, H: Experimentelle Untersuchungen über den Zusammenhang von Augendrucksteigerung und Gesichtsfeldschädigung. Ophthalmologica 130:357, 1955.
31. Duke-Elder, S: The problems of simple glaucoma. Trans Ophthal Soc UK 82:307, 1962.
32. Lampert, PW, Vogel, MH, Zimmerman, LE: Pathology of the optic nerve in experimental acute glaucoma. Electron microscopic studies. Invest Ophthal 7:199, 1968.
33. Quigley, HA, Green, WR: The histology of human glaucoma cupping and optic nerve damage: clinicopathologic correlation in 21 eyes. Ophthalmology 86:1803, 1979.
34. Quigley, HA, Addicks, EM: Regional differences in the structure of the lamina cribrosa and their relationship to glaucomatous optic nerve damage. Arch Ophthal 99:137, 1981.
35. Shaffer, RN: The role of the astroglial cells in glaucomatous disc cupping. Doc Ophthal 26:516, 1969.

36. Shaffer, RN, Hetherington, J Jr: The glaucomatous disc in infants. A suggested hypothesis for disc cupping. Trans Am Acad Ophthal Otol 73:929, 1969.
37. Schwartz, B: Cupping and pallor of the optic disc. Arch Ophthal 89:272, 1973.
38. Kornzweig, AL, Eliasoph, I, Feldstein, M: Selective atrophy of the radial peripapillary capillaries in chronic glaucoma. Arch Ophthal 80:696, 1968.
39. Daicker, B: Selective atrophy of the radial peripapillary capillaries and visual field defects in glaucoma. Albrecht v Graefes Arch Klin Exp Ophthal 195:27, 1975.
40. Hayreh, SS: Pathogenesis of cupping of the optic disc. Br J Ophthal 58:863, 1974.
41. Emery, JM, Landis, D, Paton, D, Boniuk, M, Craig, JM: The lamina cribrosa in normal and glaucomatous human eyes. Trans Am Acad Ophthal Otol 78:290, 1974.
42. Vrabee, F: Glaucomatous cupping of the human optic disk. A neurohistologic study. Albrecht v Graefes Arch Klin Exp Ophthal 198:223, 1976.
43. Quigley, HA, Addicks, EM: Chronic experimental glaucoma in primates. II. Effect of extended intraocular pressure elevation on optic nerve head and axonal transport. Invest Ophthal Vis Sci 19:137, 1980.
44. Ernest, JT, Archer, D: Fluorescein angiography of the optic disk. Am J Ophthal 75:973, 1973.
45. Laux, U, Marquardt, R: Dye-filling pattern in routine serial angiograms. Klin Monatsbl Augenheilk 175:786, 1979.
46. Schwartz, B, Kern, J: Age, increased ocular and blood pressures, and retinal and disc fluorescein angiogram. Arch Ophthal 98:1980, 1980.
47. Tso, MOM, Shih, CY, McLean, IW: Is there a blood-brain barrier at the optic nerve head? Arch Ophthal 93:815, 1975.
48. Hayreh, SS: Optic disc changes in glaucoma. Br J Ophthal 56:175, 1972.
49. Swietliczko, I, David, NJ: Fluorescein angiography in experimental ocular hypertension. Am J Ophthal 70:351, 1970.
50. Rosen, ES, Boyd, TAS: New method of assessing choroidal ischemia in open-angle glaucoma and ocular hypertension. Am J Ophthal 70:912, 1970.
51. Raitta, C, Sarmela, T: Fluorescein angiography of the optic disc and the peripapillary area in chronic glaucoma. Acta Ophthalmologica 48:303, 1970.
52. Blumenthal, M, Best, M, Galin, MA, Toyofuku, H: Peripapillary choroidal circulation in glaucoma. Arch Ophthal 86:31, 1971.
53. Hayreh, SS: The pathogenesis of optic nerve lesions in glaucoma. Trans Am Acad Ophthal Otol 81:197, 1976.
54. Oosterhuis, JA, Boen-Tan, TN: Choroidal fluorescence in the normal human eye. Ophthalmologica 162:246, 1971.
55. Evans, PY, Shimizu, K, Limaye, S, Deglin, E, Wruck, J: Fluorescein cineangiography of the optic nerve head. Trans Am Acad Ophthal Otol 77:260, 1973.
56. Best, M, Toyofuku, H: Ocular hemodynamics during induced ocular hypertension in man. Am J Ophthal 74:932, 1972.
57. Hitchings, RA, Spaeth, GL: Fluorescein angiography in chronic simple and low-tension glaucoma. Br J Ophthal 61:126, 1977.
58. Alterman, M, Henkind, P: Radial peripapillary capillaries of the retina. II. Possible role in Bjerrum scotoma. Br J Ophthal 52:26, 1968.
59. Blumenthal, M, Gitter, KA, Best, M, Galin, MA: Fluorescein angiography during induced ocular hypertension in man. Am J Ophthal 69:39, 1970.
60. Blumenthal, M, Best, M, Galin, MA, Gitter, KA: Ocular circulation: analysis of the effect of induced ocular hypertension on retinal and choroidal blood flow in man. Am J Ophthal 71:819, 1971.
61. Archer, DB, Ernest, JT, Krill, AE: Retinal, choroidal, and papillary circulations under conditions of induced ocular hypertension. Am J Ophthal 73:834, 1972.
62. Spaeth, GL: Fluorescein angiography: its contributions towards understanding the mechanisms of visual loss in glaucoma. Trans Am Ophthal Soc 73:491, 1975.

63. Spaeth, GL: The Pathogenesis of Nerve Damage in Glaucoma: Contributions of Fluorescein Angiography, Grune & Stratton, New York, 1977.
64. Schwartz, B, Rieser, JC, Fishbein, SL: Fluorescein angiographic defects of the optic disc in glaucoma. Arch Ophthal 95:1961, 1977.
65. Sonty, S, Schwartz, B: Two-point fluorophotometry in the evaluation of glaucomatous optic disc. Arch Ophthal 98:1422, 1980.
66. Fishbein, SL, Schwartz, B: Optic disc in glaucoma. Topography and extent of fluorescein filling defects. Arch Ophthal 95:1975, 1977.
67. Adam, G, Schwartz, B: Increased fluorescein filling defects in the wall of the optic disc cup in glaucoma. Arch Ophthal 98:1590, 1980.
68. Loebl, M, Schwartz, B: Fluorescein angiographic defects of the optic disc in ocular hypertension. Arch Ophthal 95:1980, 1977.
69. Talusan, E, Schwartz, B: Specificity of fluorescein angiographic defects of the optic disc in glaucoma. Arch Ophthal 95:2166, 1977.
70. Talusan, ED, Schwartz, B, Wilcox, LM Jr: Fluorescein angiography of the optic disc. A longitudinal follow-up study. Arch Ophthal 98:1579, 1980.
71. Tsukahara, S: Hyperpermeable disc capillaries in glaucoma. Adv Ophthal 35:65, 1978.
72. Wirtschafter, JD, Rizzo, FJ, Smiley, BC: Optic nerve axoplasm and papilledema. Surv Ophthal 20:157, 1975.
73. Minckler, DS, Tso, MOM: A light microscopic, autoradiographic study of axoplasmic transport in the normal rhesus optic nerve head. Am J Ophthal 82:1, 1976.
74. Minckler, DS, Bunt, AH, Johanson, GW: Orthograde and retrograde axoplasmic transport during acute ocular hypertension in the monkey. Invest Ophthal Vis Sci 16:426, 1977.
75. Taylor, AC, Weiss, P: Demonstration of axonal flow by the movement of tritium-labeled protein in mature optic nerve fibers. Proc Natl Acad Sci USA 54:1521, 1965.
76. Weiss, P, Pillai, A: Convection and fate of mitochondria in nerve fibers: axonal flow as vehicle. Proc Natl Acad Sci USA 54:48, 1965.
77. Anderson, DR, Hendrickson, A: Effect of intraocular pressure on rapid axoplasmic transport in monkey optic nerve. Invest Ophthal 13:771, 1974.
78. Minckler, DS, Tso, MOM, Zimmerman, LE: A light microscopic, autoradiographic study of axoplasmic transport in the optic nerve head during ocular hypotony, increased intraocular pressure, and papilledema. Am J Ophthal 82:741, 1976.
79. Quigley, HA, Anderson, DR: The dynamics and location of axonal transport blockade by acute intraocular pressure elevation in primate optic nerve. Invest Ophthal 15:606, 1978.
80. Minckler, DS, Bunt, AH, Klock, IB: Radioautographic and cytochemical ultrastructural studies of axoplasmic transport in the monkey optic nerve head. Invest Ophthal Vis Sci 17:33, 1978.
81. Quigley, HA, Guy, J, Anderson, DR: Blockade of rapid axonal transport. Effect of intraocular pressure elevation in primate optic nerve. Arch Ophthal 97:525, 1979.
82. Quigley, HA, Anderson, DR: Distribution of axonal transport blockade by acute intraocular pressure elevation in the primate optic nerve head. Invest Ophthal Vis Sci 16:640, 1977.
83. Gaasterland, D, Tanishima, T, Kuwabara, T: Axoplasmic flow during chronic experimental glaucoma. I. Light and electron microscopic studies of the monkey optic nervehead during development of glaucomatous cupping. Invest Ophthal Vis Sci 17:838, 1978.
84. Quigley, HA, Flower, RW, Addicks, EM, McLeod, DS: The mechanism of optic nerve damage in experimental acute intraocular pressure elevation. Invest Ophthal Vis Sci 19:505, 1980.
85. Minckler, DS, Bunt, AH: Axoplasmic transport in ocular hypotony and papill-

edema in the monkey. Arch Ophthal 95:1430, 1977.

86. Tso, MOM: Axoplasmic transport in papilledema and glaucoma. Trans Am Acad Ophthal Otol 83:771, 1977.

87. Anderson, DR, Hendrickson, AE: Failure of increased intracranial pressure to affect rapid axonal transport at the optic nerve head. Invest Ophthal Vis Sci 16:423, 1977.

88. Levy, NS, Adams, CK: Slow axonal protein transport and visual function following retinal and optic nerve ischemia. Invest Ophthal 14:91, 1975.

89. Levy, NS: The effect of interruption of the short posterior ciliary arteries on slow axoplasmic transport and histology within the optic nerve of the rhesus monkey. Invest Ophthal 15:495, 1978.

90. Radius, RL: Optic nerve fast axonal transport abnormalities in primates. Occurrence after short posterior ciliary artery occlusion. Arch Ophthal 98:2018, 1980.

91. Radius, RL, Anderson, DR: Breakdown of the normal optic nerve head blood-brain barrier following acute elevation of intraocular pressure in experimental animals. Invest Ophthal Vis Sci 19:244, 1980.

92. Radius, RL, Schwartz, EL, Anderson, DR: Failure of unilateral carotid artery ligation to affect pressure-induced interruption of rapid axonal transport in primate optic nerves. Invest Ophthal Vis Sci 19:153, 1980.

93. Ernest, JT: Pathogenesis of glaucomatous optic nerve disease. Tr Am Ophthal Soc 73:366, 1975.

94. Sipperley, J, Anderson, DR, Hamasaki, D: Short-term effect of intraocular pressure elevation on the human electroretinogram. Arch Ophthal 90:385, 1973.

95. Bartl, G: The electroretinogram and the visual evoked potential in normal and glaucomatous eyes. Albrecht v Graefes Arch Klin Exp Ophthal 207:243, 1978.

96. Weiter, J, Fine, BS: A histologic study of regional choroidal dystrophy. Am J Ophthal 83:741, 1977.

97. Hayreh, SS: Anterior Ischemic Optic Neuropathy, Springer-Verlag, New York, 1975.

98. Quigley, H, Anderson, DR: Cupping of the optic disc in ischemic optic neuropathy. Trans Am Acad Ophthal Otol 83:755, 1977.

99. Hitchings, RA: The optic disc in glaucoma, III: diffuse optic disc pallor with raised intraocular pressure. Br J Ophthal 62:670, 1978.

100. Radius, RL, Maumenee, AE: Optic atrophy and glaucomatous cupping. Am J Ophthal 85:145, 1978.

101. Jampol, LM, Board, RJ, Maumenee, AE: Systemic hypotension and glaucomatous changes. Am J Ophthal 85:154, 1978.

102. Quigley, HA, Anderson, DR: The histologic basis of optic disk pallor in experimental optic atrophy. Am J Ophthal 83:709, 1977.

103. Henkind, P, Bellhorn, R, Rabkin, M, Murphy, ME: Optic nerve transection in cats. II. Effect on vessels of optic nerve head and lamina cribrosa. Invest Ophthal Vis Sci 16:442, 1977.

104. Radius, RL, Anderson, DR: The mechanism of disc pallor in experimental optic atrophy. A fluorescein angiographic study. Arch Ophthal 97:532, 1979.

105. Brownstein, S, Font, RL, Zimmerman, LE, Murphy, SB: Nonglaucomatous cavernous degeneration of the optic nerve. Report of two cases. Arch Ophthal 98:354, 1980.

106. Bengtsson, B: The variation and covariation of cup and disc diameters. Acta Ophthalmologica 54:804, 1976.

107. Schwartz, B: Cupping and pallor of the optic disc. Arch Ophthal 89:272, 1973.

108. Armaly, MF: Genetic determination of cup/disc ratio of the optic nerve. Arch Ophthal 78:35, 1967.

109. Schwartz, JT, Reuling, FH, Garrison, RJ: Acquired cupping of the optic nerve head in normotensive eyes. Br J Ophthal 59:216, 1975.

110. Fishman, RS: Optic disc asymmetry. A sign of ocular hypertension. Arch Ophthal 84:590, 1970.

111. Holm, OC, Becker, B, Asseff, CF, Podos, SM: Volume of the optic disk cup. Am J Ophthal 73:876, 1972.
112. Hollows, FC, McGuiness, R: The size of the optic cup. Trans Ophthalmol Soc Aust NZ 19:33, 1966.
113. Armaly, MF, Sayegh, RE: The cup/disc ratio. The findings of tonometry and tonography in the normal eye. Arch Ophthal 82:191, 1969.
114. Armaly, MF: The optic cup in the normal eye. I. Cup width, depth, vessel displacement, ocular tension and outflow facility. Am J Ophthal 68:401, 1969.
115. Becker, B: Cup/disk ratio and topical corticosteroid testing. Am J Ophthal 70:681, 1970.
116. Snydacker, D: The normal optic disc. Ophthalmoscopic and photographic studies. Am J Ophthal 58:958, 1964.
117. Schwartz, B, Reinstein, NM, Lieberman, DM: Pallor of the optic disc. Quantitative photographic evaluation. Arch Ophthal 89:278, 1973.
118. Kolker, AE, Hetherington, J Jr: Becker-Shaffer's Diagnosis and Therapy of the Glaucomas, 4th ed, CV Mosby Co, St Louis, 1976, p 134.
119. Tomlinson, A, Phillips, CI: Ovalness of the optic cup and disc in the normal eye. Br J Ophthal 58:543, 1974.
120. Portney, GL: Qualitative parameters of the normal optic nerve head. Am J Ophthal 76:655, 1973.
121. Portney, GL: Photogrammetric categorical analysis of the optic nerve head. Trans Am Acad Ophthal Otol 78:275, 1974.
122. Shields, MB: Problems in recognizing non-glaucomatous optic nerve head cupping. Pers Ophthal 2:129, 1978.
123. Shields, MB: Gray crescent in the optic nerve head. Am J Ophthal 89:238, 1980.
124. Kirsch, RE, Anderson, DR: Identification of the glaucomatous disc. Trans Am Acad Ophthal Otol 77:143, 1973.
125. Kirsch, RE, Anderson, DR: Clinical recognition of glaucomatous cupping. Am J Ophthal 75:442, 1973.
126. Weisman, RL, Asseff, CF, Phelps, CD, Podos, SM, Becker, B: Vertical elongation of the optic cup in glaucoma. Trans Am Acad Ophthal Otol 77:157, 1973.
127. Read, RM, Spaeth, GL: The practical clinical appraisal of the optic disc in glaucoma: the natural history of cup progression and some specific disc-field correlations. Trans Am Acad Ophthal Otol 78:255, 1974.
128. Spaeth, GL, Hitchings, RA, Sivalingam, E: The optic disc in glaucoma: pathogenetic correlation of five patterns of cupping in chronic open-angle glaucoma. Trans Am Acad Ophthal Otol 81:217, 1976.
129. Hitchings, RA, Spaeth, GL: The optic disc in glaucoma. I. Classification. Br J Ophthal 60:778, 1976.
130. Radius, RL, Maumenee, AE, Green, WR: Pit-like changes of the optic nerve head in open-angle glaucoma. Br J Ophthal 62:389, 1978.
131. Pederson, JE, Anderson, DR: The mode of progressive disc cupping in ocular hypertension and glaucoma. Arch Ophthal 98:490, 1980.
132. Portney, GL: Photogrammetric analysis of the three-dimensional geometry of normal and glaucomatous optic cups. Trans Am Acad Ophthal Otol 81:239, 1976.
133. Chandler, PA, Grant, WM: Glaucoma, 2nd ed, Lea & Febiger, Philadelphia, 1977.
134. Cher, I, Robinson, LP: "Thinning" of the neural rim of the optic nerve-head. An altered state, providing a new ophthalmoscopic sign associated with characteristics of glaucoma. Trans Ophthal Soc UK 93:213, 1973.
135. Cher, I, Robinson, LP: Thinning of the neural rim: A simple new sign on the optic disc related to glaucoma—statistical considerations. Aust J Ophthal 2:27, 1974.
136. Sommer, A, Pollack, I, Maumenee, AE: Optic disc parameters and onset of glaucomatous field loss. I. Methods and progressive changes in disc morphology. Arch Ophthal 97:1444, 1979.

137. Herschler, J, Osher, RH: Baring of the circumlinear vessel. An early sign of optic nerve damage. Arch Ophthal 98:865, 1980.
138. Drance, SM, Fairclough, M, Butler, DM, Kottler, MS: The importance of disc hemorrhage in the prognosis of chronic open angle glaucoma. Arch Ophthal 95:226, 1977.
139. Susanna, R, Drance, SM, Douglas, GR: Disc hemorrhages in patients with elevated intraocular pressure. Occurrence with and without field changes. Arch Ophthal 97:284, 1979.
140. Hitchings, RA, Spaeth, GL: Chronic retinal vein occlusion in glaucoma. Br J Ophthal 60:694, 1976.
141. Radius, RL: Thickness of the retinal nerve fiber layer in primate eyes. Arch Ophthal 98:1625, 1980.
142. Sommer, A, Miller, NR, Pollack, I, Maumenee, AE, George, T: The nerve fiber layer in the diagnosis of glaucoma. Arch Ophthal 95:2149, 1977.
143. Sommer, A, Pollack, I, Maumenee, AE: Optic disc parameters and onset of glaucomatous field loss. II. Static screening criteria. Arch Ophthal 97:1449, 1979.
144. Quigley, HA, Miller, NR, George, T: Clinical evaluation of nerve fiber layer atrophy as an indicator of glaucomatous optic nerve damage. Arch Ophthal 98:1564, 1980.
145. Radius, RL, Anderson, DR: The histology of retinal nerve fiber layer bundles and bundle defects. Arch Ophthal 97:948, 1979.
146. Newman, NM: Ophthalmoscopic observation of the retinal nerve fiber layer. Trans Am Acad Ophthal Otol 83:786, 1977.
147. Primrose, J: The incidence of the peripapillary halo glaucomatosus. Trans Ophthal Soc UK 89:585, 1969.
148. Wilensky, JT, Kolker, AE: Peripapillary changes in glaucoma. Am J Ophthal 81:341, 1976.
149. Kohn, AN, Moss, AP, Podos, SM: Relative afferent pupillary defects in glaucoma without characteristic field loss. Arch Ophthal 97:294, 1979.
150. Jensen, PE, Kalina, RE: Congenital anomalies of the optic disk. Am J Ophthal 82:27, 1976.
151. Harrington, DO: The Visual Fields, 3rd ed, CV Mosby Co, St Louis, 1971, p 227.
152. Kindler, P: Morning glory syndrome: unusual congenital optic disk anomaly. Am J Ophthal 69:376, 1970.
153. Brown, GC, Shields, JA, Goldberg, RE: Congenital pits of the optic nerve head. II. Clinical studies in humans. Ophthalmology 87:51, 1980.
154. Theodossiadis, G: Evolution of congenital pit of the optic disk with macular detachment in photocoagulated and nonphotocoagulated eyes. Am J Ophthal 84:620, 1977.
155. Trobe, JD, Glaser, JS, Cassady, JC: Optic atrophy. Differential diagnosis by fundus observation alone. Arch Ophthal 98:1040, 1980.
156. Trobe, JD, Glaser, JS, Cassady, J, Herschler, J, Anderson, DR: Nonglaucomatous excavation of the optic disc. Arch Ophthal 98:1046, 1980.
157. Lichter, PR, Henderson, JW: Optic nerve infarction. Am J Ophthal 85:302, 1978.
158. Portney, GL, Roth, AM: Optic cupping caused by an intracranial aneurysm. Am J Ophthal 84:98, 1977.
159. Shaffer, RN, Ridgway, WL, Brown, R, Kramer, SG: The use of diagrams to record changes in glaucomatous disks. Am J Ophthal 80:460, 1975.
160. Lichter, PR: Variability of expert observers in evaluating the optic disc. Trans Am Ophthal Soc 74:532, 1976.
161. Schwartz, JT: Methodologic differences and measurement of cup-disc ratio. An epidemiologic assessment. Arch Ophthal 94:1101, 1976.
162. Gloster, J, Parry, DG: Use of photographs for measuring cupping in the optic disc. Br J Ophthal 58:850, 1974.
163. Delori, FC, Gragoudas, ES, Francisco, R, Pruett, RC: Monochromatic ophthalmoscopy and fundus photography. Arch Ophthal 95:861, 1977.

164. Miller, NR, George, TW: Monochromatic (red-free) photography and ophthalmoscopy of the peripapillary retinal nerve fiber layer. Invest Ophthal Vis Sci 17:1121, 1978.
165. Frisen, L: Photography of the retinal nerve fibre layer: an optimised procedure. Br J Ophthal 64:641, 1980.
166. Cohan, BE: Multiple-slit illumination of the optic disc. Arch Ophthal 96:497, 1978.
167. Schwartz, B, Kern, J: Scanning microdensitometry of optic disc pallor in glaucoma. Arch Ophthal 95:2159, 1977.
168. Rosenthal, AR, Falconer, DG, Barrett, P: Digital measurement of pallor-disc ratio. Arch Ophthal 98:2027, 1980.
169. Cohan, BE, Pearch, AC, Anderson, SA: Comparison of photo slit lamp and fundus camera photography of the optic disc. Arch Ophthal 97:1462, 1979.
170. Allen, L: Stereoscopic fundus photography with the new instant positive print films. Am J Ophthal 57:539, 1964.
171. Donaldson, DD: A new camera for stereoscopic fundus photography. Arch Ophthal 73:253, 1965.
172. Donaldson, DD, Prescott, R, Kennedy, S: Simultaneous stereoscopic fundus camera incorporating a single optical axis. Invest Ophthal Vis Sci 19:289, 1980.
173. Saheb, NE, Drance, SM, Nelson, A: The use of photogrammetry in evaluating the cup of the optic nervehead for a study in chronic simple glaucoma. Can J Ophthal 7:466, 1972.
174. Rosenthal, AR, Kottler, MS, Donaldson, DD, Falconer, DG: Comparative reproducibility of the digital photogrammetric procedure utilizing three methods of stereophotography. Invest Ophthal Vis Sci 16:54, 1977.
175. Donaldson, DD, Grant, WM: Stereoscopic comparator with primary use for optic discs. Arch Ophthal 96:503, 1978.
176. Halberg, GP: Charting and scoring the optic disc. Arch Ophthal 82:149, 1969.
177. Schwartz, B: New techniques for the examination of the optic disc and their clinical application. Trans Am Acad Ophthal Otol 81:227, 1976.
178. Kottler, MS, Rosenthal, AR, Falconer, DG: Analog vs. digital photogrammetry for optic cup analysis. Invest Ophthal 15:651, 1976.
179. Krohn, MA, Keltner, JL, Johnson, CA: Comparison of photographic techniques and films used in stereophotogrammetry of the optic disk. Am J Ophthal 88:859, 1979.
180. Schirmer, KE: Simplified photogrammetry of the optic disc. Arch Ophthal 94:1997, 1976.
181. Johnson, CA, Keltner, JL, Krohn, MA, Portney, GL: Photogrammetry of the optic disc in glaucoma and ocular hypertension with simultaneous stereo photography. Invest Ophthal Vis Sci 18:1252, 1979.
182. Schirmer, KE, Kratky, V: Stereochronoscopy of the optic disc with stereoscopic cameras. Arch Ophthal 98:1647, 1980.
183. Gloster, J: The colour of the optic disc. Doc Ophthal 26:155, 1969.
184. Davies, EWG: Quantitative assessment of colour of the optic disc by a photographic method. Exp Eye Res 9:106, 1970.
185. Berkowitz, JS, Balter, S: Colorimetric measurements of the optic disk. Am J Ophthal 69:385, 1970.
186. Cohen, JS, Stone, RD, Hetherington, J Jr, Bullock, J: Glaucomatous cupping of the optic disk by ultrasonography. Am J Ophthal 82:24, 1976.

Chapter 5

VISUAL FIELDS

VISUAL FIELDS

I. THE NORMAL VISUAL FIELD

A helpful way to begin the study of visual fields and the methods by which they are measured is to consider Traquair's[1] classic analogy of "an island of vision surrounded by a sea of blindness" (Fig. 5.1):

A. Boundary

The shoreline of the island is the *peripheral limits* of the visual field, which normally measure from fixation approximately 60° above and nasally, 70 to 75° below, and 100 to 110° temporally.[2] This boundary, which is referred to as an *isopter*, creates a characteristic horizontal oval shape in the normal visual field. The shape of the field is usually of greater diagnostic significance than the size, since the latter is more easily influenced by the stimulus value of test objects.

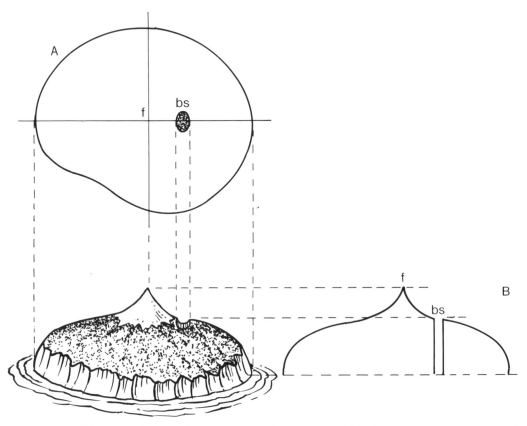

Figure 5.1.   The normal visual field is depicted as Traquair's[1] "island of vision surrounded by a sea of blindness," with projections showing the peripheral limits (**A**) and the profile (**B**); fixation (**f**) corresponds to the foveola of the retina, and the blind spot (**bs**), to the optic nerve head.

B. Contour

The peaks and valleys on the island are *areas of increased or decreased vision* within the peripheral limits of the visual field:

1. The area of maximum visual acuity in the normal field is at the point of fixation, which corresponds to the *foveola* of the retina. The visual sensitivity drops off fairly precipitously around fixation, then tapers down more gradually until it again falls abruptly at the peripheral limits.

2. Within the boundaries of the normal visual field is an area called the *blind spot*, which corresponds to the region of the *optic nerve head*. It is located approximately 15° temporal to fixation and has *two portions* (Fig. 5.2):[3]

   a. An *Absolute scotoma* corresponds to the area of the optic nerve head and is seen as a vertical oval. This portion is independent of the test object stimulus value.

   b. A *relative scotoma* surrounds the absolute portion and corresponds to peripapillary retina, which has reduced visual sensitivity, especially inferiorly and superiorly. This portion of the blind spot is dependent on stimulus value and varies with different testing methods

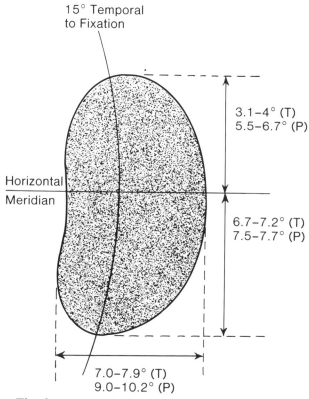

Figure 5.2. The location and dimensions of the normal blind spot as determined by Armaly[3] with a 1/1,000 test object on the tangent screen (**T**) and an I2e target on the Goldmann perimeter (**P**). Paired values represent means of two testing periods with the same population.

(average normal values are shown in Fig. 5.2). If the temporal margin of the relative blind spot comes close to the corresponding isopter, the two boundaries may artifactually become confluent, creating *false baring of the blind spot* (Fig. 5.3). Furthermore, because the reduced sensitivity of peripapillary retina is greater in the upper and lower poles, test objects with small stimulus value may cause vertical elongation of the blind spot, which can break through the isopter causing *true baring of the blind spot* (Fig. 5.3b).

II. INSTRUMENTS AND TECHNIQUES

A detailed consideration of the instruments and techniques used in visual field testing is beyond the scope of this study guide, but is

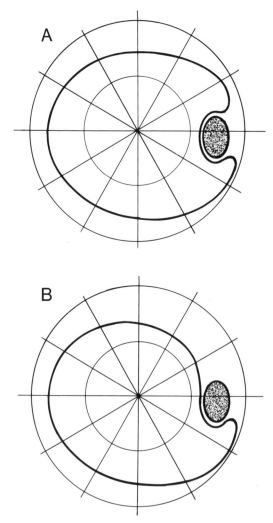

Figure 5.3. False baring (**A**) and true baring (**B**) of the blind spot (modified from Armaly[3]).

available in several excellent textbooks of clinical perimetry.[1, 2, 4, 5] The following discussion is limited to the fundamental aspects of this subject.

Just as a cartographer maps the boundaries and topography of an island, so the perimetrist can measure both the peripheral limits of a visual field and the relative visual acuity of areas within those limits. This is accomplished by two fundamental techniques: kinetic and static.

A. Kinetic Techniques

This involves *moving* the test object from a non-seeing area and recording the point at which it is first seen in relation to fixation. The procedure might be compared to studying an island by aerial reconnaissance, since it demonstrates the *boundaries* of the visual field, both for the absolute limits and for areas of relative difference in visual acuity within the field. As previously noted, the boundaries or contour lines are called *isopters.* The size and shape of a particular isopter depends, in part, on the stimulus value of the corresponding test object. Two basic types of screens are used for kinetic visual field testing:

1. *The tangent screen* is a *flat* square of black felt or flannel on which 30° of the visual field can be studied.[6] It has been recommended that the test be performed in mesopic lighting of approximately 7 foot-candles[7] with the patient seated 1 or 2 m from the screen. With the patient fixing on a white button in the center of the screen, the examiner moves a test object from the periphery toward fixation until the patient indicates recognition of the target. The procedure is repeated at various intervals around fixation until the isopter has been mapped. The stimulus value of the test object varies according to its size and color, and the corresponding isopter is designated by the ratio of target diameter to distance between patient and target, with both expressed in millimeters, *e.g.,* "2/1000 white" for a 2 mm white test object at 1 m (when the color is not indicated it is understood to be white).

This technique has the advantages of low cost and simplicity of operation and is said to be capable of eliciting 90% of field defects in general.[2] However, reproducibility of the fields, which is essential in managing patients with glaucoma, is limited by variations in background lighting and stimulus value of the targets and by difficulty in monitoring fixation. Furthermore, it does not include the peripheral field, where early glaucomatous defects may appear.

2. *Perimeters.* With these instruments, both the *central* and *peripheral* fields of vision can be examined. The screen of a perimeter may be either an *arc* or a *bowl.* The latter is preferable for glaucoma examinations, and the prototype is the the *Goldmann perimeter.*[8] Other similar instruments have been compared with the Goldmann unit with variable results.[9] The bowl of the Goldmann perimeter has

a radius of 300 mm and extends 95° to each side of fixation. The target is projected onto the bowl, and the stimulus value can be varied by changing the: 1) size (designated by 0, I, II, III, IV, V), 2) intensity (1, 2, 3, 4), or 3) light transmission (a, b, c, d, e) of the target. The latter variable merely provides finer intensity adjustment for the stimulus. An isopter might be designated as "I-2-e," which indicates a test object size of ¼ mm², an intensity of 10 millilamberts, and 100% transmission of the light source. The patient's fixation can be monitored by the examiner through a telescope in the center of the bowl. This instrument can be used for both kinetic and static visual field testing.

B. Static Techniques

Static techniques involve the presentation of *stationary* test objects. In general, static perimetry is superior to kinetic methods for finding glaucomatous defects. The static techniques are performed in two basic ways.

1. *Suprathreshold static presentation* is an "on-off" technique in which a test object that is just above the anticipated threshold for the corresponding portion of the visual field is momentarily presented, and the points at which the patient fails to recognize the target are noted. It is a way of "spot checking" for areas of relative or absolute blindness, usually within the central visual field. The technique may be performed with the *tangent screen*, by rotating a disc-shaped test object from the black to the white side, or by using a self-illuminating target with an on-off switch. It may also be used with the *perimeter* by turning the projected target light on and off. The use of the latter technique in glaucoma screening will be discussed later in this chapter.

2. *Threshold static* (profile) *perimetry.* To continue the analogy of Traquair's island of vision, profile perimetry might be compared to observing the topography of an island from a boat in the surrounding sea. In other words, it measures the relative *intensity thresholds* for the visual acuity within the field of vision. The prototype instrument for this technique is the Tübingen perimeter,[10, 11] which consists of a bowl-type screen and stationary test objects with variable light intensity. The technique involves gradually increasing the target light from subthreshold intensity and recording the intensity at which the patient first indicates recognition of the target. A series of such points can be plotted either 1) along one *meridian*, radiating from fixation or 2) in a *circular* manner along a fixed eccentricity from fixation (Fig. 5.4). The circular plot may be displayed either on a flat abscissa or a circular chart (Fig. 5.4).[2, 4, 5]

A variation of the profile static technique has been called *acuity profile perimetry*, in which the patient is required to distinguish different target shapes, rather than simply indicate the presence of the object. It has been suggested that the technique may have particular value in detecting optic nerve disease.[12]

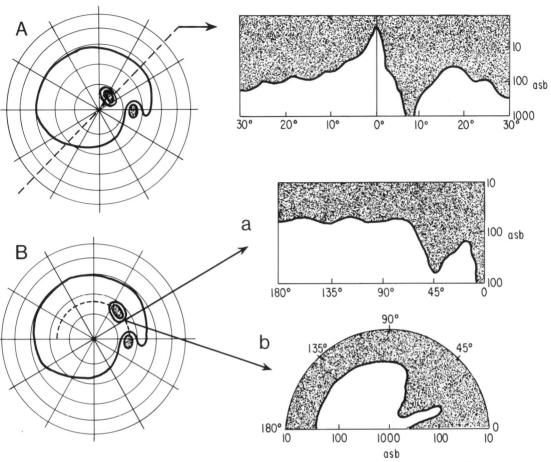

Figure 5.4. Threshold static (profile) perimetry. **A:** Meridian static perimetry. **B:** Circular static perimetry on flat abscissa (**a**) and circular chart (**b**). The dotted lines indicate the cuts through the fields that are being displayed in profile.

Threshold static perimetry has been shown to be more sensitive than kinetic perimetry in detecting glaucomatous field loss[13] and is a useful adjunct in detecting subtle changes. However, in addition to the time requirement, profile perimetry is limited, as are all forms of visual field testing, by the patient's ability to give reliable responses. One study showed that variability of response with repeated testing increased in areas of decreased retinal sensitivity, whether this was due to a more peripheral retinal position in the normal eye or a glaucomatous scotoma.[14] For this reason, the authors suggested that subtle field changes may not be a reliable indication of change and that more reliance should be placed on the grossest defects.

C. Specific Techniques

Within the context of glaucoma detection and management, visual field testing has two basic aspects: 1) *screening techniques* to detect the presence of glaucomatous field loss, and 2) *in-depth techniques* to more accurately determine the extent of the damage and to follow the fields for evidence of progressive change.

1. *Screening techniques*

a. *Selective perimetry* (Armaly-Drance technique) is an example of a screening technique for glaucoma. It utilizes the Goldmann perimeter with suprathreshold static perimetry to test for central field defects[15] and both suprathreshold static and kinetic perimetry to examine the peripheral field, with emphasis on the nasal[16] and temporal[17] periphery (Fig. 5.5). An evaluation of the technique in 106 normal individuals and 49 with glaucomatous defects revealed a high sensitivity and specificity, which made it suitable for clinical and survey screening.[16, 18] Similar techniques have been devised for the detection of both glaucomatous and neurological defects.[19]

b. Rapid screening devices and automatic perimeters are also available for glaucoma screening and are discussed later in this chapter.

2. *In-Depth techniques.* When a glaucomatous field defect is suspected by use of a screening technique, the physician has two choices. The patient can be asked to return another day either for a repeat screening field or an in-depth study. In many cases, however, it is more practical to proceed with the in-depth test at the time the defect is detected. The conversion from a screening to an in-depth field study is facilitated with the Armaly-Drance technique, since both are performed on the Goldmann perimeter with identical or similar target settings. The principle of in-depth field testing is to map out the size and shape of all *scotomas* (a field defect within an isopter) as well as *complete isopters*, using both the central threshold target and two or more additional targets of greater stimulus value. The basic principles to be used in both in-depth testing and screening techniques are considered below.

D. Basic Principles

The *basic principles* of visual field testing include the following considerations.[20, 21]

1. *Presentation of test object*

a. To minimize the patient's anticipation of when or where the next test object will appear, the presentation should be *random*, rather than consecutively along one isopter, and the *time between stimuli* should be *varied* slightly.

b. To avoid patient anxiety when testing in a non-seeing area, return periodically to a previously seen area.

c. Kinetic targets should be moved at a *consistent rate* of approximately 5°/sec in the periphery and slower centrally. Always move the test object from a *non-seeing to a seeing area*, i.e., from the center of the blind spot or of a scotoma, and from the periphery toward fixation when outlining the isopter.

d. *Suprathreshold static targets* should be presented for a consistent duration of time; usually ½ to 1 sec. Test objects should be

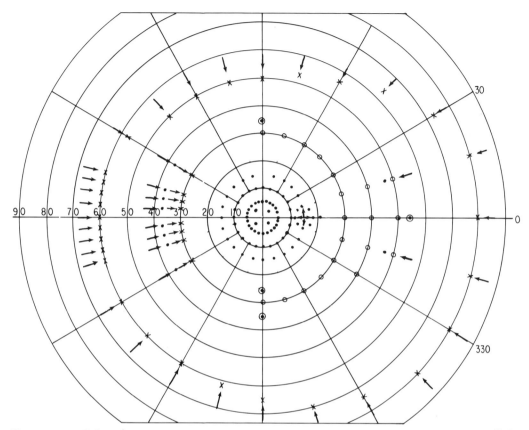

Figure 5.5. Selective perimetry on Goldmann perimeter (Armaly-Drance technique[15–18]). With refractive correction in place, determine central suprathreshold target at 25° from fixation (◉) by starting with I2e target and increasing stimulus value (I3e, I4e, II4e, III4e, IV4e, V4e) until the target is first seen. Using the suprathreshold target, familiarize patient with testing procedure by static presentation in each quadrant within 5° (●). Then outline blind spot with kinetic technique (arrows, ●) and "spot check" with static presentation along each 15° meridian at 5°, 10°, and 15° from fixation (●). Recheck each missed spot once at conclusion of each circle. Two misses in one spot constitutes a positive finding. Test peripheral limits of central suprathreshold target along temporal isopter (arrows, ●) and nasal isopter (arrows, ×) by kinetic presentation. Remove refractive correction and determine peripheral suprathreshold target (◉) using same sequence of stimulus values as for central target. Test temporal field with static presentation (○). Outline peripheral isopter by kinetic presentation of peripheral suprathreshold target (arrows, ×).

just above threshold for the area being tested. A modified target for static presentation has been suggested in which brightness increases toward the center of the object, according to a sine curve.[22] This is said to have the advantage of minimizing the effect of form sense on the visual field examination.[22]

    2. *Illumination*

        a. Background illumination is usually mesopic (approximately 7 foot-candles) to stimulate both rods and cones. With bowl perimeters, photometric adjustment should be made with the patient in place, since facial coloring affects luminosity.

b. The most important principle regarding illumination is to keep both target and background *constant and reproducible* from one examination to the next.

3. *Physiologic factors that influence visual fields* should be compensated for if possible or otherwise should be considered when interpreting the fields. These factors include the following:

a. *Clarity of ocular media*

(1). *Cataracts*, especially if associated with *miosis*, can cause or exaggerate central or peripheral field defects, which could be mistaken for the development or progression of glaucomatous field loss. In a study of 90 eyes with open-angle glaucoma and cataracts, 41% had loss of a partial or complete scotoma after cataract extraction.[23] Threshold sensitivity was correlated with visual acuity levels in 74 patients with varying degrees of cataracts to quantitate the extent of isopter depression for five standard stimuli on the Goldmann perimeter.[24] These data are available for use in determining the significance of field change in a patient with glaucoma and cataracts (reader is referred to original article).[24]

(2). Reduced clarity of the ocular media from other causes, such as corneal disturbance or vitreous opacities, may also affect the visual fields.

b. *Pupil size. Miosis* alone may depress central and peripheral isopters and exaggerate field defects. For this reason, the pupil size should be recorded with each field, and the influence of miosis should be considered when a field change is detected. Mydriasis has minimal influence on the visual field, other than the reduced accommodation that may result from a topical mydriatic-cycloplegic.

c. *Refractive errors* primarily influence the *central* field.

(1). *Myopia* does not require correction when using a 300 mm perimeter, unless the refractive error exceeds 3 diopters. *Posterior staphylomas* can create areas of relative myopia, called refraction scotomas, which may be confused with glaucomatous field defects, but can usually be eliminated with an appropriate refractive correction.

(2). *Hyperopia* should be corrected for central fields when using perimeters. Age tables are available to aid in determining the appropriate correction for *presbyopia*. A contact lens provides the best correction for the *aphakic eye*,[25] although spectacle correction can be used for the central 25 to 30° with no correction for the peripheral field.

(3). *Astigmatism* should be corrected unless the cylinder is under 1 diopter, in which case it can be included as its spherical equivalent.

d. *Increasing age* is also associated with a reduction in threshold sensitivity.[26, 27] This effect of age, especially on the superior paracentral portion of the visual field, may be accelerated by intraocular pressure elevation.[27]

4. *Psychological factors*, including the patient's understanding of the test and his alertness, concentration, fixation, and cooperation,[26] as well as the skill of the perimetrist,[28] also influence the results of visual field testing.

E. Additional Instruments

1. *Rapid screening devices* have been developed to aid in the detection of glaucoma patients. The *Harrington-Flocks screener* utilizes the flash presentation of multiple dot patterns, and the patient is asked to indicate the number of dots seen.[29] The device was found to be reliable in a study of 1500 screening tests.[30] The *Friedmann Visual Field Analyzer* is a similar instrument, which involves the static presentation of single or multiple test objects that can be varied in intensity.[31, 32] Studies have also demonstrated the reliability of this device for mass screening programs.[33, 34] More recently, *television* has been used for mass screening of visual fields by employing the *multiple dot pattern* technique.[35] The value of this method has yet to be established.

2. *Automatic perimeters* are currently being developed which utilize *computers* to program visual field test sequences.[36–46] These instruments range in complexity from relatively simple bowl-type perimeters, with a limited array of suprathreshold static targets, to highly sophisticated instruments that are capable of kinetic and static visual field analysis. Some computerized perimeters may also be modified to display profile sensitivity along a meridian of the visual field.[44] The primary value of automatic perimeters at the present time appears to be as screening devices in detecting field loss, and preliminary studies have shown favorable comparisons with standard manual kinetic and static perimetry.[36–43] However, the rapidly expanding technology of computerized perimeters promises an ever increasing role for these instruments in the testing of visual fields.

3. *Miscellaneous devices*

a. *Visual evoked responses* (VER) have been studied in patients with glaucomatous field loss. Under stimulation with a pattern reversal of light and dark squares, a delayed response has been correlated with visual field loss.[47, 48] Using transscleral stimulation, a good linear correlation between amplitude of VER and amount of field loss was found,[49] and it has been suggested that alterations in the VER may provide the earliest reliable evidence of optic pathway impairment due to elevated intraocular pressure.[50]

b. *Laser scotometry* has been described as a technique for mapping out blind spots directly on the retina, by moving the focusing beam of the laser away from the center of a non-seeing area until the patient indicates visualization of the beam.[51]

F. Recording and Scoring Visual Field Data

The complex nature of visual field defects makes it difficult to reduce the information to simple descriptions or numbers. Therefore, storage of the data in its raw form, *i.e.*, as transferred directly from the testing screen, is usually the most practical means of record keeping. However, when it is necessary to estimate the percentage of functional visual field loss, a system is available (the *Esterman grids*), in which the field is divided into 100 blocks of varying size according to functional value, with each representing 1%.[52, 53] In addition, techniques are being developed to convert visual field data into forms that will facilitate computer storage and analysis.[54–56]

III GLAUCOMATOUS FIELD DEFECTS

A. The Anatomic Basis of Glaucomatous Field Defects

1. *Retinal nerve fiber distribution.* As the axons traverse the nerve fiber layer from the ganglion cell bodies to the optic nerve head, they are distributed in a characteristic pattern (Fig. 5.6). Most fibers reach the nerve head by a direct route, except those that are temporal to the macula, which arch above or below the fovea. These *arcuate nerve fibers* do not cross the horizontal line temporal to the fovea, thereby

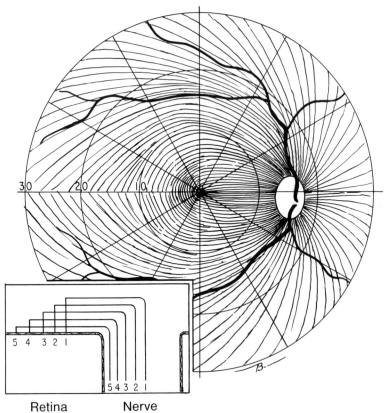

Retina   Nerve

Figure 5.6. Anatomy of retinal nerve fiber distribution. Inset depicts cross-sectional view of axonal arrangement. Peripheral fibers run closer to choroid and exit in periphery of optic nerve, while fibers originating closer to the nerve head are situated closer to the vitreous and occupy a more central portion of the nerve.

creating a temporal or *median raphe.* [57] As bundles of nerve fibers are destroyed in glaucomatous optic atrophy, the resulting visual field defect will correspond to this pattern of axon distribution in the retinal nerve fiber layer.

2. *Axon distribution within the optic nerve head.* Primate studies indicate that the arcuate nerve fibers occupy the superior and inferior temporal portions of the optic nerve head.[58] Axons originating in the peripheral retina lie closer to the ganglion cell layer and occupy the more peripheral region of the nerve head, while fibers from ganglion cells closer to the disc lie nearer to the vitreous and enter the nerve head more centrally (Fig. 5.6).[58] The arcuate nerve fibers and the related superior and inferior temporal portions of the optic nerve head are the most sensitive to glaucomatous damage, accounting for the early loss in the corresponding regions of the visual fields. Macular fibers spread over approximately one-third of the distal optic nerve, primarily temporally, and intermingle with extramacular fibers,[59] which may explain the retention of central vision during early glaucomatous optic atrophy.

B. ''The Glaucoma Field''

It is not possible to define "the glaucoma field." The changes in visual function, which will continually worsen as long as the intraocular pressure is too high, are complex and only partially understood. Nevertheless, the following features constitute our general understanding of this dynamic process of visual destruction in glaucoma.

C. Early Glaucomatous Field Defects

1. *Generalized reduction in visual threshold* appears to be one of the earliest detectable alterations in the visual field of a patient with glaucoma. Although the diagnostic value of this change is limited by its non-specific nature, which probably reflects a lack of sufficiently sensitive testing methods, it should be looked for and noted in the course of visual field testing and analysis. The following are some of the ways in which *generalized reduction in visual threshold* may become manifest:

a. *Isopter contraction.* In a study of patients with elevated intraocular pressures who eventually developed glaucomatous field defects, the peripheral (I4e) isopter area was significantly smaller prior to visual field loss, and both peripheral and central (I2e) isopter areas correlated linearly with the increase in cup-disc ratio coincident with field loss.[60] However, this isopter contraction is produced by so many factors that it is said to be of limited diagnostic value.[61, 62]

b. *Baring of the blind spot*, due to depression of central isopters, is also considered to be an early glaucomatous field change. However, it can be produced in normal individuals with threshold targets and is not a pathognomonic sign of glaucoma.[62]

c. *Angioscotomata* are long, branching scotomata above and

below the blind spot, which are presumed to result from shadows created by the large retinal vessels and are felt to be an early glaucomatous field defect.[63]

2. *Scatter* (or localized minor disturbances) is defined as variable threshold responses to repeated testing of the same area. It has been found to frequently precede a definitive field defect in the area where the defect subsequently appeared.[64]

D. Definitive Glaucomatous Field Defects

The following group of visual field defects are more characteristic of glaucoma than the aforementioned changes, although they are not pathognomonic. They are all related to underlying disturbances in retinal nerve fiber bundles.

1. *Arcuate nerve fiber bundle defects.*[65, 66]

a. The *arcuate* or *Bjerrum* (pronounced "Bee yer' um") *area* within the visual field extends above and below fixation from the blind spot to the median raphe, and corresponds to the previously discussed arcuate retinal nerve fibers. The nasal extreme of the arcuate area along the median raphe may come within 1° of fixation and extend nasally for 10 to 20° (Fig. 5.7a). Early visual loss in glaucoma commonly occurs within this arcuate area, which correlates with the predilection of the inferior and superior temporal poles of the optic nerve head for early glaucomatous damage. Furthermore, defects in the superior arcuate area usually occur before those in the inferior area,[67] corresponding to the greater tendency for early glaucomatous cupping in the inferior temporal pole of the optic nerve head.

b. As field defects develop within the arcuate areas, they may present in several characteristic patterns[68, 69]:

(1). The earliest defect in the arcuate area is usually a *paracentral scotoma*, which may have a central absolute defect, surrounded by a relative scotoma (Fig. 5.7b).

(2). Rarely, the early arcuate defect arises from the blind spot and tapers to a point in a slightly curved course (Fig. 5.7c). This is referred to as a *Seidel scotoma.*

(3). As isolated scotomata in the arcuate area enlarge and coalesce, they form an arching scotoma that eventually fills the entire arcuate area from the blind spot to the median raphe (Fig. 5.7d). This is referred to as an *arcuate* or *Bjerrum* scotoma. With further progression, a double arcuate (or ring) scotomata will develop (Fig. 5.7e).

c. *Differential diagnosis of arcuate scotomata.* Although the arcuate defect is probably the most reliable early form of glaucomatous field loss, it is not pathognomonic, and the following additional causes must be considered, especially when the field and disc changes do not seem to correlate[65, 66, 70]:

(1). *Chorioretinal lesions* (juxtapapillary choroiditis and retinochoroiditis,[71] myopia with peripapillary atrophy, and atypical retinitis pigmentosa[72]).

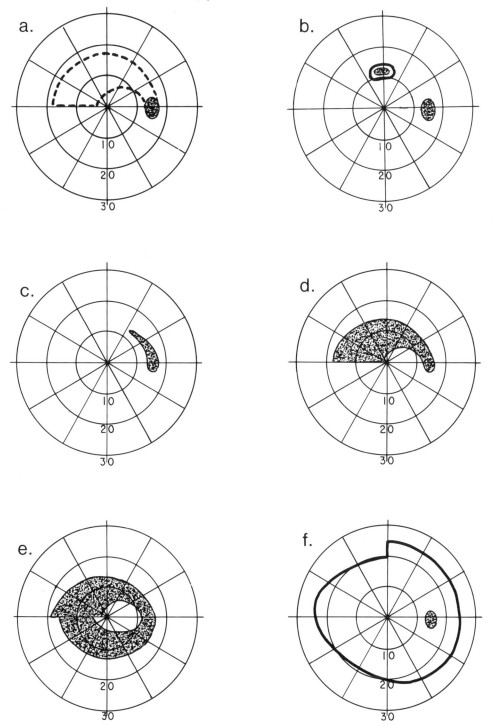

Figure 5.7. Arcuate nerve fiber bundle defects. **a:** The arcuate (or Bjerrum) area is shown within the dotted lines. **b:** Superior paracentral scotoma, with central absolute defect surrounded by a relative scotoma. **c:** Seidel scotoma. **d:** Complete arcuate (Bjerrum) scotoma. **e:** Double arcuate (ring) scotoma with superior central nasal step. **f:** Vertical step (or hemianopic offset).

(2). *Optic nerve head lesions* (drusen,[73] retinal artery plaques, papilledema, coloboma, optic nerve pit, optic atrophy, papillitis, and central retinal artery occlusion).

(3). *Anterior optic nerve lesions* (carotid and ophthalmic artery occlusion, ischemic infarct, cerebral arteritis, retrobulbar neuritis, electric shock, and exophthalmos).

(4). *Posterior lesions of the visual pathway* (pituitary adenoma, opticochiasmatic arachnoiditis, meningioma of the dorsum sella or optic foramen, and progressive external ophthalmoplogia[74]).

2. *Nasal steps.* The loss of retinal nerve fibers rarely proceeds at the same rate in the upper and lower portions of an eye. Consequently, a step-like defect is frequently created where the nerve fibers meet along the *median raphe.* Since the superior field is involved somewhat more frequently than the inferior in the early stages of glaucoma, the nasal step more often results from a greater defect above the horizontal midline, which is referred to as a superior nasal step (Fig. 5.7e). However, the opposite is not uncommon. *Two forms* of nasal steps have been described[75]:

a. *A central nasal step* is created at the nasal termination of unequal double arcuate scotomata (Fig. 5.7e).

b. *The peripheral nasal step (of Rönne)* results from unequal

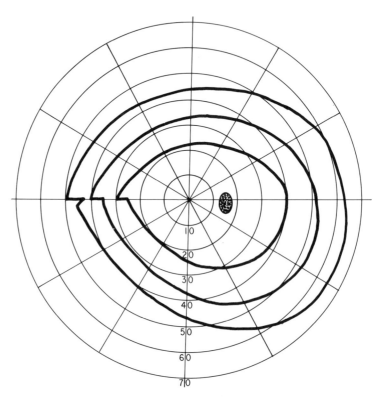

Figure 5.8. Peripheral nasal step (of Rönne), showing effect of distance from fixation on shape of nasal step.

contraction of the peripheral isopters due to loss of corresponding bundles of peripheral arcuate nerve fibers (Fig. 5.8). It may begin as an isolated scotoma in the nasal periphery.[76] The shape of the peripheral nasal step differs according to its distance from fixation (Fig. 5.8), and is not necessarily found in all isopters.[68, 69] In early stages of glaucomatous field loss, the peripheral nasal step may be the only detectable defect,[75–78] emphasizing the importance of testing the peripheral field, especially nasally.

3. *A vertical step* (or heminanopic offset) is a less common feature of glaucomatous field loss, although it has been reported to occur in up to 20% of cases.[79] This defect more often appears on the *nasal* side of the vertical midline (Fig. 5.7f). However, studies of normal subjects have also revealed greater sensitivity temporal to the hemianopic border, and it has been suggested that a small peripheral step at the vertical midline should arouse suspicion of glaucoma only if the defect is located temporally.[80, 81] In addition, the presence of a hemianopic field defect should always arouse suspicion of a *neurological* lesion.[82]

4. A *temporal sector* field defect represents a loss of nerve fibers nasal to the optic nerve head, where the axons converge on the disc by a direct route.[68, 69] This defect usually appears later in the course of glaucomatous field loss,[83] although it was the only defect in 2.7% of the eyes in one study.[84]

E. Advanced Glaucomatous Field Defects

The natural history of progressive glaucomatous field loss is eventual development of complete double arcuate scotomas with extension to the peripheral limits in all areas except temporally. This results in a *central island* and *temporal island* of vision in advanced glaucoma. With continued damage, these islands of vision progressively diminish in size until the tiny central island is totally extinguished, which may occur abruptly. It was once thought that the sudden hypotony of glaucoma surgery might accelerate this final loss of a small central island, although studies have not supported this concept.[85, 86] The temporal island of vision is more resistant and may persist long after central vision is lost. However, it too will eventually be destroyed if the intraocular pressure is not controlled, leaving the patient with no light perception.

F. Visual Field Changes with Acute Pressure Elevation

1. The preceding discussion has dealt with field changes that are associated primarily with chronic glaucoma. When the intraocular pressure elevation is sudden and marked, as in *acute angle-closure glaucoma*, the associated field changes have been variously reported as general depression, early loss of central vision, arcuate scotomata, enlargement of the blind spot, or no detectable defect.[87] After the acute attack is brought under control, the fields may return to normal, while other patients may have reduced color vision, generalized

decreased sensitivity with static perimetry, or constriction of isopters, especially superiorly.[88]

2. When the intraocular pressure is *artificially elevated*, either by compression of the globe[89-91] or administration of topical steroids,[92-96] typical glaucomatous field defects[89-95] or constriction of central isopters[96] occur in some eyes. The changes are reversible when the IOP returns to normal.[93-95] This response to artificial pressure elevation is said to occur more commonly in glaucoma patients,[89, 90] especially those with low-tension glaucoma,[92] although one study found no significant difference between glaucoma and non-glaucoma patients.[91]

G. Response of Field Defects to Reduced Pressure

It is reported that visual acuity and field may improve if the intraocular pressure is reduced in the early stages of glaucoma.[61, 97] However, this is the exception, since most glaucomatous field defects are irreversible.

IV. THE CORRELATION BETWEEN OPTIC NERVE HEAD AND VISUAL FIELD DEFECTS

Several large studies have been conducted to determine whether established or impending field loss can be predicted by the appearance of the optic nerve head.

A. Established Field Loss

The reported ability to correctly predict the presence of *established field loss* on the basis of disc appearance ranges from 66 to 85%,[98-103] while 80 to 97% accuracy is reported in predicting the absence of field loss.[99, 101, 102] In most cases, disc changes precede detectable field loss,[103] with *extensive or focal absence of neural rim tissue*, especially at the inferior or superior poles, being the most reliable indicator of visual field disturbance.[101, 104, 105] However, field loss may occur before the pallor reaches the disc margin,[106] and unusual cases have been reported with field damage despite round, symmetric cups.[101] The nature of optic nerve head cupping can also be used to predict, in many cases, the type of field loss (Fig. 5.9).[106] For example, when the disc is cupped to the inferior rim, a field defect in the superior arcuate area would be anticipated.

B. Impending Field Loss

Predicting *impending field loss* by the appearance of the optic nerve head is even more difficult. No single parameter or combination of parameters in glaucomatous optic atrophy has been found to be totally satisfactory for this purpose. Defects in the *retinal nerve fiber layer* are reported to correlate most closely with future field loss, and further investigation in this area appears to be warranted.[107, 108]

C. Conclusion

In *conclusion*, while the correlation between optic nerve head and visual field defects in glaucoma is not perfect, it is close enough that

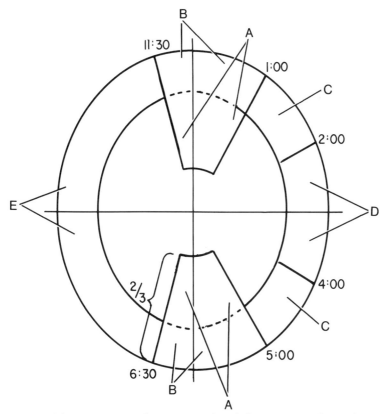

Figure 5.9. Theoretic map of optic nerve head showing correlation between defect of nerve head and visual field loss.[106] **A:** Central "Bjerrum's rhomboid," corresponding to proximal arcuate scotoma. **B:** Peripheral "Bjerrum's rhomboid," corresponding to distal arcuate scotoma. **C:** Inferior and superior temporal rims, corresponding to peripheral nasal constriction. **D:** Temporal rim, corresponding to central island. **E:** Nasal rim, corresponding to temporal island. (Modified from Read and Spaeth[106]).

failure to establish a correlation should prompt a search for other underlying disease processes, such as neurological disorders. Nevertheless, the absence of a perfect correlation indicates that both disc and field examinations are essential in managing the glaucoma patient.[109] Optic nerve head changes possibly have their greatest value in the early stages of glaucoma, while progressive visual field loss becomes the more useful guide to therapy in advanced cases.[103]

V. OTHER VISUAL DISTURBANCES IN GLAUCOMA

A. Color Vision

Reduced sensitivity to colors has been described in various forms of glaucoma,[110–112] although reports differ regarding the nature of the color vision disturbance, and the diagnostic value of this test for glaucoma has yet to be established.

B. Flickering Stimuli

The *frequency* at which the flickering of a light is first detected (flicker fusion frequency) is reported to be below normal in glaucomatous eyes.[2] In addition, glaucoma patients were found to have reduced sensitivity for *contrast* between light and dark stimuli when presented as a diffuse flickering field or a counterphase flickering grating.[113]

C. Sinusoidal Gratings

The ability to recognize the presence of light and dark bands in a sinusoidal grating can be used as a subtle test of central visual acuity.[114] Impaired detection has been reported in patients with glaucoma[114, 115] and in some individuals with elevated intraocular pressure but no detectable optic nerve head or visual field change.[114] However, another study showed that age significantly influenced the test scores and that there was no significant difference between age-matched normals and glaucoma patients.[116]

D. Dark Adaptation

Dark adaptation, tested with chromatic stimuli, has been reported to be abnormal in individuals with elevated intraocular pressures but normal optic nerve heads and visual fields.[117]

E. Dichoptic Testing

Dichoptic testing involves the presentation of one-half of a test object to one eye and the other half to the fellow eye as an aid in determining the location of a defect in the visual pathway. Preliminary tests in open-angle glaucoma patients indicate abnormal responses.[118]

F. Visual Evoked Responses

Visual evoked responses may also be abnormal in patients with glaucoma, and were discussed earlier in this chapter.

References

1. Scott, GI: Traquair's Clinical Perimetry, 7th ed. CV Mosby Co, St Louis, 1957, p 1.
2. Harrington, DO: The Visual Fields. A Textbook and Atlas of Clinical Perimetry, 3rd ed. CV Mosby Co, St Louis, 1971, pp 25, 100.
3. Armaly, MF: The size and location of the normal blind spot. Arch Ophthal 81:192, 1969.
4. Reed, H, Drance, SM: The Essentials of Perimetry Static and Kinetic, 2nd ed. Oxford University Press, London, 1972, p 66.
5. Tate, GW, Jr, Lynn, JR: Principles of Quantitative Perimetry: Testing and Interpreting the Visual Field. Grune & Stratton, New York, 1977.
6. Chamlin, M: Methodology and techniques in visual field studies. Surv Ophthal 13:97, 1968.
7. Portney, GL, Rubenzer, MA: Comparisons of glaucomatous visual fields using the black tangent screen and the Goldmann perimeter. Surv Ophthal 17:164, 1972.
8. Goldmann, VH: Ein selbstregistrierendes Projektionskugelperimeter. Ophthalmologica 109:71, 1945.

9. Portney, GL, Hanible, JE: A comparison of four projection perimeters. Am J Ophthal 81:678, 1976.
10. Harms, H: Entwicklungsmöglichkeiten der Perimetrie. Albrecht von Graefes Arch fur Ophthalmol 150:28, 1950.
11. Harms, H, Aulhorn, E: Vergleichends Untersuchungen über den Wert der quantitativen Perimetrie, Skiaskotometrie und Verschmelzungsfrequenz für die Erkennung beginnender Gesichtsfeldstörungen beim Glaukom. Doc Ophthal 13:303, 1959.
12. Johnson, CA, Keltner, JL, Balestrery, FG: Acuity profile perimetry. Description of technique and preliminary clinical trials. Arch Ophthal 97:684, 1979.
13. Portney, GL, Krohn, MA: The limitations of kinetic perimetry in early scotoma detection. Ophthalmology 85:287, 1978.
14. Donovan, HC, Weale, RA, Wheeler, C: The perimeter as a monitor of glaucomatous changes. Br J Ophthal 62:705, 1978.
15. Armaly, MF: Ocular pressure and visual fields. A ten-year follow-up study. Arch Ophthal 81:25, 1969.
16. Rock, WJ, Drance, SM, Morgan, RW: A modification of the Armaly visual field screening technique for glaucoma. Can J Ophthal 6:283, 1971.
17. Drance, SM, Brais, P, Fairclough, M, Bryett, J: A screening method for temporal visual defects in chronic simple glaucoma. Can J Ophthal 7:428, 1972.
18. Rock, WJ, Drance, SM, Morgan, RW: Visual field screening in glaucoma. An evaluation of the Armaly technique for screening glaucomatous visual fields. Arch Ophthal 89:287, 1973.
19. Trobe, JD, Acosta, PC: An algorithm for visual fields. Surv Ophthal 24:665, 1980.
20. Goldmann, VH: Grundlagen exakter Perimetrie. Ophthalmologica 109:57, 1945.
21. Lynn, JR: Examination of the visual field in glaucoma. Invest Ophthal 8:76, 1969.
22. Crick, RP, Crick, JCP: Sine bell stimulus perimeter. Glaucoma 2:393, 1980.
23. Bigger, JF, Becker, B: Cataracts and open-angle glaucoma. Am J Ophthal 7:335, 1971.
24. Radius, RL: Perimetry in cataract patients. Arch Ophthal 96:1574, 1978.
25. Krohn, DL, Breitfeller, JM, Shen, YT: Peripheral fields in aphakic glaucoma: soft contact lens versus spectacle correction. Glaucoma 2:514, 1980.
26. Drance, SM, Berry, V, Hughes, A: Studies in the reproducibility of visual field areas in normal and glaucomatous subjects. Can J Ophthal I:14, 1966.
27. Pinkerton, RMH: The Bjerrum area in ocular hypertension. Invest Ophthal 8:91, 1969.
28. Trobe, JD, Acosta, PC, Shuster, JJ, Krischer, JP: An evaluation of the accuracy of community-based perimetry. Am J Ophthal 90:654, 1980.
29. Harrington, DO, Flocks, M: Multiple pattern method of visual field examination. JAMA 157:645, 1955.
30. Roberts, W: The multiple-pattern tachystoscopic visual field screener in glaucoma. Arch Ophthal 58:244, 1957.
31. Friedman, A: The assessment of the efficacy of glaucoma control by static perimetry, or 'point' analysis of clinical visual thresholds. Trans Ophthal Soc UK 82:381, 1962.
32. Friedmann, AI: Serial analysis of changes in visual field defects, employing a new instrument, to determine the activity of diseases involving the visual pathways. Ophthalmologica 152:1, 1966.
33. Greve, EL, Verduin, WM: Mass visual field investigation in 1834 persons with supposedly normal eyes. Albrecht Graefes Arch Klin Exp Ophthal 183:286, 1972.
34. Boles Carenini, B, Liuzzi, L, Cembrano, S, Musso, M: Friedmann visual field analyzer: efficacy in the screening of glaucomatous visual field defects. Glaucoma 2:488, 1980.
35. Flocks, M, Rosenthal, AR, Hopkins, JL: Mass visual screening via television. Ophthalmology 85:1141, 1978.

36. Keltner, JL, Johnson, CA, Balestrery, FG: Suprathreshold static perimetry. Initial clinical trials with the fieldmaster automated perimeter. Arch Ophthal 97:260, 1979.
37. Johnson, CA, Keltner, JL, Balestrery, FG: Suprathreshold static perimetry n in glaucoma and other optic nerve disease. Ophthalmology 86:1278, 1979.
38. Johnson, CA, Keltner, JL: Automated suprathreshold static perimetry. Am J Ophthal 89:731, 1980.
39. Dannheim, F: Clinical experiences with a semi-automated perimeter. Int Ophthal 2:11, 1980.
40. Heijl, A: Automatic perimetry in glaucoma visual field screening. A clinical study. Graefes Archiv Ophthalmologie 200:21, 1976.
41. Heijl, A, Drance, SM, Douglas, GR: Automatic perimetry (COMPETER). Ability to detect early glaucomatous field defects. Arch Ophthal 98:1560, 1980.
42. Heijl, A, Drance, SM: Computerized profile perimetry in glaucoma. Arch Ophthal 98:2199, 1980.
43. Li, SG, Spaeth, GL, Scimeca, HA, Schatz, NJ, Savino, PJ: Clinical experiences with the use of an automated perimeter (Octopus) in the diagnosis and management of patients with glaucoma and neurologic diseases. Ophthalmology 86:1302, 1979.
44. Holmin, C, Krakau, CET: Computerized meridian perimetry. A preliminary report. Acta Ophthal 58:33, 1980.
45. Fankhauser, F, Spahr, J, Bebie, H: Some aspects of the automation of perimetry. Surv Ophthal 22:131, 1977.
46. Portney, GL, Krohn, MA: Automated perimetry: background, instruments and methods. Surv Ophthal 22:271, 1978.
47. Cappin, JM, Nissim, S: Visual evoked responses in the assessment of field defects in glaucoma. Arch Ophthal 93:9, 1975.
48. Huber, C, Wagner, T: Electrophysiological evidence for glaucomatous lesions in the optic nerve. Ophthal Res 10:22, 1978.
49. Levy, NS, Korhnak, L: The monocularly elicited visual evoked response in chronic glaucoma. Ann Ophthal 10:551, 1978.
50. Neetens, A: Predictability of impending functional damage after IOP rise. Glaucoma 2:477, 1980.
51. Kelley, JS, Hoover, RE, Robin, A, Kincaid, M: Laser scotometry in drusen and pits of the optic nerve head. Ophthalmology 86:442, 1979.
52. Esterman, B: Grid for scoring visual fields. I. Tangent screen. Arch Ophthal 77:780, 1967.
53. Esterman, B: Grid for scoring visual fields. II. Perimeter. Arch Ophthal 79:400, 1968.
54. Wirtschafter, JD, Prater, BN: A simplified stimulus value notation using preferred stimulus combinations for Goldmann quantitative perimetry. Surv Ophthal 23:177, 1978.
55. Trost, DC, Woolson, RF, Hayreh, SS: Quantification of visual fields for statistical analysis. Arch Ophthal 97:2175, 1979.
56. Drasdo, N, Peaston, WC: Sampling systems for visual field assessment and computerised perimetry. Br J Ophthal 64:705, 1980.
57. Vrabec, FR: The temporal raphe of the human retina. Am J Ophthal 62:926, 1966.
58. Minckler, DS: The organization of nerve fiber bundles in the primate optic nerve head. Arch Ophthal 98:1630, 1980.
59. Hoyt, WF, Luis, O: Visual fiber anatomy in the infrageniculate pathway of the primate. Arch Ophthal 68:94, 1962.
60. Hart, WM, Yablonski, M, Kass, MA, Becker, B: Quantitative visual field and optic disc correlates early in glaucoma. Arch Ophthal 96:2209, 1978.
61. Armaly, MF: The visual field defect and ocular pressure level in open angle glaucoma. Invest Ophthal 8:105, 1969.
62. Drance, SM: The early field defects in glaucoma. Invest Ophthal 8:84, 1969.
63. Colenbrander, MC: The early diagnosis of glaucoma. Ophthalmologica 162:276, 1971.

64. Werner, EB, Drance, SM: Early visual field disturbances in glaucoma. Arch Ophthal 95:1173, 1977.
65. Harrington, DO: The Bjerrum scotoma. Trans Am Ophthal Soc 62:324, 1964.
66. Harrington, DO: The Bjerrum scotoma. Am J Ophthal 59:646, 1965.
67. Drance, SM: The visual field of low tension glaucoma and shock-induced optic neuropathy. Arch Ophthal 95:1359, 1977.
68. Drance, SM: The glaucomatous visual field. Br J Ophthal 56:186, 1972.
69. Drance, SM: The glaucomatous visual field. Invest Ophthal 11:85, 1972.
70. Harrington, DO: Differential diagnosis of the arcuate scotoma. Invest Ophthal 8:96, 1969.
71. Martin, WG, Brown, GC, Parrish, RK, Kimball, R, Naidoff, MA, Benson, WE: Ocular toxoplasmosis and visual field defects. Am J Ophthal 90:25, 1980.
72. Trobe, JD, Bergsma, DR: Atypical retinitis pigmentosa masquerading as a nerve fiber bundle lesion. Am J Ophthal 79:681, 1975.
73. Savino, PJ, Glaser, JS, Rosenberg, MA: A clinical analysis of pseudopapilledema. II. Visual field defects. Arch Ophthal 97:71, 1979.
74. Trobe, JD, Watson, RT: Retinal degeneration without pigment alterations in progressive external ophthalmoplegia. Am J Ophthal 83:372, 1977.
75. LeBlanc, RP, Becker, B: Peripheral nasal field defects. Am J Ophthal 72:415, 1971.
76. Werner, EB, Beraskow, J: Peripheral nasal field defects in glaucoma. Ophthalmology 86:1875, 1979.
77. Armaly, MF: Visual field defects in early open angle glaucoma. Trans Am Ophthal Soc 69:147, 1971.
78. Armaly, MF: Selective perimetry for glaucomatous defects in ocular hypertension. Arch Ophthal 87:518, 1972.
79. Lynn, JR: Correlation of pathogenesis, anatomy, and patterns of visual loss in glaucoma. *In* Symposium on Glaucoma. CV Mosby Co, St Louis, 1975, p 151.
80. Damgaard-Jensen, L: Vertical steps in isopters at the hemiopic border—in normal and glaucomatous eyes. Acta Ophthalmologica 55:111, 1977.
81. Damgaard-Jensen, L: Demonstration of peripheral hemiopic border steps by static perimetry. Acta Ophthalmologica 55:815, 1977.
82. Trobe, , JD: Chromophobe adenoma presenting with a hemianopic temporal arcuate scotoma. Am J Ophthal 77:388, 1974.
83. Brais, P, Drance, SM: The temporal field in chronic simple glaucoma. Arch Ophthal 88:518, 1976.
84. Phelps, CD: Perimetry. Ann Ophthal 10:1527, 1978.
85. Chandler, PA, Grant, WM: Glaucoma, 2nd ed. Lea & Febiger, Philadelphia, 1979, pp 98–99.
86. Lichter, RR, Ravin, JG: Risks of sudden visual loss after glaucoma surgery. Am J Ophthal 78:1009, 1974.
87. Radius, RL, Maumenee, AE: Visual field changes following acute elevation of intraocular pressure. Trans Am Acad Ophthal Otol 83:61, 1977.
88. McNaught, EI, Rennie, A, McClure, E, Chisholm, IA: Pattern of visual damage after acute angle-closure glaucoma. Trans Ophthal Soc UK 94:406, 1974.
89. Drance, SM: Studies in the susceptibility of the eye to raised intraocular pressure. Arch Ophthal 68:478, 1962.
90. Tsamparlakis, JC: Effects of transient induced elevation of the intraocular pressure on the visual field. Br J Ophthal 48:237, 1964.
91. Scott, AB, Morris, A: Visual field changes produced by artificially elevated intraocular pressure. Am J Ophthal 63:308, 1967.
92. Armaly, MF: Effect of corticosteroids on intraocular pressure and fluid dynamics. III. Changes in visual function and pupil size during topical dexamethasone application. Arch Ophthal 71:636, 1964.
93. Kolker, AE, Becker, B, Mills, DW: Intraocular pressure and visual fields: effects of corticosteroids. Arch Ophthal 72:772, 1964.
94. Nordmann, J, Lobstein, A, Gerhard, JP, Benck, P: Le test a la cortisone dans le glaucome simple a champ visuel normal. Ophthalmologica 150:46, 1965.
95. LeBlance, RP, Stewart, RH, Becker, B: Corticosteroid provocative testing. Invest

Ophthal 9:946, 1970.

96. Hart, WM Jr, Becker, B: Visual field changes in ocular hypertension. A computer-based analysis. Arch Ophthal 95:1176, 1977.

97. Heilmann, K: On the reversibility of visual field defects in glaucomas. Trans Am Acad Ophthal Otol 78:304, 1974.

98. Aulhorn, E, Harms, H: Papillenveränderung und Gesichtsfeldstörung beim Glaukom. Ophthalmologica 139:279, 1960.

99. Shutt, HKR, Boyd, TAS, Salter, AB: The relationship of visual fields, optic disc appearances and age in non-glaucomatous and glaucomatous eyes. Can J Ophthal 2:83, 1967.

100. Drance, SM: Correlation between optic disc changes and visual field defects in chronic open-angle glaucoma. Trans Am Acad Ophthal Otol 81:224, 1976.

101. Hoskins, HD Jr, Gelber, EC: Optic disk topography and visual field defects in patients with increased intraocular pressure. Am J Ophthal 8:284, 1975.

102. Hitchings, RA, Spaeth, GL: The optic disc in glaucoma, II: correlation of the appearance of the optic disc with the visual field. Br J Ophthal 61:107, 1977.

103. Drance, SM: The disc and the field in glaucoma. Ophthalmology 85:209, 1978.

104. Gloster, J: Quantitative relationship between cupping of the optic disc and visual field loss in chronic simple glaucoma. Br J Ophthal 62: 665, 1978.

105. Bengtsson, B, Holmin, C, Krakau, CET: Characteristics of manifest glaucoma in the early stages. Glaucoma 2:351, 1980.

106. Read, RM, Spaeth, GL: The practical clinical appraisal of the optic disc in glaucoma: the natural history of cup progression and some specific disc-field correlations. Trans Am Acad Ophthal Otol 78:255, 1974.

107. Sommer, A, Miller, NR, Pollack, I, Maumenee, AE, George, T: The nerve fiber layer in the diagnosis of glaucoma. Arch Ophthal 95:2149, 1977.

108. Sommer, A, Pollack, I, Manmenee, AE: Optic disc parameters and onset of glaucomatous field loss. II. Static screening criteria. Arch Ophthal 97:1449, 1979.

109. Armaly, MF: The correlation between appearance of the optic cup and visual function. Trans Am Acad Ophthal Otol 73:898, 1969.

110. Osiecka-Pilecka, H, Jaworowska, H, Wojcicka-Mazurowska, L: The examination of colour thresholds of central vision in glaucoma. Klinika Oczna 36:355, 1966.

111. Zimmermann, U: Disturbances of colour sense during glaucoma. Klin Monatsbl Augenheilkd 148:845, 1966.

112. Koliopoulos, JX: Acquired color vision deficiency in open-angle glaucoma. Glaucoma 1:155, 1979.

113. Atkin, A, Bodis-Wollner, I, Wolkstein, M, Moss, A, Podos, SM: Abnormalities of central contrast sensitivity in glaucoma. Am J Ophthal 88:205, 1979.

114. Arden, GB, Jacobson, JJ: A simple grating test for contrast sensitivity: preliminary results indicate value in screening for glaucoma. Invest Ophthal Vis Sci 17:23, 1978.

115. Wolkstein, M, Atkin, A, Bodis-Wollner, I: Contrast sensitivity in retinal disease. Ophthalmology 87:1140, 1980.

116. Sokol, S, Domar, A, Moskowitz, A: Utility of the Arden grating test in glaucoma screening: high false-positive rate in normals over 50 years of age. Invest Ophthal Vis Sci 19:1529, 1980.

117. Goldthwaite, D, Lakowski, R, Drance, SM: A study of dark adaptation in ocular hypertensives. Can J Ophthal 11:55, 1976.

118. Enoch, JM: Quantitative layer-by-layer perimetry. Invest Ophthal Vis Sci 17:208, 1978.

Section Two

Clinical Forms of Glaucoma

Chapter 6

A CLASSIFICATION OF THE GLAUCOMAS

In Section One, we considered the common parameters shared by the many forms of glaucoma, which include the intraocular pressure and the influence of elevated pressure on the optic nerve head and visual field. In the present section, we will look at the specific clinical and histopathologic features that characterize the individual glaucomas. With possible rare exceptions, all of these conditions have *increased resistance to aqueous outflow*, which leads to the intraocular pressure elevation. However, the glaucomas differ according to the mechanism responsible for the increased resistance. Most classification schemes are based on the underlying cause of the altered resistance to aqueous outflow, as well as the clinical appearance of the anterior chamber angle. The nucleus of these classification systems is the concept of primary vs. secondary glaucoma and the presence of an open or closed anterior chamber angle.

I. PRIMARY VS. SECONDARY GLAUCOMA

The concept of "primary" and "secondary" glaucoma that will be used in this study guide relates to the mechanism responsible for the increased resistance to aqueous outflow.

A. Primary Glaucomas

These forms of glaucoma are not consistently associated with obvious systemic or other ocular disorders that might account for the alteration in the resistance to aqueous outflow. They are typically bilateral and are generally believed to have a genetic basis.

B. Secondary Glaucomas

These conditions are characterized by associated ocular or systemic abnormalities that appear to be responsible for the alteration in resistance to aqueous outflow. They may be either unilateral or bilateral and inherited or acquired.

C. Developmental Glaucomas

A third group of glaucomas, that are occasionally distinguished from the primary and secondary categories, are those in which a

developmental abnormality of the anterior chamber angle is responsible for the increased resistance to aqueous outflow. One of these
conditions is classified as *primary congenital glaucoma*, because
systemic or other ocular abnormalities are not consistently present.
The remainder of the *developmental glaucomas* have *associated
anomalies*, but these additional abnormalities are not always responsible for the obstruction to aqueous outflow.

II. OPEN-ANGLE VS. ANGLE-CLOSURE GLAUCOMA

In 1938, Barkan[1] classified glaucoma into two major anatomic
categories on the basis of the gonioscopic appearance of the anterior
chamber angle. He called the two groups "deep-chamber and shallow-
chamber types of glaucoma." Today these are generally referred to
as *open-angle* and *angle-closure* glaucomas, respectively.

A. Open-angle Glaucoma

As the name implies, this occurs in eyes with a deep anterior
chamber and an open anterior chamber angle (Fig. 6.1). The mechanism of increased resistance to aqueous outflow in these cases is a
direct alteration in the structures involved with aqueous drainage.

1. *Primary open-angle glaucoma.* In this condition, the actual alteration responsible for the increased resistance to aqueous outflow is
uncertain, but the many theories are reviewed in Chapter 7.

2. *Secondary open-angle glaucomas.* Among these disorders, several mechanisms of outflow obstruction may be seen (Fig. 6.2).

   a. *Pre-trabecular.* In some cases, aqueous outflow may be prevented by various types of *membranes* across the inner surface of the
trabecular meshwork in an otherwise open anterior chamber angle.

   b. *Trabecular.* In other situations, the obstruction to aqueous
outflow results from alterations within the trabecular meshwork,
either by the *accumulation of material*, such as cells, pigment granules, fibrin, etc., or by *structural alterations* in the trabeculae, such as
edema or fibrosis.

   c. *Post-trabecular.* Still other conditions are due to aqueous
outflow obstruction distal to the trabecular meshwork, either in
Schlemm's canal, the scleral outlet channels, or the episcleral veins.

B. Angle-closure Glaucoma

In these forms of glaucoma, the anterior chamber is shallow and
aqueous outflow is blocked by the root of the iris, which lies in
apposition to the trabecular meshwork (Fig. 6.1). The aqueous drainage system may be otherwise normal, although concomitant damage
to these structures may also be present.

1. *Primary angle-closure glaucoma.* In this disorder, the factors
which lead to closure of the anterior chamber angle are only partially
understood and are considered in Chapter 8.

2. *Secondary angle-closure glaucomas.* Among these forms of glaucoma, a number of conditions have been recognized, which may

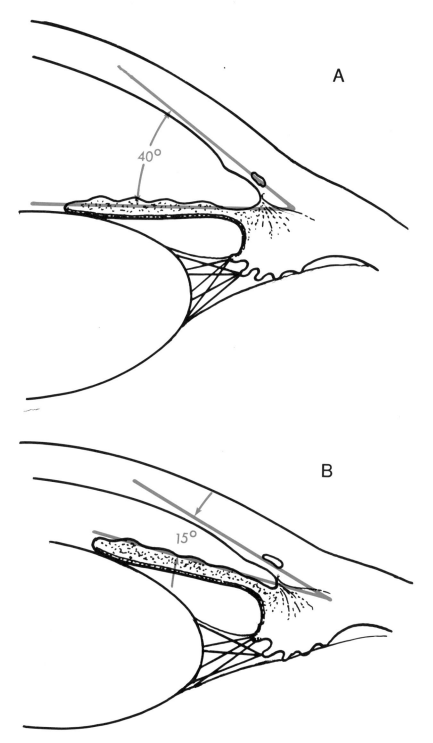

Figure 6.1. The angle of the anterior chamber (red lines) is formed by the cornea and iris: **A:** the typical configuration in open-angle forms of glaucoma; **B:** the narrow angle that typically precedes most forms of angle-closure glaucoma.

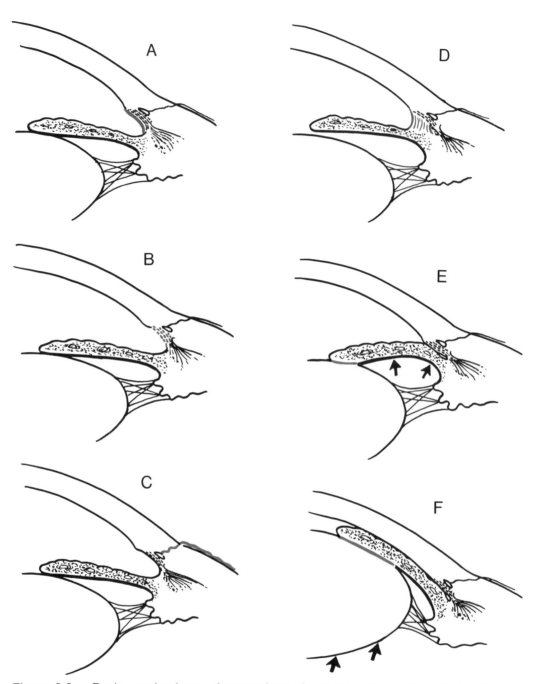

Figure 6.2. Basic mechanisms of secondary glaucomas (the site of obstruction to aqueous outflow is shown in red). Open-angle forms of secondary glaucoma may be of the pre-trabecular (**A**), trabecular (**B**), or post-trabecular type (**C**). Angle-closure forms of secondary glaucoma may be of the anterior ''pulling'' type (**D**) or of the posterior ''pushing'' type. The latter may occur with (**E**) or without (**F**) pupillary block (arrows indicate location of force pushing iris or lens-iris diaphragm forward).

either pull or push the peripheral iris into the anterior chamber angle (Fig. 6.2).

a. *Angle "pulled" closed.* In some cases, the peripheral iris is pulled into apposition with the trabecular meshwork by the *contracture* of structures in the anterior chamber angle, such as membranes or inflammatory precipitates.

b. *Angle "pushed" closed.* In other circumstances, the iris is pushed into the anterior chamber angle by *increased pressure behind the iris.* This may result directly from a forward shift of the lens-iris diaphragm due to space occupying changes such as a tumor, hemorrhage, ciliary body congestion, or choroidal detachment. In other cases, the peripheral iris may bow forward due to increased resistance to flow from the posterior to the anterior chamber, which is referred to as *pupillary block.* The latter condition may result from a slight forward shift in the lens-iris diaphragm or from synechiae between the iris and lens.

III. CLASSIFICATION SYSTEM

The classification scheme used in this study guide is based on the aforementioned concepts of primary, secondary, and developmental glaucoma. While the open-angle and angle-closure aspects are useful in classifying the primary glaucomas, they are of less value with regard to the secondary glaucomas, since many of these may involve more than one mechanism of outflow obstruction, depending on the stage of the disease. For example, neovascular glaucoma may have intraocular pressure elevation due to a fibrovascular membrane across the open anterior chamber angle in the early stages, while contracture of the membrane may lead to closure of the angle late in the disease process. For this reason, a classification based on the underlying condition which leads to aqueous outflow obstruction will be used for the secondary glaucomas.

A. Primary Glaucomas

1. Primary open-angle glaucoma.
2. Primary angle-closure glaucoma.

B. Developmental glaucomas

1. Primary congenital glaucoma.
2. Developmental glaucomas with associated anomalies

C. Secondary glaucomas

1. Glaucomas associated with intraocular tumors.
2. Glaucomas associated with primary disorders of the corneal endothelium.
3. Pigmentary glaucoma.
4. Glaucomas associated with disorders of the lens.
5. Glaucomas associated with retinal disorders.

6. Glaucomas associated with ocular inflammation.
7. Glaucomas associated with intraocular hemorrhage.
8. Glaucomas associated with ocular trauma.
9. Glaucomas following ocular surgery.
10. Steroid-induced glaucoma.
11. Glaucomas associated with elevated episcleral venous pressure.

References

1. Barkan, O: Glaucoma: Classification, causes, and surgical control. Results of microgonioscopic research. Am J Ophthal 21:1099, 1938.

Chapter 7

PRIMARY OPEN-ANGLE GLAUCOMA

PRIMARY OPEN-ANGLE GLAUCOMA

I. TERMINOLOGY

As previously discussed, it is not possible to define any form of glaucoma strictly on the basis of intraocular pressure. The concept that two standard deviations above the mean represents the upper limit of "normal" intraocular pressure is invalid due to the non-Gaussian distribution of pressures in the general population. The commonly used figure of 21 mmHg, therefore, should be thought of as only a rough approximation when used in definitions of glaucoma. Many eyes do not develop glaucomatous damage of the optic nerve head or visual field, at least not for long periods of time, despite intraocular pressures well above 21 mmHg, while others undergo characteristic disc and field changes at pressures even in the teens. For this reason, the following terms will be found in the literature:

A. Primary Open-angle Glaucoma

There is general agreement that this disorder, in its *typical* form, is defined by the following three criteria:

1. An intraocular pressure consistently above 21 mmHg in at least one eye.

2. An open, normal appearing anterior chamber angle with no apparent ocular or systemic abnormality that might account for the elevated intraocular pressure.

3. Typical glaucomatous visual field and/or optic nerve head damage, as described in Chapters 5 and 4, respectively.

Synonymous terms that also appear in the literature include "open-angle glaucoma," "chronic open-angle glaucoma," "chronic simple glaucoma," and "open-angle glaucoma with damage."

B. Ocular Hypertension

There is considerably less agreement regarding the patient who has the first two criteria noted above, *i.e.*, an elevated pressure for which there is no apparent cause, but who has normal optic nerve heads and visual fields.[1-4] The problem is that there are no absolute indicators as to when or if an individual with elevated pressures will develop glaucomatous disc or field damage.

Many physicians refer to this condition as "ocular hypertension,"[2,4] although others point out disadvantages of the term. Some feel it does not connote the potential seriousness of the situation and may lead to a false sense of security on the part of both patient and physician. Furthermore, it is hard to know whether the terminology should arbitrarily be changed to "glaucoma" when the intraocular pressure reaches a level at which treatment for pressure alone is felt to be indicated.

Chandler and Grant[1] prefer the term *"early open-angle glaucoma without damage"* for this condition, while Shaffer[3] suggests *"glaucoma suspect."* The latter term usually encompasses additional risk factors for glaucoma, including suspicious optic nerve heads and narrow anterior chamber angles.

Whatever term one chooses to use for this condition, the most important point is that both physician and patient must be fully aware of its potential consequences. Later in this chapter, we will consider the management of such patients.

C. Low-tension Glaucoma

At the other end of the spectrum from ocular hypertension is a small group of patients who have typical glaucomatous damage of the visual fields and/or optic nerve heads, but intraocular pressures consistently 21 mmHg or less.[5-9] This may be a variation of primary open-angle glaucoma,[5-7] although some feel the mechanism of optic atrophy in the two conditions is not the same.[8] At any rate, the predominant feature in populations of low-tension glaucoma patients is *cardiovascular abnormalities* (discussed later in this chapter) which could lead to an imbalance between the intraocular pressure and perfusion pressure of the optic nerve head. Hayreh[10] suggests that low-tension glaucoma differs from *anterior ischemic optic neuropathy* only in that the latter is a more acute process.

Drance and co-workers[6,7] describe *two forms* of low-tension glaucoma:

1. A *nonprogressive* form is usually associated with a transient episode of vascular shock.

2. A *progressive* form is believed to result from chronic vascular insufficiency of the optic nerve head.

It is important in the differential diagnosis of low-tension glaucoma to determine whether the intraocular pressure is consistently low around the clock and to rule out non-glaucomatous causes of disc and field changes as discussed in Chapters 4 and 5. The treatment of this form of glaucoma is typically difficult and will be considered separately at the end of this chapter.

II. EPIDEMIOLOGY

A. Frequency Among the Glaucomas

Although primary open-angle glaucoma is clearly the *most common* single form of glaucoma, it is difficult to precisely establish the ratio of individuals with this disorder to the total number of patients with all forms of glaucoma. In one survey of 4231 individuals between the ages of 40 and 75 years, 39 glaucoma patients were detected, of whom 13 (*i.e.*, one-third of the glaucoma population or 0.28% of the general population) had primary open-angle glaucoma.[11] This figure, however, may differ considerably from one population to the next.

B. Prevalence Within General Populations

Several large surveys have been conducted to determine the number of patients with ocular hypertension and primary open-angle glaucoma (or glaucoma in general) within a population at a given time.[11-14] The prevalence of glaucoma is less than 1% in most studies. However, reports vary considerably, which probably reflects differences in diagnostic criteria, screening techniques, and characteristics of the particular population. Nevertheless, most surveys show that the prevalence of ocular hypertension is considerably higher than that of glaucoma, even when all forms of glaucoma are included, which some investigators take as evidence that elevated intraocular pressure does not invariably lead to glaucoma.[15]

C. Incidence of Primary Open-Angle Glaucoma Among Ocular Hypertensives

Numerous studies have been conducted to determine the rate of occurrence of primary open-angle glaucoma within populations of untreated ocular hypertensives (Table 7.1).[16-23] Most studies span an observation period of 5 to 10 years, during which time the incidence of patients developing field loss was roughly 1% per year. However, there are large differences in the results of these studies, which suggest variable degrees of susceptibility among populations of ocular hypertensives. It should also be kept in mind that "normotensive" individuals may develop glaucoma. In some cases this may represent low-tension glaucoma, while other patients may initially have intraocular pressures below 21 mmHg, but later have a rise in pressure and develop primary open-angle glaucoma.[24, 25]

D. Natural History of Field Loss in Primary Open-Angle Glaucoma.

Leydhecker[26] noted in a large population study that the prevalence of field loss was the same as the prevalence of ocular hypertension in a population 20 years younger. From this he concluded that approximately 20 years elapse between the onset of pressure elevation and

Table 7.1
Incidence of Primary Open-angle Glaucoma Among Ocular Hypertensives

Investigator(s)	No. Ocular Hypertensives (Patients)	Observation Period (Years)	No. Developed Open-Angle Glaucoma (Patients)
Perkins[16]	124	5–7	4 (3.2%)
Walker[17]	109	11	11 (11%)
Wilensky et al[18]	50	Avg. 6	3 (6%)
Norskov[19]	68	5	0
Linner[20]	92	10	0
Kitazawa et al[21]	75	Avg. 9.5	7 (9.3%)
David et al[22]	61	Avg. 3.3 Range 1–11	10 (16.4%)
Hart et al[23]	92	5	33 (35%)

field loss. This concept may be subject to considerable error, however, since the study did not show that the same individuals with elevated pressures were the ones who subsequently developed field loss. Lichter and Shaffer[27] found that field loss in a population of 378 ocular hypertensives, observed for a period averaging 12¾ years, occurred earlier than Leydhecker suggested, despite the fact that most were being treated during this time. Furthermore, once field loss has occurred, further damage tends to progress more rapidly than in the fellow undamaged eye exposed to the same intraocular pressure,[28] which simply reflects the increased susceptibility of the damaged eye.

III. RISK FACTORS

The preceding discussion underscores the problem in recognizing early primary open-angle glaucoma before optic nerve head or visual field damage has become apparent. For this reason, the clinician must be familiar with other features, or risk factors, that are commonly associated with the disease, in order to identify those cases that require closer observation or the initiation of therapy. The relative prognostic significance of these risk factors will be considered later in this chapter.

A. General Features of Patients

The first set of risk factors to consider are the following general features of patients with primary open-angle glaucoma:

1. *Age*. All studies agree that the prevalence of primary open-angle glaucoma increases with the age of the population being considered. For example, in one general population survey of 3000 individuals, the prevalence of primary open-angle glaucoma and low-tension glaucoma by age group was 0.22% among 40 to 49 year olds, 0.10% for 50 to 59, 0.57% for 60 to 69, 2.81% for 70 to 79, and 14.29% for patients 80+ years of age.[29] Age, therefore, becomes an increasingly significant risk factor with each decade.

It is important to emphasize, however, that primary open-angle glaucoma is by no means limited to those over 40 years of age. In one study, 25% of glaucoma patients 10 to 35 years old had this form of glaucoma.[30] Another study of 13 primary open-angle glaucoma patients under 40 years of age, four of whom were in their teens, emphasized the unusual severity of the disease in younger patients and stressed the need for applanation tonometry in all individuals old enough to permit the study.[31]

2. *Race*. Several studies have shown that primary open-angle glaucoma is more prevalent, develops at an earlier age, and is more severe in *blacks* as compared to whites.[32-36] In one large population survey, the prevalence of the disease was approximately 1.4% in Jamaicans.[35] Furthermore, non-whites are said to have seven to eight times more blindness from glaucoma than whites.[36] In another study, 25 black and 47 white ocular hypertensives were followed 1 to 12 years, during which time glaucomatous damage developed in 18.1% of the former

and 5.4% of the latter group.[34] A possible explanation for this racial difference might be that the high incidence of sickle cell anemia among blacks increases the potential for optic nerve head ischemia. However, this theory was not supported by a study that found sickle trait in only 2 of 40 blacks undergoing filtering surgery for primary open-angle glaucoma.[37]

3. *Sex*. The prognostic significance of sex is less clear than that of age and race, although some studies suggest a higher prevalence among men.[12, 13, 38]

4. *Related systemic diseases*.

a. *Diabetes mellitus*. The prevalence of primary open-angle glaucoma and ocular hypertension is several times higher in the diabetic population than in the general population according to most surveys.[39, 40] In addition, the prevalence of diabetes or a positive glucose tolerance test is higher in patients with primary open-angle glaucoma[40, 41] or a high intraocular pressure response to topical steroids.[40, 42]

b. *Thyroid disorders*. One study suggested that primary open-angle glaucoma patients have an increased prevalence of various thyroid disturbances,[43] while another investigation revealed low normal protein bound iodine and radioactive iodine uptake.[44] However, baseline thyroxine, thyrotropin (TSH), and triiodothyronine (T_3) resin uptake levels in patients with primary open-angle glaucoma did not differ from normal values.[45]

c. *Other endocrine disorders* have not been associated with primary open-angle glaucoma, but may influence the intraocular pressure and, therefore, should be considered in the diagnosis and management of glaucoma. For example, elevated intraocular pressure has occurred in patients with Cushing's syndrome, with normalization of pressure after treatment of the systemic disease.[46, 47] One study showed that relatives of such patients were often positive topical steroid responders (discussed later in this chapter) and suggested this as the mechanism of the pressure rise.[47] Pituitary dysfunction may be associated with instability of intraocular pressure[48] and aqueous humor dynamics,[49] and elevated estrogen or progesterone may lower the intraocular pressure,[50] while male hormones may raise it.[51]

d. *Cardiovascular abnormalities*, as noted earlier in this chapter, are common features in populations with *low-tension glaucoma*. Reported associated findings include hemodynamic crises[5–7] and hypercoagulability (*e.g.*, increased platelet adhesiveness and euglobulin lysis time[5, 6]), although another study revealed no statistically significant hypercoagulability in low-tension glaucoma.[52] Reports of alterations in systemic blood pressure are also conflicting.[5, 6, 8, 53] Hypercholesterolemia is reported to be higher in low-tension glaucoma.[54]

There are also conflicting reports regarding systemic blood pressure in patients with *primary open-angle glaucoma*. Some studies revealed no significant deviation from the general population[55–57] while at least one investigation showed a significant increase in systemic blood pressure.[53] An increased incidence of acute blood loss has also been reported in patients with primary open-angle glaucoma,[55] and a preliminary study suggested an association between open-angle glaucoma in Caucasians and the rhesus D(+) blood group.[58]

5. *Family history*. Primary open-angle glaucoma is generally believed to have a *genetic* basis, although the exact hereditary mode is unknown. Indirect evidence, such as the topical steroid response, suggests the mode is most likely *polygenic* or *multifactorial*.

Of more immediate concern to the clinician, however, is the increased prevalence of primary open-angle glaucoma among close relatives of glaucoma patients. This figure varied from approximately 5% in one study[59] to 19% in another,[60] although a third investigation revealed only four ocular hypertensives among 100 close relatives.[61] Another survey, however, found a family history of glaucoma in 50% of patients with open-angle glaucoma,[62] and a positive family history is generally considered to be a significant prognostic indicator.

6. *Symptoms*. Primary open-angle glaucoma is characterized by an absence of symptoms until late in the disease when advanced peripheral field loss may be recognized. It is for this reason that periodic examinations are needed to detect the condition in its early stages.

B. Clinical Features

The second set of risk factors to be considered are those which are discovered during the basic glaucoma examination:

1. *Refractive error*. There is an increased prevalence of primary open-angle glaucoma among *myopes*,[63] although one study of ocular dimensions found a shallower anterior chamber depth and thicker lens diameter in primary open-angle glaucoma patients as compared to normal controls.[64]

2. *Intraocular pressure*. The risk of developing glaucomatous damage is related to the level of intraocular pressure. One study of 307 patients revealed the following prevalence of optic nerve head damage in each pressure group[65]:

IOP (mmHg)	% with Nerve Damage
25–29	7
30–34	14
35–39	52
40–44	61
45–49	73
50–54	83
55–59	83
≥60	70

It has also been suggested that the *trend* in the intraocular pressure over a period of time may have more prognostic value than an individual pressure reading.[66] Among ocular hypertensives, those whose pressures increase with time are felt to have a greater risk of developing glaucomatous damage.[66]

3. The *slit lamp examination* is typically normal, although patients

with cornea guttata are reported to frequently have abnormal tono-graphic values,[67] and preliminary specular microscopic studies of patients with chronic glaucoma have revealed abnormal corneal en-dothelium.[68] Whether the cornea is truly abnormal in this disease and whether it is a primary or secondary phenomenon is unknown.

4. *Gonioscopy*. The fundamental techniques of gonioscopy and the normal appearance of the anterior chamber angle were considered in Chapter 2. By definition, the anterior chamber angle is open and grossly normal in eyes with primary open-angle glaucoma, and the primary importance of gonioscopy with regard to this disease is to rule out other forms of glaucoma.

5. *Funduscopic examination*.

a. *The optic nerve head*. The size of the physiologic cup before glaucomatous damage occurs may have prognostic significance. Al-though Armaly[69] found that the cup/disc ratio was not related to a family history of primary open-angle glaucoma, Chandler and Grant[70] state that a wide, deep physiologic cup tolerates increased intraocular pressure poorly and the tendency is to enlargement and total cupping. This concept was supported by a study in which 102 ocular hyper-tensives were observed for 5 years, and the 27 patients who developed field loss during this time had significantly larger vertical cup/disc ratios than those who did not develop field loss.[71] In another study, eyes that were falsely suspected of having field loss on the basis of the optic nerve head appearance had a high incidence of subsequent field loss.[72]

The greatest diagnostic value of observing the optic nerve head comes when the first definite evidence of progressive glaucomatous damage is detected.[73] These features were considered in detail in Chapter 4, and the importance of close observation for these changes in glaucoma suspects is re-emphasized.

b. *The retina*. It was also noted in Chapter 4 that changes in the retinal nerve fiber layer may be seen in association with glaucomatous optic atrophy and may even precede apparent changes in the nerve head.[74]

6. *Visual field*. The early manifestations of glaucomatous field loss were discussed in Chapter 5. Once damage to the visual field has occurred in one eye, there is a high incidence of subsequent field loss in the fellow eye. This figure was reported to be 29% in 31 patients followed 3 to 7 years,[75] and 25% of 104 individuals after 5 years of follow-up in another series.[76]

IV. ADJUNCTIVE TESTS

Numerous tests have been studied in an attempt to find additional prognostic indicators of primary open-angle glaucoma. Although none of these have yet been clearly proven to be of clinical value, the physician should be familiar with some of the more frequently discussed adjunctive tests.

A. Tonography

The details of this procedure and its limitations as a clinical tool in the diagnosis of primary open-angle glaucoma were discussed in Chapter 2.

B. Water Provocative Test

Drinking a large quantity of water in a short period of time will generally lead to a rise in the intraocular pressure. Based on the theory that glaucomatous eyes have a greater pressure response to water drinking, a "provocative" test was developed for the early detection of primary open-angle glaucoma:

1. *Procedure*.[77] After an 8-hr fast, the test begins with baseline applanation tonometric readings. Indentation tonometry is unsatisfactory, since water drinking reduces ocular rigidity.[78, 79] The patient is then instructed to drink approximately 1 liter of tap water, following which applanation tonometry is performed every 15 min for 1 hr.

2. *Interpreting the results*. The maximum intraocular pressure rise usually occurs in 15 to 30 min and returns to the initial level after approximately 60 min in both normal and glaucomatous eyes.[77, 80] A rise of 8 mmHg is generally felt to be a significant response. It has also been suggested that performing tonography after a water drinking test has additional diagnostic value.[79, 81, 82]

3. *The mechanism* of intraocular pressure rise after water drinking is uncertain. One theory is that reduced serum osmolality might cause increased aqueous inflow, although studies have revealed an inconsistent correlation between the intraocular pressure and serum osmolality.[77, 83] Furthermore, tonographic studies have shown reduced aqueous outflow facility in human[84–86] and rabbit[87] eyes, although a suggestion of increased aqueous production has been observed in monkeys.[88]

4. *Clinical value*. Kronfeld[86] found that the combined water drinking test and tonography gave statistically significant lowering of aqueous outflow facility in 35 ocular hypertensives. However, the response was too small to be clinically significant for the individual patient. He concluded that the two tests in this situation added little to the information provided by tonometry. Two additional studies suggested that the water provocative test has no diagnostic value, since 22% false positives and 48% false negatives were found in one series,[89] while the other group had 24% false negatives.[90]

C. Dilation Provocative Tests

Dilation provocative tests are used primarily in eyes suspected of having potentially occludable anterior chamber angles, which will be discussed in the next chapter. However, cycloplegics and mydriatics have also been studied with regard to their influence on open-angle forms of glaucoma. Although these studies have not yet provided clinically useful diagnostic tests for primary open-angle glaucoma, it is important to understand how different eyes respond to these drugs, especially when interpreting a mydriatic provocative test for angle-closure glaucoma.

1. *The cycloplegic effect*

a. *Strong cycloplegics*, such as 1% cyclopentolate, 1% atropine, 5% homatropine, or 0.25% scopolamine, have been shown to cause a significant intraocular pressure rise (greater than 6 mmHg) in many eyes with primary open-angle glaucoma.[91] A similar response may occur in eyes with angle-closure glaucoma when an uncontrolled pressure persists despite a patent iridectomy,[92] and in non-glaucomatous eyes after several weeks of topical dexamethasone.[93] Primary open-angle glaucoma eyes are more likely to have this pressure rise if they are being treated with miotics,[94] and the mechanism of the pressure response to strong cycloplegics is felt to include inhibition of the miotic effect and direct inhibitory action on the ciliary muscle.[94, 95]

One reported test (the fluorescein angiographic provocative test) combines repeated instillations of a strong cycloplegic agent with water-drinking to study perfusion of the optic nerve head by fluorescein angiography before and during periods of induced ocular hypertension.[96]

b. A *weak cycloplegic*, such as 1% tropicamide, has been found to cause a significant pressure rise in open-angle glaucoma eyes only when the eye is on miotic therapy, suggesting the mechanism is competition with the miotic.[97]

2. The *mydriatic action* of cycloplegic-mydriatic agents is also felt to be a cause of elevated intraocular pressure in some eyes with open anterior chamber angles.[98–100] This occurs only when there is an associated shower of pigment in the anterior chamber, and the mechanism is felt to be temporary obstruction of the trabecular meshwork by pigment granules. This occurs predominantly in eyes with the exfoliation syndrome, pigmentary glaucoma, or open-angle glaucoma with other causes of heavy pigmentation in the anterior chamber angle.[98–100]

D. Therapeutic Trials

Based on a theory that eyes with primary open-angle glaucoma respond to anti-glaucoma drugs with a greater intraocular pressure response than is the case with non-glaucomatous eyes, the following attempts have been made to develop prognostic tests:

1. *Epinephrine test*. There is evidence that patients with primary open-angle glaucoma may be particularly sensitive to epinephrine.[101] Such individuals reportedly have a greater intraocular pressure drop and more frequent cardiac arrythmias in response to topical epinephrine than patients with secondary glaucoma.[101] It has been theorized that the mechanism of this increased responsiveness is an epinephrine-stimulated rise in intraocular cyclic adenosine monophosphate to which the primary open-angle glaucoma patient may be unusually sensitive.[102, 103]

Based on this apparent sensitivity to epinephrine, a test was devised in which 1 to 2% epinephrine twice daily was administered, and a pressure drop of more than 5 mmHg over a 1 to 7 day period was considered a "response."[104] (A subsequent study indicated that the pressure drop 4 hr after a single dose could also be used as the indicator of response.[105]) In a 5 to 10 year follow-up of 80 ocular hypertensives, 85% of those who developed field loss were positive responders, while only 28% without field loss had shown the positive response.[104] However, in another study the positive response was found in 53% of 32 ocular hypertensives and 56% of 18 open-angle glaucoma patients with field loss.[106] Further study is needed to confirm the prognostic value of this test.

2. *Other therapeutic trials* that have been suggested include the *pilocarpine test*, in which an intraocular pressure drop of more than 4 mmHg at the peak of the diurnal curve is felt to suggest glaucoma,[107, 108] and the *acetazolamide test*, which is used to estimate the coefficient of aqueous outflow facility based on applanation intraocular pressure measurements after the drug is given intravenously.[109] However, neither of these tests have confirmed clinical value.

3. *A uniocular therapeutic trial* of a topical anti-glaucoma drug is a valuable clinical adjunct in helping to decide when to institute medical therapy, simply because it reveals the effectiveness in pressure reduction and the side effects that can be expected with that particular medication.[110] It has been suggested that this information can be obtained, at least in part, during a 4-hr office trial with 2% pilocarpine.[111]

E. Response to Induced IOP Elevation

The influence of transient, artificially-induced intraocular pressure elevation on the visual field also provides a possible approach to the early identification of primary open-angle glaucoma patients.[112, 113] However, long-term investigations are needed to establish the value of this test as a prognostic indicator.

F. Micellaneous Observations

Preliminary studies suggested that primary open-angle glaucoma populations have significantly more non-tasters of phenylthiourea[114] or phenylthiocarbamide, but this was not confirmed in a subsequent study.[115] It was also reported that patients with primary open-angle glaucoma have a higher prevalence of the histocompatibility (HLA) antigens, HLA-B12 and HLA-B7,[116] although numerous studies have subsequently shown no significant correlation between HLA antigens and glaucoma.[117-124]

V. THEORIES OF MECHANISM

As in virtually all forms of glaucoma, elevation of intraocular pressure in primary open-angle glaucoma is due to *obstruction of aqueous outflow*. However, the precise mechanism(s) of outflow obstruction in this condition has not been fully explained, despite the fact that it has been studied more than in any other type of glaucoma. The following data from these studies provide only suggestions of what the final answer may hold:

A. Histopathologic Observations

Histopathologic observations provide the most likely source for the eventual explanation of aqueous outflow obstruction in primary open-angle glaucoma. However, the interpretation of these findings must take into consideration additional influences, such as age, the secondary effects of prolonged intraocular pressure elevation, the alterations that medical and surgical treatment of the glaucoma might have induced, and artifacts created by tissue processing.

1. *Trabecular meshwork.* Grant[125] demonstrated that the largest proportion of resistance to aqueous outflow in enucleated normal human eyes could be eliminated by incising the trabecular meshwork. Whether this tissue is the site of abnormal resistance in primary open-angle glaucoma has not been determined, but the following observations have been reported:

a. The *collagen* of the trabecular beams is fragmented, with thickening of the glass membrane and increased curly collagen,[126] diffuse nodular proliferation of extracellular long-spacing collagen and coiling of fiber bundles,[127] and changes in orientation and osmophilia of the fibers.[128] However, similar changes are seen in association with aging and one study found the changes correlated more closely with age than with reduction in outflow facility.[129] It has been suggested that the changes in primary open-angle glaucoma may represent an exaggeration of the normal aging process.[130]

b. The *endothelial cells* lining the trabeculae appear to be more active than in normotensive eyes,[127] and are reported to show proliferation with foamy degeneration and basement membrane thickening.[126, 128] One theory holds that changes in the endothelial cells of the trabecular meshwork result in a greater exposure of other trabecular elements to aqueous, which causes a degeneration of these elements.[131]

c. The *intertrabecular spaces*, as might be anticipated from the general thickening of the trabeculae, are *narrowed*.[128, 130] In addition, they may contain red blood cells, pigment, and dense amorphous material.[128] It has also been reported that *acid mucopolysaccharides* are more abundant in the meshwork of human eyes with open-angle glaucoma.[132] A scanning electron microscopic study of 10 trabeculectomy specimens revealed an unknown substance coating the meshwork, which was felt to be sufficient to obstruct aqueous outflow.[133] However, this finding has not been confirmed by other investigators.[134, 135]

d. The *juxtacanilicular connective tissue* just beneath the inner wall endothelium of Schlemm's canal has been noted by several observers to contain a layer of *amorphous, osmophilic material*.[129, 136-]

[138] This has been described as moderately electron-dense, non-fibril-lar material[129] with characteristics of basement membrane and curly collagen[138] and cytochemical properties of chondroitin sulfate protein complex.[129]

   e. *Giant vacuoles*, as described in Chapter 2, are found in the inner wall endothelium of Schlemm's canal in normal eyes and are felt to be related to aqueous transport. In eyes with primary open-angle glaucoma, the giant vacuoles have been reported to be decreased or absent,[128, 138–140] although other investigators were unable to support these findings.[141]

   2. *Collapse of Schlemm's canal* will also increase resistance to aqueous outflow and has been proposed as the mechanism of outflow obstruction in primary open-angle glaucoma.[142–144] The collapse represents a bulge of trabecular meshwork into the canal, which might result from alterations in the meshwork and/or relaxation of the ciliary muscle. In support of this theory, some histopathologic studies have revealed a narrowed Schlemm's canal with adhesions between the inner and outer walls.[128, 142, 143]

   3. The *intrascleral channels* could also be a site of increased resistance to aqueous outflow in primary open-angle glaucoma. Histopathologic observations have revealed attenuation of the channels, which may be due to a swelling of mucopolysaccharides in the adjacent sclera.[126] Krasnov[145] has suggested that intrascleral blockage may be the mechanism of outflow obstruction in approximately half of the eyes with primary open-angle glaucoma. However, it has been reported that removal of tissue overlying Schlemm's canal does not improve outflow facility until the canal is actually entered,[142] suggesting that removal of this material may be relieving a blockade of the canal.

B. Corticosteroid Sensitivity

   There is evidence that patients with primary open-angle glaucoma are unusually sensitive to corticosteroids and that this steroid sensitivity may be related to the intraocular pressure elevation. We will consider first the evidence for the increased sensitivity and then look at theories of how this may lead to a pressure rise.

   1. *Topical corticosteroid response*. It has been well documented that chronic corticosteroid therapy, especially with topical administration, can lead to elevated intraocular pressures. In a small percentage of the general population, the magnitude of this pressure rise is sufficient to cause a severe form of secondary glaucoma, which will be considered in Chapter 20. The present discussion will be limited to prospective studies of topical steroid response in various populations.

   Several large population studies have been performed in which a potent topical corticosteroid, such as 0.1% betamethasone or 0.1% dexamethasone, was given three to four times daily for 3 to 6 weeks. These studies all agree that a significant number of individuals will respond with variable degrees of intraocular pressure elevation. The studies differ considerably, however, with regard to many important aspects of this pressure response.

   a. The *distribution* of pressure responses in *general populations* was found in some studies to be trimodal, with approximately two-thirds having a low response (usually defined as a rise of less than 5 mmHg), one-third showing an intermediate response (6–15 mmHg rise), and 4 to 5% having a rise greater than 15 mmHg.[146–148] However, a study of monozygotic and like-sex dizygotic twins did not reveal a trimodal distribution.[149] Furthermore, when the topical corticosteroid test was repeated in the same population, individuals did not always give the same response each time.[150]

   b. *Primary open-angle glaucoma* populations have been shown to have a greater number of individuals with a high intraocular pressure response to topical corticosteroids, although the actual reported percentage of high responders varies according to the criteria used to define this group.[146, 148] *Ocular hypertensives* also have a greater incidence of high responders,[151] and a significant number of high responders are reported to have reversible glaucomatous field defects.[152] Another study, however, found that the pressure response among glaucoma suspects was not significantly different from that in a normal population.[153] Primary angle-closure glaucoma eyes that had undergone prophylactic peripheral iridectomies were also reported to resemble normals in their topical corticosteroid response.[154]

   c. *Inheritance* of the topical corticosteroid response and how this may relate to primary open-angle glaucoma have been matters of particular controversy. Becker[146, 155] postulated an autosomal recessive mode for the corticosteroid response and suggested that the gene is either closely related or identical to that for primary open-angle glaucoma, which he felt had an autosomal recessive inheritance. Armaly[148] agreed that the two conditions might be genetically related, but proposed a polygenic inheritance for primary open-angle glaucoma with the gene for the topical corticosteroid response being one of the genes involved. Francois and co-workers[156] were also unable to confirm Becker's recessive theory in a study of the topical corticosteroid responsiveness among normal subjects with no family history of glaucoma and normals who had relatives with glaucoma. Levene and co-workers[153] agreed that the topical corticosteroid response is genetically determined, but found that it relates in a similar manner to glaucoma and normal eyes. Still other investigators could not even substantiate that the corticosteroid response was entirely genetic. In the previously mentioned twin heritability study, Schwartz and co-workers[149, 157–159] found a low estimate of heritability that did not support a predominant role of inheritance in the response to corticosteroids, and suggested that non-genetic factors play the major role. In addition, Spaeth[160] found that eyes with angle recession responded to topical corticosteroids with a higher pressure rise than the fellow, nontraumatized eye, suggesting that the steroid response may not be solely genetic.

   2. *Plasma cortisol studies* provide other evidence that patients with

primary open-angle glaucoma may be unusually sensitive to corticosteroids.

a. One investigation showed higher than normal *plasma cortisol* levels in primary open-angle glaucoma patients,[161] although this observation was not confirmed in another study.[162]

b. Of greater interest is the response of primary open-angle glaucoma patients to *plasma cortisol suppression*. This test consists of measuring plasma cortisol before and after the oral administration of dexamethasone. The normal response is a reduction in plasma cortisol of 35% or more approximately 9 hr after administration of the corticosteroid, due to suppression of trophic hormones. Reports of plasma cortisol suppression in primary open-angle glaucoma patients differ, with one study showing less suppression,[161, 163] which did not appear to be genetically determined,[164] while another investigation revealed no significant difference from non-glaucomatous individuals.[162, 165]

c. *Pretreatment with diphenylhydantoin* (Dilantin) normally prevents plasma cortisol suppression, presumably by enhancing liver enzyme degradation of the dexamethasone before it suppresses the release of trophic hormones from the pituitary. However, in 89% of primary open-angle glaucoma patients, diphenylhydantoin did not prevent the plasma cortisol suppression.[162] The mechanism of plasma cortisol suppression despite pretreatment with diphenylhydantoin in patients with primary open-angle glaucoma does not appear to be due to an alteration in liver enzyme degradation of dexamethasone,[166] but rather to an *increased sensitivity* to lower levels of circulating steroids.[167] The corticosteroid sensitivity in primary open-angle glaucoma patients appears to be relatively specific, since oral dexamethasone does not have an abnormal effect on baseline thyroid function tests or thyroid stimulating hormone suppression in these individuals.[168]

d. *The relationship of topical corticosteroid response* to plasma cortisol suppression has also been investigated, and a correlation between high topical corticosteroid responders and reduced plasma cortisol suppression has been demonstrated.[165, 169, 170] In addition, approximately half of the high topical corticosteroid responders from a general population study had plasma cortisol suppression despite pretreatment with diphenylhydantoin. The latter individuals also more closely resembled primary open-angle glaucoma patients on the basis of other parameters, such as a larger cup/disc ratio and an abnormal glucose tolerance test.[162] However, a 5-year prospective study failed to show that plasma cortisol suppression can predict the development of primary open-angle glaucoma among high topical steroid responders.[171]

3. *Lymphocyte transformation inhibition* studies may offer yet a third source of evidence for increased corticosteroid sensitivity in patients with primary open-angle glaucoma, although reports are also conflicting on this subject.

Lymphocytes from peripheral blood can be transformed from the usual state of relative metabolic inactivity to a metabolically active state by mitogenic agents such as phytohemagglutinin. The degree of transformation can be measured by the uptake of tritiated thymidine into DNA. *Corticosteroids inhibit* the lymphocyte transformation, and the degree of inhibition can be taken as a measure of sensitivity to corticosteroids. Such studies have revealed increased corticosteroid sensitivity among patients with primary open-angle glaucoma,[172, 173] although other investigators failed to confirm these findings.[174, 175] The effect of ouabain on lymphocyte transformation is normal in primary open-angle glaucoma patients and high topical corticosteroid responders, suggesting that steroid sensitivity, if it exists, is specific and not the general vulnerability of "sick cells."[176]

4. *Relationship of intraocular pressure elevation to corticosteroid sensitivity.* If patients with primary open-angle glaucoma are unusually sensitive to corticosteroids, as much of the aforementioned evidence would suggest, by what mechanism(s) might this lead to elevated intraocular pressure? Furthermore, does this mechanism(s) only function in response to exogenously administered corticosteroids, or do normal circulating corticosteroids also adversely influence the intraocular pressure in primary open-angle glaucoma patients? Attempts to answer these questions include the following *theories*:

a. It has been suggested that an abnormal response of the *hypothalamic-pituitary-adrenal axis* in primary open-angle glaucoma patients may be related to alterations in aqueous humor dynamics in response to corticosteroids.[170]

b. It may be that corticosteroids influence the intraocular pressure by altering *cyclic adenosine monophosphate (AMP)*. Corticosteroids have a permissive effect on the β-adrenergic stimulation of adenyl cyclase, the enzyme responsible for the synthesis of cyclic AMP.[177] How this relates to aqueous humor dynamics is uncertain, although primary open-angle glaucoma patients and high topical steroid responders appear to be unusually sensitive to cyclic AMP. Evidence for this increased sensitivity has been observed in studies of lymphocyte transformation, as previously described, which is normally inhibited by cyclic AMP. Theophylline inhibits the enzyme, phosphodiesterase, which destroys cyclic AMP, and primary open-angle glaucoma patients reportedly require less theophylline than control subjects to stimulate inhibition of lymphocyte transformation.[178]

c. It has also been reported that intraocular pressure elevation associated with corticosteroid sensitivity may be related to *mucopolysaccharides* in the trabecular meshwork.[170] When polymerized, mucopolysaccharides becomes hydrated, swell, and obstruct aqueous outflow. Catabolic enzymes, released from lysosomes, depolymerize the mucopolysaccharides, and corticosteroids stabilize the lysosome membrane, preventing release of the enzyme.

d. Yet another possible effect of steroids on intraocular pressure may be related to the *phagocytic activity of endothelial cells* lining the trabecular meshwork. As discussed in Chapter 2, these cells are normally phagocytic, and it may be that they function to "clean" the aqueous of debris before it reaches the inner wall endothelium of Schlemm's canal. Failure to do so might result in a build-up of material that could account for the amorphous layer in the juxtacanilicular connective tissue, as previously described. Corticosteroids suppress phagocytosis, and it may be that the trabecular endothelium in primary open-angle glaucoma patients is unusually sensitive even to endogenous corticosteroids.[180]

C. Immunologic Aspects

Increased γ-globulin[181] and plasma cells[182] in the trabecular meshwork of eyes with primary open-angle glaucoma have been reported, and a high percentage of patients with this disease were found in one study to have positive anti-nuclear antibodies reactions.[183] These reports suggested a possible immunologic mechanism in the pathogenesis of primary open-angle glaucoma. However, subsequent assays for specific immunoglobulins in the trabecular meshwork of eyes with primary open-angle glaucoma revealed no difference from non-glaucomatous eyes.[184, 185] Furthermore, a second study of anti-nuclear antibodies in open-angle glaucoma patients and normal controls revealed no significant difference in positive reactions.[186] Cell-mediated immunity, as indicated by leukocyte migration inhibition *in vitro*, has also been studied in patients with primary open-angle glaucoma and revealed no unusual sensitivity to ocular antigens.[187] The absence of a correlation between HLA antigens and primary open-angle glaucoma was discussed earlier in this chapter. At the present time, therefore, the bulk of the evidence is against an immunogenic mechanism in primary open-angle glaucoma.

VI. MANAGEMENT

The present discussion will be limited to the basic principles of deciding when to begin treatment and what type of therapy to use. The details of the drugs and surgical procedures will be considered in Section Three.

A. When to Treat

In the typical case of primary open-angle glaucoma with established visual field and/or optic nerve head damage, treatment to reduce the intraocular pressure is clearly indicated whatever the pressure may be. A long-term follow-up study of such cases confirmed the generally accepted belief that intraocular pressure reduction is important in preventing visual loss in glaucoma.[188]

However, in the case of elevated intraocular pressure with normal optic nerve heads and visual fields, the answer is less clear. As discussed earlier in this chapter, not all such patients appear destined to develop glaucomatous damage, and there is no way of predicting with certainty which ones will go on to manifest the full picture of primary open-angle glaucoma. Prospective studies have indicated that significant *risk factors* include elevated intraocular pressure, abnormalities of the optic nerve head, advancing age, a family history of glaucoma, and cardiovascular disorders.[18, 189–191] However, no single risk factor or group of factors have yet been shown to predict the future development of glaucomatous damage with reasonable accuracy.[192, 193]

For lack of a precise indicator of future glaucomatous damage, it is suggested that patients with moderate intraocular pressure elevations be followed without treatment, but with periodic visual field and optic nerve head examinations.[194] However, most ophthalmologists will initiate therapy at a certain intraocular pressure level despite normal discs and fields. Goldmann[195] begins medical therapy at 25 mm Hg, while Chandler and Grant[70] suggest 30 mmHg as a guideline for initiating treatment in the absence of apparent damage. It has also been pointed out that central retinal vein occlusion is more common in individuals with elevated intraocular pressures, and these authors suggest that patients over 65 years of age should be treated to keep their pressures below 25 mmHg.[196] Clearly, any arbitrary pressure level should be adjusted for each patient on the basis of that individual's risk factors. In doubtful cases, a *trial of therapy* in one eye may be helpful. Although it has not been proven that eyes with primary open-angle glaucoma are more sensitive to anti-glaucoma drugs, a good pressure reduction with minimal side effects might argue in favor of continuing the therapy.

B. How to Treat

Once the decision has been made to begin treatment, the next questions are what form of therapy should be used and what should be the guidelines for successful therapy?

1. *Medical therapy.* Primary open-angle glaucoma is basically a medical disease, in that surgery is usually reserved for cases that cannot be controlled with drugs. The basic principle of medical therapy is to use the least amount of medicine that will control the glaucoma with the fewest side effects. To this end, it is customary to begin with a low dose of topical medication and to increase the concentration and/or advance to combinations of drugs until the desired pressure level is reached. It is good practice to treat only one eye initially in symmetric cases, so the fellow eye can be used as a control in determining the efficacy of therapy. Opinions differ regarding the "initial drug of choice."[197–199] The relative advantages and disadvantages of the various anti-glaucoma drugs are considered in Section Three.

It is not possible to predict what intraocular pressure level will be adequate to prevent progressive glaucomatous damage in each individual case. In general, a pressure below 20 mmHg is recommended in eyes with early field or disc damage,[200] while a pressure below 18 mmHg appears to be desirable for advanced cases.[200, 201] However, the main guide to therapy is the appearance of the optic nerve heads and visual fields, and progressive change in these parameters demands further pressure reduction regardless of what the present level may be.

2. *Surgical therapy.* Surgical intervention is usually indicated whenever there is progressive glaucomatous damage despite *"maximum tolerable medical therapy."* In some cases, this may mean that all available forms of anti-glaucoma drugs in their highest concentrations are being used, although other cases of medical failure are due to *drug intolerances* or poor *compliance* with the recommended therapy. In one study, eleven of 40 randomly selected primary open-angle glaucoma patients failed to comply with their medical therapy.[202] Factors related to poor compliance included males, no other medical disease, glaucoma not ranked most troubling when other disorders were present, side effects with medication, and failure to relate glaucoma to blindness.

In advanced cases with total cupping of the disc and a small, central field, it is no longer possible to use progressive disc and field change as a guide to surgical intervention, and reliance must be placed on the intraocular pressure. In a study of 101 such eyes, Kolker[201] reported loss of central vision in 30% of those with average pressures above 22 mmHg and recommended that serious consideration be given to glaucoma filtering surgery when the pressure is consistently above this level.

Loss of central vision may occur after glaucoma surgery as well as during medical therapy, and in one study it occurred with equal frequency with these two modalities of treatment.[201] Another investigation suggested surgery had less field loss, although the statistical significance of these findings was not certain.[203] When progressive field loss does occur despite good pressure levels following surgery, it is frequently due to vascular insufficiency of the optic nerve head.[204]

The procedure most often used for primary open-angle glaucoma is one of the many forms of filtering surgery. The details of these and other available surgical modalities are discussed in Section Three.

C. Treatment of Low-tension Glaucoma

Damage to the optic nerve head and visual field may progress even at low normal intraocular pressures in this condition. Indeed, there is no firm evidence that treating the intraocular pressure improves the prognosis, and the most important aspect of management may be the treatment of any *cardiovascular abnormality*, e.g., gastrointestinal lesions, anemia, congestive heart failure, transient ischemic attacks, and cardiac arrythmias, to ensure maximum perfusion of the optic nerve head.[8] Nevertheless, most clinicians try to keep the intraocular pressure as low as possible with medication, and Sugar[205] has advocated filtering surgery in one eye for progressive field loss, and in the second eye only if it is successful in the first. In another study, however, surgery did not help.[206]

References

1. Chandler, PA, Grant, WM: 'Ocular hypertension' vs open-angle glaucoma. Arch Ophtha 95:585, 1977.
2. Kolker, AE, Becker, B: 'Ocular hypertension' vs open-angle glaucoma: a different view. Arch Ophthal 95:586, 1977.
3. Shaffer, R: 'Glaucoma suspect' or 'ocular hypertension'? Arch Ophthal 95:588, 1977.
4. Phelps, CD: Ocular hypertension: to treat or not to treat? Arch Ophthal 95:588, 1977.
5. Drance, SM: Some factors in the production of low tension glaucoma. Br J Ophthal 56:229, 1972.
6. Drance, SM, Sweeney, VP, Morgan, RW, Feldman, F: Studies of factors involved in the production of low tension glaucoma. Arch Ophthal 89:457, 1973.
7. Drance, SM, Morgan, RW, Sweeney, VP: Shock-induced optic neuropathy. A cause of nonprogressive glaucoma. N Engl J Med 288:392, 1973.
8. Chumbley, LC, Brubaker, RF: Low-tension glaucoma. Am J Ophthal 81:761, 1976.
9. Levene, RZ: Low tension glaucoma: a critical review and new material. Surv Ophthal 24:621, 1980.
10. Hayreh, SS: Anterior Ischemic Optic Neuropathy. Springer-Verlag, New York, 1975, p 22.
11. Hollows, FC, Graham, PA: Intra-ocular pressure, glaucoma, and glaucoma suspects in a defined population. Br J Ophthal 50:570, 1966.
12. Segal, P, Skwierczynska, J: Mass screening of adults for glaucoma. Ophthalmologica 153:336, 1967.
13. Kahn, HA, Leibowitz, HM, Ganley, JP, Kini, MM, Colton, T, Nickerson, RS, Dawber, TR: The Framingham eye study. I. Outline and major prevalence findings. Am J Epidemiol 106:17, 1977.
14. Leske, MC, Rosenthal, J: Epidemiologic aspects of open-angle glaucoma. Am J Epidemiol 109:250, 1979.
15. Graham, PA: Epidemiology of simple glaucoma and ocular hypertension. Br J Ophthal 56:223, 1972.
16. Perkins, ES: The Bedford glaucoma survey. I. Long-term follow-up of borderline cases. Br J Ophthal 57:179, 1973.
17. Walker, WM: Ocular hypertension. Follow-up of 109 cases from 1963 to 1974. Trans Ophthal Soc UK 94:525, 1974.
18. Wilensky, JT, Podos, SM, Becker, B: Prognostic indicators in ocular hypertension. Arch Ophthal 91:200, 1974.
19. Norskov, K: Routine tonometry in ophthalmic practice. II. Five-year follow-up. Acta Ophthal 48:873, 1970.
20. Linner, E: Ocular hypertension. I. The clinical course during ten years without therapy, aqueous humour dynamics. Acta Ophthal 54:707, 1976.
21. Kitazawa, Y, Horie, T, Aoki, S, Suzuki, M, Nishioka, K: Untreated ocular hypertension. A long-term prospective study. Arch Ophthal 95:1180, 1977.
22. David, R, Livingston, DG, Luntz, MH: Ocular hypertension—a long-term follow-up of treated and untreated patients. Br J Ophthal 61:668, 1977.
23. Hart, WM Jr, Yablonski, M, Kass, MA, Becker, B: Multivariate analysis of the risk of glaucomatous visual field loss. Arch Ophthal 97:1455, 1979.
24. Armaly, MF: Ocular pressure and visual fields. A ten-year follow-up study. Arch Ophthal 81:25, 1969.
25. Perkins, ES: The Bedford glaucoma survey. II. Rescreening of normal population. Br J Ophthal 57:186, 1973.
26. Leydhecker, W: Zur verbreitung des glaucoma simplex in der scheinbar gesunden, augenarztlich nicht behandelten bevolkerung. Doc Ophthal 13:359, 1959.
27. Lichter, PR, Shaffer, RN: Ocular hypertension and glaucoma. Trans Pacific Coast Oto-Ophthal Soc 54:63, 1973.
28. Harbin, TS Jr, Podos, SM, Kolker, AE, Becker, B: Visual field progression in

open-angle glaucoma patients presenting with monocular field loss. Trans Am Acad Ophthal Otol 81:253, 1976.

29. Wright, JE: The Bedford glaucoma survey. *In* Glaucoma (Symposium), L. B. Hunt, ed. E & S Livingston, Ltd, Edinburgh, 1966, p 12.

30. Goldwyn, R, Waltman, SR, Becker, B: Primary open-angle glaucoma in adolescents and young adults. Arch Ophthal 84:579, 1970.

31. Mandell, AI, Elfervig, J: Open-angle glaucoma in patients under forty years of age. Pers Ophthal 1:215, 1977.

32. Sasovetz, D: Open-angle glaucoma in blacks: a review. J Natl Med Assn 69:705, 1977.

33. Wilensky, JT, Gandhi, N, Pan, T: Racial influences in open-angle glaucoma. Ann Ophthal 10:1398, 1978.

34. David, R, Livingston, D, Luntz, MH: Ocular hypertension: a comparative follow-up of black and white patients. Br J Ophthal 62:676, 1978.

35. Wallace, J, Lovell, HG: Glaucoma and intraocular pressure in Jamaica. Am J Ophthal 67:93, 1969.

36. Hiller, R, Kahn, HA: Blindness from glaucoma. Am J Ophthal 80:62, 1975.

37. Schwartz, AL, Helfgott, MA: The incidence of sickle trait in blacks requiring filtering surgery. Ann Ophthal 9:957, 1977.

38. Kahn, HA, Milton, RC: Alternative definitions of open-angle glaucoma. Effect on prevalence and associations in the Framingham Eye Study. Arch Ophthal 98:2172, 1980.

39. Armstrong, JR, Daily, RK, Dobson, HL, Girard, LJ: The incidence of glaucoma in diabetes mellitus. A comparison with the incidence of glaucoma in the general population. Am J Ophthal 50:55, 1960.

40. Becker, B: Diabetes mellitus and primary open-angle glaucoma. Am J Ophthal 71:1, 1971.

41. Marre, VE, Marre, M: A contribution to glaucoma in the presence of diabetes mellitus. Klin Montabl Augenheilkd 153:396, 1968.

42. Armaly, MF: Dexamethasone ocular hypertension and eosinopenia, and glucose tolerance test. Arch Ophthal 78:193, 1967.

43. McLenachan, J, Davies, DM: Glaucoma and the thyroid. Br J Ophthal 49:441, 1965.

44. Becker, B, Kolker, AE, Ballin, N: Thyroid function and glaucoma. Am J Ophthal 61:997, 1966.

45. Krupin, T, Jacobs, LS, Podos, SM, Becker, B: Thyroid function and the intra-ocular pressure response to topical corticosteroids. Am J Ophthal 83:643, 1977.

46. Neuner, HP, Dardenne, U: Ocular changes in the Cushing syndrome. Klin Mbl Augenheilkd 152:570, 1968.

47. Haas, JS, Nootens, RH: Glaucoma secondary to benign adrenal adenoma. Am J Ophthal 78:497, 1974.

48. Abdel-Aziz, M, Labib, MA: The relationship of the intraocular pressure and the hormonal disturbance. II. The pituitary gland. Bull Ophthal Soc Egypt 62:61, 1969.

49. Caygill, WM: Aqueous humor dynamics following pituitary irradiation in diabetic patients with retinopathy. Am J Ophthal 71:826, 1971.

50. Treister, G, Mannor, S: Intraocular pressure and outflow facility. Effect of estrogen and combined estrogen-progestin treatment in normal human eyes. Arch Ophthal 83:311, 1970.

51. Abdel-Aziz, M, Labib, MA: The relationship of the intra-ocular pressure to hormonal disturbance. IV. The gonads. Bull Ophthal Soc Egypt 62:83, 1969.

52. Joist, JH, Lichtenfeld, P, Mandell, AI, Kolker, AE: Platelet function, blood coagulability, and fibrinolysis in patients with low tension glaucoma. Arch Ophthal 94:1893, 1976.

53. Leighton, DA, Phillips, CI: Systemic blood pressure in open-angle glaucoma, low tension glaucoma, and the normal eye. Br J Ophthal 56:447, 1972.

54. Winder, AF: Circulating lipoprotein and blood glucose levels in association with low-tension and chronic simple glaucoma. Br J Ophthal 61:641, 1977.

55. Morgan, RW, Drance, SM: Chronic open-angle glaucoma and ocular hypertension. An epidemiological study. Br J Ophthal 5:211, 1975.
56. Kahn, HA, Leibowitz, HM, Ganley, JP, Kini, MM, Colton, T, Nickerson, RS, Dawber, TR: The Framingham eye study. II. Association of ophthalmic pathology with single variables previously measured in the Framingham Heart Study. Am J Epidemiology 106:33, 1977.
57. Bengtsson, B: Findings associated with glaucomatous visual field defects. Acta Ophthalmologica 58:20, 1980.
58. David, R, Jenkins, T: Genetic markers in glaucoma. Br J Ophthal 64:227, 1980.
59. Perkins, ES: Family studies in glaucoma. Br J Ophthal 58:529, 1974.
60. Kolker, AE: Glaucoma family study. Ten-year follow-up (preliminary report). Israel J Med Sci 8:1357, 1972.
61. Cameron, D, Crombie, AL, Jackson, CRS: Results of a survey restricted to relatives of known cases in Edinburgh. In Glaucoma (Symposium) 1965, L. B. Hunt, ed, E & S Livingston Ltd, Edinburgh, 1966.
62. Shin, DH, Becker, B, Kolker, AE: Family history in primary open-angle glaucoma. Arch Ophthal 95:598, 1977.
63. Schlossman, A: Myopia with glaucoma. Contact Intraocul Lens Med J 1:84, 1975.
64. Tomlinson, A, Leighton, DA: Ocular dimensions and the heredity of open-angle glaucoma. Br J Ophthal 58:68, 1974.
65. Pohjanpelto, EJ, Palva, JP: Ocular hypertension and glaucomatous optic nerve damage. Acta Ophthal 52:194, 1974.
66. Schwartz, B, Talusan, AG: Spontaneous trends in ocular pressure in untreated ocular hypertension. Arch Ophthal 98:105, 1980.
67. Buxton, JN, Preston, RW, Riechers, R, Guilbault, N: Tonography in cornea guttata. A preliminary report. Arch Ophthal 77:602, 1967.
68. Hiles, DA, Biglan, AW, Fetherolf, EC: Central corneal endothelial cell counts in children. Am Intra-Ocular Implant Soc J 5:292, 1979.
69. Armaly, MF: Genetic determination of cup/disc ratio of the optic nerve. Arch Ophthal 78:35, 1967.
70. Chandler, PA, Grant, WM: Lectures on Glaucoma. Lea & Febiger, Philadelphia, 1965, p 13.
71. Yablonski, ME, Zimmerman, TJ, Kass, MA, Becker, B: Prognostic significance of optic disk cupping in ocular hypertensive patients. Am J Ophthal 89: 585, 1980.
72. Susanna, R, Drance, SM: Use of discriminant analysis. I. Prediction of visual field defects from features of the glaucoma disc. Arch Ophthal 96: 1568, 1978.
73. Hitchings, RA, Wheller, CA: The optic disc in glaucoma. IV. Optic disc evaluation in the ocular hypertensive patient. Br J Ophthal 64:232, 1980.
74. Sommer, A, Miller, NR, Pollack, I, Maumenee, AE, George, T: The nerve fiber layer in the diagnosis of glaucoma. Arch Ophthal 95:2149, 1977.
75. Kass, MA, Kolker, AE, Becker, B: Prognostic factors in glaucomatous visual field loss. Arch Ophthal 94:1274, 1976.
76. Susanna, R, Drance, SM, Douglas, GR: The visual prognosis of the fellow eye in uniocular chronic open-angle glaucoma. Br J Ophthal 62:327, 1978.
77. Spaeth, GL: The water drinking test. Indications that factors other than osmotic considerations are involved. Arch Ophthal 77:50, 1967.
78. Vucicevic, ZM, Ralston, J, Burns, WP, Gaffney, HP: Influence of the water drinking test on scleral rigidity. Arch Ophthal 82:761, 1969.
79. Vucicevic, ZM, Scheie, HG, Berry, A, Yaros, M, Frauenhoffer, C: The importance and accuracy of the water drinking test and tonography. Ann Ophthal 7:39, 1975.
80. Armaly, MF: Water-drinking test. I. Characteristics of the ocular pressure response and the effect of age. Arch Ophthal 83:169, 1970.
81. Becker, B, Christensen, RE: Water-drinking and tonography in the diagonsis of glaucoma. Arch Ophthal 56:321, 1956.
82. Becker, B: Tonography in the diagnosis of simple (open angle) glaucoma. Trans Am Acad Ophthal Otol 65:156, 1961.

83. Kimura, R: Clinical studies on glaucoma. Report III. The diagnostic significance of the water-drinking test. Acta Soc Ophthal Jpn 71:2133, 1967.

84. Ballin, N, Becker, B: Provocative testing for primary open-angle glaucoma in "senior citizens." Invest Ophthal 6:126, 1967.

85. Armaly, MF, Sayegh, RE: Water-drinking test. II. The effect of age on tonometric and tonographic measures. Arch Ophthal 83:176, 1970.

86. Kronfeld, PC: Water drinking and outflow facility. Invest Ophthal 14:49, 1975.

87. Thorpe, RM, Kolker, AE: A tonographic study of water loading in rabbits. Arch Ophthal 77:238, 1967.

88. Casey, WJ: Intraocular pressure and facility in monkeys after water drinking. A study in the Cynomolgus monkey, *Macaca irus*. Arch Ophthal 74:841, 1965.

89. Roth, JA: Inadequate diagnostic value of the water-drinking test. Br J Ophthal 58:55, 1974.

90. Rasmussen, KE, Jorgensen, HA: Diagnostic value of the water-drinking test in early detection of simple glaucoma. Acta Ophthal 54:160, 1976.

91. Harris, LS: Cycloplegic-induced intraocular pressure elevations. A study of normal and open-angle glaucomatous eyes. Arch Ophthal 79:242, 1968.

92. Harris, LS, Galin, MA: Cycloplegic provocative testing. Arch Ophthal 81: 356, 1969.

93. Harris, LS, Galin, MA, Mittag, TW: Cycloplegic provocative testing after topical administration of steroids. Arch Ophthal 86:12, 1971.

94. Harris, LS, Galin, MA: Cycloplegic provocative testing. Effect of miotic therapy. Arch Ophthal 81:544, 1969.

95. Barany, E, Christensen, RE: Cycloplegia and outflow resistance in normal human and monkey eyes and in primary open-angle glaucoma. Arch Ophthal 77:757, 1967.

96. Spaeth, GL, Vacharat, N: Provocative tests and chronic simple glaucoma. I. Effect of atropine on the water-drinking test: intimations of central regulatory control. II. Fluorescein angiography provocative test: a new approach to separation of the normal from the pathological. Br J Ophthal 56:205, 1972.

97. Portney, GL, Purcell, TW: Influence of tropicamide on intraocular pressure. Ann Ophthal 7:31, 1975.

98. Kristensen, P: Mydriasis-induced pigment liberation in the anterior chamber associated with acute rise in intraocular pressure in open-angle glaucoma. Acta Ophthal 43:714, 1965.

99. Kristensen, P: Pigment liberation test in open-angle glaucoma. Acta Ophthal 46:586, 1968.

100. Valle, O: The cyclopentolate provocative test in suspected or untreated open-angle glaucoma. III. The significance of pigment for the result of the cyclopentolate provocative test in suspected or untreated open-angle glaucoma. Acta Ophthal 54:654, 1976.

101. Becker, B, Montgomery, SW, Kass, MA, Shin, DH: Increased ocular and systemic responsiveness to epinephrine in primary open-angle glaucoma. Arch Ophthal 95:789, 1977.

102. Shin, DH, Kass, MA, Becker, B: Intraocular pressure response to topical epinephrine and HLA-B12. Arch Ophthal 96:1012, 1978.

103. Palmberg, PF, Hajek, S, Cooper, D, Becker, B: Increased cellular responsiveness to epinephrine in primary open-angle glaucoma. Arch Ophthal 95:855, 1977.

104. Becker, B, Shin, DH: Response to topical epinephrine. A practical prognostic test in patients with ocular hypertension. Arch Ophthal 94:2057, 1976.

105. Kass, MA, Becker, B: A simplified test of epinephrine responsiveness. Arch Ophthal 96:999, 1978.

106. Drance, SM, Saheb, NE, Schulzer, M: Response to topical epinephrine in chronic open-angle glaucoma. Arch Ophthal 96:1001, 1978.

107. Hollwich, F: Test a la pilocarpine dans le diagnostic precoce du glaucome. Ann Oculist 206:909, 1973.

108. Hollwich, F: The pilocarpine-test for the early diagnosis of glaucoma. Klin Montabl Augenheilk 163:115, 1973.

109. Nissen, OI, Kjer, P, Olsen, L: A comparison between an acetazolamide test and

weight tonography in pathological and apathological circulation of the aqueous humor. Invest Ophthal 15:844, 1976.

110. Drance, SM: The uniocular therapeutic trial in the management of elevated intraocular pressure. Surv Ophthal 25:203, 1980.
111. Rothkoff, L, Biedner, B, Biger, Y, Blumenthal, M: A proposed pilocarpine therapeutic test. Arch Ophthal 96:1380, 1978.
112. Goldmann, H: Open-angle glaucoma. Br J Ophthal 56:242, 1972.
113. Langham, ME: The temporal relation between intraocular pressure and loss of vision in chronic simple glaucoma. Glaucoma 2:427, 1980.
114. Becker, B, Morton, WR: Phenylthiourea taste testing and glaucoma. Arch Ophthal 72:323, 1964.
115. Kalmus, H, Lewkonia, I: Relation between some forms of glaucoma and phenylthiocarbamide testing. Br J Ophthal 57:503, 1973.
116. Shin, DH, Becker, B, Waltman, SR, Palmberg, PF, Bell, CE, Jr: The prevalence of HLA-B12 and HLA-B7 antigens in primary open-angle glaucoma. Arch Ophthal 95:224, 1977.
117. Ritch, R, Podos, SM, Henley, W, Moss, A, Southern, AL, Fotino, M: Lack of association of histocompatibility antigens with primary open-angle glaucoma. Arch Ophthal 96:2204, 1978.
118. Shaw, JF, Levene, RZ, Sowell, JG: The incidence of HLA antigens in black primary open-angle glaucoma patients. Am J Ophthal 86:501, 1978.
119. Damgaard-Jensen, L, Kissmeyer-Nielsen, F: HLA histocompatibility antigens in open-angle glaucoma. Acta Ophthal 56:384, 1978.
120. Scharf, J Gideoni, O, Zonis, S, Barzilai, A: Histocompatibility antigens (HLA) and open angle glaucoma. Ann Ophthal 10:914, 1978.
121. David, R, Maier, G, Baumgarten, I, Abrahams, C: HLA antigens in glaucoma and ocular hypertension. Br J Ophthal 63:293, 1979.
122. Rosenthal, AR, Payne, R: Association of HLA antigens and primary open-angle glaucoma. Am J Ophthal 88:479, 1979.
123. Ticho, U, Cohen, T, Brautbar, C: Absence of association between HLA antigens and primary open angle glaucoma in Israel. Israel J Med Sci 15:124, 1979.
124. Kass, MA, Palmberg, P, Becker, B, Miller, JP: Histocompatibility antigens and primary open-angle glaucoma. A reassessment. Arch Ophthal 96:2207, 1978.
125. Grant, WM: Futher studies on facility of flow through the trabecular meshwork. Arch Ophthal 60:523, 1958.
126. Ashton, N: The exit pathway of the aqueous. Trans Ophthal Soc UK 80:397, 1960.
127. Speakman, JS, Leeson, TS: Site of obstruction to aqueous outflow in chronic simple glaucoma. Br J Ophthal 46:321, 1962.
128. Zatulina, NI: Electron-microscopy of trabecular tissue in far-advanced stage of simple open-angle glaucoma. Oftal Z 28:117, 1973.
129. Segawa, K: Electron microscopic changes of the trabecular tissue in primary open-angle glaucoma. Ann Ophthal 11:49, 1979.
130. Fine, BS, Yanoff, M, Stone, RA: A clnicopathologic study of four cases of primary open-angle glaucoma compared to normal eyes. Am J Ophthal 91:88, 1981.
131. Chi, HH, Teng, CC, Katzin, HM: Experimental implants of sclera into the anterior chamber. Am J Ophthal 46:534, 1958.
132. Armaly, MF, Wang, Y: Demonstration of acid mucopolysaccharides in the trabecular meshwork of the Rhesus monkey. Invest Ophthal 14:507, 1975.
133. Chaudhry, HA, Dueker, DK, Simmons, RJ, Bellows, AR, Grant, WM: Scanning electron microscopy of trabeculectomy specimens in open-angle glaucoma. Am J Ophthal 88:78, 1979.
134. Maglio, M, McMahon, C, Hoskins, D, Alvaredo, J: Potential artifacts in scanning electron microscopy of the trabecular meshwork in glaucoma. Am J Ophthal 90:645, 1980.
135. Quigley, HA, Addicks, EM: Scanning electron microscopy of trabeculectomy specimens from eyes with open-angles glaucoma. Am J Ophthal 90:854, 1980.

136. Rohen, JW: Fine structural changes in the trabecular meshwork of the human eye in different forms of glaucoma. Klin Montabl Augenheilk 163:401, 1973.
137. Zimmerman, LE: The outflow problem in normal and pathologic eyes. Trans Am Acad Ophthal Otol 70:767, 1966.
138. Rodrigues, MM, Spaeth, GL, Silvalingam, E, Weinreb, S: Value of trabeculectomy specimens in glaucoma. Ophthal Surg 9:29, 1978.
139. Tripathi, RC: Ultrastructure of the trabecular wall of Schlemm's canal. (A study of normotensive and chronic simple glaucomatous eyes.) Trans Ophthal Soc UK 89:449, 1969.
140. Tripathi, RC: Ultrastructure of Schlemm's canal in relation to aqueous outflow. Exp Eye Res 7:335, 1968.
141. Fink, AI, Felix, MD, Fletcher, RC: Schlemm's canal and adjacent structures in glaucomatous patients. Am J Ophthal 74:893, 1972.
142. Nesterov, AP: Role of the blockade of Schlemm's canal in pathologenesis of primary open-angle glaucoma. Am J Ophthal 70:691, 1970.
143. Nesterov, AP, Batmanov, YE: Trabecular wall of Schlemm's canal in the early stage of primary open-angle glaucoma. Am J Ophthal 78:639, 1974.
144. Moses, RA, Grodzki, WJ Jr, Etheridge, EL, Wilson, CD: Schlemm's canal: the effect of intraocular pressure. Invest Ophthal Vis Sci 20:61, 1981.
145. Krasnov, MM: Sinusotomy. Foundations, results, prospects. Trans Am Acad Ophthal Otol 76:368, 1972.
146. Becker, B, Hahn, KA: Topical cortiscosteroids and heredity in primary open-angle glaucoma. Am J Ophthal 57:543, 1964.
147. Armaly, MF: The heritable nature of dexamethasone-induced ocular hypertension. Arch Ophthal 75:32, 1966.
148. Armaly, MF: Inheritance of dexamethasone hypertension and glaucoma. Arch Ophthal 77:747, 1967.
149. Schwartz, JT, Reuling, FH, Feinleib, M, Garrison, RJ, Collie, DJ: Twin study on ocular pressure after topical dexamethasone. I. Frequency distribution of pressure response. Am J Ophthal 76:126, 1973.
150. Palmberg, PF, Mandell, A, Wilensky, JT, Podos, SM, Becker, B: The reproducibility of the intraocular pressure response to dexamethasone. Am J Ophthal 80:844, 1975.
151. Dean, GO Jr, Deutsch, AR, Hiatt, RL: The effect of dexamethasone on borderline ocular hypertension. Ann Ophthal 7:193, 1975.
152. LeBlanc, RP, Stewart, RH, Becker, B: Corticosteroid provocative testing. Invest Ophthal 9:946, 1970.
153. Levene, R, Wigdor, A, Edelstein, A, Baum, J: Topical corticosteroid in normal patients and glaucoma suspects. Arch Ophthal 77:593, 1967.
154. Kitazawa, Y: Primary angle-closure glaucoma. Corticosteroid responsiveness. Arch Ophthal 84:724, 1970.
155. Becker, B: The genetic problem of chronic simple glaucoma. Ann Ophthal 3:351, 1971.
156. Francois, J, Heintz-De Bree, C, Tripathi, RC: The cortisone test and the heredity of primary open-angle glaucoma. Am J Ophthal 62:844, 1966.
157. Schwartz, JT, Reuling, FH, Feinleib, M, Garrison, RJ, Collie, DJ: Twin heritability study of the effect of corticosteroids in intraocular pressure. J Med Gen 9:137, 1972.
158. Schwartz, JT, Reuling, FH Jr, Feinleib, M, Garrison, RJ, Collie, DJ: Twin heritability study of the corticosteroid response. Trans Am Acad Ophthal Otol 77:126, 1973.
159. Schwartz, JT, Reuling, FH, Feinleib, M, Garrison, RJ, Collie, DJ: Twin study on ocular pressure following topically applied dexamethasone. II. Inheritance of variation in pressure response. Arch Ophthal 90:281, 1973.
160. Spaeth, GL: Traumatic hyphema, angle recession dexamathasone hypertension, and glaucoma. Arch Ophthal 78:714, 1967.
161. Schwartz, B, Levene, RZ: Plasma cortisol differences between normal and glaucomatous patients before and after dexamethasone suppression. Arch

Ophthal 87:369, 1972.

162. Krubin, T, Podos, SM, Becker, B: Effect of diphenylhydantoin on dexamethosone suppression of plasma cortisol in primary open-angle glaucoma. Am J Ophthal 71:997, 1971.

163. Rosenberg, S, Levene, R: Suppression of plasma cortisol in normal and glaucomatous patients. Arch Ophthal 92:6, 1974.

164. Levene, RZ, Schwartz, B, Workman, PL: Heritability of plasma cortisol. Arch Ophthal 87:389, 1972.

165. Becker, B, Ramsey, CK: Plasma cortisol and the intraocular pressure response to topical corticosteroids. Am J Ophthal 69:999, 1970.

166. Podos, SM, Becker, B, Beaty, C, Cooper, DG: Diphenylhydantoin and cortisol metabolism in glaucoma. Am J Ophthal 74:498, 1972.

167. Becker, B, Podos, SM, Asseff, CF, Cooper, DG: Plasma cortisol suppression in glaucoma. Am J Ophthal 75:73, 1973.

168. Krupin, T, Jacobs, LS, Podos, SM, Becker, B: Thyroid function and the intraocular pressure response to topical corticosteroids. Am J Ophthal 83:643, 1977.

169. Levene, RZ, Schwartz, B: Depression of plasma cortisol and the steroid ocular pressure response. Arch Ophthal 80:461, 1968.

170. Schwartz, B: Hypothalmic-pituitary-adrenal axis and steroid glaucoma. Klin Montabl Augenheilk 161:280, 1972.

171. Kass, MA, Krupin, T, Becker, B: Plasma cortisol suppression test used to predict the development of primary open-angle glaucoma. Am J Ophthal 82:496, 1976.

172. Bigger, JF, Palmberg, PF, Becker, B: Increased cellular sensitivity to glucocorticoids in primary open-angle glaucoma. Invest Ophthal 11:832, 1972.

173. Foon, KA, Yuen, K, Ballintine, EJ, Rosenstreich, DL: Analysis of the systemic corticosteroid sensitivity of patients with primary open-angle glaucoma. Am J Ophthal 83:167, 1977.

174. BenEzra, D, Ticho, U, Sachs, U: Lymphocyte sensitivity to glucocorticoids. Am J Ophthal 82:866, 1976.

175. Sowell, JG, Levene, RZ, Bloom, J, Bernstein, M: Primary open-angle glaucoma and sensitivity to corticosteroids in vitro. Am J Ophthal 84:715, 1977.

176. Palmberg, PF, Rachlin, D, Becker, B: Differential sensitivity at the cellular level in primary open-angle glaucoma: prednisolone and ouabain. Invest Ophthal 15:403, 1976.

177. Kass, MA, Shin, DH, Becker, B: The ocular hypotensive effect of epinephrine in high and low corticosteroid responders. Invest Ophthal 16:530, 1977.

178. Zink, HA, Palmberg, PF, Bigger, JF: Increased sensitivity to theophylline associated with primary open-angle glaucoma. Invest Ophthal 12:603, 1973.

179. Francois, J, Victoria-Troncoso, V: Mucopolysaccharides and pathogenesis of cortisone glaucoma. Klin Montabl Augenheilk 165:5, 1974.

180. Bill, A: The drainage of aqueous humor. Invest Ophthal 14:1, 1975.

181. Becker, B, Keates, EU, Coleman, SL: Gamma-globulin in the trabecular meshwork of glaucomatous eyes. Arch Ophthal 68:643, 1962.

182. Becker, B, Unger, HH, Coleman, SL: Plasma cells and gamma-globulin in trabecular meshwork of eyes with primary open-angle glaucoma. Arch Ophthal 70:38, 1963.

183. Waltman, SR, Yarian, D: Antinuclear antibodies in open-angle glaucoma. Invest Ophthal 13:695, 1974.

184. Shields, MB, McCoy, RC, Shelburne, JD: Immunoflourescent studies on the trabecular meshwork in open-angle glaucoma. Invest Ophthal 15:1014, 1976.

185. Rodrigues, MM, Katz, SI, Foidart, JM, Spaeth, GL: Collagen, factor VIII antigen, and immunoglobulins in the human aqueous drainage channels. Ophthalmology 87:337, 1980.

186. Felberg, NT, Leon, SA, Gasparini, J, Spaeth, GL: A comparison of antinuclear antibodies and DNA-binding antibodies in chronic open-angle glaucoma. Invest Ophthal Vis Sci 16:757, 1977.

187. Henley, WL, Okas, S, Leopold, IH: Cellular immunity in chronic ophthalmic disorders. 4. Leukocyte migration inhibition in diseases associated with glaucoma. Am J Ophthal 76:60, 1973.

188. Quigley, HA, Maumenee, AE: Long-term follow-up of treated open-angle glaucoma. Am J Ophthal 87:519, 1979.
189. Drance, SM: Chronic open angle glaucoma—present and future. The second Spaeth lecture. Can J Ophthal 12:251, 1977.
190. Drance, SM, Schulzer, M, Douglas, GR, Sweeney, VP: Use of discriminant analysis. II. Identification of persons with glaucomatous visual field defects. Arch Ophthal 96:1571, 1978.
191. Kass, MA, Hart, WM Jr, Gordon, M, Miller, JP: Risk factors favoring the development of glaucomatous visual field loss in ocular hypertension. Surv Ophthal 25:155, 1980.
192. Armaly, MF, Krueger, DE, Maunder, L, Becker, B, Hetherington, J Jr, Kolker, AE, Levene, RZ, Maumenee, AE, Pollack, IP, Shaffer, RN: Biostatistical analysis of the collaborative glaucoma study. I. Summary report of the risk factors for glaucomatous visual-field defects. Arch Ophthal 98:2163, 1980.
193. Armaly, MF: Lessons to be learned from the collaborative glaucoma study. Surv Ophthal 25:139, 1980.
194. Phelps, CD: The "no treatment" approach to ocular hypertension. Surv Ophthal 25:175, 1980.
195. Goldmann, H: An analysis of some concepts concerning chronic simple glaucoma. Am J Ophthal 80:409, 1975.
196. Luntz, MH, Schenker, HI: Retinal vascular accidents in glaucoma and ocular hyptension. Surv Ophthal 25:163, 1980.
197. Levene, RZ: Indications for medical treatment of ocular hypertension and the initial use of pilocarpine. Surv Ophthal 25:183, 1980.
198. Podos, SM, Ritch, R: Epinephrine as the initial therapy in selected cases of ocular hypertension. Surv Ophthal 25:188, 1980.
200. Richardson, KT: Medical control of the glaucomas. Br J Ophthal 56:272, 1972.
201. Kolker, AE: Visual prognosis in advanced glaucoma: A comparison of medical and surgical therapy for retention of vision in 101 eyes with advanced glaucoma. Tr Am Ophthal Soc 75:539, 1977.
202. Bloch, S, Rosenthal, AR, Friedman, L, Caldarolla, P: Patient compliance in glaucoma. Br J Ophthal 61:531, 1977.
203. Smith, RJH: Medical versus surgical therapy in glaucoma simplex. Br J Ophthal 56:277, 1972.
204. Werner, EB, Drance, SM: Progression of glaucomatous field defects despite successful filtration. Can J Ophthal 12:275, 1977.
205. Sugar, HS: Low tension glaucoma: A practical approach. Ann Ophthal 11:1155, 1979.
206. Bloomfield, S: The results of surgery for low-tension glaucoma. Am J Ophthal 36:1067, 1953.

Chapter 8

PRIMARY ANGLE-CLOSURE GLAUCOMA

PRIMARY ANGLE-CLOSURE GLAUCOMA

I. TERMINOLOGY

Several forms of primary angle-closure glaucoma are recognized on the basis of clinical presentation and mechanism of angle closure. A variety of terms have been applied to these entities, which has led to some confusion regarding nomenclature. The following *classification of primary angle-closure glaucoma*, which will be used in this chapter, provides a brief introduction to the subject. Details of mechanism and clinical appearance will be considered later in the chapter.

A. Pupillary Block Glaucoma

In this category of primary angle-closure glaucoma, the initiating event is felt to be a functional block between the pupillary portion of the iris and the anterior lens surface,[1] which is associated with mid-dilation of the pupil.[2] This functional block causes a build-up of aqueous in the posterior chamber, which leads to a forward shift of the peripheral iris and closure of the anterior chamber angle (Fig. 8.1).[1-3] Three forms of pupillary block glaucoma may be distinguished on the basis of symptoms and clinical findings:

1. *Acute angle-closure glaucoma.* In many cases of pupillary block glaucoma, the symptoms are sudden and severe, with marked pain, blurred vision, and a red eye. This clinical entity was once referred to as "congestive" glaucoma.[4]

2. *Subacute angle-closure glaucoma.*[5] This clinical entity is felt to have the same pupillary block mechanism as the acute form, but symptoms are either mild or absent. The condition has also been called intermittent, prodromal, or subclinical,[6] and was probably once lumped with the "non-congestive" glaucomas.[4] However, the latter term also included open-angle glaucoma and has been largely abandoned since Barkan[4] classified the glaucomas on the basis of an open or closed anterior chamber angle. Patients with subacute angle-closure glaucoma may have repeated subacute or subclinical attacks before finally having an acute attack or developing peripheral anterior synechiae with chronic pressure elevation.[5]

3. *Chronic angle-closure glaucoma.* In this condition, portions of the anterior chamber angle are permanently closed by *peripheral anterior synechiae*, and the intraocular pressure is chronically elevated.[6, 7] The synechial closure may result from a prolonged acute attack or repeated subacute attacks of angle-closure glaucoma. A variation of this condition has been called shortening of the angle,[8] or creeping angle-closure[9] glaucoma.

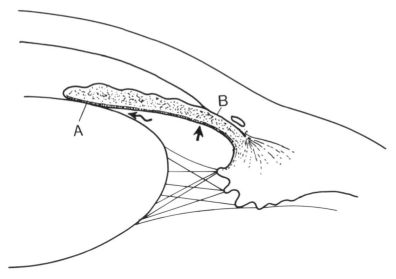

Figure 8.1. Pupillary block glaucoma. A functional block between the lens and iris (**A**) leads to increased pressure in the posterior chamber (**arrows**) with forward shift of the peripheral iris and closure of the anterior chamber angle (**B**).

B. Plateau Iris[10, 11]

In a very small percentage of patients with primary angle-closure glaucoma, the mechanism appears to be an abnormal anatomical configuration of the anterior chamber angle, which leads to occlusion of the trabecular meshwork by peripheral iris in association with dilation of the pupil. This situation differs from pupillary block glaucoma in that closure of the anterior chamber angle is apparently due to an infolding of iris into the angle in association with pupillary dilation, but without a significant pupillary block component (Fig. 8.2). The condition has been divided into the "plateau iris configuration" and "plateau iris syndrome,"[12] which will be explained later in this chapter.

C. Combined Mechanism (Mixed) Glaucoma

In some eyes there appears to be both an open-angle and an angle-closure mechanism to the glaucoma. The diagnosis is usually made after a primary acute angle-closure glaucoma attack in which the intraocular pressure remains elevated after a peripheral iridectomy, despite an open, normal appearing angle. In one study this was seen in 6 of 267 (2.2%) eyes that underwent peripheral iridectomy for presumed angle-closure glaucoma.[13]

II. EPIDEMIOLOGY

Primary angle-closure glaucoma is considerably less common than primary open-angle glaucoma, although a precise ratio between the

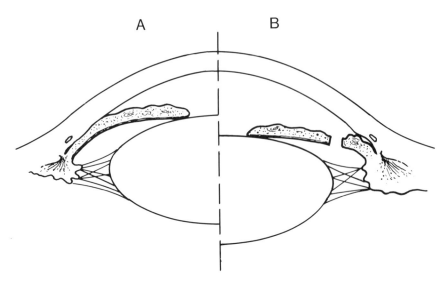

Figure 8.2. Pupillary block glaucoma (**A**) contrasted with plateau iris syndrome (**B**). In the latter situation, note the deep central anterior chamber, the flat iris plane, patent iridectomy, and bunching up of peripheral iris in the anterior chamber angle.

two conditions has not been clearly established. Studies of the anterior chamber angle within general populations suggest an approximate prevalence for individuals who may be at risk of developing angle-closure glaucoma. In a study of over 2500 consecutive individuals, about 5% had suspiciously narrow angles, but only 0.64% were considered to have critically narrow anterior chamber angles.[14] Another investigation of 947 eyes of Caucasians revealed 1.1% with angles so narrow that the iris touched the trabecular endothelial surface and 6% with anterior convexity of the peripheral iris that produced an easily occluded angle recess.[15]

III. GENERAL FEATURES OF PATIENTS

The prevalence of primary angle-closure glaucoma is influenced by the following factors:

A. Age

The depth and volume of the anterior chamber diminish with age,[16] so that the percent of individuals with critically narrow angles is higher in older age groups.[15] The prevalence of primary angle-closure glaucoma also increases with age, although it peaks earlier in life than primary open-angle glaucoma (in approximately the sixth decade[17]) and has been reported in children.[18]

B. Race

1. Primary angle-closure glaucoma is *less common* among *blacks,* and is more often of the *chronic* form when it does occur.[19-21] The

explanation for this difference is uncertain. One study suggested it might be due to a thinner average lens thickness,[20] although another investigation revealed the anterior chamber depth in Nigerian blacks to be equivalent to that of whites.[22] It has also been suggested that the weaker response to mydriatics observed among African blacks could indicate that darker irides are less able to exert the force which may lead to pupillary block.[23]

2. Some groups of the *Mongolian* race are reported to have a *higher prevalence* of primary angle-closure glaucoma. Among North Canadian Eskimos, this was found to be 0.58% in general and 2.9% in those over 40 years of age.[24] Angle-closure glaucoma was found to have a reduced prevalence in American Indians and was often secondary to a swollen lens when it did occur in this group.[21]

C. Sex

There is a statistically significant predominance of *females* in populations with primary angle-closure glaucoma, which is felt to be due to the shallower anterior chamber among women in general.[16, 17, 22, 24]

D. Refractive Error

The depth and volume of the anterior chamber are also related to the degree of ametropia, with smaller dimensions in hyperopes.[16]

E. Family History

The potential for primary angle-closure glaucoma is generally believed to be inherited. In one study, 20% of 95 relatives of angle-closure glaucoma patients were felt to have potentially occludable angles.[25] However, aside from a few reported families in which many members developed angle-closure glaucoma, the family history is not very useful in predicting a future angle-closure attack.[26]

IV. CLINICAL FEATURES

The examination of a patient with regard to the question of primary angle-closure glaucoma has several facets. During the course of every ocular evaluation, the physician should look for anatomical features that might predispose to an angle-closure attack. When suspicious findings are noted, further diagnostic measures are usually needed to determine the presence of or the potential for angle-closure glaucoma. In other situations, the patient may present with signs and symptoms suggestive of angle-closure glaucoma, and the correct diagnosis will depend on an understanding of the symptoms, predisposing circumstances, and physical findings of the disease, as well as the differential diagnosis. These various aspects will now be considered.

A. Predisposing Anatomical Features

The following clinical features describe the appearance of eyes that are anatomically predisposed to develop primary angle-closure glaucoma:

1. The *intraocular pressure* is normal or only slightly elevated unless synechial closure has begun to develop from prior angle-closure attacks. One study, however, found a larger than normal amplitude in the diurnal intraocular pressure curve, which the authors felt might have prognostic value.[27] *Tonography* also characteristically reveals normal outflow facility before or between attacks, unless synechial damage has begun to develop.[2]

2. *External examination.* Since the intraocular pressure does not provide a clue regarding the potential for developing an angle-closure attack, other parameters must be sought. The most useful of these is the anatomy of the anterior chamber angle. Although this is best evaluated with the slit lamp and goniolens, it has been shown that estimation of the anterior chamber depth with *oblique flashlight illumination* (Fig. 8.3) can be a useful screening measure.[28]

3. *Slit lamp examination.* The central anterior chamber depth may be estimated during examination with the slit lamp, and techniques for making this measurement have been proposed.[29, 30] Of more diagnostic value within the context of angle-closure glaucoma, however, is the depth of the *peripheral anterior chamber.*[31] van Herick and co-workers[32] developed a technique for making this estimation

A

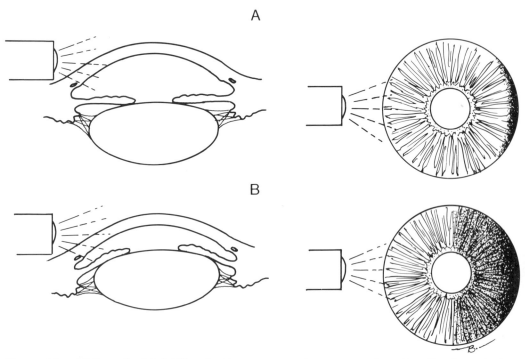

B

Figure 8.3. Oblique flashlight illumination as a screening measure for estimating the anterior chamber depth. **A:** with a deep chamber, nearly the entire iris is illuminated. **B:** when the iris is bowed forward, only the proximal portion is illuminated, and a shadow is seen in the distal half.

by comparing the peripheral anterior chamber depth to the thickness of the adjacent cornea (Fig. 8.4). When the depth is less than ¼ corneal thickness, the anterior chamber angle is usually dangerously narrow.[32]

4. *Gonioscopy.* Whenever the peripheral anterior chamber is felt to be shallow (van Herick slit lamp Grade 1 or 2), careful gonioscopic examination of the angle is required. Numerous *grading systems* have been suggested in an attempt to correlate gonioscopic appearance with potential for angle-closure:

a. Scheie[33] proposed a system based on the extent of *anterior*

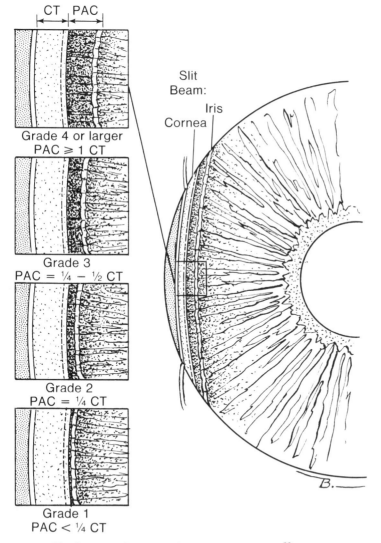

CT PAC

Slit
Beam:

Iris

Cornea

Grade 4 or larger
PAC ≥ 1 CT

Grade 3
PAC = ¼ − ½ CT

Grade 2
PAC = ¼ CT

Grade 1
PAC < ¼ CT

B.

Figure 8.4.   Slit lamp technique of van Herick *et al*,[32] for estimating the depth of the peripheral anterior chamber (**PAC**) by comparing it to the adjacent corneal thickness (**CT**).

chamber angle structures that can be visualized (Fig. 8.5). He noted a high risk of angle closure in eyes with Grade III or IV angles.

Scheie Classification	Gonioscopic Appearance
Wide open	All structures visible
Grade I narrow	Hard to see over iris root into recess
Grade II narrow	Ciliary band obscured
Grade III narrow	Posterior trabeculum obscured
Grade IV narrow (closed)	Only Schwalbe's line visible

b. Shaffer[34] suggested using the *angular width* of the angle recess as the criterion for grading the angle and attempted to correlate this with the potential for angle-closure (Fig. 8.6).

Shaffer Classification	Clinical Interpretation
Wide open (20–45°)	Closure improbable
Moderately narrow	Closure possible
Extremely narrow (10°)	Closure probable
Partially or totally closed	Closure present

c. Other authors feel that any single criterion does not fully describe the anterior chamber angle. Becker[35] proposed combining an estimation of the anterior chamber angle width and the height of the iris insertion, while Spaeth[15, 36] suggested an evaluation of the

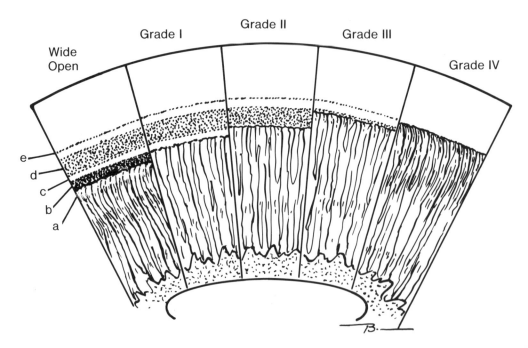

Figure 8.5. Scheie's[33] gonioscopic classification of the anterior chamber angle, based on the extent of visible angle structures: **a:** root of the iris; **b:** ciliary body band; **c:** scleral spur; **d:** trabecular meshwork; **e:** Schwalbe's line. (See details in text.)

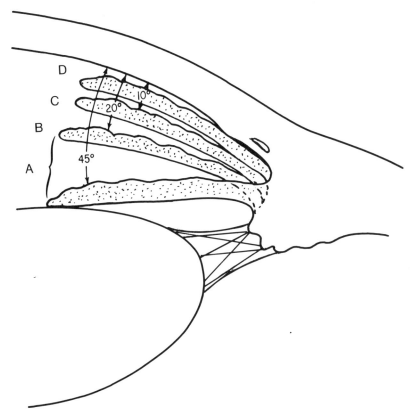

Figure 8.6. Shaffer's[34] gonioscopic classification of the anterior chamber angle, based on the angular width of the angle recess: **A:** wide open; **B:** moderately narrow; **C:** extremely narrow; **D:** partially or totally closed. (See interpretations in text.)

following *three variables* (Fig. 8.7):

Spaeth Classification	
Criteria	*Designations*
Angular width of angle recess	0–40°
Configuration of peripheral iris	q, r, s,
"Insertion" of iris root	A–E

d. Other clinicians prefer descriptive words and drawings over arbitrary classifications. In the final analysis, the greatest value in each of the aforementioned grading systems is the awareness they provide of the multiple parameters that must be considered in evaluating the anterior chamber angle and in interpreting one's findings.

B. Adjunctive Tests

Having decided that a patient has suspiciously narrow anterior chamber angles, the physician is now faced with a difficult decision. If it could be predicted that the patient would one day have an attack

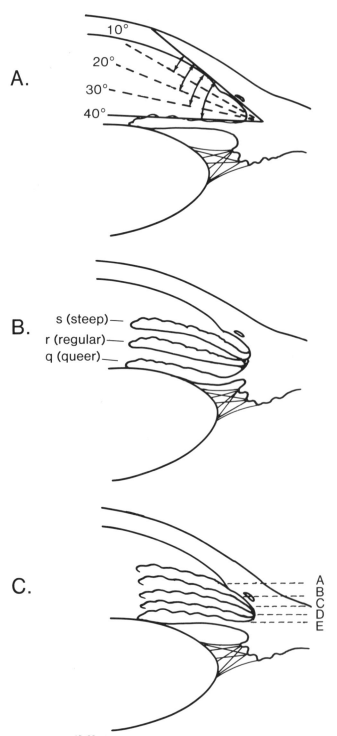

Figure 8.7. Spaeth's[15, 36] gonioscopic classification of the anterior chamber angle, based on three variables: **A:** angular width of the angle recess; **B:** configuration of the peripheral iris; and **C:** apparent insertion of the iris root.

of angle-closure glaucoma, the appropriate course in most cases would be prophylactic peripheral iridectomies. The results of one study suggest that optic nerve damage occurs in the early time period after intraocular pressure rise, supporting the value of detection and surgery prior to an attack.[17] Unfortunately, however, it is usually not possible to predict with certainty, on the basis of the anterior chamber angle appearance, which patients will eventually suffer a glaucomatous attack. For this reason, adjunctive tests have been devised to improve the detection rate of primary angle-closure glaucoma patients.

1. *Provocative tests.* A variety of tests have been designed to precipitate an angle-closure attack, with the rationale that it is better for this to occur in the physician's office, where it can be treated promptly, than in a situation where it might go unrecognized or where medical attention might not be readily available. It is important that a provocative test be as physiologic as possible in an effort to create a situation that might occur under natural circumstances.

a. *Mydriatic provocative tests.* A short acting topical mydriatic (*e.g.*, 0.5% tropicamide) is instilled, and a rise in intraocular pressure of 8 mmHg or more is considered to be a positive test. However, gonioscopic confirmation of angle closure is essential, since mydriatics and cycloplegics can also cause pressure rises in eyes with open anterior chamber angles, as discussed in Chapter Seven.

b. *Dark room provocative test.* Mydriasis is induced by placing the patient in a dark room for 60 to 90 min. It is important that the patient remain awake during this time to avoid the miosis of sleep. A positive test again is taken as a pressure rise of 8 mmHg or more with gonioscopic confirmation of angle closure. Exposure to light should be kept to a minimum during the post-dark room studies to avoid reversing the pressure-inducing mechanism.[37] It has also been reported that using a 30% decrease in the tonographic facility of outflow as an additional parameter increased the positive yield from 30 to 67%.[38]

c. *Prone provocative test.* The patient is placed in a prone position for 60 min, and a pressure rise of 8 mmHg or more is taken as a positive response.[39] The mechanism of angle closure with this test is uncertain, but it is apparently not related to mydriasis.[40] One theory holds that angle closure during prone provocative testing is due to pupillary block associated with a slight forward shift of the lens, although no significant shallowing of the anterior chamber could be demonstrated in patients with positive prone provocative tests.[41]

The prone provocative test was compared to the mydriatic and dark room tests in 76 angle-closure glaucoma eyes and was found to yield 71% positive responses before peripheral iridectomy and 6.5% after surgery in contrast to 58 and 1.4%, respectively, for the mydriatic test, and 48 and 6.5% with the dark room test.[42] In another study of 19 patients with a diagnosis of narrow angle glaucoma, the percentage of positive provocative tests was approximately 50% with either the prone or the dark room test alone, compared to 11 and 16% with phenylephrine or cyclopentolate mydriatic provocative testing, respectively.[40] If both a prone test and a dark room test is performed separately on the same patient, the yield is almost 90% positives.[40]

The reported routine at the Massachusetts Eye and Ear Infirmary for patients with narrow angles considered capable of closing or narrow angles with a history suggestive of prior attacks is a prone/dark room provocative test, which is repeated every 6 months as long as it is negative.[43]

d. *Pilocarpine/phenylephrine test.*[44-47] Two percent pilocarpine and 10% phenylephrine are instilled simultaneously every minute for three applications to achieve a mid-dilated pupil. If this does not achieve a positive response (intraocular pressure rise greater than 8 mmHg) in 2 hr, the test is repeated. If the second test is also negative after 90 min, it is terminated with 0.5% thymoxamine, and a mydriatic provocative test with 0.5% tropicamide is performed on another day. In a study of 119 high risk patients, 74 had positive responses with the initial pilocarpine/phenylephrine test, while nine more had positive responses to tropicamide, and only one of the remaining 36 developed angle-closure glaucoma during an average 3-year follow-up.[44]

e. Another provocative test utilizes *annular compression* with a 16-mm suction cup to produce forward shift of the lens-iris diaphragm.[48]

f. Still others feel that no currently available provocative test is suitable and stress instead the importance of an accurate history and physical examination as the best guide to management.[49]

2. Another suggested adjunctive test for identifying angle-closure glaucoma suspects is *ultrasonography* for measuring the anterior chamber depth.[50] HLA antigens were studied in 35 angle-closure glaucoma patients, and no correlation was found.[51]

C. Precipitating Factors

In an eye that is anatomically predisposed to develop angle-closure, the following factors may precipitate an attack.

1. *Factors which produce mydriasis.*

a. *Dim illumination.* A common history is the onset of an acute attack when the patient is in a dark room, such as a theater or restaurant. It has been reported that the incidence of angle-closure glaucoma increases in the winter, although a direct association with hours of sunshine and an inverse association with cloud amount was also noted, which the authors thought might be related to the contrast between day and evening levels of illumination.[52]

b. *Emotional stress.* Occasionally an acute angle-closure attack will follow severe emotional stress. It may be that this is related to the mydriasis of increased sympathetic tone, although the exact mechanism is not fully understood.

c. *Drugs.* Mydriatics may also precipitate a primary angle-closure attack in an anatomically predisposed eye:

(1). *Anticholinergics* (*e.g.*, atropine, cyclopentolate, tropicamide, etc.) create a particularly high risk when administered topically.[53, 54] In one study, 0.5% cyclopentolate precipitated attacks in 9 of 21 (43%) high risk eyes, while 0.5% tropicamide did the same in 19 of 58 (33%) eyes.[55] Systemic atropine can also create a hazard, especially when large doses are used during surgery, and it has been suggested that high risk eyes should be protected with topical pilocarpine before, during, and after surgery.[56] However, miosis can also precipitate angle-closure attacks, and an alternative approach to managing the high risk eye might be close observation during the postoperative period. Other systemic drugs with weaker anticholinergic properties (*e.g.*, anti-histaminic, anti-parkinsonism, anti-psychotic, and gastrointestinal spasmolytic drugs) also present a risk proportional to the pupillary effect.[54]

(2). *Adrenergics.* The mydriatic effect of topical *epinephrine* may precipitate an angle-closure attack in the predisposed eye. *Phenylepherine* can also precipitate an attack, although it was found to be safer than cyclopentolate or tropicamide for dilating high risk eyes.[55] In addition, systemic drugs with adrenergic properties (*e.g.*, vasoconstrictors, central nervous system stimulants, appetite depressants, bronchodilators, and hallucinogenic agents) may also present a risk in the predisposed eye.[54]

2. *Factors which produce miosis.* As previously noted, miosis may occasionally lead to an acute attack of primary angle-closure glaucoma. This has been observed following the miosis induced by reading or bright lights. It is uncertain whether the mechanism is an increase in the relative pupillary block due to a wider zone of contact between iris and lens or relaxation of the lens zonules, allowing a forward shift of the iris-lens diaphragm. Angle closure may also be precipitated by *strong miotics*, such as the cholinesterase inhibitors (*e.g.*, diisopropyl fluorophosphate and echothiophate iodide), and it has been speculated that this is either due to the miosis or congestion of the uveal tract. Chandler[2] favors the former theory, since he noted that an acute rise in intraocular pressure following the use of a miotic did not occur in an eye with a peripheral iridectomy.

3. Vasodilators were once felt to create a risk of precipitating angle-closure attacks, but this has subsequently been disproven.[54, 57]

D. Symptoms

Primary angle-closure glaucoma, in marked contrast to primary open-angle glaucoma, is characterized by profound symptoms. However, there is a wide spectrum regarding the severity of these symptoms:

1. *Subacute angle-closure glaucoma.* This form of the disease may have no recognizable symptoms. Studies have suggested that intermittent partial angle closure may occur without clinical symptoms[58] and may be one of the causes of ocular hypertension.[59] In other cases,

the patient may notice a dull ache behind the eye and/or slight blurring of vision. A symptom that is particularly typical of the subacute acute is *colored halos around lights.* This is felt to result from an alteration in the cornea, which causes it to act as a diffraction grating, producing a blue-green central and yellow-red peripheral halo.[14] These symptoms, which more often occur at night after the patient has been in a dark room, will often spontaneously clear by the following morning, presumably due to the miosis of sleep.

2. *Acute angle-closure glaucoma.* This condition is characterized by pain, redness, and blurred vision.[14] The *pain* is typically a severe, deep ache, which follows the trigeminal distribution and may be associated with nausea, vomiting, bradycardia, and profuse sweating. The *conjunctival hyperemia* is usually both a ciliary flush and peripheral conjunctival congestion. The *blurred vision*, which is typically marked, is felt to be due to stretching of the corneal lamellae initially and later to edema of the cornea.

E. Clinical Findings During an Acute Attack

1. The *central visual acuity* is significantly reduced, and the *intraocular pressure* is markedly elevated, usually in a range of 40 to 60 mmHg or more.

2. *External examination.* Characteristic findings include the previously noted conjunctival hyperemia, a cloudy cornea, and an irregular (usually vertically oval), mid-dilated, fixed pupil. The pupillary change is thought to result from paralysis of the sphincter, which is apparently due to a reduction in circulation induced by the elevated intraocular pressure,[60-62] and possibly to degeneration of the ciliary ganglion.[63]

3. *Slit lamp examination.* This confirms the corneal edema, which frequently must be cleared by topical application of glycerin before the anterior chamber can be studied. The anterior chamber is shallow, but typically is formed centrally with anterior *bowing of the mid-peripheral iris*, often making contact with peripheral cornea. Aqueous flare may be present due to increased protein concentration.[64] Other findings may include pigment dispersion, sector atrophy of the iris, and glaukomflecken, which are irregular white opacities in the anterior portion of the lens.

4. *Gonioscopy.* It is essential to confirm the diagnosis by demonstrating a *closed anterior chamber angle.* If gonioscopy is not possible due to persistent corneal edema, gonioscopy of the fellow eye may provide useful information if it reveals an extremely narrow angle. In a study of 10 eyes with angle-closure glaucoma, the Koeppe lens was felt to be more reliable than the Goldmann three-mirror or Zeiss four-mirror lenses in determining whether the angle was open or closed, because it caused no artifactual widening of the angle and allowed the best view over a convex iris.[65, 66] Peripheral anterior synechiae may also be present, and the techniques and importance of making this determination will be discussed later in this chapter.

5. *Fundus examination.* The *optic nerve head* may be hyperemic and edematous in the early stages of the attack. Monkeys exposed to high intraocular pressures usually developed congestion of the optic nerve head within 12 to 15 hr, which persisted for 4 to 5 days. The disc then became pale, and glaucomatous cupping was observed after 9 to 10 days.[67] In a study of human eyes with a history of angle-closure glaucoma, pallor but no cupping was seen in eyes following acute attacks, while both pallor and cupping occurred in chronic cases.[68]

6. *Visual fields.* As discussed in Chapter 5, visual field changes associated with acute elevation of intraocular pressure typically show non-specific constriction. In one study of 25 patients with acute angle-closure glaucoma that had been surgically corrected, the most common field defect was constriction of the upper field,[69] while another revealed nerve fiber bundle defects in 7 of 18 acute and 9 of 11 chronic cases.[68]

F. Differential Diagnosis

The sudden onset of pain, redness, and blurred vision, which characterizes the acute primary angle-closure glaucoma attack, may also be seen with other forms of glaucoma, creating a differential diagnostic problem:

1. *Open-angle glaucomas* may occasionally present as an acute attack, especially when secondary to events such as inflammation, hemorrhage, or rubeosis iridis. These cases are usually readily distinguished from primary angle-closure glaucoma on the basis of the gonioscopic appearance and associated findings. However, in the eye with an elevated intraocular pressure and a narrow anterior chamber angle, it may be difficult to distinguish between primary angle-closure glaucoma and primary open-angle glaucoma with narrow angles. A *thymoxamine test* has been suggested for this situation.[70] Thymoxamine is an α-adrenergic blocker, which produces miosis by relaxation of the dilator muscle without effecting the ciliary musculature. Topical thymoxamine 0.5% can often open a narrow or appositionally-closed angle, but will not alter the intraocular pressure in an eye with open-angle glaucoma.[70]

2. *Secondary angle-closure glaucomas* may present even more difficult diagnostic problems, especially when the initiating event is posterior to the lens-iris diaphragm, where early detection can be difficult. The following are some of the ocular disorders that may lead to secondary angle closure (the details of these conditions will be considered in subsequent chapters):

    a. Central retinal vein occlusion (Chapter 15).

    b. Ciliary body swelling, inflammation, or cysts (Chapters 16, 19).

    c. Ciliary block (malignant) glaucoma (Chapter 19).

    d. Posterior segment tumors (Chapter 11).

    e. Contracting fibrous tissue (Chapter 19).

f. Scleral buckling procedures and panretinal photocoagulation (Chapter 15).

g. Nanophthalmos (Chapter 15).

h. Corneal thickening (Chapter 12).

V. THEORIES OF MECHANISM

A. Relative Pupillary Block

As noted earlier in this chapter, the most common mechanism leading to primary angle-closure glaucoma appears to be increased resistance to aqueous flow from the posterior to the anterior chamber between the iris and lens. This concept was suggested by Curran[1, 71] and Banziger[3] in the early 1920s, and advanced by the teachings of Chandler,[2] who noted that an eye with a shallow anterior chamber has a wider zone of contact between the surfaces of the iris and lens (Fig. 8.1). He postulated that the musculature of the iris exerts a backward pressure against the lens which increases the resistance to flow of aqueous into the anterior chamber. This increases the pressure in the posterior chamber, causing the thin peripheral iris to bulge into the anterior chamber angle. Gonioscopic studies by Mapstone[72, 73] suggest that this angle closure may occur in two stages, with the first being iridocorneal contact anterior to the trabecular meshwork, followed by apposition of the iris to the meshwork as the pressure rises (Fig. 8.8). There is considerable clinical evidence which strongly favors the basic concept of pupillary block, the most convincing of which is the excellent response to peripheral iridectomy, which presumably works by circumventing the block (Fig. 8.9).[2]

1. *Anatomical factors predisposing to pupillary block.* Several anatomical aspects of the eye combine to produce a *shallow anterior chamber.* These include a thicker, more anteriorly placed *lens*, a smaller diameter and shorter posterior curvature of the *cornea*, and a shorter axial length of the *globe.*[74-79] In addition, Spaeth[15] observed that relatives of patients with angle-closure glaucoma tended to have a more *anterior insertion of the iris* into the ciliary body, a *narrower angular approach* to the recess of the anterior chamber angle, and a more *anterior peripheral convexity* of the iris than the average eye. All of the above parameters are variably influenced by *hyperopia,* increasing *age,* and *genetics.*

2. *The significance of pupillary dilation.* Chandler,[2] emphasized that a *mid-dilated pupil* of 3.5 to 6 mm is the critical degree of dilation that seems to bring on the acute attack. He felt this might be due to continued pupillary block combined with sufficient relaxation of peripheral iris to allow its forward displacement into the anterior chamber. In addition, Mapstone[80] proposed a mathematical model in which the combined pupil-blocking forces of the dilator and sphincter muscles and the stretching force of the iris were greatest with a mid-dilated pupil (Fig. 8.10). Factors which may precipitate an angle-closure attack by dilating the pupil were discussed earlier in this chapter.

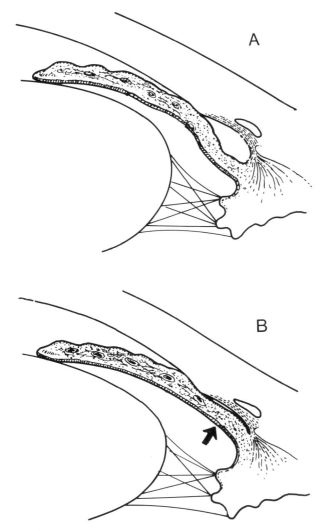

Figure 8.8. Two stages of anterior chamber angle closure in pupillary block glaucoma according to Mapstone.[72, 73] **A:** iridocorneal contact in early stage of angle closure, and **B:** iridotrabecular contact in advanced stage (**arrow** indicates pressure effect in posterior chamber).

B. Plateau Iris

A second basic mechanism leading to primary angle-closure glaucoma appears to result from an abnormal anatomical configuration of the anterior chamber angle. It is far less common than the pupillary block mechanism and is usually recognized after a peripheral iridectomy for presumed pupillary block glaucoma has failed. *Two variations* of plateau iris have been described.[12]

1. *Plateau iris configuration.* This diagnosis is made pre-operatively, based on the gonioscopic findings of a closed anterior chamber angle, but a *flat iris plane* (as opposed to the forward bowing of

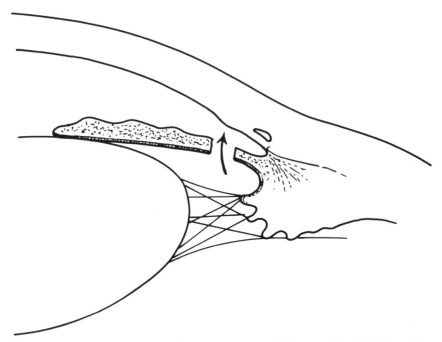

Figure 8.9. The strongest evidence in support of the pupillary block mechanism of angle-closure glaucoma is the excellent response to peripheral iridectomy, which circumvents the block (**arrow**).

peripheral iris with the pupillary block mechanism) and a normal central anterior chamber depth. Relative pupillary block plays a significant role in this situation, and most of these cases are cured by peripheral iridectomy.

2. *Plateau iris syndrome.* This constitutes a small percentage of eyes with the plateau iris configuration and represents the true plateau iris mechanism. The peripheral iris bunches up in the anterior chamber angle when the pupil is dilated, presumably due in part to an anterior insertion of the iris (Fig. 8.2). This diagnosis is made postoperatively when angle closure recurs with pupillary dilation despite a patent iridectomy and deep central anterior chamber. These cases are treated with pilocarpine.

C. Other Factors

Other factors that reportedly may contribute to the mechanism of primary angle-closure glaucoma include 1) an anomalous position or swelling of the ciliary body and ciliary processes,[81] 2) increased trabecular meshwork outflow in combination with pupillary block, which pulls the iris on to the cornea,[82] 3) direct lens-block angle-closure due to a forward movement of the lens,[83] which may in some cases be related to vitreous liquefaction with posterior pooling of aqueous and forward displacement of the lens-iris diaphragm,[84] and 4) increased vitreous hydration following a sudden increase in intraocular pressure.[85]

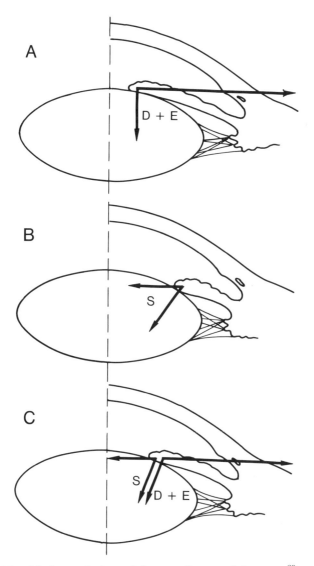

Figure 8.10. Mathematical model according to Mapstone[80] attempts to explain the importance of a mid-dilated pupil in the pupillary block mechanism: **A:** in miosis, the dilator muscle (**D**) and the stretching effect of the iris (**E**) have their greatest pupil-blocking (posterior vector) force. **B:** in mydriasis, the sphincter muscle (**S**) has its greatest pupil-blocking force. **C:** In mid-dilation, the combined effect of **S** and **D + E** creates the maximum pupil-blocking force.

D. Chronic Angle-closure Glaucoma

Peripheral anterior synechiae may eventually develop with prolonged or recurrent acute or subacute attacks, leading to chronic angle-closure glaucoma. In addition, a more insidious form has been recognized in which the angle slowly closes from the periphery toward Schwalbe's line.[6, 8, 9] The synechial closure usually begins superiorly, where the angle is normally narrowest, and progresses inferiorly.[7] This condition has been referred to as *shortening of the angle*[8] or *creeping angle-closure.*[9] These cases are frequently cured by peripheral iridectomy if detected early enough, but occasionally require filtering surgery.

VI. MANAGEMENT

The details regarding drugs and surgical procedures used in the treatment of primary angle-closure glaucoma are considered in Section Three. The present discussion will be limited to the general approach and basic concepts of the management.

A. Medical Therapy

Although the vast majority of eyes with primary angle-closure glaucoma are managed surgically, it is desirable to first bring the glaucoma under medical control. In the case of an acute attack, this constitutes a medical emergency and is approached in *two stages*: 1) reduce the intraocular pressure and 2) break the angle closure:

1. *Reduction of intraocular pressure.* Miotic therapy is frequently ineffective when the intraocular pressure is high, presumably because the pressure-induced ischemia of the iris leads to paralysis of the sphincter muscle.[60-62] For this reason, the first line of defense is to administer drugs that will promptly lower the intraocular pressure:

a. *Carbonic anhydrase inhibitors* (*e.g.*, acetazolamide 500 mg intramuscularly, intravenously, or orally) will, in many cases, sufficiently lower the pressure for the miotic to be effective.[86]

b. *Hyperosmotics* are often used in conjunction with the acetazolamide. This may be given orally as *glycerol* or *isosorbide* or, if the patient is too nauseated to tolerate oral medication, it may be given intravenously as *mannitol* or *urea*.

c. The topical administration of *timolol* has also been reported to be a valuable alternative when systemic medication is contraindicated.[87]

d. *Corneal indentation.* Anderson[88] has described an office maneuver which may obviate the need for a hyperosmotic to break an attack of acute angle-closure glaucoma. After gonioscopically confirming the diagnosis of angle-closure glaucoma, the central cornea is indented with a soft instrument, such as a cotton-tipped applicator, for several 30-sec intervals. This opens the anterior chamber angle by forcing aqueous from the central to the peripheral portion of the anterior chamber and eventually reduces the intraocular pressure (Fig. 8.11). A carbonic anhydrase inhibitor and pilocarpine are still needed to keep the angle open and prevent another attack before surgery.

2. *Miotic therapy.* Once the intraocular pressure has been reduced, a miotic is instilled to break the pupillary block and open the anterior chamber angle.

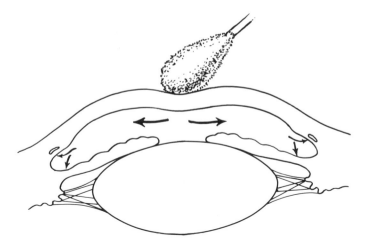

Figure 8.11. Corneal indentation with a soft instrument, such as a cotton-tipped applicator, may lower the intraocular pressure during a primary angle-closure attack by forcing aqueous from the central to the peripheral anterior chamber (**arrows**), thereby temporarily opening the chamber angle and re-establishing aqueous outflow (Anderson[88]).

a. *Pilocarpine.* A single drop of pilocarpine approximately 3 hours after administration of acetazolamide[86, 87] or timolol[88] has been reported to effectively break the angle-closure attack. This is also safer than copious use of the drug since it reduces the chances of pilocarpine toxicity. Since the concentration of the pilocarpine does not appear to be important in this situation,[88] a low dosage of 1 to 2% is preferable.

b. *Thymoxamine* has theoretic advantages over pilocarpine, since the mechanism of miosis is relaxation of the dilator muscle, which permits its use during high pressures and reduces the posterior vector force caused by sphincter contracture.[89, 90] However, others have not found thymoxamine alone to be effective in the treatment of angle-closure glaucoma.[91] Furthermore, the drug is not presently commercially available in the United States.

c. Strong miotics, such as eserine and echothiophate iodide, are generally contraindicated in acute angle-closure glaucoma, since they may aggravate the situation by producing vascular congestion or increasing the pupillary block.

B. Surgical Management

Once the intraocular pressure has been brought under control medically (or all efforts at medical control have been exhausted), the surgeon is then faced with *two decisions*: 1) when to operate and 2) what procedure to use:

1. *When to operate.*

a. In the uncommon event that the elevated pressure can not be controlled medically, Chandler and Grant[92] advise considering surgery within the next few hours, especially if vision is failing. The surgical risks are considerably higher under these circumstances, and Anderson[88] notes that Kolker has recommended corneal indentation to lower the pressure in such cases before surgery.

b. If the intraocular pressure does respond to medical therapy, the eye should be re-examined gonioscopically to determine the mechanism of the pressure reduction:

(1). An open anterior chamber angle without corneal indentation by the goniolens suggests that the angle-closure attack has been broken. In this situation, there is less urgency as to when to operate, although surgeons differ as to when they will proceed with surgery. Some do so within the next several hours, while others may wait a day or two. If surgery is delayed, topical steroids to quieten the eye may be beneficial.

(2). If the angle is still closed, it may be that the pressure reduction is due to the carbonic anhydrase inhibitor and hyperosmotic and that the attack has not actually been broken. Since the high pressure may recur as the effects of these medications begin to wear off, consideration should be given to surgery within the next few hours.

2. *What operation to use.* The eye with primary angle-closure glaucoma typically responds well to a *peripheral iridectomy.* However, follow-up studies indicate that approximately 25% of these eyes will eventually require the addition of medication to control the pressure and some will need *filtering surgery.*[13, 93-95] There is some controversy as to whether eyes requiring filtering surgery can be identified prior to the initial procedure, but the following techniques have been proposed for this purpose:

a. *Chamber deepening procedures.* Most cases that need a filtering operation have *peripheral anterior synechiae* involving more than half of the angle.[95, 96] Forbes[97, 98] has described a procedure in which the degree of synechial closure can be determined pre-operatively by indenting the central cornea with a Zeiss four-mirror gonioprism. This forces aqueous into the peripheral portion of the anterior chamber, thereby deepening it and facilitating visualization of the angle (Fig. 8.12). Similar approaches have been suggested for use at the time of surgery. Chandler and Simmons[96] deepen the anterior chamber with saline and study the angle with a Koeppe goniolens before proceeding with the surgery, while Shaffer[99] performs the same maneuver after making an iridectomy. These procedures may also be performed with the Goldman gonioprism and the operating microscope.

b. *Other diagnostic adjuncts.* It has also been suggested that *tonography* may be helpful by indicating the amount of residual outflow obstruction after the angle-closure attack has been medically broken,[100] and one study indicated that *visual field loss* prior to surgery is an indication to proceed with a filtering procedure.[101] The duration of the acute attack does not appear to be a reliable indicator as to whether a filtering operation is needed instead of a peripheral iridectomy.[101, 102]

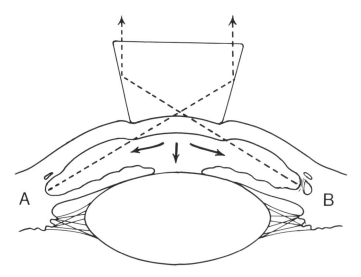

Figure 8.12. Indentation gonioscopy with a Zeiss four-mirror gonioprism deepens the peripheral anterior chamber by displacing aqueous from the central chamber (**arrows**). This facilitates gonioscopic examination of the chamber angle before surgery to distinguish between appositional (**A**) and synechial (**B**) closure of the angle (Forbes[97, 98]).

c. Many surgeons feel that it is not possible to predict which eyes will require filtering surgery (other than possibly by visual field loss[101]), and recommend a peripheral iridectomy in nearly all cases, with the addition of medication or further surgery as required.[13, 93, 94, 101, 102] The importance of close follow-up during the early postoperative period has been emphasized.[94]

3. A *prophylactic peripheral iridectomy* is generally recommended in two situations relative to primary angle-closure glaucoma:

a. *The fellow eye.* Several large studies have shown that approximately 50 to 75% of the patients who develop primary angle-closure glaucoma in one eye will have an attack in the fellow, unoperated eye within 5 to 10 years despite miotic prophylaxis,[103–108] whereas such an attack after an iridectomy is rare.[106, 109] For this reason, most surgeons recommend a prophylactic peripheral iridectomy in the fellow eye of patients who have had an angle-closure attack. Rare exceptions to this include a deeper anterior chamber in the fellow eye due to anisometropia or a dislocated lens or an elderly patient controlled for years on miotics.[92] As an alternative approach, it has been suggested that fellow eyes with negative provocative tests, which was 23% in one series, might be followed closely without surgery.[110]

b. A *positive provocative test* for angle-closure glaucoma or a strong history of a previous angle-closure attack (with consistent physical findings) is also taken by most surgeons as an indication to recommend a prophylactic peripheral iridectomy.

References

1. Curran, EJ: A new operation for glaucoma involving a new principle in the aetiology and treatment of chronic primary glaucoma. Arch Ophthal 49:131, 1920.
2. Chandler, PA: Narrow-angle glaucoma. Arch Ophthal 47:695, 1952.
3. Banziger, T: The mechanism of acute glaucoma and the explanation for the effectiveness of iridectomy for the same. Ber Deutsch Ophthal Ges 43:43, 1922.
4. Barkan, O: Glaucoma: Classification, causes, and surgical control. Results of microgonioscopic research. Am J Ophthal 21:1099, 1938.
5. Chandler, PA, Trotter, RR: Angle-closure glaucoma. Subacute types. Arch Ophthal 53:305, 1955.
6. Pollack, IP: Chronic angle-closure glaucoma. Diagnosis and treatment in patients with angles that appear open. Arch Ophthal 85:676, 1971.
7. Bhargava, SK, Leighton, DA, Phillips, CI: Early angle-closure glaucoma. Distribution of iridotrabecular contact and response to pilocarpine. Arch Ophthal 89:369, 1973.
8. Gorin, G: Shortening of the angle of the anterior chamber in angle-closure glaucoma. Am J Ophthal 49:141, 1960.
9. Lowe, RF: Primary creeping angle-closure glaucoma. Br J Ophthal 48:544, 1964.
10. Tornquist, R: Angle-closure glaucoma in an eye with a plateau type of iris. Acta Ophthal 36:413, 1958.
11. Shaffer, RN: Gonioscopy, ophthalmoscopy, and perimetry. Trans Am Acad Ophthal Otol 64:112, 1960.
12. Wand, M, Grant, WM, Simmons, RJ, Hutchinson, BT: Plateau iris syndrome. Trans Am Acad Ophthal Otol 83:122, 1977.
13. Hyams, SW, Keroub, C, Pokotilo, E: Mixed glaucoma. Br J Ophthal 61:105, 1977.
14. Kolker, A, Hetherington, J Jr: Becker-Shaffer's Diagnosis and Therapy of the Glaucomas, 4th ed. CV Mosby Co, St Louis, 1976, p 183.
15. Spaeth, GL: The normal development of the human anterior chamber angle: A new system of descriptive grading. Trans Ophthal Soc UK 91:709, 1971.
16. Fontana, ST, Brubaker, RF: Volume and depth of the anterior chamber in the normal aging human eye. Arch Ophthal 98:1803, 1980.
17. Hillman, JS: Acute closed-angle glaucoma: An investigation into the effect of delay in treatment. Br J Ophthal 63:817, 1979.
18. Appleby, RS Jr, Kinder, RSL: Bilateral angle-closure glaucoma in a 14-year old boy. Arch Ophthal 86:449, 1971.
19. Alper, MG, Laubach, JL: Primary angle-closure glaucoma in the American Negro. Arch Ophthal 79:663, 1968.
20. Clemmesen, V, Luntz, MH: Lens thickness and angle-closure glaucoma. A comparative oculometric study in South African Negroes and Danes. Acta Ophthal 54:193, 1976.
21. Wilensky, J: Racial influences in glaucoma. Ann Ophthal 9:1545, 1977.
22. Olurin, O: Anterior chamber depths of Nigerians. Ann Ophthal 9:315, 1977.
23. Emiru, VP: Response to mydriatics in the African. Br J Ophthal 55:538, 1971.
24. Drance, SM: Angle closure glaucoma among Canadian Eskimos: Can J Ophthal 8:252, 1973.
25. Spaeth, GL: Gonioscopy: uses old and new. The inheritance of occludable angles. Ophthalmology 85:222, 1978.
26. Lichter, PR, Anderson, DR, ed: Discussions on Glaucoma. Grune & Stratton, New York, 1977, p 139.
27. Shapiro, A, Zauberman, H: Diurnal changes of the intraocular pressure of patients with angle-closure glaucoma. Br J Ophthal 63:225, 1979.
28. Vargas, E, Drance, SM: Anterior chamber depth in angle-closure glaucoma. Clinical methods of depth determination in people with and without the disease. Arch Ophthal 90:438, 1973.
29. Smith, RJH: A new method of estimating the depth of the anterior chamber. Br J Ophthal 63:215, 1979.

30. Jacobs, IH: Anterior chamber depth measurement using the slit-lamp microscope. Am J Ophthal 88:236, 1979.
31. Chan, RY, Smith, JA, Richardson, KT: Anterior segment configuration correlated with Shaffer's grading of anterior chamber angle. Arch Ophthal 99:104, 1981.
32. van Herick, W, Shaffer, RN, Schwartz, A: Estimation of width of angle of anterior chamber. Incidence and significance of the narrow angle. Am J Ophthal 68:626, 1969.
33. Scheie, HG: Width and pigmentation of the angle of the anterior chamber. A system of grading by gonioscopy. Arch Ophthal 58:510, 1957.
34. Shaffer, RN: Symposium: Primary Glaucomas. III. Gonioscopy, ophthalmoscopy and perimetry. Trans Am Acad Ophthal Otol 62:112, 1960.
35. Becker, S: Clinical Gonioscopy—A Text and Stereoscopic Atlas. CV Mosby Co, St Louis, 1972.
36. Spaeth, GL: Distinguishing between the normally narrow, the suspiciously shallow, and the particularly pathological, anterior chamber angle. Pers Ophthal 1:205, 1977.
37. Gloster, J, Poinoosawmy, D: Changes in intraocular pressure during and after the dark-room test. Br J Ophthal 57:170, 1973.
38. Foulds, WS: Observations on the facility of aqueous outflow in closed-angle glaucoma. Br J Ophthal 43:613, 1959.
39. Hyams, SW, Friedman, BZ, Neumann, E: Elevated intraocular pressure in the prone position. A new provocative test for angle-closure glaucoma. Am J Ophthal 66:661, 1968.
40. Harris, LS, Galin, MA: Prone provocative testing for narrow angle glaucoma. Arch Ophthal 87:493, 1972.
41. Neumann, E, Hyams, SW: Gonioscopy and anterior chamber depth in the prone-position provocative test for angle-closure glaucoma. Ophthalmologica 167:9, 1973.
42. Friedman, Z, Neumann, E: Comparison of prone-position, dark-room, and mydriatic tests for angle-closure glaucoma before and after peripheral iridectomy. Am J Ophthal 74:24, 1972.
43. Wand, M: Provocative tests in angle-closure glaucoma: a brief review with commentary. Ophthal Surg 5:32, 1974.
44. Mapstone, R: Provocative tests in closed-angle glaucoma. Br J Ophthal 60:115, 1976.
45. Mapstone, R: Normal response to pilocarpine and phenylephrine. Br J Ophthal 61:510, 1977.
46. Mapstone, R: Outflow changes in positive provocative tests. Br J Ophthal 61:634, 1977.
47. Mapstone, R: Partial angle closure. Br J Ophthal 61:525, 1977.
48. Nesterov, AP, Kiselev, GA, Devlikamova, ER: New compression tests in glaucoma. II. Posterior annular compression test. Acta Ophthal 51:749, 1973.
49. Lowe, RF: Primary angle-closure glaucoma. A review of provocative tests. Br J Ophthal 51:727, 1967.
50. Bellows, JG: Ultrasonic diagnostic techniques in glaucoma. Ann Ophthal 10:91, 1978.
51. Gieser, DK, Wilensky, JT: HLA antigens and acute angle-closure glaucoma. Am J Ophthal 88:232, 1979.
52. Hillman, JS, Turner, JDC: Association between acute glaucoma and the weather and sunspot activity. Br J Ophthal 61:512, 1977.
53. Grant, WM: Action of drugs on movement of ocular fluids. Ann Rev Pharmacol 9:85, 1969.
54. Grant, WM: Ocular complications of drugs. Glaucoma. JAMA 207:2089, 1969.
55. Mapstone, R: Dilating dangerous pupils. Br J Ophthal 61:517, 1977.
56. Schwartz, H, Apt, L: Mydriatic effect of anticholinergic drugs used during reversal of nondepolarizing muscle relaxants. Am J Ophthal 88:609, 1979.

57. Whitworth, CG, Grant, WM: Use of nitrate and nitrite vasodilators by glaucomatous patients. Arch Ophthal 71:492, 1964.
58. Mapstone, R: One model of outflow damage. Br J Ophthal 63:322, 1979.
59. Mapstone, R: Mechanisms in ocular hypertension. Br J Ophthal 63:325, 1979.
60. Charles, ST, Hamasaki, DI: The effect of intraocular pressure on the pupil size. Arch Ophthal 83:729, 1970.
61. Rutkowski, PC, Thompson, HS: Mydriasis and increased intraocular pressure. I. Pupillographic studies. Arch Ophthal 87:21, 1972.
62. Anderson, DR, Davis, EB: Sensitivities of ocular tissues to acute pressure-induced ischemia. Arch Ophthal 93:267, 1975.
63. Kapoor, S, Sood, M: Glaucoma-induced changes in the ciliary ganglion. Br J Ophthal 59:573, 1975.
64. Bessiere, M, Rebeller, JL, Maurain, C, Danton, JM: Pre- and post-operative study of the aqueous humour protein in the primary glaucomas. D'Ophthalmologie 34:67, 1974.
65. Campbell, DG: A comparison of diagnostic techniques in angle-closure glaucoma. Am J Ophthal 88:197, 1979.
66. Campbell, DG: Angle-closure glaucoma, an update. Pers Ophthal 4:123, 1980.
67. Zimmerman, LE, de Venecia, G, Hamasaki, DI: Pathology of the optic nerve in experimental acute glaucoma. Invest Ophthal 6:109, 1967.
68. Douglas, GR, Drance, SM, Schulzer, M: The visual field and nerve head in angle-closure glaucoma. A comparison of the effects of acute and chronic angle closure. Arch Ophthal 93:409, 1975.
69. McNaught, EI, Rennie, A, McClure, E, Chisholm, IA: Pattern of visual damage after acute angle-closure glaucoma. Trans Ophthal Soc UK 94:406, 1974.
70. Wand, M, Grant, WM: Thymoxamine test. Differentiating angle-closure glaucoma from open-angle glaucoma with narrow angles. Arch Ophthal 96:1009, 1978.
71. Feibel, RM: Edward J. Curran and the concept of relative pupillary block. Surv Ophthal 25:270, 1981.
72. Mapstone, R: One gonioscopic fallacy. Br J Ophthal 63:221, 1979.
73. Mapstone, R: The mechanism and clinical significance of angle closure. Glaucoma 2:249, 1980.
74. Tornquist, R: Corneal radius in primary acute glaucoma. Br J Ophthal 41:421, 1957.
75. Lowe, RF: Causes of shallow anterior chamber in primary angle-closure glaucoma. Ultrasonic biometry of normal and angle-closure glaucoma eyes. Am J Ophthal 67:87, 1969.
76. Phillips, CI: Aetiology of angle-closure glaucoma. Br J Ophthal 56:248, 1972.
77. Lowe, RF, Clark, BAJ: Posterior corneal curvature. Correlations in normal eyes and in eyes involved with primary angle-closure glaucoma. Br J Ophthal 57:464, 1973.
78. Tomlinson, A, Leighton, DA: Ocular dimensions in the heredity of angle-closure glaucoma. Br J Ophthal 57:475, 1973.
79. Kerman, BM, Christensen, RE, Foos, RY: Angle-closure glaucoma: a clinico-pathologic correlation. Am J Ophthal 76:887, 1973.
80. Mapstone, R: Mechanics of pupil block. Br J Ophthal 52:19, 1968.
81. Mizuno, K, Kimura, R, Muroi, S: Cycloscopy of angle-closure glaucoma. Albrecht Graefes Arch Klin Exp Ophthal 204:247, 1977.
82. Mapstone, R: The syndrome of closed-angle glaucoma. Br J Ophthal 60:120, 1976.
83. Hung, PT, Chou, LH: Provocation and mechanism of angle-closure glaucoma after iridectomy. Arch Ophthal 97:1862, 1979.
84. Christensen, L, Irvine, AR Jr: Pathogenesis of primary shallow chamber angle closure glaucoma. Arch Ophthal 75:490, 1966.
85. Robbins, RM, Galin, MA: Vitreous response in glaucoma. Am J Ophthal 76:921, 1973.

86. Ganias, F, Mapstone, R: Miotics in closed-angle glaucoma. Br J Ophthal. 59:205, 1975.
87. Airaksinen, PJ, Saari, KM, Tiainen, TJ, Jaanio, EAT: Management of acute closed-angle glaucoma with miotics and timolol. Br J Ophthal 63:822, 1979.
88. Anderson, DR: Corneal indentation to relieve acute angle-closure glaucoma. Am J Ophthal 88:1091, 1979.
89. Rutkowski, PC, Fernandez, JL, Galin, MA, Halasa, AH: Alpha-adrenergic receptor blockade in the treatment of angle-closure glaucoma. Trans Am Acad Ophthal Otol 77:137, 1973.
90. Halasa, AH, Rutkowski, PC: Thymoxamine therapy for angle-closure glaucoma. Arch Ophthal 90:177, 1973.
91. Wand, M, Grant, WM: Thymoxamine hydrochloride: an alpha-adrenergic blocker. Surv Ophthal 25:75, 1980.
92. Chandler, PA, Grant, WM: Glaucoma, 2ed. Lea & Febiger, Philadelphia, 1979, p 140.
93. Krupin, T, Mitchell, KB, Johnson, F, Becker, B: The long-term effects of iridectomy for primary acute angle-closure glaucoma. Am J Ophthal 86:506, 1978.
94. Playfair, TJ, Watson, PG: Management of acute primary angle-closure glaucoma: a long-term follow-up of the results of peripheral iridectomy used as an initial procedure. Br J Ophthal 63:17, 1979.
95. Iwata, K: A new indentation gonioscope and evaluation of peripheral iridectomy in angle-closure glaucoma. Glaucoma 3:546, 1980.
96. Chandler, PA, Simmons, RJ: Anterior chamber deepening for gonioscopy at time of surgery. Arch Ophthal 74:177, 1965.
97. Forbes, M: Gonioscopy with corneal indentation. A method for distinguishing between appositional closure and synechial closure. Arch Ophthal 76:488, 1966.
98. Forbes, M: Indentation gonioscopy and efficacy of iridectomy in angle-closure glaucoma. Trans Am Ophthal Soc 72:488, 1974.
99. Shaffer, RN: Operating room gonioscopy in angle closure glaucoma surgery. Trans Am Ophthal Soc 55:59, 1957.
100. Williams, DJ, Gills, JP Jr, Hall, GA: Results of 233 peripheral iridectomies for narrow-angle glaucoma. Am J Ophthal 65:548, 1968.
101. Playfair, TJ, Watson, PG: Management of chronic or intermittent primary angle-closure glaucoma: a long-term follow-up of the results of peripheral iridectomy used as an initial procedure. Br J Ophthal 63:23, 1979.
102. Murphy, MB, Spaeth, GL: Iridectomy in primary angle-closure glaucoma. Classification and differential diagnosis of glaucoma associated with narrowness of the angle. Arch Ophthal 91:114, 1974.
103. Lowe, RF: Acute angle-closure glaucoma. The second eye: An analysis of 200 cases. Br J Ophthal 46:641, 1962.
104. Benedikt, O: Prophylactic iridectomy in the partner eye after angle closure glaucoma. Klin Monatsbl Augenheilkd 156:80, 1970.
105. Ritzinger, I, Benedikt, O, Dirisamer, F: Surgical or conservative prophylaxis of the partner eye after primary acute angle bloc glaucoma. Klin Monatsbl Augenheilkd 164:645, 1974.
106. Wollensak, J, Ehrhorn, J: Angle block glaucoma and prophylactic iridectomy in the eye without symptoms. Klin Monatsbl Augenheilkd 167:791, 1975.
107. Imre, G, Bogi, J: The fellow eye in acute angle-closure glaucoma. Klin Monatsbl Augenheilk 169:264, 1976.
108. Snow, JT: Value of prophylactic peripheral iridectomy on the second eye in angle-closure glaucoma. Trans Ophthal Soc UK 97:189, 1977.
109. Lowe, RF: Primary angle-closure glaucoma. A review 5 years after bilateral surgery. Br J Ophthal 57:457, 1973.
110. Hyams, SW, Friedman, Z, Keroub, C: Fellow eye in angle-closure glaucoma. Br J Ophthal 59:207, 1975.

Chapter 9

PRIMARY CONGENITAL GLAUCOMA

PRIMARY CONGENITAL GLAUCOMA

I. A CLASSIFICATION OF CHILDHOOD GLAUCOMAS

There is no universal agreement regarding a classification system or terminology for the diverse group of glaucomas that may occur in childhood. The following simplified scheme is based on the clinical and histopathologic appearance of these disorders and will be used, for purposes of discussion, in this text.

A. Developmental Glaucoma Without Associated Ocular or Systemic Anomalies

There is a form of childhood glaucoma in which obstruction to aqueous outflow is due to a developmental abnormality of the anterior chamber angle. The disease appears to be *inherited* and is a *primary* glaucoma in the sense that no systemic or other ocular defect is typically present. (The concept of "primary" and "secondary" glaucomas used in this text is discussed in Chapter 6.) Although it is not always recognized at birth, the glaucoma is a *congenital* disorder, because the underlying anomaly presumably develops during gestation.

This form of childhood glaucoma is commonly called *primary congenital glaucoma*[1, 2] or *primary congenital open-angle glaucoma.*[3] The present chapter will be limited to a discussion of this glaucoma. Other names that have been used for the condition relate primarily to age of onset[2, 4] or clinical appearance and will be considered later in the chapter.

B. Developmental Glaucomas with Associated Ocular or Systemic Anomalies

There are other glaucomas of childhood which also have developmental abnormalities of the anterior chamber angle as the cause of aqueous outflow obstruction, but which are characterized by additional ocular and/or systemic anomalies. These conditions are inherited and congenital, although some may not be clinically recognized until late childhood or even early adulthood. It should be emphasized that there is no clear division between primary congenital glaucoma and some of the developmental glaucomas with associated anomalies, and it is possible that these conditions may represent a spectrum of disease. Nevertheless, the latter group of childhood glaucomas will be discussed separately in Chapter 10.

C. Glaucomas Secondary to Ocular or Systemic Disease

In a third group of childhood glaucomas, the aqueous outflow system is obstructed secondarily by a disorder which may have originated elsewhere in the eye or as a systemic disease. The fundamental defect may be inherited, such as a neoplasia or a dislocated lens, or it may be an acquired condition, including inflammation, trauma, or a complication of surgery. In general, children may be subjected to nearly all of the problems that can cause secondary glaucoma in adults, and it is difficult to clearly separate these glaucomas on the basis of childhood and adult afflictions. Therefore, these forms of glaucoma, as they relate to both children and adults, will be considered in subsequent chapters in this section.

II. EMBRYOLOGY OF THE ANTERIOR OCULAR SEGMENT

A basic understanding of the related embryology is helpful preparation for a discussion of developmental disorders. Therefore, we will consider the embryology of the anterior ocular segment at this time. Theories of abnormal development in primary congenital glaucoma will be discussed later in this chapter, while those relating to the developmental glaucomas with associated anomalies will be considered in Chapter 10.

A. General Development

According to classic teaching, the anterior ocular segment is formed by the following three primordial tissues[5]:

1. *Surface ectoderm* gives rise to the *lens*, which develops as an invagination during the third week of gestation and separates from the surface ectoderm by the sixth week. *Corneal epithelium* also arises from this primordial layer.

2. *Neural ectoderm* forms the optic cup, the margins of which reach the lens equator by the sixth week and later give rise to the *epithelium of the iris.*

3. An *undifferentiated mass of mesoderm* comes to lie just anterior to the margin of the optic cup by the sixth week and subsequently gives rise to the structures of the anterior chamber.

B. Theory of Mesodermal Development

Traditionally, it has been felt that the undifferentiated mesoderm gives rise to many of the anterior ocular segment structures according to the following scheme:

1. *Three waves* of tissue come forward from the mesodermal mass between the surface ectoderm and lens during the seventh and eighth weeks of intrauterine life to form the following structures (listed in order of appearance):

    a. Corneal endothelium, which later secretes Descemet's membrane.

    b. Corneal stroma.

    c. Stroma of the iris.

2. The same cellular mass that gives rise to the aforementioned waves of tissue is generally felt to be involved in the formation of the *anterior chamber angle.* This development begins in the seventh or eighth week of gestation, but it is not complete until just before birth. Many *theories* have been advanced regarding the tissue changes that

lead to formation of the anterior chamber angle:

a. *Atrophy*, which implies cell death.[5] However, subsequent studies have failed to show dead or dying cells.[6, 7]

b. *Resorption* by adjacent tissue.[8]

c. *Cleavage* into an anterior and posterior layer as a result of different growth patterns.[6] Other investigators have suggested that the cleavage is an artifact of tissue fixation.[7, 9]

d. *Rarefaction*, which implies a rearrangement of the tissue and a coalescence of spaces to eventually form the trabecular meshwork.[7]

C. Theory of Neural Crest Cell Development

More recent evidence suggests that neural crest cells give rise to a continuous layer of tissue, which extends from the corneal endothelium to the trabecular meshwork endothelium and onto the surface of the iris.[10] This layer loses its continuity between the seventh and eighth month of gestation,[11, 12] and appears to contribute to the trabecular meshwork, corneal stroma and endothelium, and the stroma of the iris.[10] Neural crest cells also contribute to the development of bones, including those of the face, as well as dental papillae, cartilage, and meninges, which may explain the association of developmental glaucomas with malformations of these structures,[10] which will be discussed in the next chapter.

III. GENERAL FEATURES

A. Frequency

Although primary congenital glaucoma is the most common glaucoma of childhood, it occurs much less frequently than the primary glaucomas that are seen in adults. It has been estimated that the average ophthalmic practice will have only one case of primary congenital glaucoma every 5 years.[4]

B. Age of Onset

Primary congenital glaucoma is usually diagnosed at birth or shortly thereafter, and most cases are recognized in the first year of life.[4] However, the condition may become apparent at any time throughout childhood or even in young adults, and various names have been used, based on the age of onset.

1. *Infantile glaucoma*. This term has been applied to those cases which appear during the first few years of life.[2, 4] If the intraocular pressure is elevated at this age, the eye may become enlarged, which led to the terms, *"buphthalmos"* (cow's eye) and *"hydrophthalmia,"* as synonyms for infantile glaucoma, although these are not recommended.[3]

2. *Juvenile glaucoma*. This form of primary congenital glaucoma appears later in childhood or in early adulthood.[1] *Three years of age* is generally taken as the division between infantile and juvenile glaucoma, because it is at approximately this age that the eye no longer expands in response to elevated intraocular pressure.[1, 3]

C. Heredity

Although it is generally believed that primary congenital glaucoma has a genetic basis, reports are conflicting regarding the precise mode of inheritance. An *autosomal recessive* mode with incomplete or variable penetrance has been suspected,[4] but a study of the pedigrees of 64 families led to the hypothesis that most cases are caused by *multifactorial inheritance.*[13] In studies of identical twins, congenital glaucoma was usually present in both siblings,[13, 14] although only one member was afflicted in one pair of monozygotic twins,[15] suggesting that non-genetic factors may also be involved.

Reports are conflicting as to whether parents of children with primary congenital glaucoma have an increased prevalence of abnormal anterior chamber angles and topical corticosteroid responses.[16, 17] Chromosomal abnormalities are not a feature of primary congenital glaucoma, although they have been reported in variations of this disease.[18, 19] No statistically significant differences in HLA histocompatibility antigens were found in one study of patients with primary congenital glaucoma as compared to controls.[20]

D. Bilateral

Primary congenital glaucoma is typically *bilateral*, although a significant intraocular pressure elevation may occur in only one eye in 25 to 30% of the cases.

IV. CLINICAL FEATURES

A. History

There is a *classic triad* of manifestations, any one of which should arouse suspicion of glaucoma in an infant or young child:

1. *Epiphora* (excessive tearing).

2. *Photophobia* (hypersensitivity to light), which is due to corneal edema, and is manifest by the child hiding his face in bright lighting, or even in ordinary lighting in severe cases.

3. *Blepharospasm* (squeezing the eyelids) is seen with epiphora and photophobia and is another manifestation of irritation from the corneal edema.

B. External Examination

Changes in the cornea (especially in the first few years of life) provide strong additional support to the diagnosis:

1. *Corneal diameter.* The average horizontal corneal diameter at birth is under 10.5 mm.[4] *Distention of the globe* in response to elevated intraocular pressure (buphthalmos) leads to enlargement of the cornea, especially at the corneoscleral junction, and a diameter over 12 mm in the first year of life is highly suspicious.[4] Grossly, this is more obvious in the unilateral case.

2. *Corneal edema.* Initially, this may be a direct result of the elevated intraocular pressure, producing a corneal haze that clears with normalization of the pressure. In more advanced cases, tears in

Descemet's membrane lead to a dense opacification of the corneal stroma, which does not always clear completely with reduction of the intraocular pressure.

C. Tonometry

Any of the aforementioned findings demand a thorough examination to rule out congenital glaucoma. Since the pressure is often measured during general anesthesia, the possible influence of the anesthesia on intraocular pressure (see Chapter 3) must be considered. The normal pressure in an infant under halothane anesthesia is said to be approximately 9 to 10 mmHg,[21, 22] and a pressure of 20 mmHg or more should arouse suspicion.[21] It has also been reported that children can be successfully examined under chloral hydrate sedation and, using this approach, the pressures by Mackay-Marg tonometry in 17 non-glaucomatous eyes ranged from 11 to 17 mmHg.[23] However, the most reliable method of measuring the the intraocular pressure is probably with the child awake, if cooperation permits, and the Perkins tonometer has been found to be particularly suitable in this situation.[24] In one study, the mean intraocular pressure in unanesthetized newborns was 11.4 ± 2.4 mmHg.[25] In the normal, alert child, the pressure is the same as in adults.

D. Slit-lamp Examination

This is best performed with a portable slit-lamp, with or without general anesthesia, and may reveal:

1. *Tears in Descemet's membrane* (Haab's striae) may be single or multiple and typically occur in the horizontal meridian or concentric to the limbus, peripherally. They are usually associated with corneal edema, although this may clear when the tears are repaired by endothelial overgrowth.

2. The *anterior chamber* is characteristically *deep*, especially when distention of the globe is present.

3. The *iris* is typically normal, although it may have stromal hypoplasia with loss of the crypts.

E. Gonioscopy

Evaluation of the anterior chamber angle is essential for the accurate interpretation of primary congenital glaucoma. The instruments and techniques of gonioscopy were discussed in Chapter 2. In performing gonioscopy on infants and children under anesthesia, a *Koeppe goniolens* is recommended.

1. The *normal anterior chamber angle in childhood* differs significantly from that of adults, and the gonioscopist must be familiar with these differences in order to recognize the abnormal state. The most characteristic feature of the child's anterior chamber angle is the *uveal meshwork*, which has the appearance of a smooth, homogeneous membrane, extending from peripheral iris to Schwalbe's line, during the first year of life, and becomes coarser and more pigmented with

the passing years.[3] In addition, the peripheral iris tends to be thinner and flatter.[3]

2. In *primary congenital glaucoma*, the typical gonioscopic appearance is an *open angle*, with a *high insertion of the iris root*, which forms a scalloped line. *Abnormal tissue*, with a chagreened, glistening appearance may be seen in the angle, and appears to pull the peripheral iris anteriorly. Although the angle is usually avascular, loops of vessels from the major arterial circle may be seen above the iris root, which has been called the "Loch Ness monster phenomenon."[8] In addition, the peripheral iris may be covered by a fine, fluffy tissue that has been referred to as "Lister's morning mist."[8]

3. As previously noted, the clinical features of primary congenital glaucoma seem to merge with other forms of developmental glaucoma. A gonioscopic assessment of over 100 eyes with developmental glaucoma led to the following classification (the surgical significance of these findings will be discussed later in the chapter)[26]:

a. "*Mesodermal anomalies of the angle*" is the commonest gonioscopic appearance and is characterized by an open angle, a flat iris (*i.e.*, no deformation of the peripheral iris), and variable amounts of abnormal angle tissue ranging from aggregations of pigmented tissue, through thickened, pigmented uveal meshwork, to homogenous sheets of golden-brown tissue.

b. A "*cicatrized angle*," was described as having grayish or golden-brown vascularized tissue, terminating in a scalloped border above the iris root. Finger-like processes of this tissue extended onto the peripheral iris and tented the iris anteriorly, leaving a concave configuration between the processes.

c. Varying degrees of "*iridocorneal dysgenesis*" were also described. However, while these conditions may be in a broad spectrum of disease with primary congenital glaucoma, they are clinically and histopathologically distinct entities and will be considered separately in Chapter Ten.

F. Funduscopy

The *optic nerve head* in normal newborns is typically pink but may have slight pallor, and a small physiologic cup is usually present.[27] Glaucomatous cupping is said to proceed more rapidly in infants than in adults,[28, 29] which may be due to a more vulnerable circulation in the infant optic nerve head.[29] The morphology of glaucomatous optic atrophy in childhood glaucoma resembles that seen in adult eyes, with a preferential loss of neural tissue in the vertical poles.[30] A child's eye does differ from that of the adult, however, in that the scleral canal in children enlarges in response to elevated intraocular pressure, especially in the horizontal meridian, causing further enlargement of the cup in addition to that resulting from the actual loss of neural tissue.[30]

Cupping of the optic nerve head in infants may be reversible if the pressure is lowered early enough.[29, 31] This was once thought to be the result of an initial loss of astroglial tissue.[29] However, a subsequent study suggested that incomplete development of connective tissue in the lamina cribrosa allows compression or posterior movement of the optic disc tissue in response to elevated intraocular pressure, with an elastic return to normal when the pressure is lowered.[31] Transient, reversible cupping following normalization of intraocular pressure was documented in a patient with juvenile-onset glaucoma, although the optic nerve head resumed its preoperative excavated appearance within the first postoperative month despite a normal tension.[32]

G. Visual fields

When tested after the child becomes old enough for a reliable study, the visual fields are identical to these in adult-onset glaucoma, with an initial predilection for the arcuate areas.[30]

H. Visual acuity

Good vision may be achieved if the intraocular pressure is controlled before optic atrophy occurs. Occasionally, however, the acuity is poor despite adequate pressure control. In some cases this is due to optic nerve damage, corneal clouding, or irregular astigmatism.[30, 33] Other children may have normal appearing optic nerve heads and clear media but develop amblyopia from anisometropia or strabismus.[28, 34] Retinal detachment is also an occasional cause of poor visual results.[35]

I. Ultrasonography

Ultrasonography has also been suggested as a diagnostic method for documenting progression of infantile glaucoma by recording changes in the axial length of the globe,[36] although the value of this study has not yet been established.

V. THEORIES OF MECHANISM

Although it is generally agreed that the mechanism of intraocular pressure elevation in primary congenital glaucoma is an abnormal tissue in the anterior chamber angle which obstructs aqueous outflow, there is no universal agreement as to the nature of the tissue or the developmental alteration that leads to its formation. Most theories of mechanism for primary congenital glaucoma parallel the basic concepts regarding the normal development of the anterior chamber angle, as previously discussed:

1. Mann[5] postulated that *incomplete atrophy* of anterior chamber mesoderm resulted in the abnormal tissue.

2. Barkan[8] suggested that *incomplete resorption* of the mesodermal cells by adjacent tissue led to the formation of a *membrane* across the anterior chamber angle. This "membrane" became known as *Barkan's membrane*, although its existence has not been proved histologically. In one study, two cases were reported to have an

apparent membrane by gonioscopy and the dissecting microscope, but electron microscopy showed this to be uveal meshwork.[37]

3. Allen et al.[6] postulated that *incomplete cleavage* of mesoderm in the anterior chamber angle results in the congenital defect.

4. Worst[9] proposed a combined theory, which included *elements of the atrophy and resorption concepts*, but rejected the cleavage theory. He suggested that incomplete development of the scleral spur leads to a high insertion of the longitudinal portion of the ciliary muscle on the trabeculum. In addition, a single layer of endothelial cells is felt to cover the anterior chamber angle during gestation, and its abnormal retention in primary congenital glaucoma is felt to constitute Barkan's membrane.

5. Maumenee[38, 39] also observed the *abnormal anterior insertion of the ciliary musculature* into the trabecular meshwork, and reasoned that this might compress the scleral spur forward and externally, thus narrowing Schlemm's canal. He also noted the absence of Schlemm's canal in some histopathologic specimens and suggested that this might be a cause of aqueous outflow obstruction in congenital glaucoma,[39] although others feel this may be a secondary change.[37]

6. Smelser and Ozanics[7] explained primary congenital glaucoma as a *failure of anterior chamber angle mesoderm to become properly rearranged* into the normal trabecular meshwork. Electron microscopic studies favor this theory by showing dense uveal meshwork.[37, 40, 41] One report also described a thick, constant layer of amorphous material beneath the internal endothelium of Schlemm's canal.[41] A histologic study of a pair of eyes with congenital glaucoma suggested that the trabecular meshwork was compressed by ectopic trabecular pillars bridging the anterior chamber angle.[19] This case, however, may belong in the category of developmental glaucomas with associated anomalies. Structural changes of the trabecular meshwork have also been found in eyes with juvenile glaucoma associated with goniodysgenesis.[42]

7. Kupfer and Kaiser-Kupfer[10] suggested that the defects in several forms of congenital glaucoma may represent *abnormal development of neural crest cells*. This theory could explain many secondary developmental glaucomas, since the neural crest cells, as previously noted, are also involved with other ocular structures as well as bones, dental papilla, cartilage, and meninges.

VI. DIFFERENTIAL DIAGNOSIS

Some of the clinical features of primary congenital glaucoma are also found in other conditions, and these must be considered in the differential diagnosis.

A. Excessive Tearing

Excessive tearing in the infant is most commonly caused by obstruction of the lacrimal drainage system. The epiphora of nasolacrimal duct obstruction is distinguished from that of infantile-onset glaucoma in that the former condition almost always has purulent discharge and is not associated with photophobia or blepharospasm. Epiphora, photophobia, or blepharospasm may also result from a variety of other disorders of the anterior ocular segment.

B. Corneal Changes

1. A *large cornea* may represent congenital megalocornea without glaucoma, and an enlarged globe may be due to *high myopia.* It has been emphasized, however, that infantile-onset glaucoma may be a cause of progressive myopia and should be suspected in these cases.[43]

2. *Tears in Descemet's membrane* may result from birth trauma. These tears are usually vertical or oblique in contrast to those of congenital glaucoma, which tend to be horizontal or concentric with the limbus.

3. *Corneal opacification* in infancy may be associated with a variety of disorders:[44]

a. Congenital malformations, such as sclerocornea and dermoid tumors.

b. Congenital hereditary corneal dystrophies.

c. Birth trauma.

d. Inflammatory processes.

e. Inborn errors of metabolism, including the mycopolysaccharidoses and cystinosis. In the latter condition, corneal opacification is usually not seen before one year of age, although fine crystals in the cornea may be seen by slit lamp before this time.

C. Other Childhood Glaucomas

The differential diagnosis of primary congenital glaucoma should also include developmental glaucomas with associated anomalies, as well as the childhood glaucomas secondary to ocular or systemic disease, all of which will be discussed in subsequent chapters.

VII. MANAGEMENT

Primary congenital glaucoma is almost always managed surgically, with medical therapy being used only occasionally, usually as a temporizing measure. The present discussion will be limited to the concepts of management, while details of the operative procedures will be considered in Section Three.

A. Surgical Techniques

The *primary surgical techniques* are designed to eliminate the resistance to aqueous outflow created by the abnormal tissue in the anterior chamber angle. This can be accomplished by either an internal (goniotomy) or external (trabeculotomy) approach.

1. *Goniotomy.* Barkan[45, 46] described a technique in which the abnormal tissue (presumably Barkan's membrane) is incised under

direct visualization with the aid of a goniolens. In one study of 65 eyes, followed for an average of 11 years, 44% were controlled by goniotomy alone,[47] while only one-third of another series were controlled following an initial goniotomy.[48] Repeated goniotomies, however, increase the success rate. In a study of 120 eyes, 79 were controlled after the first goniotomy, and an additional 23 were controlled with a second or third goniotomy.[4] The severity of the glaucoma also influences the success rate, with the worst prognosis occurring in infants with elevated pressure and cloudy corneas at birth. The most favorable outcome is seen in infants operated between the second and eighth month, while goniotomy is less effective with increasing age after the first year of life, or when the corneal diameter exceeds 14 mm.[4]

2. *Trabeculotomy.* Harms and Dannheim[49] described a technique in which Schlemm's canal is identified by external dissection, and the trabecular meshwork (including the abnormal angle tissue) is incised by passing a probe into the canal and then rotating it into the anterior chamber. One advantage of this procedure is that it can be performed in eyes with cloudy corneas, which is not the case with goniotomy. While some surgeons employ the technique only in cases with corneal opacification or when multiple goniotomies have failed, others prefer it as the initial procedure in primary congenital glaucoma. McPherson[50] reported success in 12 of 15 such cases. However, as with goniotomy, success is related to the severity and duration of the glaucoma. In one series, trabeculotomy controlled all the eyes with "mesodermal anomalies of the angle," but less than one-third of those with "cicatrized angle" or "iridocorneal dysgenesis."[26] (These terms were defined earlier in this chapter, under "Clinical Features.") In another study, success with trabeculotomy was better when the size of Schlemm's canal was closer to normal, which correlated with the diameter of the cornea and height of the intraocular pressure.[51]

3. When multiple goniotomies and/or trabeculotomies have failed, the surgeon usually resorts to a filtering procedure, such as a trabeculectomy. In some desperate situations in which all else has failed, cyclocryotherapy may be useful.

B. Follow-up

The *follow-up* has several important facets. In the early postoperative period, close observation is required regarding success of the procedure. Corneal edema may persist for weeks after successful reduction of the intraocular pressure, and changes in the optic nerve head provide the most important indicator of the course of the disease.[34] As previously discussed, poor vision may result from amblyopia despite adequate pressure control, and the child must also be followed and treated for this. Finally, sequelae of primary congenital glaucoma can occur at any age, and these patients must be followed throughout their life.

References

1. Kwitko, ML: Glaucomas in Infants and Children. Appleton-Century-Crofts, New York, 1973, p 185.
2. Kolker, AE, Hetherington, J Jr: Becker-Shaffer's Diagnosis and Therapy of the Glaucomas, 4th ed. CV Mosby Co, St Louis, 1976, p 276.
3. Walton, DS: Primary Congenital Open-Angle Glaucoma. In Glaucoma, by Chandler, PA, Grant, WM, eds. Lea & Febiger, Philadelphia, 1979, p 329.
4. Shaffer, RN, Weiss, DI: Congenital and Pediatric Glaucomas. CV Mosby Co, St Louis, 1970, p 37.
5. Mann, IC: The Development of the Human Eye, University Press, Cambridge, 1928.
6. Allen, L, Burian, HM, Braley, AE: A new concept of the development of the anterior chamber angle. Its relationship to developmental glaucoma and other structural anomalies. Arch Ophthal 53:783, 1955.
7. Smelser, GK, Ozanics, V: The development of the trabecular meshwork in primate eyes. Am J Ophthal 70:366, 1971.
8. Barkan, O: Pathogenesis of congenital glaucoma. Gonioscopic and anatomic observation of the angle of the anterior chamber in the normal eye and in congenital glaucoma. Am J Ophthal 40:1, 1955.
9. Worst, JGF: The Pathogenesis of Congenital Glaucoma. An Embryological and Goniosurgical Study. Charles C Thomas, Springfield, Ill, 1966.
10. Kupfer, C, Kaiser-Kupfer, MI: Observations on the development of the anterior chamber angle with reference to the pathogenesis of congenital glaucomas. Am J Ophthal 88:424, 1979.
11. Kupfer, C, Ross, K: The development of outflow facility in human eyes. Invest Ophthal 10:513, 1971.
12. Hansson, HA, Jerndal, T: Scanning electron microscopic studies on the development of the iridocorneal angle in human eyes. Invest Ophthal 10:252, 1971.
13. Merin, S, Morin, D: Heredity of congenital glaucoma. Br J Ophthal 56:414, 1972.
14. Rasmussen, DH, Ellis, PP: Congenital glaucoma in identical twins. Arch Ophthal 84:827, 1970.
15. Fried, K, Sachs, R, Krakowsky, D: Congenital glaucoma in only one of identical twins. Ophthalmologica 174:185, 1977.
16. Kaufman, PL, Kolker, AE: Ocular findings and corticosteroid responsiveness in parents of children with primary infantile glaucoma. Invest Ophthal 14:46, 1975.
17. Jerndal, T, Munkby, M: Corticosteroid response in dominant congenital glaucoma. Acta Ophthal 56:373, 1978.
18. Dar, et al: Congenital glaucoma associated with chromosomal abnormalities. A case report. J Ped Ophthal 10:173, 1973.
19. Broughton, WL, Fine, BS, Zimmerman, LE: Congenital glaucoma associated with a chromosomal defect. A histologic study. Arch Ophthal 99:481, 1981.
20. Hvidberg, A, Kessing, V, Svejgaard, A: HLA histocompatibility antigens in primary congenital glaucoma. Glaucoma 1:134, 1979.
21. Dominquez, A, Banos, MS, Alvarez, MG, Contra, GF, Quintela, FB: Intraocular pressure measurement in infants under general anesthesia. Am J Ophthal 78:110, 1974.
22. Grote, P: Augeninnendruckmessungen bei Kleinkindern ohne Glaukam in Halothanmaskennarkose. Ophthalmologica 171:202, 1975.
23. Judisch, GF, Anderson, S, Bell, WE: Chloral hydrate sedation as a substitute for examination under anesthesia in pediatric ophthalmology. Am J Ophthal 89:560, 1980.
24. Van Buskirk, EM, Palmer, EA: Office assessment of young children for glaucoma. Ann Ophthal 11:1749, 1979.
25. Radtke, ND, Cohen, BF: Intraocular pressure measurement in the newborn. Am J Ophthal 78:501, 1974.
26. Luntz, MH: Congenital, infantile, and juvenile glaucoma. Ophthalmology 86:793, 1979.

27. Khodadoust, AA, Ziai, M, Biggs, SL: Optic disc in normal newborns. Am J Ophthal 66:502, 1968.
28. Shaffer, RN: New concepts in infantile glaucoma. Can J Ophthal 2:243, 1967.
29. Shaffer, RN, Hetherington, J Jr: The glaucomatous disc in infants. A suggested hypothesis for disc cupping. Trans Am Acad Ophthal Otol 73:929, 1969.
30. Robin, AL, Quigley, HA, Pollack, IP, Maumenee, AE, Maumenee, IH: An analysis of visual acuity, visual fields, and disk cupping in childhood glaucoma. Am J Ophthal 88:847, 1979.
31. Quigley, HA: The pathogenesis of reversible cupping in congenital glaucoma. Am J Ophthal 84:358, 1977.
32. Robin, AL, Quigley, HA: Transient reversible cupping in juvenile-onset glaucoma. Am J Ophthal 88:580, 1979.
33. Morin, JD, Bryars, JH: Causes of loss of vision in congenital glaucoma. Arch Ophthal 98:1575, 1980.
34. Rice, NSC: Management of infantile glaucoma. Br J Ophthal 56:294, 1972.
35. Cooling, RJ, Rice, NSC, McLeod, D: Retinal detachment in congenital glaucoma. Br J Ophthal 64:417, 1980.
36. Buschmann, W, Bluth, K: Ultrasonographic follow-up examination of congenital glaucoma. Albrecht Graefes Arch Klin Exp Ophthal 192:313, 1974.
37. Anderson, DR: Pathology of the glaucomas. Br J Ophthal 56:146, 1972.
38. Maumenee, AE: The pathogenesis of congenital glaucoma. A new theory. Am J Ophthal 47:827, 1959.
39. Maumenee, AE: Further observations on the pathogenesis of congenital glaucoma. Am J Ophthal 55:1163, 1963.
40. Sampaolesi, R, Argento, C: Scanning electron microscopy of the trabecular meshwork in normal and glaucomatous eyes. Invest Ophthal Vis Sci 16:302, 1977.
41. Maul, E, Strozzi, L, Munoz, C, Reyes, C: The outflow pathway in congenital glaucoma. Am J Ophthal 89:667, 1980.
42. Rodrigues, MM, Spaeth, GL, Weinreb, S: Juvenile glaucoma associated with goniodysgenesis. Am J Ophthal 81:786, 1976.
43. Marcon, IM: Evolutionary myopia and congenital glaucoma. Glaucoma 3:557, 1980.
44. Ching, FC: Corneal opacification in infancy. Med Coll Virginia Quart 8:230, 1972.
45. Barkan, O: Operation for congenital glaucoma. Am J Ophthal 25:552, 1942.
46. Barkan, O: Goniotomy for the relief of congenital glaucoma. Br J Ophthal 32:701, 1948.
47. Schlieter, F, Nathrath, P, Nicolai, R: Follow-up examination long after surgical treatment of congenital glaucomas. Klin Monatsbl Augenheilkd 164:317, 1974.
48. Kiffney, GT, Meyer, GW, McPherson, SD Jr: The surgical management of congenital glaucoma. South Med J 53:989, 1960.
49. Harms, H, Dannheim, R: Trabeculotomy results and problems. In Microsurgery in Glaucoma, Mackenson, G, ed. S Karger, Basel, 1970, p 121.
50. McPherson SD Jr: Results of external trabeculotomy. Am J Ophthal 76:918, 1973.
51. Grote, P: In vivo measurements of the latitude of Schlemm's canal in buphthalmos. Albrecht Graefes Arch Klin Exp Ophthal 209:257, 1979.

Chapter 10

DEVELOPMENTAL GLAUCOMAS WITH ASSOCIATED ANOMALIES

DEVELOPMENTAL GLAUCOMAS WITH ASSOCIATED ANOMALIES

The disorders to be discussed in this chapter all have systemic and/ or ocular developmental abnormalities. Glaucoma may occur with each of these conditions and is usually due to associated developmental defects of the anterior chamber angle.

I. MESODERMAL DYSGENESES OF THE ANTERIOR OCULAR SEGMENT

A. Classification

Several developmental anomalies have been described which have traditionally been felt to represent a dysgenesis of *mesoderm* in the anterior ocular segment. As noted in Chapter 9, however, more recent evidence suggests that much of the tissue involved in the normal development of the anterior ocular segment, and that which may be defective in the abnormalities in question, is of *neural crest* origin. Therefore, the term "mesodermal" may not accurately apply to these disorders. Nevertheless, the commonly used terms will be retained for purposes of discussion in this text.

These conditions involve primarily the cornea, anterior chamber angle, iris, and lens. In some cases, the defects are predominantly in the *peripheral* anterior ocular segment, while others are limited to *central* abnormalities. Rare cases may have both peripheral and central involvement, which led to the suggestion that the entire spectrum of anomalies be lumped under the term, "anterior chamber cleavage syndrome".[1] However, the vast majority of peripheral and central defects occur as separate, unrelated entities, and the following three-part classification has been recommended[2-4]

1. Peripheral mesodermal dysgeneses of the anterior ocular segment
    a. Prominent Schwalbe's ring
    b. Axenfeld's anomaly
    c. Rieger's anomaly and syndrome
    d. Other peripheral mesodermal defects of the anterior ocular segment
2. Central mesodermal dysgeneses of the anterior ocular segment
    a. Posterior Keratoconus
    b. Peters' anomaly
    c. Congenital corneal leukomas and staphylomas
3. Combined Rieger's syndrome and Peters' anomaly

B. Peripheral Mesodermal Dysgeneses of the Anterior Ocular Segment

1. *Prominent Schwalbe's ring.* It has been estimated that between 8%[3] and 15%[5] of the general population have a prominent Schwalbe's

ing. By slit lamp biomicroscopy, this feature appears as a thin, white line, parallel to the limbus at the level of Descemet's membrane in the peripheral cornea. The finding is occasionally referred to as *posterior corneal embryotoxon*, a term originally used by Axenfeld.[6] However, as will be discussed next, the condition he described had additional anterior chamber angle abnormalities. In the vast majority of cases, a prominent Schwalbe's ring is an anatomical variant in an otherwise normal eye, although it is also seen in many, but not all, eyes with mesodermal dysgenesis of the anterior chamber angle. Therefore, its discovery by slit lamp biomicroscopy should be followed by a gonioscopic examination to rule out possible disease.

2. *Axenfeld's anomaly.* In 1920, Axenfeld[6] reported a condition in which strands of iris traversed the anterior chamber angle from peripheral iris to a prominent Schwalbe's ring. This abnormality, which Axenfeld called posterior corneal embryotoxon, became known as Axenfeld's anomaly. It is generally defined as having an otherwise normal iris, which distinguishes it from a similar disorder described by Rieger.[7] However, Axenfeld also noted a subtle defect in the stroma of the iris in his original case, and it may be that the conditions described by Axenfeld and Rieger represent a spectrum of disease, any portion of which may be associated with developmental glaucoma. For this reason, the two disorders will be considered together under the arbitrary heading of Rieger's anomaly and syndrome.

3. *Rieger's anomaly and syndrome.* Rieger,[7] in 1935, reported cases with anterior chamber angle abnormalities similar to those described by Axenfeld, associated with stromal hypoplasia of the iris and pupillary abnormalities (Fig. 10.1). This condition became known as *Rieger's anomaly.* Some cases also have facial and dental anomalies, which has been called *Rieger's syndrome.* Table 10.1 summarizes the peripheral mesodermal dysgeneses of the anterior ocular segment.

a. *General features.* Most cases are familial with autosomal dominant transmission.[2, 3] There is no race or sex predilection, and the disease is typically bilateral.

b. *Clinical features.* The following findings apply to both Axenfeld's and Rieger's variations, with exceptions as noted.

(1). *Slit lamp examination.* The cornea is characteristically clear, aside from the prominent Schwalbe's ring, although subtle abnormalities in size and shape have been described.[3] Specular microscopy has revealed normal corneal endothelium.[8] In Rieger's variations, the iris has stromal hypoplasia with occasional holes through the pigment epithelial layer. Pupillary defects include dyscoria, corectopia, and ectropion uveae (Fig. 10.1). Abnormalities of the iris were once felt to be stationary,[3] although several cases with progressive change, not related to glaucoma or miotic therapy, have now been reported.[9–11]

(2). *Gonioscopy.* The common feature in this spectrum of disease is the previously described strands of iris in the anterior chamber angle (Fig. 10.1). These may be few and delicate or numerous

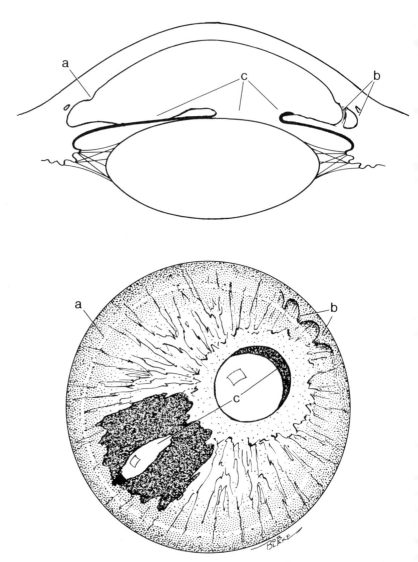

Figure 10.1. Peripheral mesodermal dysgenesis of the anterior ocular segment: **a:** prominent Schwalbe's ring; **b:** iridocorneal adhesions and defect of the trabecular meshwork (seen in Axenfeld's and Rieger's anomalies); **c:** corectopia, ectropion uvea, and stromal hypoplasia with hole formation of the iris (typical of Rieger's anomaly).

and broad. Although they characteristically run from peripheral iris to the prominent Schwalbe's ring, they have also been reported to extend as far centrally as the collarette or pupillary margin of the iris.[2]

   (3). *Systemic features of Rieger's syndrome.* These include a typical *facial configuration* characterized by a broad, flat nasal bridge, frequent telecanthus (wide interorbital distance), occasional hypertelorism (wide intercanthal distance), flattening of the midface due to

Table 10.1
Peripheral Mesodermal Dysgeneses of the Anterior Ocular Segment

	Prominent Schwalbe's Ring	Chamber Angle Anomalies	Abnormalities of the Iris	Facial and Dental Anomalies
Prominent Schwalbe's ring (posterior embryotoxon)	X			
Axenfeld's Anomaly	X	X		
Rieger's Anomaly	X	X	X	
Rieger's syndrome	X	X	X	X

maxillary hypoplasia, and a protruding lower lip.[3, 12] *Dental anomalies* are equally common features and consist of hypodontia (decreased number of teeth) and microdontia (reduced crown size).[3] Hypospadias[10] and redundant periumbilical skin[10, 12] have also been described.

(4). *Glaucoma.* Approximately half of the cases in either Axenfeld's or Rieger's variations will have glaucoma, although a slightly higher incidence is seen in the latter conditions.[2, 3] The glaucoma is usually recognized during infancy or childhood, with the diagnosis generally being made between the ages of 5 and 30 years.[2] The presence of glaucoma does not always correlate with the extent of gonioscopically visible adhesions in the anterior chamber angle.[3]

c. *Theories of mechanism.* Histopathologic reports ar e scant, but most described a prominent Schwalbe's ring connected to peripheral iris by varying adhesions.[2, 13] In one histopathologic case report, it appeared that tissue strands in the anterior chamber angle, which resembled uveal meshwork in structure, were compressing the trabecular meshwork.[14] Other studies have revealed various developmental abnormalities of the trabecular meshwork and Schlemm's canal, which may be mild[15] or severe.[3, 13, 16] In some cases, the mechanism of glaucoma may be the developmental abnormalities of trabecular meshwork and Schlemm's canal,[3] while others appear to be due, at least in part, to the adhesions in the anterior chamber angle.[13, 14] Changes in the iris include stromal hypoplasia[3, 13, 16] and ectropion uvea,[13, 16] and several reports have described a thin layer of abnormal tissue covering portions of the iris.[3, 15, 17]

d. *Differential diagnosis.* The peripheral mesodermal dysgeneses of the anterior ocular segment may occasionally be confused with the following conditions:

(1). *Iridocorneal endothelial syndrome* (see Chapter 12). The iris and anterior chamber angle abnormalities in this spectrum of disease resemble those of Rieger's syndrome, but the additional features of corneal endothelial disease, unilaterality, absence of family history, and onset in adulthood clearly separate these two conditions.

(2). *Posterior polymorphous dystrophy* (see Chapter 12). One variation of this disorder also has changes in the iris and anterior chamber angle similar to those of Rieger's syndrome, but the differentiation is again made on the basis of corneal disease and clinical recognition usually in later childhood or early adulthood.

(3). *Aniridia* (discussed later in this chapter). This condition is distinguished from the mesodermal dysgeneses by the rudimentary iris and occasional corneal and lenticular disease.

(4). *Congenital iris hypoplasia.* It has been reported that patients may have congenital hypoplasia of the iris without the anterior chamber angle defects of Rieger's anomaly or syndrome or any other ocular abnormality.[18]

(5). *Oculodentodigital dysplasia.* The dental anomalies in this condition are similar to those seen in Rieger's syndrome. In addition these patients may have occasional mild stromal hypoplasia of the iris,[3] mesodermal changes in the anterior chamber angle,[19] and microphthalmia. Glaucoma may rarely occur in this syndrome.[19]

(6). *Ectopia lentis et pupillae.* This autosomal recessive condition is characterized by bilateral displacement of the lens and pupil,[20] with the two structures typically going in opposite directions. The corectopia in this disorder may resemble that of Rieger's syndrome, but the absence of anterior chamber angle defects is a differential feature.

(7). *Iridoschisis.* In this condition, there is bilateral separation and dissolution of the stromal layers of the iris, which may be associated with glaucoma.[9] However, it differs from other abnormalities of the iris by an onset in the sixth or seventh decade of life.

e. *Management.* The glaucoma in any form of mesodermal dysgenesis of the anterior ocular segment usually requires surgical intervention when the onset is in early childhood. The procedures most often used are goniotomy, trabeculotomy, and filtering surgery. The individual with a later onset of glaucoma may respond to medical therapy, especially with drugs that reduce aqueous production.

4. *Other peripheral mesodermal defects of the anterior ocular segment.* There are additional reported cases in which abnormal development of the anterior chamber angle is associated with other anomalies, including iris hypoplasia and juvenile-onset glaucoma with autosomal dominant inheritance,[21] cataracts in two brothers with no other family history of a similar disorder,[22] and unilateral uveal ectropion with congenital or late infantile-onset glaucoma.[23] These cases differ only slightly from the more typical conditions described by Axenfeld and Rieger and may represent parts of a spectrum of developmental abnormalities in which primary congenital glaucoma and Rieger's syndrome are at the opposite extremes. Dysembryogenesis of the cornea, iris, and anterior chamber angle has also been described in infants with trisomy 13–15.[24]

C. Central Mesodermal Dysgeneses of the Anterior Ocular Segment

1. *Posterior keratoconus* is a rare disorder, characterized by thinning of the central corneal stroma, with excessive curvature of the posterior corneal surface and variable overlying stromal haze.[2,]

An ultrastructural study revealed a multilaminar Descemet's membrane with abnormal anterior banding and localized posterior excrescences.[26] It has been suggested that this condition may be the mildest form in a spectrum of central mesodermal anomalies of the anterior ocular segment.[3] Glaucoma is rarely associated with posterior keratoconus.[2]

2. **Peters' anomaly.** In 1897, von Hippel[27] reported a case of buphthalmos with bilateral central corneal opacities and adhesions from these defects to the iris. Peters, beginning in 1906,[28] described similar cases of what has become generally known as Peters' anomaly.

a. *General features.* Most cases are hereditary with recessive transmission. The defect is present at birth and is usually bilateral.

b. *Clinicopathologic features.* The hallmark of Peters' anomaly is a central defect in Descemet's membrane and corneal endothelium with thinning and opacification of the corresponding area of corneal stroma.[29-32] Adhesions extend from the borders of this defect to the central iris. Bowman's membrane may also be absent centrally.[31, 32] The disorder has been *sub-divided* into *three groups* (Fig. 10.2), each of which may have more than one pathogenic mechanism[30]:

(1). *Not associated with keratolenticular contact or cataract.* In these cases, the defect in Descemet's membrane may represent primary failure of corneal endothelial development.[31] However, rare cases may be secondary to intrauterine inflammation,[33] which was originally postulated by von Hippel[27] and gave rise to the term "von Hippel's internal corneal ulcer."

(2). *Associated with keratolenticular contact or cataract.* Most histopathologic studies suggest that the lens developed normally and was then secondarily pushed forward against the cornea by one of several mechanisms, causing the loss of Descemet's membrane.[30, 31, 34] It is also possible that some cases may result from incomplete separation of the lens vesicle from surface ectoderm.

(3). *Associated with Rieger's syndrome.* This rare condition will be discussed later in this chapter.

c. *Glaucoma.* Approximately half of the patients with Peters' anomaly will develop glaucoma, and this is frequently present at birth.[3] The mechanism of the glaucoma is uncertain, since the anterior chamber angle is usually grossly normal by clinical examination. One histopathologic report of the eye of a young child with Peters' anomaly described changes in the trabecular meshwork that are characteristic of aging.[35] In cases of Peters' anomaly associated with the anterior chamber angle abnormalities of Rieger's syndrome, the mechanism of glaucoma is presumably the same as in the latter condition, as discussed earlier in this chapter.

d. *Differential diagnosis.* Central mesodermal dysgenesis of the anterior ocular segment must be distinguished from other causes of central corneal opacities in infants, which include primary congenital glaucoma, birth trauma, the mucopolysaccharidoses, and congenital hereditary corneal dystrophy.

e. *Management.* All infants and children with cloudy corneas

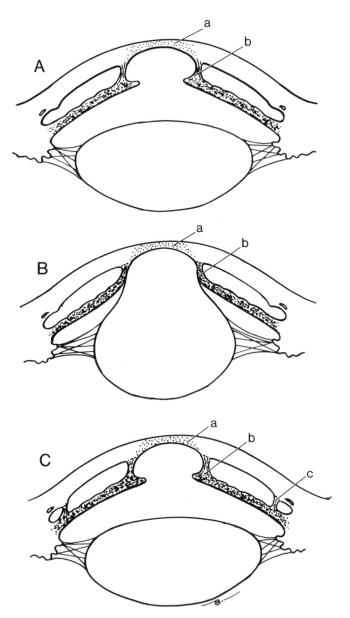

Figure 10.2. Peter's anomaly with central corneal defect (**a**) and adhesions (**b**) from corneal defect to central iris, showing three forms according to Townsend *et al.*[30] **A:** without keratolenticular contact or cataract; **B:** with keratolenticular contact or cataract; **C:** with peripheral defects of Rieger's anomaly (**c**).

must be examined carefully for the possibility of associated glaucoma. The glaucoma usually requires surgical intervention, and a trabeculectomy may offer the best chance of success. Penetrating keratoplasty is also frequently necessary.

3. *Congenital corneal leukomas and staphylomas.* These cases may represent the more severe forms of central mesodermal dysgenesis of the anterior ocular segment and are frequently associated with glaucoma.[3]

D. Combined Rieger's Syndrome and Peters' Anomaly

In 1962, Zimmerman presented a case to the Verhoeff Society in which a prominent Schwalbe's ring and malformation of the filtration angle was associated with iris adhesions to both central and peripheral corneal defects.[1] Although the association of central and peripheral developmental defects of the anterior ocular segment is rare, other cases have subsequently been reported.[3, 30, 31, 32, 36] In addition, anterior segment dysgenesis and keratolenticular adhesion have been described in association with aniridia.[37]

II. GLAUCOMA ASSOCIATED WITH ANIRIDA

A. Aniridia[38]

1. *General features.* Aniridia is a bilateral condition, which may be inherited by autosomal dominant transmission, although some cases occur spontaneously,[38] and patients with chromosomal abnormalities have also been reported.[39, 40]

2. *Clinical Features.* The hallmark of aniridia is the *congenital absence of a normal iris.* The name "aniridia," however, is a misnomer, since the iris is only partially absent, with a rudimentary stump of variable width (Fig. 10.3). Aniridia is associated with multiple ocular defects, some of which are present at birth, while others may develop later in childhood or early adulthood. In addition, some cases of aniridia may be associated systemic abnormalities.

 a. *Associated ocular defects.*

 (1). *Cornea.* In a high percentage of cases, a corneal pannus and opacity begins in the peripheral cornea in early life and advances toward the center of the cornea with increasing age. Microcornea[41] and keratolenticular adhesions[37] have also been reported.

 (2). *Lens.* Localized congenital opacities are common but usually insignificant. However, progressive cataracts may lead to significant visual impairment by approximately the third decade of life. The lens may also be subluxed,[41] or congenitally absent.[42]

 (3). *Foveal hypoplasia.* This is a frequent finding and presumably accounts for the characteristic *poor visual acuity* and *nystagmus* of aniridia, since some aniridic patients may have reasonably good vision and no nystagmus despite the absence of large amounts of iris.[43]

 (4). *Other ocular defects.* Aniridia has also been reported in association with choroidal colobomas,[38] persistent pupillary membranes,[44] sclerocornea in a patient with the Hallerman-Streiff syndrome,[40] small optic nerve heads,[38] strabismus,[43] and ptosis.[42, 45]

 (5). *Glaucoma.* This common feature of aniridia is discussed below.

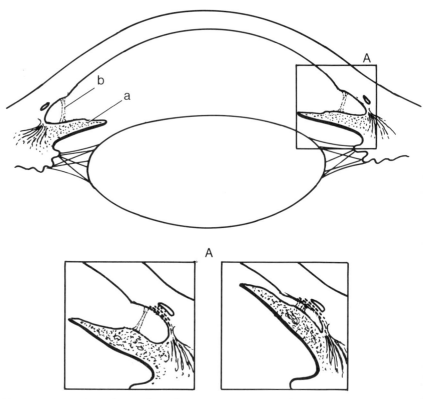

Figure 10.3. Aniridia with rudimentary iris (**a**) and fine tissue strands (**b**) extending across the anterior chamber angle. Insets (**A**) show theory of progressive angle closure by contracture of tissue strands as proposed by Grant and Walton.[46]

    b. *Associated systemic abnormalities.* Some patients with aniridia, especially the sporadic cases, will have a *Wilms tumor* or other genitourinary anomalies. *Mental retardation* may also occur in association with aniridia.

    3. *A classification* of four phenotypes of aniridia has been proposed on the basis of ocular features and associated systemic abnormalities[43]:

    a. Associated with foveal hypoplasia, nystagmus, corneal pannus, and glaucoma.

    b. Iris changes predominate and visual acuity may be normal.

    c. Associated with mental retardation.

    d. Associated with Wilms tumor and other genitourinary anomalies.

B. Glaucoma in Aniridia

    Glaucoma occurs in 50 to 75% of patients with aniridia, but usually does not appear before late childhood or adolescence.[38, 46]

1. *Theories of Mechanism.* The development of glaucoma in an eye with aniridia appears to correlate with the gonioscopic appearance of the anterior chamber angle.[38, 46]

a. In infancy, the angle is usually open and unobstructed, although some eyes may have strands of tissue with occasional fine blood vessels extending from the iris root to the trabecular meshwork or higher. The presence of congenital anomalies in the filtration angle appears to be more common in patients with chromosomal defects and may lead to glaucoma early in life.

b. During the first 5 to 15 years of life, many eyes with aniridia will undergo progressive change in the anterior chamber angle as the rudimentary stump of iris comes to lie over the trabecular meshwork. The progressive obstruction of the anterior chamber angle may be due to contracture of the tissue strands between the peripheral iris and angle wall (Fig. 10.3).[46] In eyes with mild intraocular pressure elevation, the obstruction to aqueous outflow may be limited to the superior quadrant, while in most eyes with more advanced glaucoma, the iris stroma covers much of the trabecular meshwork.

2. *Management.* Conventional medical therapy may control the intraocular pressure initially, but eventually proves to be inadequate in most cases. Filtering surgery is often unsuccessful, while cyclo-cryotherapy has been shown to have lasting benefit in some cases. Goniotomy is of no value in advanced cases, but preliminary experience suggests that early goniotomy to separate the strands between the iris and the trabecular meshwork may prevent the development of glaucoma.[38, 46]

III. GLAUCOMAS ASSOCIATED WITH CONGENITAL SYNDROMES

Glaucoma may be a feature of many congenital syndromes. The present discussion will be limited to those syndromes that represent multiple-system developmental anomalies.

A. Lowe's (Oculocerebrorenal) Syndrome[47]

1. *General features.* Lowe's syndrome is a sex-linked disorder characterized by mental retardation, renal rickets, aminoaciduria, hypotonia, acidemia, and irritability.

2. *Ocular features.* The two principal ocular abnormalities are *cataracts*, which are usually bilateral and occur in nearly all cases, and *glaucoma*, which is seen in approximately two-thirds of the patients. The mechanism of the glaucoma is related to faulty development of the filtration angle. Gonioscopy reveals only minor anatomic defects, including poor visualization of the scleral spur and a narrow ciliary band. Goniotomy is reported to be beneficial in some cases. Other ocular findings include microphthalmia, strabismus, nystagmus, miosis, and iris atrophy.

B. Chromosomal Anomalies[47]

1. *Trisomy 21* (Down's syndrome). This condition is characterized by mental retardation and a typical facies. Ocular findings include epicanthus, nystagmus, strabismus, keratoconus, cataracts, and congenital glaucoma.

2. *Trisomy D (13–15) syndrome.* The principal systemic features include mental retardation, deafness, heart disease, and motor seizures. The condition is usually not compatible with life, although milder forms have been reported.[48] Ocular findings include microphthalmia, coloboma with cartilage, congenital cataracts, retinal dysplasia, and hyperplastic primary vitreous.[24] In addition, dysembryogeneses of the anterior chamber angle has been described.[24] Glaucoma may be present as a result of several of these developmental defects.

3. *Turners Syndrome* (XO). These patients are typically short-statured, post-adolescent females with sexual infantilism and multiple systemic anomalies. Ocular findings include ptosis, epicanthus, cataract, strabismus, blue sclera, corneal nebulae, and color blindness.[49] Developmental glaucoma is rarely associated.

C. Stickler's Syndrome

Stickler's syndrome (hereditary progressive arthro-ophthalmopathy). This autosomal dominant connective tissue dysplasia is characterized by ocular, orofacial, and generalized skeletal abnormalities.[50] The *Pierre-Robin anomaly*, of mandibular hypoplasia, glossoptosis, and cleft palate may be seen in some patients. The most common ocular manifestations are high myopia, open-angle glaucoma, cataracts, vitreoretinal degeneration, and retinal detachment.[51] Neovascular glaucoma has also been reported in association with Stickler's syndrome.[52] The mechanism of the open-angle glaucoma is unknown. It can usually be controlled medically, although miotics should be avoided if possible, due to the potential for retinal detachment.

D. Hallerman-Streiff Syndrome

Micrognathia and dwarfism in this condition may be associated with ocular findings, including cataracts and microphthalmos. Glaucoma may also be present in association with absorption of lens material.

E. Rubenstein's Broad-thumb Syndrome

These individuals have mental retardation with characteristically large thumbs and big toes. Some may have glaucoma of the infantile type.

F. Ehlers Danlos Syndrome

This connective tissue disorder is characterized by loose skin and joints. The blood vessels are fragile, and spontaneous hemorrhage and dissecting aortic aneurysms may occur. Glaucoma has been reported among the multiple ocular anomalies.

G. Oculodentodigital Dysplasia

The systemic features of this disorder are hypoplastic dental enamel, microdontia, bilateral syndactyly and a characteristic thin nose. Multiple ocular anomalies have been described, including glaucoma. The mechanism of the glaucoma is uncertain, although some have mild mesodermal abnormalities of the anterior chamber angle,[19] and one case of chronic angle closure glaucoma associated with bilateral microcornea has been reported.[53]

H. Hurler's Syndrome

This prototype of the mucopolysaccharidoses is an autosomal recessive disease with central nervous system, skeletal, and visceral abnormalities. The typical ocular finding is corneal clouding. Glaucoma has also been reported and was felt to result from mucopolysaccharide-containing cells in the aqueous outflow system.[54]

IV. PHAKOMATOSES

A. Terminology

In 1932, Van der Hoeve[55] coined the term, "phakomatosis," meaning "motherspot" or "birthmark," to denote a group of disorders that are characterized by *hamartomas*, or congenital tumors arising from tissue that is normally found in the involved area. These hamartomas primarily involve the *eye*, *skin*, and *nervous system.* Other systems may be involved to a lesser degree, including the pulmonary, cardiovascular, gastrointestinal, renal, and skeletal systems.[56] In some cases, the anomalies are present at birth, while others become manifest later in life. Only those phakomatoses that may be associated with glaucoma will be discussed in this text.

B. Sturge-Weber Syndrome (Encephalotrigeminal Angiomatosis)

1. *General features.* The hamartoma in this condition arises from *vascular tissue* and produces a characteristic *port wine hemangioma* of the skin along the trigeminal distribution and an *ipsilateral leptomeningeal angioma.* The angiomata are present at birth and are usually unilateral, although bilateral cases also occur. The nervous system involvement frequently causes seizure disorders, hemispheric motor or sensory defects and intellectual deficiency. A characteristic radiographic finding is cortical calcifications that develop after several years and appear as double densities or "railroad tracks." There is no race or sex predilection, and no hereditary pattern has been established.

2. *Ocular features*

a. *Glaucoma.* In approximately half of the cases in which the port-wine stain involves both the ophthalmic and maxillary divisions of the trigeminal nerve, glaucoma will be present. This is always on the side of the cutaneous lesion.

(1). *Theories of mechanism.* The cause of glaucoma in the

Sturge-Weber syndrome is a controversial issue. Weiss[57] described two mechanisms, the more common of which occurs in infants, with a *developmental anomaly* of the anterior chamber angle similar to that of primary congenital glaucoma. The other type appears later in life and is associated with an open anterior chamber angle and small *arteriovenous fistulas* in the episcleral vessels. Phelps,[58] however, observed episcleral hemangiomas in all cases and *elevated episcleral venous pressure* when this parameter could be studied, but saw no abnormalities of the anterior chamber angle. One histopathologic report described hemangiomas of the choroid and episclera, as well as a partial mesodermal anomaly of the anterior chamber angle.[59]

(2). *Management.* Medical therapy may suffice to control the glaucoma which occurs in later life, while the infantile form usually requires surgical intervention.[57] Since it is not certain whether glaucoma is due to anterior chamber angle anomalies or elevated episcleral venous pressure, a combined trabeculotomy-trabeculectomy may offer the best hope of success, by treating both possible sources of elevated intraocular pressure.[60] Complications of surgery in this condition include massive choroidal effusion,[60, 61] and expulsive hemorrhage.[59]

b. *Choroidal hemangioma* is another ocular feature of the Sturge-Weber syndrome. The possible relationship to the postoperative uveal effusion has not been established.

C. von Recklinghausen's Neurofibromatosis

1. *General features.* The principal systemic lesions in this condition involve the skin and include *cafe' au lait spots*, which are flat hyperpigmented lesions with well-circumscribed borders, and *neurofibromas*, that appear as soft, flesh-colored, pedunculated masses. The latter lesions arise from Schwann cells. Central nervous system involvement is uncommon, although neurofibromas may develop from cranial nerves, especially the acoustic nerve. The condition is inherited by an autosomal dominant mode with variable expressivity.

2. *Ocular features*

a. *Neurofibromas.* These lesions may also involve the eyelids, conjunctiva, iris, ciliary body, and choroid. In addition, retinal hamartomas and gliomas of the optic nerve are occasionally present.

b. *Glaucoma.* Intraocular pressure elevation is more likely to occur in neurofibromatosis when the lids are involved with neurofibromas. Several mechanisms of glaucoma have been described[62, 63]

(1). Infiltration of the angle with neurofibromatous tissue.

(2). Closure of the anterior chamber angle due to neurofibromas thickening of the ciliary body and choroid.

(3). Fibrovascular membrane resembling neovascular glaucoma.

(4). Failure of normal anterior chamber angle development.

3. *Management.* In treating the glaucoma, medical measures should be attempted first, since surgical approaches are often not satisfactory

D. von Hippel-Lindau Disease

This phakomatosis is characterized by *angiomatosis* of the retina and, in a small percentage of cases, the cerebellum. Most cases are not familial. Glaucoma may occur as a late sequelae due to rubeosis iridis or iridocyclitis.

E. Nevus of Ota (Congenital Oculodermal Melanosis)

This condition is not included in all reported classifications of the phakomatoses, but does fit the broader definition of the disease group.

1. *General features.* The hamartoma in this condition represents an abnormally large accumulation of *melanocytes* in ocular tissues, as well as the skin in the distribution of the trigeminal nerve. It is nearly always unilateral with a preponderance of females and a tendency toward dark races.[64] Degeneration to *malignant melanomas* may occur in Caucasian patients, but rarely in non-Caucasians.[65-67]

2. *Glaucoma.* In the few case reports of glaucoma associated with the nevus of Ota, additional features were present which could have caused the glaucoma.[66, 68] However, evidence of chronic glaucoma has been observed in a patient with the nevus of Ota, whose involved eye had unusually heavy pigmentation of the trabecular meshwork with no other apparent cause for the glaucoma.[69]

References

 1. Reese, AB, Ellsworth, RM: The anterior chamber cleavage syndrome. Arch Ophthal 75:307, 1966.
 2. Waring, GO III, Rodrigues, MM, Laibson, PR: Anterior chamber cleavage syndrome. A stepladder classification. Surv Ophthal 20:3, 1975.
 3. Alkemade, PPH: Dysgenesis Mesodermalis of the Iris and the Cornea. Assen, Netherlands, Charles C Thomas, Springfield, Ill, 1969.
 4. Shields, MB: Mesodermal Dysgeneses of the Anterior Ocular Segment. *In* The Secondary Glaucomas, Ritch, R, Shields, MB, eds, CV Mosby Co, St Louis (in press).
 5. Burian, HM, Braley, AE, Allan, L: External and gonioscopic visibility of the ring of Schwalbe and the trabecular zone. An interpretation of the posterior corneal embryotoxon and the so-called congenital hyaline membranes on the posterior corneal surface. Trans Am Ophthal Soc 51:389, 1955.
 6. Axenfeld, T: Embryotoxon corneae posterius. Ber Deutsch Ophthalmol Ges 42:301, 1920.
 7. Rieger, H: Beitrage zur Kenntnis seltener Mibbildungen der Iris. II. Uber Hypoplasie des Irisvorderblattes mit Verlagerung und Entrundung der Pupille. Albrecht Graefes Arch Klin Exp Ophthal 133:602, 1935.
 8. Hirst, LW, Quigley, HA, Stark, WJ, Shields, MB: Specular microscopy in iridocorneal endothelial syndrome. Am J Ophthal 89:11, 1980.
 9. Cross, HE, Maumenee, AE: Progressive spontaneous dissolution of the iris. Surv Ophthal 18:186, 1973.
10. Judisch GF, Phelps, CD, Hanson, J: Rieger's syndrome. A case report with a 15-year follow-up. Arch Ophthal 97:2120, 1979.
11. Gregor, Z, Hitchings, RA: Rieger's anomaly: a 42-year follow-up. Br J Ophthal 64:56, 1980.
12. Cross, HE, Jorgenson, RJ, Levin, LS, Kelly, TE: The Rieger syndrome: an autosomal dominant disorder with ocular, dental and systemic abnormalities. Pers Ophthal 3:3, 1979.
13. Sugar, HS: Juvenile glaucoma with Axenfeld's syndrome. A histologic report.

Am J Ophthal 59:1012, 1965.

14. Broughton, WL, Fine, BS, Zimmerman, LE: Congenital glaucoma associated with a chromosomal defect. A histologic study. Arch Ophthal 99:481, 1981.

15. Delmarcelle, Y, De Clerck, P, Pivont, A: Glaucome congenital associe a des malformations oculaires et somatiques dans deux generations successives. Bull Soc Belge Ophthal 120:638, 1958.

16. Wolter, JR, Sandall, GS, Fralick, FB: Mesodermal dysgenesis of the anterior eye: With a partially separated posterior embryotoxon. J Pediatr Ophthal 4:41, 1967.

17. Troeber, R, Rochels, R: Histologic findings in Rieger's mesodermal dysgenesis of the iris. Albrecht Graefes Arch Klin Ophthal 213:169, 1980.

18. Rubel, E: Angeborene Hypoplasie bzw. Aplasie des Irisvorderblattes. Klin Monatsbl Augenheilkd 51:174, 1913.

19. Judisch, GF, Martin-Casals, A, Hanson, JW, Olin, WH: Oculodentodigital dysplasia. Four new reports and a literature review. Arch Ophthal 97:878, 1979.

20. Cross, HE: Ectopia lentis et pupillae. Am J Ophthal 88:381, 1979.

21. Jerndal, T: Goniodysgenesis and hereditary juvenile glaucoma. Acta Ophthal 107:(Suppl):1, 1980.

22. Henkind, P, Friedman, AH: Iridogoniodysgenesis with cataract. Am J Ophthal 72:949, 1971.

23. Gramer, E, Krieglstein, GK: Infantile glaucoma in unilateral uveal ectropion. Albrecht Graefes Arch Klin Exp Ophthal 211:215, 1979.

24. Hoepner, J, Yanoff, M: Ocular anomalies in trisomy 13–15: an analysis of 13 eyes with two new findings. Am J Ophthal 74:729, 1972.

25. Wolter, JR, Haney, WP: Histopathology of keratoconus posticus circumscriptus. Arch Ophthal 69:357, 1963.

26. Krachmer, JH, Rodrigues, MM: Posterior keratoconus. Arch Ophthal 96:1867, 1978.

27. Hippel, E: Ueber Hydrophthalmus congenitus nebst Bemerkungen uber die Verfarbung der Cornea durch Blutfarbstoff. Pathologisch–anatomische Untersuchung. Albrecht Graefes Arch Klin Exp Ophthal 44:539, 1897.

28. Peters, A: Ueber angeborene Defektbildung der Descemetschen Membran. Klin Monatsbl Augenheilkd 44:27, 1906.

29. Townsend, WM: Congenital corneal leukomas. I. Central defect in Descemet's membrane. Am J Ophthal 77:80, 1974.

30. Townsend, WM, Font, RL, Zimmerman, LE: Congenital corneal leukomas. II. Histopathologic findings in 19 eyes with central defect in Descemet's membrane. Am J Ophthal 77:192, 1974.

31. Stone, DL, Kenyon, KR, Green, WR, Ryan, SJ: Congenital central corneal leukoma (Peters' anomaly). Am J Ophthal 81:173, 1976.

32. Nakanishi, I, Brown, SI: The histopathology and ultrastructure of congenital, central corneal opacity (Peters' anomaly). Am J Ophthal 72:801, 1971.

33. Polack, FM, Graue, EL: Scanning electron microscopy of congenital corneal leukomas (Peters' anomaly). Am J Ophthal 88:169, 1979.

34. Heckenlively, J, Kielar, R: Congenital perforated cornea in Peters's anomaly. Am J Ophthal 88:63, 1979.

35. Kupfer, C, Kuwabara, T, Stark, WJ: The histopathology of Peters' anomaly. Am J Ophthal 80:653, 1975.

36. Scheie, HG, Yanoff, M: Peters' anomaly and total posterior coloboma of retinal pigment epithelium and choroid. Arch Ophthal 87:525, 1972.

37. Beauchamp, GR: Anterior segment dysgenesis keratolenticular adhesion and aniridia. J Pediatr Ophthal Strabismus 17:55, 1980.

38. Walton, DS: Glaucoma in aniridia. *In* The Secondary Glaucomas, Ritch, R, Shields, MB, eds. CV Mosby Co, St Louis (in press).

39. Hittner, HM, Riccardi, VM, Francke, U: Aniridia caused by a heritable chromosome 11 deletion. Ophthalmology 86:1173, 1979.

40. Schanzlin, DJ, Goldberg, DB, Brown, SI: Hallermann-Streiff syndrome associated with sclerocornea, aniridia, and a chromosomal abnormality. Am J Ophthal 90:411, 1980.

41. David, R, MacBeath, L, Jenkins, T: Aniridia associated with microcornea and

subluxated lenses. Br J Ophthal 62:118, 1978.

42. Shields, MB, Reed, JW: Aniridia and congenital ptosis. Ann Ophthal 7:203, 1975.

43. Elsas, FM, Maumenee, IH, Kenyon, KR, Yoder, F: Familial aniridia with preserved ocular function. Am J Ophthal 83:718, 1977.

44. Hamming, N, Wilensky, J: Persistent pupillary membrane associated with aniridia. Am J Ophthal 86:118, 1978.

45. Bergamini, L, Ferraris, F, Gandiglio, G, Inghirami, L: Su di una singolare sindrome neuro-oftalmologica congenita e familiare (ptosi palpebrale, aniridia, cataratta, nistagmo, subatrofia ottica). Rivista Oto-Neuro-Oftalmologica 41:81, 1966.

46. Grant, WM, Walton, DS: Progressive changes in the angle in congenital aniridia with development of glaucoma. Am J Ophthal 78:842, 1974.

47. Kwitko, M, Friedman, AH: Glaucomas associated with congenital syndromes. In The Secondary Glaucomas, Ritch, R, Shields, MB, Eds. CV Mosby Co, St. Louis (in press).

48. Lichter, PR, Schmickel, RD: Posterior vortex vein and congenital glaucoma in a patient with trisomy 13 syndrome. Am J Ophthal 80:939, 1975.

49. Lessell, S, Forbes, AP: Eye signs in Turner's syndrome. Arch Ophthal 76:211, 1966.

50. Stickler, GB, Belau, PG, Farrell, FJ, Jones, JD, Pugh, DG, Steinberg, AG, Ward, LE: Hereditary progressive arthro-ophthalmopathy. Mayo Clin Proc 40:433, 1965.

51. Blair, NP, Albert, DM, Liberfarb, RM, Hirose, T: Hereditary progressive arthro-ophthalmopathy of Stickler. Am J Ophthal 88:876, 1979.

52. Young, NJA, Hitchings, RA, Sehmi, K, Bird, AC: Stickler's syndrome and neovascular glaucoma. Br J Ophthal 63:826, 1979.

53. Sugar, HS: Oculodentodigital dysplasia syndrome with angle-closure glaucoma. Am J Ophthal 86:36, 1978.

54. Spellacy, E, Bankes, JLK, Crow, J, Dourmashkin, R, Shah, D, Watts, RWE: Glaucoma in a case of Hurler disease. Br J Ophthal 64:773, 1980.

55. Van der Hoeve, J: Eye symptoms in phakomatoses. Trans Ophthal Soc UK 52:380, 1932.

56. Beck, RW, Hanno, R, Callen, JP: The phakomatoses and other neurocutaneous disorders. Pers Ophthal 3:173, 1979.

57. Weiss, DI: Dual origin of glaucoma in encephalotrigeminal haemangiomatosis. Trans Ophthal Soc UK 93:477, 1973.

58. Phelps, CD: The pathogenesis of glaucoma in Sturge-Weber syndrome. Ophthalmology 85:276, 1978.

59. Christensen, GR, Records, RE: Glaucoma and expulsive hemorrhage mechanisms in the Sturge-Weber syndrome. Ophthalmology 86:1360, 1979.

60. Board, RJ, Shields, MB: Combined trabeculotomy-trabeculectomy for the management of glaucoma associated with Sturge-Weber syndrome Ophthal Surg 12:813, 1981.

61. Bellows, AR, Chylack, LT Jr, Epstein, DL, Hutchinson, BT: Choroidal effusion during glaucoma surgery in patients with prominent episcleral vessels. Arch Ophthal 97:493, 1979.

62. Grant, WM, Walton, DS: Distinctive gonioscopic findings in glaucoma due to neurofibromatosis. Arch Ophthal 79:127, 1968.

63. Wolter, JR, Butler, RG: Pigment spots of the iris and ectropion uveae. With glaucoma in neurofibromatosis. Am J Ophthal 56:964, 1963.

64. Mishima, Y, Mevorah, B: Nevus Ota and Nevus Ito in American negroes. J Invest Dermatol 36:133, 1961.

65. Albert, DM, Scheie, HG: Nevus of Ota with malignant melanoma of the choroid. Report of a case. Arch Ophthal 69:774, 1963.

66. Font, RL, Reynolds, AM, Zimmerman, LE: Diffuse malignant melanoma of the iris in the nevus of Ota. Arch Ophthal 77:513, 1967.

67. Sabates, FN, Yamashita, T: Congenital melanosis oculi. Complicated by two independent malignant melanomas of the choroid. Arch Ophthal 77:801, 1967.

68. Fishman, GRA, Anderson, R: Nevus of Ota. Report of two cases, one with open-angle glaucoma. Am J Ophthal 54:453, 1962.

69. Foulks, GN, Shields, MB: Glaucoma in oculodermal melanocytosis. Ann Ophthal 9:1299, 1977.

Chapter 11

GLAUCOMAS ASSOCIATED WITH INTRAOCULAR TUMORS

GLAUCOMAS ASSOCIATED WITH INTRAOCULAR TUMORS

In the diagnosis and management of secondary glaucomas, the physician must remain alert to the possibility that the underlying cause of the intraocular pressure elevation may represent a life-threatening disease. In the rare case of an intraocular malignancy, the emphasis of therapy shifts from prevention of blindness to preservation of life, and questions related to differential diagnosis and treatment of choice may, at times, be extremely difficult. These matters are the subject of this chapter. We will begin with neoplasia of children, as a continuation of the previous chapter, and then consider the more common forms of intraocular tumors, including malignant melanoma, metastatic malignancy, and benign neoplasia.

I. NEOPLASIA IN CHILDREN

The *phakomatoses*, which represent one group of tumors that may occur in childhood and cause secondary glaucoma, were discussed in Chapter 10. Neoplasia with glaucoma-inducing potential that are more specific for children include retinoblastoma, juvenile xanthogranuloma, and medulloepithelioma.

A. Retinoblastoma

1. *Incidence of glaucoma.* Although secondary glaucoma is not commonly recognized clinically in children with retinoblastoma, histopathologic studies suggest that it is a frequent complication of this disease.[1] In one study of 149 eyes, there was histologic evidence of a glaucoma-inducing mechanism in 50% of the cases, although an elevated intraocular pressure had been clinically recorded in only 23%.[1]

2. *Mechanisms of glaucoma.* Neovascularization of the iris is a frequent histopathologic finding in eyes with retinoblastoma,[1-3] and is the most common cause of the complicating secondary glaucoma.[1] However, both the rubeosis iridis and neovascular glaucoma are frequently overlooked clinically and should be considered in all cases of retinoblastoma.[2, 3] Two additional causes of glaucoma are pupillary block with secondary angle-closure due to massive exudative retinal detachment and obstruction of the anterior chamber angle by inflammatory cells or necrotic tumor tissue.[1]

3. *Differential diagnosis.* Conditions which simulate retinoblastoma have been called "pseudogliomas" and include retrolental fibroplasia, persistent hyperplastic primary vitreous, retinal dysplasia, Coats' disease, larval granulomatosis, and infantile retinal detachment.[4] Each of these conditions also have a high incidence of rubeosis iridis, so

that this factor is not helpful in distinguishing retinoblastoma from the pseudogliomas.[3, 4]

4. *Management.* Iris neovascularization carries a more grave prognosis in patients with retinoblastoma,[3] and the majority of affected eyes, especially when rubeosis iridis or glaucoma is present, are enucleated.

B. Juvenile Xanthogranuloma

This is a self-limiting disease of infants and young children. It is characterized by discrete, yellow, papular cutaneous lesions primarily of the head and neck as well as salmon-colored to lightly pigmented lesions of the iris.[5, 6] The latter feature is usually unilateral and may cause spontaneous hyphema. Secondary glaucoma may occur from invasion of the anterior chamber angle with histiocytes or in association with the hyphema or a secondary uveitis. Recommended treatment for eyes with juvenile xanthogranuloma and secondary glaucoma is topical and systemic corticosteroids and occasionally external beam irradiation.[7, 8]

C. Medulloepithelioma (Diktyoma).

This primary tumor of childhood arises most often from nonpigmented ciliary epithelium.[9] The clinical appearance is that of a whitish-gray mass or cyst of the iris or ciliary body. In a study of 56 cases, glaucoma was observed clinically in 26 eyes.[9] Histopathologic evidence of secondary glaucoma was seen in 18 cases, 11 of which had rubeosis iridis. Peripheral anterior synechiae and shallow anterior chambers were also commonly observed. In one report, glaucoma was associated with two white flocculi floating in the anterior chamber, delicate iris neovascularization, and a globular ciliary body mass.[10] Some medulloepitheliomas are malignant, although the mortality rate is low. While enucleation is the most common treatment, success has been reported with iridocyclectomy, and local excision has been recommended when the tumor is small and well circumscribed.[9]

D. Acute Leukemia

Acute leukemia is another cause of glaucoma secondary to neoplasia in children, and will be discussed later in this chapter under "Metastatic Malignancies."

II. MALIGNANT MELANOMA

A. Uveal Melanomas and Intraocular Pressure

The intraocular pressure in an eye with a uveal melanoma may be either elevated, normal, or slightly reduced. When the iris is involved, a high percentage of cases will have an elevated pressure,[11, 12] while eyes with a melanoma confined to the ciliary body may have a tension that is 2 to 3 mmHg lower than the fellow eye.[13] Choroidal melanomas occasionally cause secondary glaucoma, depending on the size and location of the tumor and the association of a retinal detachment.[11]

B. Clinical Features of Uveal Melanomas and Glaucoma

1. *Choroidal melanomas.* The patient may present with *acute angle-closure glaucoma,* usually associated with a retinal detachment.[11, 14, 15] The choroidal melanoma may not be detected at first if the tumor is masked by other ocular changes. The finding of a *retinal detachment* and glaucoma in the same eye should alert the clinician to the possibility of a malignant melanoma.[11] Ocular *inflammation* or intraocular *hemorrhage* may also be the initial clinical finding and may mask the underlying melanoma.[16] In addition, rubeosis iridis may be present in some cases.[11]

2. *Anterior uveal melanomas.* These tumors are usually easier to recognize, although associated changes occasionally occur, which may confuse the diagnosis:

a. *Iritis* may appear to be present, although this is frequently due to tumor cells in the anterior chamber.[12]

b. *Cyst-like structures* of the iris and ciliary body occur in some eyes with anterior uveal melanomas due to separation of the two epithelial layers by an eosinophilic exudate.[12, 17]

c. *Ocular melanosis* and *nevi* may also be present in an eye with a uveal melanoma.[12]

C. Diagnostic Adjuncts

The difficulty in detecting a uveal melanoma and distinguishing it from other intraocular tumors occasionally requires the use of special diagnostic measures.

1. *Ultrasonography* may demonstrate the presence of a choroidal or ciliary body melanoma that can not be directly visualized. However, this technique does not, with absolute certainty, distinguish a neoplasm from other masses of the posterior ocular segment.[18]

2. *Radioactive phosphorous uptake* (the 32 P test) is said to be helpful in differentiating benign from malignant lesions of the choroid.[19, 20] The study is not as useful in diagnosing tumors of the anterior uvea, although reports differ as to whether it is least accurate for the iris[19] or ciliary body.[20]

3. *Fluorescein angiography of the iris* is reported to be useful in distinguishing melanomas from benign lesions, such as leiomyomas.[21, 22]

4. *Cytologic examination* of an aqueous or vitreous aspirate may provide a histopathologic diagnosis of either a primary or metastatic malignancy.[23]

D. Differential Diagnosis

Other conditions that should be considered in an eye with glaucoma and a suspected malignant melanoma include metastatic malignancies and benign tumors or inflammatory conditions of the uvea. These disorders will be discussed later in this chapter.

E. Mechanisms of glaucoma

1. *Choroidal melanomas.* The most common mechanism of glaucoma associated with a choroidal melanoma is angle-closure due to forward displacement of the lens by a large posterior tumor, which is commonly associated with a total retinal detachment.[11] Neovascular glaucoma is a less common mechanism.[11]

2. *Anterior uveal melanomas.* The glaucomas associated with these tumors are usually open-angle forms due to obstruction of the anterior chamber angle by direct extension of the tumor or by seeding of tumor cells or melanin granules.[11, 12, 17] A specific condition has been referred to as *melanomalytic glaucoma*, in which macrophages containing melanin from a necrotic melanoma obstruct the trabecular meshwork.[11, 24, 25] In another variation of anterior uveal melanoma and glaucoma, a low grade melanoma of the iris with a nodular appearance resembling tapioca (tapioca melanoma) is reported to cause glaucoma in one third of the cases.[26] Ciliary body and anterior choroidal melanomas may also cause an angle-closure form of secondary glaucoma due to compression of the iris root into the anterior chamber angle[17] or forward displacement of the lens-iris diaphragm.[27]

F. Prognosis

When glaucoma is associated with a uveal melanoma, the prognosis appears to be worse. In a clinicopathologic study of eleven consecutive anterior uveal melanomas, three of the four with *ciliary body melanoma* and glaucoma died of metastatic diseases within 2½ years after enucleation.[12] Histologic evaluation of these eyes revealed epithelioid melanoma cells in the aqueous outflow system, which is a potential route of extraocular metastasis. It may be that diagnostic and surgical manuevers that raise the intraocular pressure accelerate this and other possible routes of extraocular dissemination.[12, 28, 29]

Patients with *choroidal melanomas* also have a more guarded prognosis when secondary glaucoma is present, since the melanoma is usually large by the time glaucoma has developed. *Melanomas of the iris* have a more benign course than those of the choroid,[30, 31] although metastasis of iris melanomas has been reported.[30, 32, 33]

G. Management

As noted above, when glaucoma is present in an eye with a uveal melanoma, the tumor is most often large or has disseminated in the anterior segment. For this reason, enucleation is usually indicated in eyes with melanoma and glaucoma with the possible exception of low grade melanomas of the iris. When enucleation is performed for malignant melanoma, especially when glaucoma is present, measures to minimize intraocular pressure elevation at the time of surgery may help to minimize the extraocular spread of tumor cells. One report described a manometric pressure regulating system for this purpose.[29]

III. METASTATIC MALIGNANCIES

A. Metastatic Carcinoma

In a study of 230 patients with autopsy-proven primary carcinomas, 12% were found to have metastasis to the eye and orbit.[34] The most common primary sites are the lung and breast, and the most common site of ocular metastasis is the posterior uvea.[34, 35] Glaucoma was detected in 7.5% of 227 cases of carcinoma metastatic to the eye and orbit,[35] and in 56% of the 26 cases in which the tumor primarily involved the anterior segment.[36] The clinical features of patients with metastatic carcinoma of the anterior uvea and glaucoma include multiple, translucent nodules on the iris, rubeosis iridis, and intraocular inflammation and hemorrhage.[36–39]

Mechanisms of glaucoma in eyes with anterior uveal metastatic carcinoma include open-angle forms in which the trabecular meshwork may be covered by sheets of tumor cells or infiltrated with neoplastic tissue.[36] Other patients have angle-closure glaucoma due to compression of the iris by the tumor or due to the formation of peripheral anterior synechae.[36] Eyes with metastatic carcinoma respond well to irradiation although chemotherapy and photocoagulation are occasionally employed.[38] If the glaucoma persists, it should be controlled medically whenever possible.

B. Malignant Melanoma

Although ocular melanomas are nearly always primary malignancies, metastatic melanomas of the eye have been reported and may occasionally cause secondary glaucoma.[23]

C. Acute Leukemia

The eye may occasionally be infiltrated with neoplastic cells in patients with acute leukemia. In one study of 39 children with acute leukemia, 28% were found to have flare or cells in the anterior chamber by slit lamp examination, although the histologic basis for this was not determined.[40] A leukemic infiltration of the anterior ocular segment leads to secondary glaucoma in some cases, which may present in association with hyphema and hypopyon.[41, 42] These patients typically have acute lymphocytic leukemia. The diagnosis can be established by cytologic examination of an aqueous aspirate, and treatment usually includes irradiation and chemotherapy.

D. Histiocytosis-X

Histiocytosis-X has also been reported to involve the anterior chamber with associated secondary glaucoma.[43]

IV. BENIGN OCULAR TUMORS

Several benign tumors of the eye may also be associated with secondary glaucoma and must be distinguished from ocular malignancies.

A. Iris Nevi

In the *Cogan-Reese* (*iris nevus*) *syndrome*, pedunculated nodules or diffuse nevi of the iris are associated with the other features of the iridocorneal endothelial syndrome, which is discussed in the next chapter.[44-48] The glaucoma in this spectrum of disease is due to the extension of a membrane across the anterior chamber angle.[47] The benign lesions of the iris in this condition have been mistaken for malignant melanomas, which has led to enucleation in some patients.[44, 45] A case has also been described in which a diffuse non-pigmented nevus of the iris caused a unilateral open-angle glaucoma by direct extension across the trabecular meshwork.[49]

B. Necrotic Melanocytoma

A *necrotic melanocytoma* of the iris has been reported to cause secondary glaucoma by dispersion of pigment into the anterior chamber angle.[50]

C. Cysts

Cysts of the iris or ciliary body may develop from separation of the epithelial layers. Multiple cysts of the ciliary body may also occur in association with multiple myeloma and syphillis.[51] In rare cases these may be extensive enough to cause forward displacement of the peripheral iris with secondary angle-closure glaucoma.

D. Phakomatoses

The *phakomatoses*, some of which may be associated with glaucoma, were discussed in Chapter 10.

References

1. Yoshizumi, MO, Thomas, JV, Smith, TR: Glaucoma-inducing mechanisms in eyes with retinoblastoma. Arch Ophthal 96:105, 1978.
2. Walton, DS, Grant WM: Retinoblastoma and iris neovascularization. Am J Ophthal 65:598, 1968.
3. Spaulding, AG: Rubeosis iridis in retinoblastoma and pseudoglioma. Tr Am Ophthal Soc 76:584, 1978.
4. Moazed, K, Albert, D, Smith TR: Rubeosis iridis in "pseudogliomas." Surv Ophthal 25:85, 1980.
5. Zimmerman, L: Ocular lesions of juvenile xanthogranuloma (nevoxanthoendothelioma). Trans Am Acad Ophthal Otol 69:412, 1965.
6. Schwartz, LW, Rodrigues, MM, Hallett, JW: Juvenile xanthogranuloma diagnosed by paracentesis. Am J Ophthal 77:243, 1974.
7. Gass, JDM: Management of juvenile xanthogranuloma of the iris. Arch Ophthal 71:344, 1964.
8. Hadden, OB: Bilateral juvenile xanthogranuloma of the iris. Br J Ophthal 59:699, 1975.
9. Broughton, WL, Zimmerman, LE: A clinicopathologic study of 56 cases of intraocular medulloepitheliomas. Am J Ophthal 85:407, 1978.
10. Jakobiec, FA, Howard, GM, Ellsworth, RM, Rosen M: Electron microscopic diagnosis of medulloepithelioma. Am J Ophthal 79:321, 1975.
11. Yanoff, M: Glaucoma mechanism in ocular malignant melanomas. Am J Ophthal 70: 898, 1970.

12. Shields, MB, Klintworth, GK: Anterior uveal melanomas and intraocular pressure. Ophthalmology 87:503, 1980.

13. Foos, RY, Hull, SN, Straatsma, BR: Early diagnosis of ciliary body melanomas. Arch Ophthal 81:336, 1969.

14. Singer, PR, Krupin, T, Smith, ME, Becker, B: Recurrent orbital and metastatic melanoma in a patient undergoing previous glaucoma surgery. Am J Ophthal 87:766, 1979.

15. Levine, DJ: Surgical reversal of acute angle closure glaucoma due to malignant melanoma: case report. Glaucoma 1:84, 1979.

16. Fraser, DJ, Font RL: Ocular inflammation and hemorrhage as initial manifestations of uveal malignant melanoma. Incidence and prognosis. Arch Ophthal 97:1311, 1979.

17. Hopkins, RE, Carriker, FR: Malignant melanoma of the ciliary body. Am J Ophthal 45:835, 1958.

18. Gitter, KA, Meyer, D, Sarin, LK: Ultrasound to evaluate eyes with opaque media. Am J Ophthal 64:100, 1967.

19. Shields, JA: Accuracy and limitations of the 32P test in the diagnosis of ocular tumors: An analysis of 500 cases. Ophthalmology 85:950, 1978.

20. Goldberg, B, Kara, GB, Previte, LR: The use of radioactive phosphorus (32P) in the diagnosis of ocular tumors. Am J Ophthal 90:817, 1980.

21. Christiansen, JM, Wetzig, PC, Thatcher, DB, Green WR: Diagnosis and management of anterior uveal tumors. Ophthal Surg 10:81, 1979.

22. Brovkina, AF, Chichua, AG: Value of fluorescein iridography in diagnosis of tumours of the iridociliary zone. Br J Ophthal 63:157, 1979.

23. Char, DH, Schwartz, A, Miller, TR, Abele, JS: Ocular metastases from systemic melanoma. Am J Ophthal 90:702, 1980.

24. Yanoff, M, Scheie, HG: Melanomalytic glaucoma. Report of a case. Arch Ophthal 84:471, 1970.

25. Van Buskirk, EM, Leure-duPree, AE: Pathophysiology and electron microscopy of melanomalytic glaucoma. Am J Ophthal 85:160, 1978.

26. Reese, AB, Mund, ML, Iwamoto, T: Tapioca melanoma of the iris. I. Clinical and light microscopy studies. Am J Ophthal 74:840, 1972.

27. Sussman, W, Weintraub, J: Acute congestive glaucoma caused by malignant melanoma. Ann Ophthal 8:665, 1976.

28. Zimmerman, LE, McLean, IW, Foster, WD: Statistical analysis of follow-up data concerning uveal melanomas, and the influence of enucleation. Ophthalmology 87:557, 1980.

29. Kramer, KK, La Piana, FG, Whitmore, PV: Enucleation with stabilization of intraocular pressure in the treatment of uveal melanomas. Ophthal Surg 11: 39, 1980.

30. Rones, B, Zimmerman, LE: The prognosis of primary tumors of the iris treated by iridectomy. Arch Ophthal 60:193, 1958.

31. Dunphy, EB, Dryja, TP, Albert, DM, Smith, TR: Melanocytic tumor of the anterior uvea. Am J Ophthal 86:680, 1978.

32. Zakka, KA, Foos, RY, Sulit, H: Metastatic tapioca iris melanoma. Br J Ophthal 63:744, 1979.

33. Sunba, MSN, Rahi, AHS, Morgan, G: Tumors of the anterior uvea. I. Metastasizing malignant melanoma of the iris. Arch Ophthal 98:82, 1980.

34. Bloch, RS, Gartner, S: The incidence of ocular metastatic carcinoma. Arch Ophthal 85:673, 1971.

35. Ferry, AP, Font, RL: Carcinoma metastatic to the eye and orbit. I. A clinicopathologic study of 227 cases. Arch Ophthal 92:276, 1974.

36. Ferry, AP, Font, RL: Carcinoma metastatic to the eye and orbit. II. A clinicopathological study of 26 patients with carcinoma metastatic to the anterior segment of the eye. Arch Ophthal 93:472, 1975.

37. Freeman, TR, Friedman, AH: Metastatic carcinoma of the iris. Am J Ophthal 80:947, 1975.

38. Frank, KW, Sugar, HS, Sherman, AI, Beckman, H, Thoms, S: Anterior segment metastases from an ovarian choriocarcinoma. Am J Ophthal 87:778, 1979.
39. Miller, B, Rush, P, Luntz, MH: Metastatic carcinoma of the iris. Ann Ophthal 12:514, 1980.
40. Abramson, A: Anterior chamber activity in children with acute leukemia. Ann Ophthal 12:553, 1980.
41. Rowan, PJ, Sloan, JB: Iris and anterior chamber involvement in leukemia. Ann Ophthal 8:1081, 1976.
42. Zakka, KA, Yee, RD, Shorr, N, Smith, GS, Pettit, TH, Foos, RY: Leukemic iris infiltration. Am J Ophthal 89:204, 1980.
43. Epstein, DL, Grant, WM: Secondary open-angle glaucoma in histiocytosis X. Am J Ophthal 84:332, 1977.
44. Cogan, DG, Reese, AB: A syndrome of iris nodules, ectopic Descemet's membrane, and unilateral glaucoma. Doc Ophthal 26:424, 1969.
45. Scheie, HG, Yanoff, M: Iris nevus (Cogan-Reese) syndrome. A cause of unilateral glaucoma. Arch Ophthal 93:963, 1975.
46. Shields, MB, Campbell, DG, Simmons, RJ, Hutchinson, BT: Iris nodules in essential iris atrophy. Arch Ophthal 94:406, 1976.
47. Campbell, DG, Shields, MB, Smith, TR: The corneal endothelium and the spectrum of essential iris atrophy. Am J Ophthal 86:317, 1978.
48. Jakobiec, FA, Yanoff, M, Mottow, L, Anker, P, Jones, IS: Solitary iris nevus associated with peripheral anterior synechiae and iris endothelialization. Am J Ophthal 83:884, 1977.
49. Nik, NA, Hidayat, A, Zimmerman, LE, Fine, BS: Diffuse iris nevus manifested by unilateral open angle glaucoma. Arch Ophthal 99:125, 1981.
50. Shields, JA, Annesley, WH Jr, Spaeth, GL: Necrotic melanocytoma of iris with secondary glaucoma. Am J Ophthal 84:826, 1977.
51. Eagle, RC Jr, Yanoff, M: Glaucoma secondary to intraocular tumors. In Glaucoma: Contemporary International Concepts, Bellows, JG, ed. Masson Publ, Inc, New York, 1979, p 339.

Chapter 12

GLAUCOMAS ASSOCIATED WITH PRIMARY DISORDERS OF THE CORNEAL ENDOTHELIUM

GLAUCOMAS ASSOCIATED WITH PRIMARY DISORDERS OF THE CORNEAL ENDOTHELIUM

There are a few forms of glaucoma which are characterized by an associated primary abnormality of the corneal endothelium. In two of these situations, the *iridocorneal endothelial syndrome* and *posterior polymorphous dystrophy*, there is a spectrum of clinical and histopathologic abnormalities, with strong evidence that the glaucoma is secondary to the corneal disease. In a third condition, *Fuchs' endothelial dystrophy*, an association with glaucoma has been suggested, but this has not been clearly established.

I. IRIDOCORNEAL ENDOTHELIAL SYNDROME

A. Terminology

The term, "iridocorneal endothelial (ICE) syndrome," was suggested by Yanoff[1] to denote a spectrum of disease that is characterized by a primary corneal endothelial abnormality. The endothelial disease is variably associated with corneal edema, anterior chamber angle changes, alterations in the iris, and secondary glaucoma. On the basis of changes in the iris and relative susceptibility of the corneal edema to intraocular pressure, the following clinical variations within the ICE syndrome have been distinguished (Table 12.1):

1. ***Progressive essential iris atrophy***. Harms,[2] in 1903, described a condition that is characterized by extreme atrophy of the iris with hole formation. Subsequent observations, which will be discussed later in this chapter, indicate that iris atrophy is not the "essential" or primary feature in this disease, and the term "*progressive iris atrophy*" is felt to be more appropriate.[3]

2. ***Chandler's syndrome***. This variation was described in 1956,[4] and differs from progressive iris atrophy in that changes in the iris

Table 12.1
Iridocorneal Endothelial (ICE) Syndrome

Major Clinical Variations	Characteristic Features
1. Progressive iris atrophy	Iris features predominate, with marked corectopia, atrophy, and hole formation.
2. Chandler's syndrome	Changes in the iris are mild to absent, while corneal edema, often at normal intraocular pressures, is typical.
3. Cogan-Reese syndrome (iris nevus syndrome)	Nodular or diffuse pigmented lesions of the iris are the hallmark, and may be seen with the entire spectrum of corneal and other iris defects.

are limited to slight corectopia and mild stromal atrophy, or may be absent altogether. In addition, the corneal edema is a more consistent feature and may occur at intraocular pressures that are normal or only slightly elevated. Intermediate variations between progressive iris atrophy and Chandler's syndrome also exist in which changes in the iris are more extensive than in the later condition, but lack the hole formation of the former variation.

3. **The Cogan-Reese syndrome**. In 1969, Cogan and Reese[5] reported two cases with pigmented nodules of the iris, associated with some features of the ICE syndrome. Subsequent studies have revealed the nodules[6, 7] or diffuse nevi[6] on the surface of the iris in the complete spectrum of the syndrome. Since some, but not all, of the iris lesions in this variation have been histologically characterized as nevi, the term *"iris nevus (Cogan-Reese) syndrome"* has been proposed.[6]

B. Clinicopathologic Features

The following features, with exceptions as noted, apply to all variations of the ICE syndrome.

1. *General features*.[8] The ICE syndrome is nearly always unilateral and has a predilection for women. The condition usually is recognized in early to middle adulthood, familial cases are rare, and there is no consistent association with systemic diseases. The most common presenting manifestations are abnormalities of the iris, reduced visual acuity, or pain. The latter two symptoms are usually due to corneal alterations, but also may result from secondary glaucoma.

2. *Corneal alterations*. A common feature of the ICE syndrome is a *corneal endothelial abnormality*, which may be seen by slit lamp biomicroscopy as a fine hammered silver appearance of the posterior cornea, similar to that of Fuchs' dystrophy. This defect may occur by itself without symptoms, or it may cause *corneal edema* with variable degrees of reduced vision and pain.[9] In some cases, the corneal edema may occur at intraocular pressures that are normal or only slightly elevated which, as previously noted, may be more typical of Chandler's variation of the ICE syndrome. Specular microscopy reveals a characteristic, diffuse abnormality of the corneal endothelial cells, with variable degrees of pleomorphism in size and shape, dark areas within the cells, and loss of the clear hexagonal margins.[10, 11] Electron microscopic study of the posterior cornea in advanced cases shows attenuated, grossly abnormal cells lining a thickened, multilayered Descemet's membrane.[9, 12-14] Typical cornea guttata, as seen in Fuchs' dystrophy, are not characteristic of the ICE syndrome.

3. *Anterior chamber angle alterations*. Peripheral *anterior synechia*, usually extending to or beyond Schwalbe's line, is another feature common to all variations of the ICE syndrome. Histologic studies reveal a *cellular membrane*, consisting of a single layer of endothelial cells and a Descemet's-like membrane, extending down from the peripheral cornea. The membrane may cover an open anterior chamber angle in some areas and may be associated with synechial closure

of the angle elsewhere in the same eye.[14-18] Secondary glaucoma usually develops as the synechiae progressively close the anterior chamber angle. However, the glaucoma does not correlate precisely with the degree of synechial closure,[8] and has been reported to occur when the entire angle was open, but covered by the cellular membrane.[18] Presumably, obstruction to aqueous outflow may result from either the membrane covering the trabecular meshwork or synechial closure of the anterior chamber angle.

4. *Iris alterations*. The abnormalities of the iris constitute the primary basis for distinguishing clinical variations within the ICE syndrome (Fig. 12.1).

a. *Progressive iris atrophy*. This variation is characterized by *marked atrophy* of the iris, associated with variable degrees of corectopia and ectropion uvea. The latter two features are usually directed toward the quadrant with the most prominent area of peripheral anterior synechia.[8, 15] Histopathology of the iris in this and all variations of the ICE syndrome includes the previously described cellular membrane on portions of the anterior iris surface, which has extended down from across the anterior chamber angle.[14, 15] The membrane is most often found in the quadrant toward which the pupil is distorted.[15] The hallmark of progressive iris atrophy is *hole formation* of the iris, which occurs in two forms[8]:

(1) *Stretch holes*. In some cases, the iris is markedly thinned in the quadrant away from the direction of pupillary distortion, and the holes develop within the area that is being stretched.

(2) *Melting holes*. In other eyes, holes develop without associated corectopia or thinning of the iris, and fluorescein angiographic studies show that this is associated with ischemia of the iris.[7]

b. *Chandler's syndrome*. In this clinical form, there is minimal corectopia and mild atrophy of the stroma of the iris.[4] In some cases, there may be no detectable change in the iris.

c. *The Cogan-Reese (iris-nevus) syndrome*. The eyes in this variation of the ICE syndrome may have any degree of iris atrophy, but are distinguished by the presence of pigmented, pedunculated nodules,[5-7] diffuse nevi,[6] or both[6] on the surface of the iris. The nodular lesions have an ultrastructure similar to that of the underlying stroma of the iris[14, 19, 20] and are always surrounded by the previously described cellular membrane.[14, 15, 19-22] The diffuse lesions have histopathologic features that are hard to distinguish between a nevus and a low grade melanoma.[6]

C. Theories of Mechanism. (Fig. 12.2)

The membrane theory of Campbell[15] holds that the abnormality of the corneal endothelium is the primary defect in the ICE syndrome. The endothelial defect causes the corneal edema and also leads to the proliferation of the cellular membrane across the anterior chamber angle and onto the surface of the iris. Contracture of this membrane, probably of the cellular portion, causes the formation of peripheral

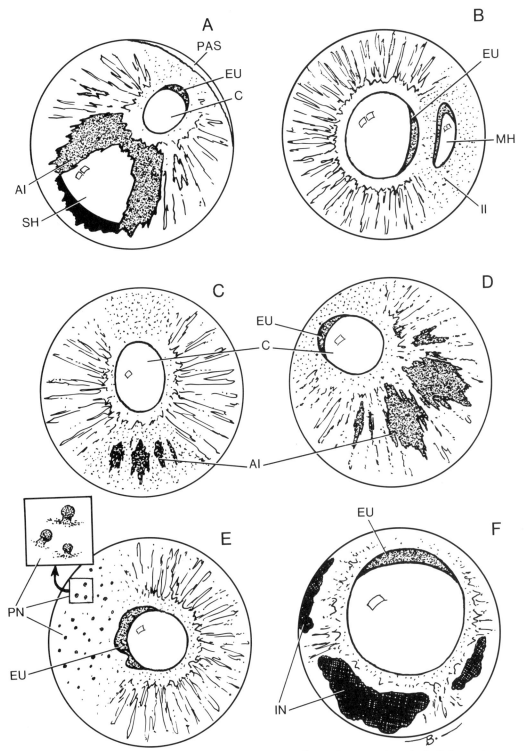

Figure 12.1. The spectrum of iris abnormalities in the iridocorneal endothelial syndrome. **A:** progressive iris atrophy with peripheral anterior synechia (**PAS**) visible on peripheral cornea, marked corectopia (**C**), ectropion uvea (**EU**) and a stretch hole (**SH**) surrounded by atrophic iris (**AI**); **B:** progressive iris atrophy with a melting hole (**MH**) surrounded by ischemic iris (**II**); **C:** Chandler's syndrome with mild corectopia and atrophy of the iris; **D:** intermediate variation with more advanced corectopia and atrophy of the iris than in the typical Chandler's syndrome, but no hole in the iris; **E** and **F:** Cogan-Reese (iris nevus) syndrome with pigmented, pedunculated nodules (**PN**) or diffuse iris nevi (**IN**).

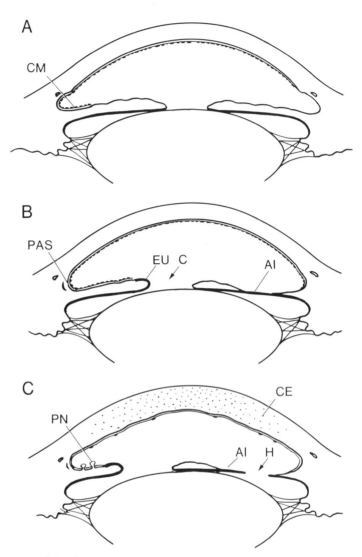

Figure 12.2. Membrane theory of Campbell for the mechanism of the iridocorneal endothelial syndrome. **A:** a cellular membrane (**CM**) extends down from abnormal corneal endothelium, across the anterior chamber angle, and onto the iris; **B:** contracture of the membrane causes formation of peripheral anterior synechiae (**PAS**), corectopia (**C**), ectropion uvea (**EU**), and atrophy of the iris (**AI**); **C:** further contracture leads to more extensive atrophy of the iris and, in some cases, holes (**H**) in the iris and pigmented nodules (**PN**). The abnormal corneal endothelium also leads to corneal edema (**CE**) in some cases.

anterior synechiae, the corectopia, and the ectropion uvea. Stretching of the iris in the direction away from the corectopia undoubtedly contributes to the atrophy and hole formation, although additional factors, such as ischemia, may also be involved.[3] The cellular membrane also is believed to be responsible for the development of the nodular lesions of the iris in the Cogan-Reese syndrome.[19, 21] It has been suggested that the membrane may encircle and pinch off portions of the iris stroma to form the nodules.[19, 21]

D. Differential Diagnosis

There are several disorders of the cornea or iris, many of which have associated glaucoma, which could be confused with the various forms of the ICE syndrome. It is helpful to think of these in the following three categories[3, 8]:

1. *Corneal endothelial disorders. Posterior polymorphous dystrophy* may have glaucoma and changes of the anterior chamber angle and iris resembling the ICE syndrome, although the corneal abnormalities, as well as other clinical features, clearly distinguish these two diseases. *Fuchs' endothelial dystrophy* has corneal changes that are clinically very similar to those of the ICE syndrome, but none of the chamber angle or iris features of the latter condition. Both of these disorders are discussed later in this chapter.

2. *Dissolution of the iris. Rieger's syndrome* has striking clinical similarities to the ICE syndrome, but the congenital nature and bilaterality, as well as the other features described in Chapter 9, help to separate the two conditions. Some advanced cases of progressive iris atrophy might resemble *aniridia*, but the bilaterality of the latter disorder is again a helpful differential feature. *Iridoschisis* is characterized by separation of superficial layers of iris stroma and may be associated with glaucoma. However, it is typically a disease of the elderly.

3. *Nodular and diffuse lesions of the iris.* Patients with the Cogan-Reese syndrome have had enucleation for presumed *melanomas* of the iris. In addition, differentiation must be made from the nodular lesions of *neurofibromatosis*, as well as nodular *inflammatory disorders*, such as sarcoidosis.

E. Management

Patients with the ICE syndrome may require treatment for corneal edema, secondary glaucoma, or both. The glaucoma can often be controlled medically in the early stages, especially with drugs that reduce aqueous production. Lowering the intraocular pressure may also control the corneal edema, although the additional use of hypertonic saline solutions and soft contact lenses may be required for the later condition. When surgical intervention is required for the glaucoma, filtering surgery is reasonably successful.[8] However, even an extremely low intraocular pressure may not relieve advanced corneal edema, and penetrating keratoplasty is usually indicated for this situation, after the glaucoma has been controlled.[9]

II. POSTERIOR POLYMORPHOUS DYSTROPHY

A. Clinicopathologic Features

1. *General features.* Posterior polymorphous dystrophy is a bilateral, familial disorder of the corneal endothelium. Inheritance is usually auto-

somal dominant, and there is no race or sex predilection. Although it is probably congenital, it typically remains asymptomatic until adulthood.[23] As with the ICE syndrome, posterior polymorphous dystrophy represents a spectrum of disorders.[24, 25] In one form, the characteristic corneal changes are associated with peripheral iridocorneal adhesions, iris atrophy, and corectopia.[24] Glaucoma occurs in approximately 15% of patients with posterior polymorphous dystrophy, both with and without the iridocorneal adhesions.

2. *Corneal alterations.* By slit lamp biomicroscopy, the posterior cornea has the appearance of blisters or vesicles at the level of Descemet's membrane. The vesicles may be linear or in groups and surrounded by an aureole of gray haze.[25] Ultrastructural studies reveal an unusually thin Descemet's membrane covered by multiple layers of collagen,[26–30] and lined by cells variably described as having features of abnormal endothelium,[28, 31] fibroblasts,[27, 29] or epithelium.[26, 30] The difference in the cells that have been reported on the posterior cornea in posterior polymorphous dystrophy may represent an evolving process of metaplasia.[29] The incompletely developed Descemet's membrane suggests that the corneal endothelium began to change in late fetal or early adolescent life[28] and subsequently deposited the additional collagen layers. Clinically, the cornea may remain clear and produce no symptoms, although *corneal edema* may develop in some cases.

3. *Anterior chamber angle and iris alterations.* A small number of patients may have broad peripheral anterior synechiae extending to or beyond Schwalbe's line, which may be associated with corectopia, ectropion uvea, and atrophy of the iris.[24, 25, 32] Histology reveals a membrane composed of epithelial-like cells and a Descemet's-like membrane extending over the anterior chamber angle and onto the iris.[17] Glaucoma may be present in some of the cases with anterior chamber angle and iris abnormalities, and has also been observed in eyes with open, normal appearing angles.[25, 32]

B. Theories of Mechanism

A membrane theory, similar to that for the ICE syndrome, has been proposed for those cases of posterior polymorphous dystrophy with iridocorneal adhesions. It is postulated that a dystrophic endothelium (or epithelium), producing a basement membrane-like material, extends across the anterior chamber angle and onto the iris, and subsequently causes the synechia formation and changes in the iris.[25] The glaucoma may be due to the iridocorneal adhesions when these are present, while cases of open-angle glaucoma may be due to a concomitant dystrophy of the trabecular endothelium or obstruction of the open angle by the previously described cellular membrane.[17]

C. Differential Diagnosis

Conditions that may be confused with posterior polymorphous dystrophy include other forms of posterior corneal dystrophy, such as Fuchs' endothelial dystrophy and congenital hereditary corneal dystrophy. When iridocorneal adhesions are present, Rieger's syndrome and the ICE syndrome should also be considered. In all of these cases, however, the typical appearance of the posterior cornea is usually sufficient to distinguish posterior polymorphous dystrophy.

D. Management

Most cases of posterior polymorphous dystrophy are asymptomatic and do not require treatment. However, corneal edema may require conservative management or penetrating keratoplasty. The glaucoma, when present, may respond to drugs that lower aqueous production. Filtering surgery generally is indicated when medical therapy is no longer adequate.

III. FUCHS' ENDOTHELIAL DYSTROPHY

A. Terminology and Clinicopathologic Features

The corneal dystrophy described by Fuchs[33] in 1910 overlaps with corneal endothelial changes that may be a result of aging or secondary to other ocular disease. It is helpful to first consider the latter situations and then to note how these may be differentiated from Fuchs' endothelial dystrophy.

1. *Influences on normal corneal endothelium*. The morphology of human corneal endothelium changes with *age*, in that the cells become larger and more irregular as the total population is progressively reduced.[34] In addition, and of particular interest to the present discussion, endothelial cell densities are reduced in human eyes with *elevated intraocular pressure* due to secondary glaucomas[35, 36] and in rabbit eyes with induced pressure elevation.[37] Corneal thickness also is slightly greater in eyes with either open-angle glaucoma or secondary glaucoma, which is most likely indirect evidence of abnormal endothelial function.[38] *Anterior uveitis* may also be associated with alterations in corneal endothelium.[36, 39]

2. *Cornea guttata*. One manifestation of the progressive changes in corneal endothelial cells, as described above, is the accumulation of collagen on the posterior surface of Descemet's membrane. Histologically, this may appear as warts or excrescences, which is the pure form of cornea guttata.[40] In other cases, however, the focal accumulations may be covered by additional basement membrane, or there may be a uniform thickening of the posterior collagen layers.[40] By slit lamp biomicroscopy, cornea guttata creates a beaten silver appearance of the central posterior cornea, similar to that seen in the ICE syndrome. However, specular microscopic study reveals a more characteristic pattern for cornea guttata, with progressive stages of severity.[41] Although the estimated prevalence varies considerably among investigators, apparently reflecting differences in diagnostic techniques and criteria, it is generally agreed that cornea guttata is a common condition, the incidence of which increases significantly with age.[42, 43]

3. *Fuchs' endothelial dystrophy*. The vast majority of individuals with cornea guttata have otherwise normal corneas with no visual impairment. A small number of patients with the same posterior corneal changes as described above, however, will develop edema of

the corneal stroma and epithelium, as described by Fuchs.[33] This is a bilateral disease with a predilection for women and an onset usually between the ages of 40 and 70 years. There is a strong familial tendency, and a study of one pedigree revealed autosomal dominant inheritance.[40] This condition may lead to severe visual reduction, often requiring penetrating keratoplasty.

B. Glaucoma

Two forms of glaucoma have been reported in association with Fuchs' endothelial dystrophy:

1. *Open-angle glaucoma.* Reports in the literature are conflicting regarding an increased incidence of open-angle glaucoma in populations of patients with Fuchs' endothelial dystrophy. It has been estimated that 10 to 15% of such patient populations have open-angle glaucoma.[44] It has also been reported that patients with cornea guttata have a high incidence of abnormal tonographic facilities of outflow.[45] However, a study of 64 families with Fuchs' endothelial dystrophy revealed only one case of open-angle glaucoma,[46] and a study of patients with cornea guttata showed a lower mean intraocular pressure in this group than in a matched population without guttata.[47]

If a secondary form of open-angle glaucoma truly exists in some cases of Fuchs' endothelial dystrophy, the mechanism of the glaucoma is only speculative at this time. One theory is that concomitant dystrophy of the trabecular endothelium may cause outflow obstruction.[44] The possibility of a genetic overlap with primary open-angle glaucoma was not supported by a study in which patients with Fuchs' endothelial dystrophy did not have the same *in vitro* lymphocyte responsiveness to corticosteroids as primary open-angle glaucoma patients.[48] As previously noted, there is evidence that elevated intraocular pressure may alter the corneal endothelium, and it may be that pressure elevation is the primary event in cases diagnosed as open-angle glaucoma associated with corneal endothelial dystrophy.

2. *Angle-closure glaucoma.* It has also been reported that patients with Fuchs' endothelial dystrophy and shallow anterior chambers may develop angle-closure glaucoma, apparently due to a gradual thickening of the cornea with eventual closure of the anterior chamber angle.[49]

C. Management

Although glaucoma is usually not present in eyes with Fuchs' dystrophy, medical efforts to further reduce the normal intraocular pressure may sometimes help to minimize the corneal edema. When glaucoma is present, the open-angle form is managed the same as primary open-angle glaucoma, while the angle-closure form requires iridectomy or filtering surgery. Prophylactic miotic therapy has not been effective in cases with impending angle closure.[49]

References

1. Yanoff, M: In discussion of Shields, MB, McCracken, JS, Klintworth, GK, Campbell, DG: Corneal edema in essential iris atrophy. Ophthalmology 86:1549, 1979.
2. Harms, C: Einseitige spontane Luckenbildung der Iris durch Atrophie ohne mechanische Zerrung. Klin Monatsbl Augenheilkd 41:522, 1903.
3. Shields, MB: Progressive essential iris atrophy, Chandler's syndrome, and the iris nevus (Cogan-Reese) syndrome: a spectrum of disease. Surv Ophthal 24:3, 1979.
4. Chandler, PA: Atrophy of the stroma of the iris. Endothelial dystrophy, corneal edema, and glaucoma. Am J Ophthal 41:607, 1956.
5. Cogan, DG, Reese, AB: A syndrome of iris nodules, ectopic Descemet's membrane, and unilateral glaucoma. Doc Ophthal 26:424, 1969.
6. Scheie, HG, Yanoff, M: Iris nevus (Cogan-Reese) syndrome. A cause of unilateral glaucoma. Arch Ophthal 93:963, 1975.
7. Shields, MB, Campbell, DG, Simmons, RJ, Hutchinson, BT: Iris nodules in essential iris atrophy. Arch Ophthal 94:406, 1976.
8. Shields, MB, Campbell, DG, Simmons, RJ: The essential iris atrophies. Am J Ophthal 85:749, 1978.
9. Shields, MB, McCracken, JS, Klintworth, GK, Campbell, DG: Corneal edema in essential iris atrophy. Ophthalmology 86:1533, 1979.
10. Hirst, LW, Quigley, HA, Stark, WJ, Shields, MB: Specular microscopy of iridocorneal endothelia syndrome. Am J Ophthal 89:11, 1980.
11. Setala, K, Vannas, A: Corneal endothelial cells in essential iris atrophy. A specular microscopic study. Acta Ophthal 57:1020, 1979.
12. Quigley, HA, Forster, DF: Histopathology of cornea and iris in Chandler's syndrome. Arch Ophthal 96:1878, 1978.
13. Richardson, TM: Corneal decompensation in Chandler's syndrome. A scanning and transmission electron microscopic study. Arch Ophthal 97:2112, 1979.
14. Eagle, RC Jr, Font, RL, Yanoff, M, Fine, BS: Proliferative endotheliopathy with iris abnormalities. The iridocorneal endothelial syndrome. Arch Ophthal 97:2104, 1979.
15. Campbell, DG, Shields, MB, Smith, TR: The corneal endothelium and the spectrum of essential iris atrophy. Am J Ophthal 86:317, 1978.
16. Rodrigues, MM, Streeten, BW, Spaeth, GL: Chandler's syndrome as a variant of essential iris atrophy. A clinicopathologic study. Arch Ophthal 96:643, 1978.
17. Rodrigues, MM, Phelps, CD, Krachmer, JH, Cibis, GW, Weingeist, TA: Glaucoma due to endothelialization of the anterior chamber angle. A comparison of posterior polymorphous dystrophy of the cornea and Chandler's syndrome. Arch Ophthal 98:688, 1980.
18. Benedikt, O, Roll, P: Open-angle glaucoma through endothelialization of the anterior chamber angle. Glaucoma 2:368, 1980.
19. Eagle, RC Jr, Font, RL, Yanoff, M, Fine, BS: The iris nevus (Cogan-Reese) syndrome: light and electron microscopic observations. Br J Ophthal 64:446, 1980.
20. Radius, RL, Herschler, J: Histopathology in the iris-nevus (Cogan-Reese) syndrome. Am J Ophthal 89:780, 1980.
21. Campbell, DG: Formation of iris nodules in primary proliferative endothelial degeneration. Presented at Association for Research in Vision and Ophthalmology, Sarasota, Florida, April 30–May 4, 1979.
22. Yanoff, M, Eagle, RC: Iridocorneal endothelial (ICE) syndrome: associated glaucoma, corneal endothelial proliferation and iris stromal abnormalities. In Glaucoma: Contemporary International Concepts, Bellows, JG, ed. Masson Publ, Inc, New York, 1979, p 323.
23. Waring, GO III, Rodrigues, MM, Laibson, PR: Corneal dystrophies. II. Endothelial dystrophies. Surv Ophthal 23:147, 1978.

24. Grayson, M: The nature of hereditary deep polymorphous dystrophy of the cornea: Its association with iris and anterior chamber dygenesis. Tr Am Ophthal Soc 72:516, 1974.
25. Cibis, GW, Krachmer, JA, Phelps, CD, Weingeist, TA: The clinical spectrum of posterior polymorphous dystrophy. Arch Ophthal 95:1529, 1977.
26. Boruchoff, SA, Kuwabara, T: Electron microscopy of posterior polymorphous degeneration. Am J Ophthal 72:879, 1971.
27. Hanselmayer, H: Zur Histopathologic der hinteren polymorphen Hornhautdystrophic nach Schlichting. II. Ultrastrukturelle Befunde, pathogenetische und pathophysiologische Bemerkungen. Albrecht Graefes Arch Klin Exp Ophthal 185:53, 1972.
28. Hanna, C, Fraunfelder, FT, McNair, JR: An ultrastructure study of posterior polymorphous dystrophy of the cornea. Ann Ophthal 9:1371, 1977.
29. Johnson, BL, Brown, SI: Posterior polymorphous dystrophy: a light and electron microscopic study. Br J Ophthal 62:89, 1978.
30. Rodrigues, MM, Sun, TT, Krachmer, J, Newsome, D: Epithelialization of the corneal endothelium in posterior polymorphous dystrophy. Invest Ophthal Vis Sci 19:832, 1980.
31. Polack, FM, Bourne, WM, Forstot, SL, Yamaguchi, T: Scanning electron microscopy of posterior polymorphous corneal dystrophy. Am J Ophthal 89:575, 1980.
32. Cibis, GW, Krachmer, JH, Phelps, CD, Weingeist, TA: Iridocorneal adhesions in posterior polymorphous dystrophy. Trans Am Acad Ophthal Otol 81:770, 1976.
33. Fuchs, E: Dystrophis epithelialis corneal. Arch Ophthal 76:478, 1910.
34. Kaufman, HE, Capella, JA, Robbins, JE: The human corneal endothelium. Am J Ophthal 61:835, 1966.
35. Vannas, A, Setala, K, Ruusuvaara, P: Endoehtlial cells in capsular glaucoma. Acta Ophthal 55:951, 1977.
36. Setala, K, Vannas, A: Endothelial cells in the glaucomato-cyclitic crisis. Adv Ophthal 36:218, 1978.
37. Melamed, S, Ben-Sira, I, Ben-Shaul, Y: Corneal endothelial changes under induced intraocular pressure elevation: a scanning and transmission electron microscopic study in rabbits. Br J Ophthal 64:164, 1980.
38. De Cevallos, E, Dohlman, CH, Reinhart, WJ: Corneal thickness in glaucoma. Ann Ophthal 8:177, 1976.
39. Waring, GO, Font, RL, Rodrigues, MM, Mulberger, RD: Alterations of Descemet's membrane in interstitial keratitis. Am J Ophthal 80:773, 1975.
40. Magovern, M, Beauchamp, GR, McTigue, JW, Fine, BS, Baumiller, RC: Inheritance of Fuchs' combined dystrophy. Ophthalmology 86:1897, 1979.
41. Laing, RA, Leibowitz, HM, Oak, SS, Chang, R, Berrospi, AR, Theodore, JA: Endothelial mosaic in Fuchs' dystrophy. A qualitative evaluation with the specular microscope. Arch Ophthal 99:80, 1981.
42. Goar, E: Dystrophy of the cornea endothelium. Am J Ophthal 17:215, 1934.
43. Lorenzetti, DWC, Uotila, MH, Parikh, N, Kaufman, HE: Central cornea guttata. Incidence in the general population. Am J Ophthal 64:1155, 1967.
44. Kolker, AE, Hetherington, J Jr: Becker, Shaffer's Diagnosis and Therapy of the Glaucomas, 4th ed. CV Mosby Co, St Louis, 1976, p 265.
45. Buxton, JN, Preston, RW, Riechers, R, Guilbault, N: Tonography in cornea guttata. A preliminary report. Arch Ophthal 77:602, 1967.
46. Krachmer, JH, Purcell, JJ Jr, Young, CW, Bucher, KD: Corneal endothelial dystrophy. A study of 64 families. Arch Ophthal 96:2036, 1978.
47. Burns, RR, Bourne, WM, Brubaker, RF: Endothelial function in patients with cornea guttata. Invest Ophthal Vis Sci 20:77, 1981.
48. Waltman, SR, Palmberg, PF, Becker, B: In vitro corticosteroid sensitivity in patients with Fuchs' dystrophy. Doc Ophthal Proc Ser 18:321, 1979.
49. Stocker, FW: The Endothelium of the Cornea and Its Clinical Implications, 2nd ed. Charles C Thomas, Springfield, Ill 1971, p 79.

Chapter 13

PIGMENTARY GLAUCOMA

PIGMENTARY GLAUCOMA

I. TERMINOLOGY

As a normal feature of maturation and aging, a variable amount of uveal pigment is chronically released and dispersed into the anterior ocular segment. This is best appreciated by observing the trabecular meshwork, which typically is not pigmented in the infant eye, but becomes progressively pigmented to variable degrees with the passage of years, presumbly due to the accumulation of the dispersed pigment in the aqueous outflow system. There is, therefore, a spectrum of ocular pigment dispersion within the general population. In addition, individuals with various forms of glaucoma will also have different degrees of pigment dispersion, although this is not believed to be a major factor in the mechanism of the glaucoma in most cases. There are several disease states of the eye, however, that are associated with an unusually heavy dispersion of pigment, which may be significantly involved in increased resistance to aqueous outflow. In 1940, Sugar[1] briefly described one such case with marked pigment dispersion and glaucoma. Sugar and Barbour[2] subsequently reported the details of this entity, which differed from other forms of pigment dispersion by typical clinical and histopathologic features. They referred to this condition as *pigmentary glaucoma*.[2] When the typical findings are encountered without associated glaucoma, the term, *pigment-dispersion syndrome*, has been advocated.[3]

II. CLINICAL FEATURES

A. General Features of Patients

The typical patient is a young, myopic male.[3, 4] The condition is seen predominantly in Caucasians.[3] A hereditary basis has been suggested,[3] but this has not been clearly established.

B. Slit-lamp Biomicroscopy and Gonioscopy

Several characteristic features are helpful in arriving at the correct diagnosis (Fig. 13.1).

1. *Pigment dispersion*. This occurs throughout the anterior ocular segment, but is seen primarily on the iris and cornea and in the anterior chamber angle.

a. Pigment granules are frequently dispersed on the *stroma of the iris*, which may give the iris a progressively darker appearance or create heterochromia in asymmetric cases.[4]

b. *Krukenberg's spindle* is an accumulation of pigment on the posterior surface of the central *cornea* in a vertical spindle-shaped pattern. Dispersed pigment is deposited on the cornea in this pattern due to aqueous convection currents and is then phagocytosed by

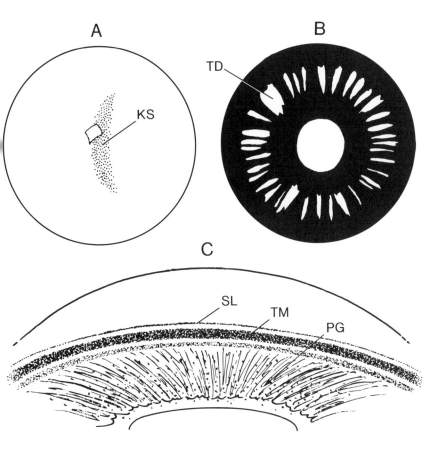

Figure 13.1. The typical clinical features of pigmentary glaucoma and the pigment-dispersion syndrome. **A:** Krukenberg's spindle (**KS**); **B:** spoke-like transillumination defects (**TD**) of the iris; **C:** gonioscopic appearance, showing dense, homogeneous pigmentation of trabecular meshwork (**TM**) and pigment accumulation along Schwalbe's line (**SL**). Note also the increased pigment granules (**PG**) on the stroma of the iris.

adjacent endothelial cells.[3] This feature is commonly seen in eyes with pigmentary glaucoma, but is neither invariable nor pathognomonic of the disease. In one study of 43 patients with Krukenberg's spindle, only two developed field loss during a follow-up that averaged 5.8 years.[5] The finding is more common in women[5] and may have a hormonal relationship.[6]

    c. *Gonioscopic findings* are highly typical, but not absolutely pathognomonic of pigmentary glaucoma. The principal feature is a dense, homogeneous band of dark brown pigment in the full circumference of the *trabecular meshwork*.[4] The dispersed pigment may also accumulate along Schwalbe's line, especially inferiorly, creating a thin, dark band that has been called Sampaolesi's line. Another gonioscopic finding, unrelated to pigment dispersion, is abundant iris processes inserting anterior to the scleral spur. These were observed in one small series of patients with pigmentary glaucoma,[7] but do not appear to be a consistent finding in this condition.

d. Pigment dispersion may also be seen on the lens capsule and zonules and within glaucoma filtering blebs.[4]

2. *Iris transillumination.* This appears to be the most diagnostic clinical feature of pigmentary glaucoma. The characteristic appearance is a radial *spoke-like* pattern in the outer portion of the iris.[8, 9] This feature can easily be seen during slit-lamp biomicroscopy by directing the light beam through the pupil, perpendicular to the plane of the iris, and observing the retinal light reflex through the defects in the iris. In some patients, however, a markedly constricted pupil may prevent an adequate retinal reflex, in which case scleral transillumination may be a better technique for observing the iris defects.

C. Clinical Course of the Glaucoma

Patients with the pigment-dispersion syndrome may go for years before developing pigmentary glaucoma or may never have a rise in intraocular pressure. In one study of 97 eyes with pigment dispersion throughout the anterior ocular segment, glaucoma was present in 42.[8] In some cases, the intraocular pressure may rise transiently in association with strenuous exercise or spontaneous changes in the pupillary diameter, presumably due to increased liberation of pigment.[10] Phenylepherine-induced mydriasis will also cause a significant shower of pigment into the anterior chamber in some, but not all, patients with pigmentary glaucoma or the pigment-dispersion syndrome, but this is not consistently associated with intraocular pressure elevation.[11] Once pigmentary glaucoma becomes established, it may be somewhat more difficult to control than primary open-angle glaucoma, although with increasing age there is a tendency for the condition to become less severe.

III. THEORIES OF MECHANISM

Two fundamental questions must be considered regarding the pathogenesis of the pigment-dispersion syndrome and the mechanism of pigmentary glaucoma: 1) What are the factors leading to the pigment dispersion? and 2) How does the dispersed pigment and/or additional features cause the glaucoma?

A. Mechanism of Pigment Dispersion

1. Histopathologic observations of the iris in eyes with the pigment-dispersion syndrome or pigmentary glaucoma have revealed changes in the *iris pigment epithelium*, which include focal atrophy and hypopigmentation,[12-14] with an apparent delay in melanogenesis,[14] and a hyperplasia of the dilator muscle.[12-14] In contrast, eyes with primary open-angle glaucoma and varying degrees of pigment dispersion had minimal hypopigmentation of the iris epithelium and

normal dilator muscle and melanogenesis.[14] These observations have led some observers to feel that a developmental abnormality of the iris pigment epithelium is the fundamental defect in the pigment-dispersion syndrome.[12-14] It has also been suggested that racial differences in the iris may account for the lower incidence of pigment dispersion among non-whites.[15]

2. Campbell[16] proposed an alternative theory for the mechanism of pigment liberation from the iris. He noted that the peripheral radial defects of the iris correspond in location and number to anterior packets of lens zonules and suggested that mechanical rubbing of these zonules against the peripheral iris leads to the dispersion of pigment. The hypothesis is supported by histologic studies showing a correlation between packets of zonules and deep grooves in the iris pigment epithelium and posterior stroma.

B. Mechanism of Intraocular Pressure Elevation

1. In 1963, Grant[17] demonstrated that *pigment granules* perfused in human autopsy eyes caused a significant obstruction to aqueous outflow. Subsequent histopathologic studies of eyes with pigmentary glaucoma revealed excessive amounts of pigment granules and cell debris in the trabecular meshwork,[14, 18, 19] associated with variable degrees of trabecular endothelial cell degeneration.[19] Based on these observations, it is generally held that dispersion of pigment into the trabecular meshwork leads to the elevation of intraocular pressure in pigmentary glaucoma.

2. An alternative theory suggests that a *primary developmental anomaly* of the anterior chamber angle may lead to aqueous outflow obstruction.[4] This is based on the previously described abundant iris processes inserting anterior to the scleral spur, which have been seen in some cases.[7, 14]

3. A third hypothesis has been that pigmentary glaucoma may be a variation of *primary open-angle glaucoma.* This theory was derived from observations that both primary open-angle glaucoma and pigmentary glaucoma may be seen in the same family.[7, 20] In addition, the previously described abundant iris processes may occur in either condition.[7] In one study, individuals with Krukenberg's spindles had topical corticosteroid responses that were similar to those seen among close relatives of patients with primary open-angle glaucoma.[20] However, patients with pigmentary glaucoma were not found to have the same corticosteroid sensitivity to *in vitro* inhibition of lymphocyte transformation as do primary open-angle glaucoma patients.[21] HLA antigen testing reportedly revealed differences between the pigment-dispersion syndrome, pigmentary glaucoma, and primary open-angle glaucoma,[22] but another study showed no significant difference among patients with pigmentary glaucoma, the pigment-dispersion syndrome, and normal controls.[23] The bulk of the current evidence suggests that pigmentary glaucoma and primary open-angle glaucoma are separate entities.

IV. DIFFERENTIAL DIAGNOSIS

As noted at the outset of this chapter, there are several disease states in which an excessive dispersion of pigment may be associated with glaucoma. These conditions constitute the differential diagnosis for pigmentary glaucoma, and include the exfoliation syndrome, some forms of uveitis, ocular melanosis and melanoma, and primary open-angle glaucoma with excessive pigment dispersion. All of these disorders are discussed in other chapters.

V. MANAGEMENT

Pigmentary glaucoma is managed basically the same as primary open-angle glaucoma. However, there may be an increased incidence of *retinal detachment* among patients with pigmentary glaucoma, and *caution with miotics* is recommended.[24] It has been suggested, however, that the miotic effect of an alpha-adrenergic blocker, such as thymoxamine, may be beneficial in keeping the iris away from the lens zonules.[16]

References

1. Sugar, HS: Concerning the chamber angle. I. Gonioscopy. Am J Ophthal 23:853, 1940.
2. Sugar, HS, Barbour, FA: Pigmentary glaucoma. A rare clinical entity. Am J Ophthal 32:90, 1949.
3. Sugar, HS: Pigmentary glaucoma. A 25-year review. Am J Ophthal 62:499, 1966.
4. Lichter, PR: Pigmentary glaucoma—current concepts. Trans Am Acad Ophthal Otol 78:309, 1974.
5. Wilensky, JT, Buerk, KM, Podos, SM: Krukenberg's spindles. Am J Ophthal 79:220, 1975.
6. Duncan, TE: Krukenberg spindles in pregnancy. Arch Ophthal 91:355, 1974.
7. Lichter, PR, Shaffer, RN: Iris processes and glaucoma. Am J Ophthal 70:905, 1970.
8. Scheie, HG, Fleischhauer, HW: Idiopathic atrophy of the epithelial layers of the iris and ciliary body. A clinical study. Arch Ophthal 59:216, 1958.
9. Donaldson, DD: Transillumination of the iris. Tr Am Ophthal Soc 72:89, 1974.
10. Schenker, HI, Lunts, MH, Kels, B, Podos, SM: Exercise-induced increase of intraocular pressure in the pigmentary dispersion syndrome. Am J Ophthal 89:598, 1980.
11. Epstein, DL, Boger, WP III, Grant, WM: Phenylephrine provocative testing in the pigmentary dispersion syndrome. Am J Ophthal 85:43, 1978.
12. Fine, BS, Yanoff, M, Scheie, HG: Pigmentary "glaucoma." A histologic study. Trans Am Acad Ophthal Otol 78:314, 1974.
13. Kupfer, C, Kuwabara, T, Kaiser-Kupfer, M: The histopathology of pigmentary dispersion syndrome with glaucoma. Am J Ophthal 80:857, 1975.
14. Rodrigues, MM, Spaeth, GL, Weinreb, S, Sivalingam, E: Spectrum of trabecular pigmentation in open-angle glaucoma: a clinicopathologic study. Trans Am Acad Ophthal Otol 81:258, 1976.
15. Richardson, TM: Pigmentary glaucoma. In Secondary Glaucomas, Ritch, R, Shields, MB, eds. CV Mosby Co, St Louis (in press).
16. Campbell, DG: Pigmentary dispersion and glaucoma. A new theory. Arch Ophthal 97:1667, 1979.
17. Grant, WM: Experimental aqueous perfusion in enucleated human eyes. Arch Ophthal 69:783, 1963.

18. Rodrigues, MM, Spaeth, GL, Sivalingam, E, Weinreb, S: Value of trabeculectomy specimens in glaucoma. Ophthal Surg 9:29, 1978.
19. Richardson, TM, Hutchinson, BT, Grant, WM: The outflow tract in pigmentary glaucoma. A light and electron microscopic study. Arch Ophthal 95:1015, 1977.
20. Becker, B, Podos, SM: Krukenberg's spindles and primary open-angle glaucoma. Arch Ophthal 76:635, 1966.
21. Zink, HA, Palmberg, PF, Sugar, A, Sugar, HS, Cantrill, HL, Becker, B, Bigger, JF: Comparison of *in vitro* corticosteroid response in pigmentary glaucoma and primary open-angle glaucoma. Am J Ophthal 80:478, 1975.
22. Becker, B, Shin, DH, Cooper, DG, Kass, MA: The pigment dispersion syndrome. Am J Ophthal 83:161, 1977.
23. Kaiser-Kupfer, MI, Mittal, KK: The HLA and ABO antigens in pigment dispersion syndrome. Am J Ophthal 85:368, 1978.
24. Delaney, WV Jr: Equatorial lens pigmentation, myopia, and retinal detachment. Am J Ophthal 79:194, 1975.

Chapter 14

GLAUCOMAS ASSOCIATED WITH DISORDERS OF THE LENS

GLAUCOMAS ASSOCIATED WITH DISORDERS OF THE LENS

Disorders of the crystalline lens are associated with several forms of glaucoma. In some cases, such as the exfoliation syndrome, a cause-and-effect relationship between the lenticular abnormality and the glaucoma is uncertain. In other situations, including some forms of dislocated lenses and cataracts, the glaucoma clearly results from the alteration of the lens.

I. EXFOLIATION SYNDROME

A. Terminology

In 1917, Lindberg[1] described cases of chronic glaucoma in which flakes of whitish material adhered to the pupillary border of the iris. Subsequent study revealed that this material is derived, at least in part, from exfoliation of the anterior lens capsule, and two types of exfoliation have now been distinguished.

1. *Capsular delamination.* In this condition, superficial layers of lens capsule separate from the deeper layers to form scroll-like margins and occasionally to float in the anterior chamber as thin, clear membranes.[2, 3] An underlying cause is usually present, such as exposure to intense heat, as seen with glassblowers,[3] inflammation,[4] trauma[2, 4] or irradiation.[4] Glaucoma is not a common feature. Dvork-Theobald[5] suggested that this condition be called *"true" exfoliation of the lens capsule* to distinguish it from the condition to be discussed next.

2. *The exfoliation syndrome.* Vogt,[6] in 1925, described what he felt to be a senile form of capsular delamination, which he called *senile exfoliation.* In addition to occurring in an older patient population, this condition differed from the other forms of exfoliation of the lens capsule in clinical appearance, as well as a more frequent association with glaucoma (*glaucoma capsulare*).[6–8] Dvorak-Theobald[5] suggested that the disease was not a true exfoliation of the lens capsule, but rather precipitates of an unknown substance in the anterior ocular segment. She recommended the term, *pseudo-exfoliation of the lens capsule*, to distinguish the condition from capsular delamination or "true" exfoliation. However, more recent ultra-structural studies have revealed that the exfoliative material is derived, at least in part, from the lens capsule, and it has been proposed that this entity be called *the exfoliation syndrome*,[9–12] and that the previously discussed form of exfoliation of the lens capsule be referred to as *capsular delamination*.[13] The following discussion deals with the exfoliation syndrome.

B. Epidemiology

Reports vary considerably regarding the prevalence of the exfoliation syndrome, apparently due to differences within the populations that have been studied. Geography may be an important factor, with higher prevalences reported in Norway, England, and Germany.[14] Race may also be important in that exfoliation in eyes with open-angle glaucoma occurred in 1.4% of whites and 20% of black patients in South Africa.[15] The reported prevalence of exfoliation in patients with glaucoma in the United States ranges from 3%[10, 11] to 12%.[16] A prospective study of 1333 persons in the southeastern United States revealed exfoliation among 3% of patients with open-angle glaucoma and in 0.9% of non-glaucomatous individuals.[17]

C. General Features of Patients

The most common age of patients with the exfoliation syndrome is late sixties and early seventies.[10, 11, 16] Most studies show no sex predilection,[10, 11, 16] although males were predominant in one series, which the author suggested might have related to radiation exposure in the environment.[18] Reports of heredity are conflicting.[14] The condition may be unilateral or bilateral, and some unilateral cases will become bilateral with time.[16]

D. Clinical Features

1. *Slit-lamp biomicroscopy.* The characteristic exfoliation material on the *anterior lens capsule,* may have three distinct zones (Fig. 14.1): 1) a translucent, central disc with occasional curled up edges, 2) a clear zone, possibly corresponding to contact with the moving iris, and 3) a peripheral granular zone, which may have radial striations.[14] The central zone is not always present, but the peripheral defect is a consistent finding, and the pupil must be dilated before the lens changes can be seen in some cases. Exfoliation material may also be found on the pupillary margin of the iris, the lens zonules and ciliary

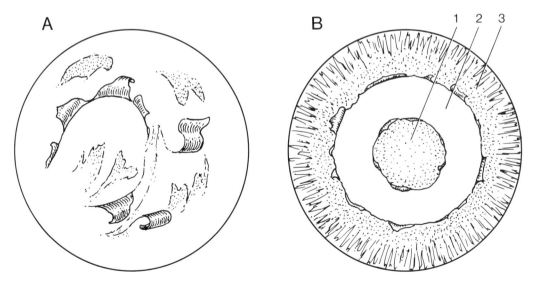

Figure 14.1. Two types of exfoliation of the anterior lens capsule. **A:** capsular delamination, characterized by thin, clear membranes separating from the anterior lens capsule and often curling at the margins. **B:** the exfoliation syndrome, with three distinct zones: (**1**) central, translucent disc; (**2**) clear zone; (**3**) peripheral granular zone, often with radial striations.

processes,[19] and on the anterior surface of the hyaloid in aphakic eyes.[20] Iris transillumination may reveal a "moth-eaten" pattern near the pupillary sphincter.[10] Cataracts occur frequently in eyes with the exfoliation syndrome,[16, 18] although this may be a function of the age of the patient population.

2. *Gonioscopy.* There is increased trabecular meshwork pigmentation, which has a more uneven distribution than that of pigmentary glaucoma and may be associated with flecks of exfoliation material.[14] Narrow anterior chamber angles occurred in a high percentage in one series,[10] although another study found normal anterior chamber depths in cases without glaucoma.[21]

3. *Course of glaucoma.* Not all patients with the exfoliation syndrome develop glaucoma, and reports vary considerably regarding the frequency of open-angle glaucoma in eyes with this condition. Some patients with bilateral exfoliation syndrome will have glaucoma in both eyes, while others will have a pressure rise in only one of the eyes with exfoliation. Less commonly, a patient with unilateral exfoliation may have open-angle glaucoma in both eyes.[16] Once glaucoma has developed in an eye with exfoliation, it is more difficult to control than cases of primary open-angle glaucoma.[22] Acute angle-closure glaucoma also occurs in a small number of cases with the exfoliation syndrome.[10, 16]

E. Differential Diagnosis

The exfoliation syndrome must be distinguished from other forms of lens exfoliation as well as other causes of pigment dispersion.

1. *Capsular delamination.* As noted earlier in this chapter, another group of disorders involve exfoliation of the anterior lens capsule and have been referred to as "true" exfoliation of the lens capsule,[5] or capsular delamination.[13] These cases differ from the exfoliation syndrome in that an underlying precipitating factor is usually present, such as trauma,[2, 4] exposure to intense heat,[3] or severe uveitis.[4] The nature of the lens exfoliation also differs, with the previously described thin, clear members separating from the anterior lens capsule and often curling at the margins (Fig. 14.1). Glaucoma is infrequent with capsular delamination.

2. *Primary familial amyloidosis.* This generalized systemic disease has numerous ocular manifestations, including glaucoma, which may be associated with a white, flaky substance on the pupillary margin of the iris and anterior lens capsule, as well as pigment deposition in the anterior chamber angle.[23]

3. *Pigment dispersion.* A variety of conditions, in addition to the exfoliation syndrome, are characterized by increased pigmentation of the trabecular meshwork. These include the pigment-dispersion syndrome and pigmentary glaucoma, some forms of anterior uveitis, melanosis and melanomas, and excessive amounts of normal pigment dispersion. These conditions can usually be distinguished from the exfoliation syndrome by observing the characteristic appearance of the anterior lens capsule in the latter disorder.

F. Theories of Mechanism

Questions that must be considered regarding the pathogenesis of the exfoliation syndrome include: 1) the nature and source of the exfoliation material, 2) the mechanism of the associated pigment dispersion, and 3) how these factors contribute to elevation of the intraocular pressure.

1. *The exfoliation material*

a. Nature. The ultrastructural appearance of the exfoliation material is that of a *fibrillar protein*,[24] arranged in an irregular meshwork and occasionally coiled as spirals.[25] Studies suggest that the material may be a mucopolysaccharide,[25, 26] basement membrane,[27] or a protein,[28] possibly of the amyloid group.[24, 29] As previously noted, there may also be clinical similarities between the exfoliation syndrome and primary familial amyloidosis,[23] and the possibility of an overlap in these two conditions exists.

b. *Source.*

(1). *Lens.* The exfoliation material occurs on and in the lens capsule,[30] and adjacent to the lens epithelium.[31] The source of the material on the lens capsule is controversial. One theory holds that it is synthesized by the subcapsular epithelial cells.[28, 31] Smaller amounts of similar fibrillar protein have been seen in the aging lens capsule, and it has been suggested that the exfoliation syndrome represents excessive accumulation of this material.[32] Other investigators argue against the lens epithelium as the source of the exfoliation material on the lens capsule since ultrastructural studies show no continuity between the capsular and epithelial material.[30] Furthermore, studies with horseradish peroxidase suggest the material could not get through the capsule.[26]

(2). *Iris.* The exfoliative material is also found in the iris in the anterior limiting layer, on the posterior aspect of the pigment epithelium, and in the vessel walls.[33] It has been suggested that the iris may be the source of the exfoliation material on the lens capsule.[12] Case studies that are felt to support this concept include an eye with an eccentric pupil in which the distribution of exfoliation material on the lens corresponded to the contact with the iris.[12] Also, cases with deposition of the typical material on the anterior hyaloid many years after intracapsular cataract extraction have been reported.[20]

(3). *Other sources.* Exfoliation material has also been found in the *non-pigmented ciliary epithelium*[34] and the *conjunctiva.*[35] The latter location appears to be another independent source of the material, rather than a secondary deposition from aqueous outflow.[36] Evidence has also been provided to suggest that *lysosomal enzymes* may be involved in the formation of the exfoliation material.[24, 37]

2. *Mechanism of pigment dispersion.* Although the production of exfoliation material appears to be the fundamental feature of the exfoliation syndrome, the associated pigment dispersion in the anterior ocular segment may have an important role in the development of the secondary glaucoma.[38] The precise mechanism of the pigment

dispersion is not fully understood. It may be that the pigment is liberated from the epithelium of the iris as a result of rubbing against the rough lens capsule. Sugar and co-workers,[12] however, feel the pigment dispersion may result from a fundamental defect of the iris.

3. *Mechanism of the glaucoma*

a. Whatever the principal sources of the exfoliation material and dispersed pigment may be, it is generally felt that these elements are involved in the development of the secondary glaucoma. Ultrastructural studies of eyes with the exfoliation syndrome have revealed both *fibrillar material* and *pigment granules* in the *trabecular meshwork*,[39-41] which may lead to obstruction of aqueous outflow. However, not all of these eyes had glaucoma,[41] suggesting that additional factors may be involved.

b. In some cases, the additional factor leading to glaucoma may be a *primary disturbance in the facility of aqueous outflow*.[42] In support of this theory are the observations that glaucoma does not develop in all eyes with exfoliation, and yet may develop in both eyes of a patient with unilateral exfoliation.[10, 11, 16, 39, 43] However, the increased incidence of glaucoma in eyes with exfoliation is felt to indicate a causal relationship between the abnormal material and the elevated intraocular pressure.[44] Furthermore, patients with the exfoliation syndrome do not have the same response to topical corticosteroids as do primary open-angle glaucoma patients.[45, 46] It appears, therefore, that the condition represents a true secondary glaucoma, but may be superimposed on primary open-angle glaucoma in some patients.

c. Another proposed mechanism of glaucoma in rare cases of the exfoliation syndrome is angle-closure glaucoma in which the exfoliative material may increase the pupillary block.[47]

G. Management

The glaucoma associated with the exfoliation syndrome is basically treated the same as primary open-angle glaucoma, although it has been emphasized that the former glaucoma is typically more difficult to control.[22] Trabeculectomy has been shown to be effective when medical therapy is no longer adequate.[48] The influence of lens removal is unclear. It has been reported that the exfoliation material diminishes and regresses after intracapsular cataract extraction,[49] while others have observed the development of the exfoliation syndrome years after intracapsular lens removal.[20, 50] Nevertheless, lens extraction is frequently indicated for improvement of visual acuity in patients with a cataract and the exfoliation syndrome, although not for the primary treatment of the glaucoma. It has been reported that cataract extraction in an eye with the exfoliation syndrome can be complicated by synechiae between the iris pigment epithelium and peripheral anterior lens capsule, which can lead to rupture of the capsule during lens removal.[51]

II. GLAUCOMAS ASSOCIATED WITH DISLOCATION OF THE LENS

A. Terminology

Several terms have been applied to the clinical situation in which the crystalline lens is displaced from its normal, central position behind the iris. *Subluxation* of the lens implies an incomplete dislocation, in which the lens is still at least partially behind the iris, but is tilted or displaced slightly in either an anterior or posterior direction or perpendicular to the optical axis. With *complete dislocation*, the entire lens may be in the anterior chamber or may have fallen posteriorly into the vitreous cavity. The term *ectopia* of the lens, or *ectopia lentis*, is also applied to cases of lens dislocation, but is nonspecific with regard to the degree of lens displacement. Subluxation or complete dislocation of the lens may be associated with a number of clinical conditions, all of which can lead to secondary glaucoma by a variety of mechanisms.

B. Clinical Features

Dislocation of the lens may be acquired or inherited.[52]

1. *Traumatic dislocation.* Trauma is the most common cause of a displaced lens.[52, 53] In one series of 166 cases, an injury was reported to account for 53% of the total.[53] The patient population with traumatic dislocation of the lens had a higher than normal percentage with serologic evidence of syphilis,[53] although a direct cause-and-effect relationship between this disease and dislocation of the lens has not been established. It may simply be that the patient who acquires syphilis is more prone to ocular trauma.[53]

2. *Spontaneous dislocation.* In some middle-aged or older individuals, dislocation of the lens may occur spontaneously, usually in association with cataract formation.[52] Spontaneous dislocation has also been reported in eyes with high myopia, uveitis, buphthalmos, or megalocornea.[52]

3. *Inherited dislocation.* It has been suggested that heritable forms of lens ectopia may be considered in three categories.[54]

  a. *Simple ectopia lentis.* Dislocation of the lens may occur as an isolated congenital anomaly, which is usually inherited by an autosomal mode with decreased penetrance.[54] The condition is typically bilateral and symmetrical, with lens dislocation generally upward and outward. Associated problems include dislocation of the lens into the anterior chamber, secondary glaucoma, and retinal detachment.

  b. *Ectopia lentis et pupillae.* This is a rare, autosomal recessive condition characterized by a small, subluxed lens, an irregular pupil that may be displaced in any direction and dilates poorly, and marked peripheral transillumination of the iris for 360°.[54, 55] These findings are usually bilateral and may be symmetric. Additional ocular problems include anterior or posterior dislocation of the lens, secondary glaucoma, and retinal detachment.

It has been suggested that simple ectopia lentis may be an incomplete expression of ectopia lentis et pupillae since both may occur in the same family and have peripheral iris transillumination.[54] In addition, some patients with ectopia lentis et pupillae may have mild systemic changes suggestive of Marfan's syndrome.[54]

   c. *Systemic diseases associated with dislocation of the lens.*

   (1). *Marfan's syndrome.* This autosomal dominant disorder is characterized by a tall, slender individual with long limbs and frequent cardiovascular disease. Lens dislocation is the most common ocular defect. It typically appears in the fourth to fifth decade of life and is rarely complete, but is usually seen as an upward subluxation. Glaucoma may result from the lens dislocation, but also occurs in association with surgical aphakia, or as an anomaly of the anterior chamber angle. Retinal detachment is also a common finding in either the phakic or aphakic eye of a patient with Marfan's syndrome.[56]

   (2). *Homocystinuria.* These patients resemble those with Marfan's syndrome in habitus and ocular problems, but differ by an autosomal recessive inheritance and frequent mental retardation. The diagnosis can be confirmed by the demonstration of homocystinuria on urine amino acid assay. The differentiation between Marfan's syndrome and homocystinuria is important since the homocystinuric patient is a greater surgical risk due to a tendency for thrombosis and emboli. The lens dislocation occurs earlier in life than in Marfan's syndrome, is more often in a downward direction, and is frequently completely dislocated into the vitreous or anterior chamber. Glaucoma is more commonly related to the lens dislocation than in Marfan's syndrome. Retinal detachment is also a frequent problem.[56]

   (3). *Weill-Marchesani syndrome.* This is the antithesis of the aforementioned conditions with respect to habitus, in that the patients are short and stocky with short limbs. However, lens dislocation occurs with equal frequency and glaucoma is even more common than in Marfan's or homocystinuria.[57] The lens in this condition is typically round, or *spherophakic*, with *loose zonules*, and glaucoma may be related to either lens dislocation[57] or a forward shift of the lens, causing pupillary-block glaucoma.[58]

   (4). Other rare congenital disorders associated with lens dislocation include Ehler's-Danlos syndrome, hyperlysemia,[59] sulfite oxidase deficiency,[60] and aniridia.[61]

C. Theories of Mechanism for Associated Glaucoma[52]

   Subluxation or complete dislocation of the lens in any of the aforementioned clinical conditions may lead to secondary glaucoma by a variety of mechanisms. In general, these mechanisms of glaucoma apply to all forms of lens ectopia.

   1. *Pupillary block.*[52, 62] The lens may block aqueous flow through the pupil if it is dislocated into the pupil or anterior chamber, or if it is subluxed or tilted forward against the iris without entering the anterior chamber. In addition, vitreous may herniate into the pupil causing pupillary block.

2. *Phacolytic glaucoma.*[63] In other cases, the lens may dislocate completely into the vitreous cavity and later undergo degenerative changes with release of material that obstructs aqueous outflow.[63] Phacolytic glaucoma is discussed later in this chapter.

3. *Other mechanisms.*[52] In cases of traumatic dislocation of the lens, *concomitant trauma* to the anterior chamber angle associated with the initial injury may be the cause of the secondary glaucoma. *Peripheral anterior synchiae* may develop from a long-standing pupillary block and produce chronic intraocular pressure elevation. In addition, a transient pressure elevation of uncertain etiology may persist for days or weeks after traumatic dislocation of the lens.

D. Management[52]

1. *Pupillary block.* This condition can occasionally be relieved by *dilating* the pupil and allowing the lens to reposit into the posterior chamber if anteriorly displaced.[64] Miotics should be avoided, since this may make the pupillary block worse. If conservative measures are not successful, an *iridectomy* (surgical or laser) may relieve the pupillary block. Cataract extraction is usually not attempted unless the lens cannot be reposited from the anterior chamber.

2. *Phacolytic glaucoma.* This is the only situation in cases of lens dislocation in which *cataract extraction* is the procedure of choice.[65] Removal of dislocated lenses is normally avoided due to the increased surgical risks, although it has been shown that subluxed lenses can be successfully removed through a pars plana approach with vitreous instruments.[66]

3. Glaucomas secondary to PAS or concomitant trauma in eyes with dislocated lenses are generally managed by standard medical measures and surgical intervention when necessary.

III. GLAUCOMAS ASSOCIATED WITH CATARACT FORMATION

A. Terminology

It has long been recognized clinically that several forms of glaucoma may occur secondary to the formation of cataracts. However, an incomplete understanding of the various mechanisms for these glaucomas has led to a plethora of terms, accompanied by considerable controversy and confusion. More recent observations have provided new explanations and terminology for several of the glaucomas that are associated with cataract formation.

1. In 1900, Gifford[67] described a form of open-angle glaucoma secondary to a *hypermature cataract.* Among the terms subsequently suggested for this condition were *phacogenetic glaucoma*[68] and *lens-induced uveitis.*[69] Flocks and co-workers[70] reported histologic findings which suggested that the glaucoma-inducing mechanism was a macrophagic response to lens material. They proposed that this condition be called *phacolytic glaucoma*, which is the term most often used today. However, Epstein and co-workers[71, 72] have provided evidence

that lens protein may be primarily responsible for the obstruction to aqueous outflow in this disorder, and the term, *lens protein glaucoma*, has been suggested.[73]

2. It was once felt that a primary toxicity of cataractous lens material caused an inflammatory reaction, which led to secondary glaucoma in some cases. The term, *phacotoxic uveitis*, has been applied to this condition, although studies have not supported the concept that liberated lens material is toxic.[74] It appears that cases incorrectly given this diagnosis are actually due to liberation of lens particles and debris following disruption of the lens capsule, and the term, *lens-particle glaucoma*, has been proposed for this entity.[73]

3. In 1922, Verhoeff and Lemaine[75] reported that a small percentage of individuals are hypersensitive to lens protein, and that rupture of the lens capsule in these cases leads to an intraocular inflammation, which they called *endophthalmitis phacoanaphylactica*. Although such cases are apparently rare, there is evidence that a true phacoanaphylaxis does occur in response to lens protein antigen,[76] with secondary inflammation and occasional open-angle glaucoma.[73]

4. A form of secondary angle-closure glaucoma may result from an *intumescent cataract*, in which the swollen lens increases a relative pupillary block with subsequent angle-closure.[77]

B. Phacolytic (Lens Protein) Glaucoma

1. *Clinical features*.[73] The typical patient presents with the *acute onset* of monocular pain and redness. There is usually a history of gradual reduction in visual acuity over the preceding months or years, and vision at the time of presentation may be reduced to inaccurate light perception only. The examination reveals a high intraocular pressure, conjunctival hyperemia, and diffuse corneal edema. It is important to note that the *anterior chamber angle is open* and usually grossly normal. A heavy flare is typically seen in the anterior chamber often associated with *iridescent particles*. The latter are reported to represent calcium oxalate crystals and may be an important diagnostic sign in phacolytic glaucoma.[78] Chunks of white material may also be seen in the aqueous and on the anterior lens capsule and corneal endothelium. The *cataract* is typically *mature* (totally opaque) or *hypermature* (liquid cortex), but may rarely be immature.[73]

A less common variation of phacolytic glaucoma is the situation in which the lens has dislocated into the vitreous and undergone phacolysis. These cases differ clinically in that the glaucoma tends to be more subacute.[73]

2. *Theories of mechanism*. It is generally accepted that part of the pathogenesis in phacolytic glaucoma is the release of *soluble lens protein* into the aqueous through microscopic defects in the lens capsule. However, theories vary as to how this protein leads to elevated intraocular pressure.

a. As previously noted, it has been postulated that *macrophages*, laden with phagocytosed lens material, block the trabecular meshwork, to produce the acute glaucoma.[70] This theory was supported by the demonstration of macrophages in the aqueous of eyes with phacolytic glaucoma, using the Millipore filtration technique for cytologic examination.[79] In addition, histologic studies of eyes with phacolytic glaucoma revealed eosinophilic "protein-like" material and macrophages in the trabecular meshwork.[80] Against this theory, however, is the observation that lens-laden macrophages in the anterior chamber do not invariably lead to elevated intraocular pressure.[73] For example, a macrophagic cellular reaction may be found in the anterior chamber aspirate following needling and aspiration of a cataract, but does not appear to obstruct aqueous outflow.[81] However, the number of macrophages in the aqueous may be greater in phacolytic glaucoma.[81]

b. An alternative theory is that *heavy molecular weight* (HMW)-*soluble protein* from the lens directly obstructs the outflow of aqueous.[71-73] Such protein has been shown to cause a significant decrease in outflow when perfused in enucleated human eyes.[71] HMW-soluble protein is known to increase in the cataractous lens,[82] and has been demonstrated in the aqueous of eyes with phacolytic glaucoma in quantities sufficient to obstruct aqueous outflow.[72] HMW protein is rare in childhood lenses,[83, 84] which may explain why phacolytic glaucoma rarely, if ever, occurs in children.

3. *Differential diagnosis.* Several forms of glaucoma may present with the sudden onset of pain and redness, creating diagnostic confusion with phacolytic glaucoma. *Acute angle-closure glaucoma*, of primary or secondary etiology, must be ruled out on the basis of the gonioscopic examination. *Open-angle glaucoma secondary to uveitis* may be more difficult to distinguish. In some cases, a paracentesis and microscopic examination of the aqueous may be helpful by demonstrating amorphous protein-like fluid and occasional macrophages in eyes with phacolytic glaucoma.[73] A therapeutic trial of topical steroids will produce only temporary remission when phacolysis is the underlying problem, which may help to distinguish it from a primary uveitis. Other conditions, such as neovascular glaucoma and trauma, may also cause a sudden intraocular pressure rise, but can usually be distinguished on the basis of history and/or clinical findings.

4. *Management.* Phacolytic glaucoma should be handled as an emergency, ultimately by intracapsular removal of the lens.[85, 86] It is desirable, however, to first bring the intraocular pressure under medical control with hyperosmotics, carbonic anhydrase inhibitors and timolol, and possibly to minimize associated inflammation with topical steroid therapy.[73] When the pressure cannot be lowered medically, it may be necessary to accomplish this at the time of surgery by gradual release of aqueous. Rupture of the fragile lens capsule may cause serious postoperative sequelae, and a sector iridectomy with use of α-chymotrypsin enzyme may help to minimize the potential complications.[73] When the capsule is ruptured, the

anterior chamber should be irrigated and all lens material removed. Following uncomplicated cataract surgery, the glaucoma usually clears and there is often a return of good vision, despite a significant preoperative reduction.

C. Lens Particle Glaucoma

1. *Clinical features.*[73] This condition is typically associated with *disruption of the lens capsule* either by extracapsular cataract extraction or penetrating injury. The onset of intraocular pressure elevation is usually soon after the primary event, and is generally proportional to the amount of *"fluffed up" lens cortical material* in the anterior chamber. Uncommon clinical variations include an onset of glaucoma many years after capsular disruption or a spontaneous rupture in the lens capsule. The latter condition may be hard to distinguish from phacolytic glaucoma, although cases of lens particle glaucoma tend to have a greater *inflammatory component*, often associated with posterior and anterior synechiae and inflammatory pupillary membranes.

2. *Theories of mechanism.* It has been demonstrated by perfusion studies with enucleated human eyes that small amounts of free particulate lens material significantly reduce outflow.[71] This is presumed to be the principal mechanism of trabecular meshwork obstruction in cases of lens particle glaucoma.[73] However, it is possible that the associated inflammation, whether in response to the surgery, trauma, or retained lens material, may also contribute to the glaucoma in this condition.

3. *Differential diagnosis.* In its typical form, the diagnosis of lens particle glaucoma is usually easy to make on the basis of history and physical findings. In atypical forms, such as delayed onset or spontaneous capsule rupture, the diagnosis might be confused with phacoanaphylaxis, phacolytic glaucoma, or other types of secondary open-angle glaucoma. When doubt exists, microscopic examination of aqueous from an anterior chamber tap may help to establish the diagnosis of lens particle glaucoma by demonstrating leukocytes and macrophages along with lens cortical material.[73]

4. *Management.* In some cases, it is possible to control the intraocular pressure medically with drugs that reduce aqueous production. Because inflammation is also present, the pupil should be dilated and topical steroids should be used, although it may be advisable to use the latter only in moderate amounts, since steroid therapy may delay absorption of the lens material.[73] The intraocular pressure will usually return to normal after the lens material has been absorbed. When the pressure cannot be adequately controlled medically, the residual lens material should be surgically removed either by irrigation if the material is loose or with vitrectomy instruments when it is adherent to ocular structures.

D. Phacoanaphylaxis

1. *Clinical features.*[73] As in the case of lens particle glaucoma, there is usually preceding disruption of the lens capsule by extracapsular

cataract surgery or penetrating injury.[87] The distinguishing feature, however, is a *latent period* during which time sensitization to lens protein occurs. A particularly likely setting for the development of phacoanaphylaxis is when lens material, especially the nucleus, is retained in the vitreous. The typical physical finding is a chronic, relentless "granulomatous-type" of inflammation centered around lens material either in the primarily involved eye or in the fellow eye after it has undergone extracapsular cataract surgery. Secondary glaucoma is only rarely a feature of phacoanaphylaxis.[73]

2. *Theories of mechanism.* It has been demonstrated in rabbits that autologous lens protein is antigenic.[76] Presumably, the lens capsule isolates the lens protein from the immune response, and only when the capsule is violated does sensitization occur. In the rabbit study cited above, there was considerable variation in the response to autologous lens antigen, which may explain the infrequency with which phacoanaphylaxis is seen clinically.[76] The cellular appearance of the immune response is characterized by polymorphonuclear leukocytes and lymphoid, epithelioid, and giant cells, usually around a nidus of lens material. It may be that the occasional glaucoma in phacoanaphylaxis is related to this cellular response in the trabecular meshwork, although lens protein or particles may also be present and could account for the glaucoma.[73]

3. *The differential diagnosis* should include other chronic forms of uveitis, especially sympathetic ophthalmia, which may occur in association with phacoanaphylaxis.[73] Microscopic examination of the aqueous may be helpful, although variations in cytology have not been fully studied in this condition, and the diagnosis may require histologic examination of the surgically removed lens material.

4. *Management.* Steroid therapy should be used to control the uveitis, with antiglaucoma medication as required. When medical measures are inadequate, the retained lens material should be surgically removed.

E. Intumescent Lens[77]

In some eyes with advanced cataract formation, the lens may swell, with progressive reduction in the anterior chamber angle. This may eventually lead to angle-closure glaucoma, either secondary to an enhanced pupillary block mechanism or by the forward displacement of the lens-iris diaphragm. In either case, the diagnosis is usually made by observing a mature, intumescent cataract associated with a central anterior chamber depth that is significantly shallower than that of the fellow eye. The treatment is initial medical reduction of the intraocular pressure with hyperosmotics, carbonic anhydrase inhibitors, and timolol, followed by intracapsular cataract extraction.

References

1. Lindberg, JF: Kliniska ov underosokingar over dipigmentaringen ov pupillenran-den. Diss Helsingfors, 1917.

2. Kraupa, E: Linsenkapselrisse ohne Wundstar. Zeitschrift fur Augenheilkunde 48:93, 1922.
3. Elschnig, A: Ablosung der Zonulalamelle bei glasblasern. Klin Monatsbl Augenheilkd 69:732, 1922.
4. Butler, TH: Capsular glaucoma. Trans Ophthal Soc UK 68:575, 1938.
5. Dvorak-Theobald, G: Pseudo-exfoliation of the lens capsule. Relation to "true" exfoliation of the lens capsule as reported in the literature and role in the production of glaucoma capsulocuticulare. Am J Ophthal 37:1, 1954.
6. Vogt, A: Ein neues Spaltlampenbild des Pupillengebietes: Hellblauer Pupillensaumfilz mit Hautchenbildung auf der Linsenvorderkapsel. Klin Monatsbl Augenheilkd 75:1, 1925.
7. Vogt, A: Weitere histologische Befunde bei seniler Vorderkapselabschilferung. Klin Monatsbl Augenheilkd 89:581, 1932.
8. Vogt, A: Vergleichende Uebersicht uber Klinik und Histologie der Alters- und Feuerlamelle der Linsenvorderkapsel. Klin Monatsbl Augenheilkd 89:587, 1932.
9. Sunde, OA: Senile exfoliation of the anterior lens capsule. Acta Ophthal 45 (Suppl):27, 1956.
10. Layden, WE, Shaffer, RN: Exfoliation syndrome. Am J Ophthal 78:835, 1974.
11. Layden, WE, Shaffer, RN: The exfoliation syndrome. Trans Am Acad Ophthal Otol 78:326, 1974.
12. Sugar, HS, Harding, C, Barsky, D: The exfoliation syndrome. Ann Ophthal 8:1165, 1976.
13. Brodrick, JD, Tate, GW Jr: Capsular delamination (true exfoliation) of the lens. Report of a case. Arch Ophthal 97:1693, 1979.
14. Layden, WE: Exfoliation Syndrome. In The Secondary Glaucomas, Ritch, R, Shields, MB, eds. CV Mosby Co, St Louis (in press).
15. Luntz, MH: Prevalence of pseudo-exfoliation syndrome in an urban South African clinic population. Am J Ophthal 74:581, 1972.
16. Roth, M, Epstein, DL: Exfoliation syndrome. Am J Ophthal 89:477, 1980.
17. Cashwell, FL, Shields, MB: The prevalence of the exfoliation syndrome in the southeastern United States, presented at Annual Meeting American Medical Association, Las Vegas, Nevada, October 1979.
18. Taylor, HR: The environment and the lens. Br J Ophthal 64:303, 1980.
19. Mizuno, K, Muroi, S: Cycloscopy of pseudoexfoliation. Am J Ophthal 87:513, 1979.
20. Sugar, HS: Onset of the exfoliation syndrome after intracapsular lens extraction. Am J Ophthal 89:601, 1980.
21. Bartholomew, RS: Anterior chamber depth in eyes with pseudoexfoliation. Br J Ophthal 64:322, 1980.
22. Olivius, E, Thorburn, W: Prognosis of glaucoma simplex and glaucoma capsulare. A comparative study. Acta Ophthal 56:921, 1978.
23. Tsukahara, S, Matsuo, T: Secondary glaucoma accompanied with primary familial amyloidosis. Ophthalmologica 175:250, 1977.
24. Dark, AJ, Streeten, BW, Cornwall, CC: Pseudoexfoliative disease of the lens: A study in electron microscopy and histochemistry. Br J Ophthal 61:462, 1977.
25. Davanger, M: The pseudo-exfoliation syndrome. A scanning electron microscopic study. I. The anterior lens surface. Acta Ophthal 53:809, 1975.
26. Davanger, M, Pedersen, OO: Pseudo-exfoliation material on the anterior lens surface. Demonstration and examination of an interfibrillar ground substance. Acta Ophthal 53:3, 1975.
27. Eagle, RC Jr, Font, RL, Fine, BS: The basement membrane exfoliation syndrome. Arch Ophthal 97:510, 1979.
28. Bertelsen, TI, Drablos, A, Flood, R: The so-called senile exfoliation (pseudoexfoliation) of the anterior lens capsule. A product of the lens epithelium. Fibrillopathia epitheliocapsularis. A microscopic, histochemical and electron microscopic investigation. Acta Ophthal 42:1096, 1964.
29. Ringvold, A, Husby, G: Pseudo-exfoliation material—an amyloid-like substance. Exp Eye Res 17:289, 1973.
30. Benedikt, O, Aubock, L, Gottinger, W, Waltinger, H: Comparative transmission

and scanning electronmicroscopical studies on lenses in so-called exfoliation syndrome. Albrecht Graefes Arch Klin Exp Ophthal 187:249, 1973.

31. Seland, JH: The ultrastructure of the deep layer of the lens capsule in fibrillo-pathia epitheliocapsularis (FEC), so-called senile exfoliation or pseudoexfoliation. A scanning electron microscopic study. Acta Ophthal 56:335, 1978.

32. Dark, AJ, Streeten, BW, Jones, D: Accumulation of fibrillar protein in the aging human lens capsule. With special reference to the pathogenesis of pseudoexfol-iative disease of the lens. Arch Ophthal 82:815, 1969.

33. Ghosh, M, Speakman, JS: The iris in senile exfoliation of the lens. Can J Ophthal 9:289, 1974.

34. Ghosh, M, Speakman, JS: The ciliary body in senile exfoliation of the lens. Can J Ophthal 8:394, 1973.

35. Speakman, JS, Ghosh, M: The conjunctiva in senile lens exfoliation. Arch Ophthal 94:1757, 1976.

36. Ringvold, A, Davanger, M: Notes on the distribution of pseudo-exfoliation material with particular reference to the uveoscleral route of aqueous humour. Acta Ophthal 55:807, 1977.

37. Mizuno, K, Hara, S, Ishiguro, S, Takei, Y: Acid phosphatase in eyes with pseudoexfoliation. Am J Ophthal 89:482, 1980.

38. Chandler, PA, Grant, WM: Glaucoma, 2nd ed. Lea & Febiger, Philadelphia, 1979, p 116.

39. Sampaolesi, R, Argento, C: Scanning electron microscopy of the trabecular meshwork in normal and glaucomatous eyes. Invest Ophthal Vis Sci 16:302, 1977.

40. Rodrigues, MM, Spaeth, GL, Sivalingam, E, Weinreb, S: Value of trabeculectomy specimens in glaucoma. Ophthal Surg 9:29, 1978.

41. Benedikt, O, Roll, P: The trabecular meshwork of a non-glaucomatous eye with the exfoliation syndrome. Electronmicroscopic study. Virchows Arch Path Anat Histol 384:347, 1979.

42. Pohjanpelto, PEJ: The fellow eye in unilateral hypertensive pseudoexfoliation. Am J Ophthal 75:216, 1973.

43. Cebon, L, Smith, RJH: Pseudoexfoliation of lens capsule and glaucoma. Case report. Br J Ophthal 60:279, 1976.

44. Aasved, H: Intraocular pressure in eyes with and without fibrillopathia epithe-liocapsularis (so-called senile exfoliation or pseudoexfoliation). Acta Ophthal 49:601, 1971.

45. Pohjola, S, Horsmanheimo, A: Topically applied corticosteroids in glaucoma capsulare. Arch Ophthal 85:150, 1971.

46. Gillies, WE: Corticosteroid-induced ocular hypertension in pseudoexfoliation of lens capsule. Am J Ophthal 70:90, 1970.

47. Herbst, RW: Angle closure glaucoma in a patient with pseudoexfoliation of the lens capsule. Ann Ophthal 8:853, 1976.

48. Gillies, WE: Trabeculotomy in pseudoexfoliation of the lens capsule. Br J Ophthal 61:297, 1977.

49. Gillies, WE: Effect of lens extraction in pseudoexfoliation of the lens capsule. Br J Ophthal 57:46, 1973.

50. Radian, AB, Radian, AL: Senile pseudoexfoliation in aphakic eyes. Br J Ophthal 59:577, 1975.

51. Dark, AJ: Cataract extraction complicated by capsular glaucoma. Br J Ophthal 63:465, 1979.

52. Chandler, PA: Choice of treatment in dislocation of the lens. Arch Ophthal 71:765, 1964.

53. Jarrett, WH: Dislocation of the lens. A study of 166 hospitalized cases. Arch Ophthal 78:289, 1967.

54. Luebbers, JA, Goldberg, MF, Herbst, R, Hattenhauer, J, Maumenee, AE: Iris transillumination and variable expression in ectopia lentis et pupillae. Am J Ophthal 83:647, 1977.

55. Townes, PL: Ectopia lentis et pupillae. Arch Ophthal 94:1126, 1976.

56. Cross, HE, Jensen, AD: Ocular manifestations in the Marfan syndrome and homocystinuria. Am J Ophthal 75:405, 1973.

57. Jensen, AD, Cross, HE: Ocular complications in the Weill-Marchesani syndrome. Am J Ophthal 77:261, 1974.

58. Willi, M, Kut, L, Cotlier, E: Pupillary-block glaucoma in the Marchesani syndrome. Arch Ophthal 90:504, 1973.

59. Smith, TH, Holland, MG, Woody, NC: Ocular manifestations of familial hyperlysinemia. Trans Am Acad Ophthal Otol 75:355, 1971.

60. Shih, VE, Abroms, IF, Johnson, JL, Carney, M, Mandell, R, Robb, RM, Cloherty, JP, Rajagopalan, KV: Sulfite oxidase deficiency. Biochemical and clinical investigations of a hereditary metabolic disorder in sulfur metabolism. N Engl J Med 297:1022, 1977.

61. David, R, MacBeath, L, Jenkins, T: Aniridia associated with microcornea and subluxated lenses. Br J Ophthal 62:118, 1978.

62. Hein, HF, Maltzman, B: Long-standing anterior dislocation of the crystalline lens. Ann Ophthal 7:66, 1975.

63. Pollard, ZF: Phacolytic glaucoma secondary to ectopia lentis. Ann Ophthal 7:999, 1975.

64. Jay, B: Glaucoma associated with spontaneous displacement of the lens. Br J Ophthal 56:258, 1972.

65. Chandler, PA: Completely dislocated hypermature cataract and glaucoma. Tr Am Ophthal Soc 57:242, 1959.

66. Treister, G, Machemer, R: Pars plana surgical approach for various anterior segment problems. Arch Ophthal 97:909, 1979.

67. Gifford, H: Danger of the spontaneous cure of senile cataracts. Am J Ophthal 17:289, 1900.

68. Zeeman, WPC: Zwei Falle von Glaucoma phacogeneticum mit anatomischem Befund. Ophthalmologica 106:136, 1943.

69. Irvine, SR, Irvine, AR Jr: Lens-induced uveitis and glaucoma. III. "Phacogenetic glaucoma": lens-induced glaucoma; mature or hypermature cataract; open iridocorneal angle. Am J Ophthal 35:489, 1952.

70. Flocks, M, Littwin, CS, Zimmerman, LE: Phacolytic glaucoma. A clinicopathologic study of one hundred thirty-eight cases of glaucoma associated with hypermature cataract. Arch Ophthal 54:37, 1955.

71. Epstein, DL, Jedziniak, JA, Grant, WM: Obstruction of aqueous outflow by lens particles and by heavy-molecular-weight soluble lens proteins. Invest Ophthal Vis Sci 17:272, 1978.

72. Epstein, DL, Jedziniak, JA, Grant, WM: Identification of heavy-molecular-weight soluble protein in aqueous humor in human phacolytic glaucoma. Invest Ophthal Vis Sci 17:398, 1978.

73. Epstein, DL: Lens-induced Open-Angle Glaucoma. In The Secondary Glaucomas, Ritch, R, Shields, MB, eds. CV Mosby Co, St Louis (in press).

74. Muller, H: Phacolytic glaucoma and phacogenic ophthalmia. (Lens induced uveitis). Trans Ophthal Soc UK 83:689, 1963.

75. Verhoeff, FH, Lemoine, AN: Endophthalmitis phacoanaphylactica. Trans Int Cong Ophthal, Wash, DC, Phila. Wm F Fell Co, 1922, p 234.

76. Rahi, AHS, Misra, RN, Morgan, G: Immunopathology of the lens. III. Humoral and cellular immune responses to autologous lens antigens and their roles in ocular inflammation. Br J Ophthal 61:371, 1977.

77. Ritch, R: Glaucoma Secondary to Lens Intumescence and Dislocation. In The Secondary Glaucomas, Ritch, R, Shields, MB, eds. CV Mosby Co, St Louis (in press).

78. Bartholomew, RS, Rebello, PF: Calcium oxalate crystals in the aqueous. Am J Ophthal 88:1026, 1979.

79. Goldberg, MF: Cytological diagnosis of phacolytic glaucoma utilizing Millipore filtration of the aqueous. Br J Ophthal 51:847, 1967.

80. Hogan, MJ, Zimmerman, LE: Ophthalmic Pathology. An Atlas and Textbook. WB Saunders, Philadelphia, 1962, p 671.

81. Yanoff, M, Scheie, HG: Cytology of human lens aspirate. Its relationship to phacolytic glaucoma and phacoanaphylactic endophthalmitis. Arch Ophthal 80:166, 1968.
82. Jedziniak, JA, Kinoshita, JH, Yates, EM, Hocker, LO, Benedek, GB: On the presence and mechanism of formation of heavy molecular weight aggregates in human normal and cataractous lenses. Exp Eye Res 15:185, 1973.
83. Spector, A, Li, S, Sigelman, J: Age-dependent changes in the molecular size of human lens proteins and their relationship to light scatter. Invest Ophthal 13:795, 1974.
84. Jedziniak, JA, Nicoli, DF, Baram, H, Benedek, GB: Quantitative verification of the existence of high molecular weight protein aggregates in the intact normal human lens by light-scattering spectroscopy. Invest Ophthal Vis Sci 17:51, 1978.
85. Chandler, PA: Problems in the diagnosis and treatment of lens-induced uveitis and glaucoma. Arch Ophthal 60:828, 1958.
86. Volcker, HE, Naumann, G: Clinical findings in phakolytic glaucoma. Klin Monatsbl Augenheilkd 166:613, 1975.
87. Perlman, EM, Albert, DM: Clinically unsuspected phacoanaphylaxis after ocular trauma. Arch Ophthal 95:244, 1977.

Chapter 15

GLAUCOMAS ASSOCIATED WITH RETINAL DISORDERS

GLAUCOMAS ASSOCIATED WITH RETINAL DISORDERS

A few types of glaucoma are associated with diseases of the retina. The most common of these is neovascular glaucoma, which is usually secondary to one of several retinal disorders, although some cases are associated with other ocular or extraocular conditions. In addition, retinal detachments and a variety of less common diseases of the vitreous, retina, or choroid may cause or occur in association with several forms of glaucoma.

I. NEOVASCULAR GLAUCOMA

A. Terminology

In 1906, Coats[1] described new vessel formation on the iris in eyes with central retinal vein occlusion. This neovascularization of the iris has become commonly known as *rubeosis iridis*, and is now recognized as a complication of many diseases of the retina and other ocular and extraocular disorders. Rubeosis iridis is frequently associated with a severe form of secondary glaucoma, which has been variably named *hemorrhagic glaucoma*, referring to the hyphema that is present in some cases, *congestive glaucoma*, describing the frequently acute nature of the condition, and *thrombotic glaucoma*, implying an underlying vascular thrombotic etiology. However, none of these terms accurately describe the glaucoma in all cases, and the more nonspecific name, *neovascular glaucoma*, as proposed by Weiss and co-workers,[2] is generally preferred.

B. Factors Predisposing to Rubeosis Iridis

Most cases of rubeosis iridis are preceded by an hypoxic disease of the retina. Diabetic retinopathy and occlusion of major retinal vessels account for over half of these with the former possibly being slightly more common.[3-5] However, many additional retinal diseases, as well as certain other ocular or extraocular disorders, have now been recognized, resulting in a long list of conditions which may predispose to the development of rubeosis iridis.

1. *Diabetic retinopathy.* In one series of patients with rubeosis iridis, one-third had diabetic retinopathy.[3] Following pars plana vitrectomy for diabetic retinopathy, rubeosis iridis is seen in 25 to 30% of the eyes, and neovascular glaucoma develops 10 to 15% of the time.[6-10] In these cases, the occurrence of rubeosis iridis is much higher in aphakic eyes,[10, 11] and postoperative intraocular pressure elevation is more common when rubeosis iridis is present before the vitrectomy.[12]

2. *Central retinal vein occlusion.* This was found to account for

28% of all rubeosis iridis in one series.[3] Many of these cases develop neovascular glaucoma within a few months after the vascular occlusive event, which has led to the term, "*90 day glaucoma.*" Rarely, rubeosis iridis and neovascular glaucoma may be associated with *central retinal artery occlusion.*[13] In addition, *branch retinal vein*[3] and *branch retinal arteriolar occlusion*[14] have been reported as rare causes of rubeosis iridis, but not neovascular glaucoma.

3. *Other retinal disorders* that may be associated with rubeosis iridis include *retinal detachment* (which is usually chronic and often overlies a *malignant melanoma*), retinoblastoma,[15] hemorrhagic retinal disorders, Coat's exudative retinopathy, retrolental fibroplasia, sickle cell retinopathy,[16] syphilitic retinal vasculitis,[17] retinoschisis,[18] and the inherited vitreoretinal degeneration of Stickler's syndrome.[19]

4. *Other ocular disorders.* *Uveitis* was said to be present in 11% of rubeotic eyes in one series.[3] However, other than the well known engorgement of normal iris vessels in response to inflammation, an association between uveitis and neovascular glaucoma has yet to be established. *End stage glaucoma* (open-angle or angle-closure) has also been said to give rise to rubeosis iridis,[3] although this is probably most often related to central retinal vein occlusion, which is commonly associated with elevated intraocular pressure.[4]

5. *Extraocular vascular disorders.* A *carotid-cavernous fistula* may cause rubeosis iridis and neovascular glaucoma as a result of decreased arterial flow and subsequent reduction in the ocular perfusion pressure, which may occur either before or after treatment of the fistula.[2, 20, 21] (In addition, a carotid-cavernous fistula may cause glaucoma by other mechanisms, which will be discussed in Chapter 20.) It has also been reported that *internal carotid artery occlusion* may create an "ophthalmic artery steal phenomenon" with associated rubeosis iridis.[22]

C. Theories of Neovasculogenesis

The mechanism(s) by which the aforementioned clinical situations lead to the development of rubeosis iridis is unknown, although the following theories have been proposed.

1. *Retinal hypoxia.* Since most, but not all, of the conditions associated with rubeosis iridis involve diminished perfusion of the retina, it may be that retinal hypoxia is at least one factor in the formation of new vessels on the iris and anterior chamber angle, as well as on the retina and optic nerve head.[23] This concept is supported by the clinical observations that rubeosis iridis in association with either proliferative diabetic retinopathy[24] or central retinal vein occlusion[25] is more likely to occur when significant capillary nonperfusion is present. A study with rhesus monkeys showed no significant difference in vitreous oxygen tension over non-perfused retina with intraretinal neovascularization as compared to normal retinal areas,[26] although vitreous body measurements may not accurately reflect retinal oxygen levels.

2. *Angiogenesis factors.* It has been demonstrated that tumors possess a diffusible factor, "*tumor angiogenesis factor,*" that is capable of eliciting new vessel growth toward the tumor.[27] Subsequent studies have suggested that human[28] and animal *retina,*[28, 29] as well as other vascular ocular tissues,[29] have similar *angiogenic activity,* which may explain why ocular neovascularization can occur in areas remote from the site of retinal capillary nonperfusion.[30] This angiogenic factor was characterized in one study as diffusible, heat-labile, and non-inflammatory,[29] and possibilities that have been considered regarding the identity of this substance include lactic acid,[31] biogenic amines,[32] and prostaglandins.[33]

It has also been speculated that vitreous may possess *vasoinhibitory factors.*[34] This is one theoretical explanation as to why vitrectomy in eyes with diabetic retinopathy is associated with a high incidence of postoperative rubeosis iridis.

3. *Chronic dilation of ocular vessels.* It has also been proposed that dilation of a vessel is the stimulus that leads to new vessel growth in response to hypoxia, or any other factor that causes a vessel to dilate.[35] According to this theory, rubeosis iridis results from local hypoxia of the iris, which causes dilation of iridic vessels and subsequent new vessel formation. This sequence may be initiated or aggravated following vitrectomy for diabetic retinopathy, when aqueous humor circulates posteriorly and loses much of its oxygen to the hypoxic retina.

4. In *summary,* it is generally believed that *hypoxia* of the retina, or possibly of other ocular tissue, is the most common initial stimulus that leads to new vessel formation, either by the release of an *angiogenic factor* or by a direct action on the vessels, such as causing *dilation.* Furthermore, there may be mechanisms that tend to oppose this neovasculogenesis, such as *vasoinhibitory factors* in the vitreous.

D. Natural History

When a patient has a predisposing factor, such as diabetic retinopathy or central retinal vein occlusion, what is the likelihood that he will develop rubeosis iridis, and what are the chances that this will lead to neovascular glaucoma? The answers to these questions are not fully known, but the following information has been reported:

1. *Diabetic retinopathy.*

a. *The prevalence of rubeosis iridis* among patients with *diabetes mellitus* was studied by Ohrt[36] and found to be 6.8% in his clinic, with a range of 0.25 to 10% in a review of six previous reports. Iris angiography may occasionally reveal new vessels near the pupillary margin before rubeosis iridis is apparent by slit lamp examination.[37] The diabetes will generally have been present for many years before rubeosis develops, and concomitant proliferative diabetic retinopathy is usually found. However, rubeosis iridis may rarely occur in an eye with non-proliferative retinopathy.[36]

b. In patient populations with *proliferative diabetic retinopathy,* rubeosis iridis is reported to occur in approximately half of the cases.[36, 38]

c. *Neovascular glaucoma* does not invariably follow the development of rubeosis iridis,[36, 38, 39, 40] and the latter condition may resolve spontaneously.[36] However, neovascular glaucoma has been reported to develop in 13 to 22% of patients with rubeosis iridis.[36, 38, 39] As previously noted, neovascular glaucoma is more likely to occur when arteriolar or capillary non-perfusion is present,[24] and is particularly common following pars plana vitrectomy for diabetic retinopathy.[6-10]

2. *Central retinal vein occlusion*

a. It is well known that eyes with central retinal vein occlusion often have pre-existing *primary open-angle glaucoma*.[40, 41] Other factors that may be associated with occlusion of the central retinal vein include systemic hypertension and increased whole blood and plasma viscosity and plasma fibrinogen.[42]

b. During the early months after a central retinal vein occlusion, *hypotony* may develop.[43, 44] The explanation for this is unclear, although the possible influences of anterior segment ischemia,[43] or an angiogenic factor[44] have been considered.

c. *Vascular changes in the iris* reportedly occur in one of three ways[43]:

(1). Transient dilation of the iridic vessels without fluorescein leakage.

(2). True rubeosis iridis with a sudden increase in intraocular pressure 8 to 15 weeks after the occlusion.

(3). True rubeosis iridis with no associated pressure elevation or a delayed rise 9 months or more following the occlusion.

d. As in diabetic retinopathy, the incidence of rubeosis iridis and neovascular glaucoma in eyes with central retinal vein occlusion is significantly correlated with the extent of *retinal capillary nonperfusion*.[25, 45, 46] In one study, the incidence of rubeosis iridis following central retinal vein occlusion was 60% when retinal ischemic was demonstrated by fluorescein angiography, compared to 1% in those with good capillary perfusion.[46] Neovascular glaucoma occurred in 14%[47] to 27%[48] of the eyes with hemorrhagic retinopathy (complete venous occlusion) following central retinal vein occlusion, but in none of the cases of venous stasis retinopathy (incomplete occlusion). Fluorescein angiography shows that virtually all eyes with extensive retinal capillary closure following central retinal vein occlusion have abnormal, leaking vessels of the iris.[49]

E. Clinicopathologic Features

To understand the events that lead from rubeosis iridis to neovascular glaucoma, as well as the rationale for the various therapeutic measures, it is helpful to consider the clinicopathologic course of the disease in the following *three stages* (Fig. 15.1):

1. *Pre-glaucoma stage* (rubeosis iridis). This stage is characterized

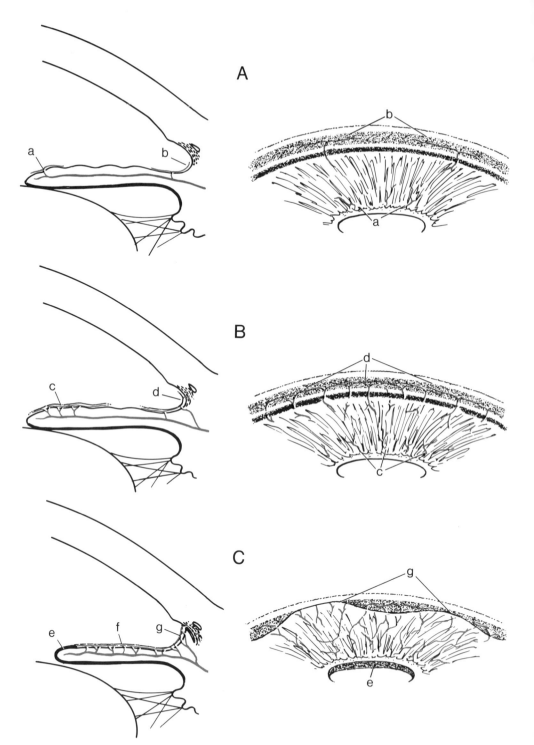

Figure 15.1. Clinicopathologic stages of neovascular glaucoma. **A:** preglaucoma stage (rubeosis iridis), characterized by new vessels on the surface of the iris (**a**) and in the anterior chamber angle (**b**); **B:** open-angle glaucoma stage, characterized by an increase in neovascularization and a fibrovascular membrane on the iris (**c**) and in the anterior chamber angle (**d**); **C:** angle-closure glaucoma stage, characterized by contracture of the fibrovascular membrane, which causes corectopia, ectropion uvea (**e**), flattening of the iris (**f**), and peripheral anterior synechiae (**g**).

by a normal intraocular pressure, unless pre-existing primary open-angle glaucoma is present.

(a). *Clinical features. Slit-lamp biomicroscopy* early in the disease process typically reveals dilated tufts of pre-existing capillaries and fine, randomly oriented vessels on the surface of the iris near the pupillary margin.[39] Even before the first new vessel formation, *fluorescein angiography* of the iris may show dilatation and leakage of pre-existing peripupillary capillaries and radial vessels.[50] The new vessels are also characterized by leakage of fluorescein.[39, 40] The neovascularization characteristically progresses from the pupillary margin toward the root of the iris.[39] *Gonioscopy* may reveal a normal anterior chamber angle, or may show a variable amount of angle neovascularization. The latter is characterized by single vascular trunks crossing the ciliary band and scleral spur and arborizing on the trabecular meshwork. Reports differ as to whether true neovascularization is first seen on the peripupillary iris[39] or in the anterior chamber angle.[50]

(b). *Histopathologic features.* The rubeosis iridis begins intrastromally and then develops on the surface of the iris.[34, 51] Silicone injection studies indicate that the new vessels on the iris arise from normal iridic arteries and drain primarily into iridic and ciliary body veins, while new vessels in the angle arise from arteries of the iris and ciliary body and connect with the peripheral neovascular network on the iris.[52] Although the clinical appearance of rubeosis iridis is said to be the same in cases of diabetes and central retinal vein occlusion,[40] the silicone injections show tighter and more evenly distributed neovascularization in the diabetic eye.[52] The silicone injection studies also show that new vessels in the angle run circumferentually in the trabecular meshwork, with branches coursing into the fibrosed Schlemm's canal and occasionally into collector channels.[52] The new vessels are characterized histologically as having thin walls[51, 53] and are arranged in irregular patterns.[51] The ultrastructure in cases of rubeosis iridis associated with sickle cell retinopathy is said to be similar to that in diabetes and retinal occlusive disease with open interendothelial cell junctions, attenuated intraendothelial cytoplasm, and pericyte formation.[54]

2. *Open-angle glaucoma stage.*

a. *Clinical features.* The rubeosis iridis is typically more florid in this stage and biomicroscopic examination of the aqueous often reveals an inflammatory reaction. By gonioscopy, th anterior chamber angle is still open, but the neovascularization is intense. The intraocular pressure is now elevated and may rise suddenly, causing the patient to present with acute onset glaucoma. Hyphema may also be present in this stage.

b. *Histopathologic features.* The hallmark of this stage is a *fibrovascular membrane* which covers the anterior chamber angle and anterior surface of the iris,[51, 53] and may even extend onto the posterior iris.[53] Chronic inflammatory changes are also typically seen on histologic examination.[51, 53] The glaucoma in this stage probably results from obstruction of the trabecular meshwork by the fibrovascular membrane, with variable contribution from the inflammation and hemorrhage. In addition, cases have been described in which endothelialization of the anterior chamber angle was associated with rubeosis iridis and glaucoma, although most of these had antecedent trauma.[55]

3. *Angle-closure glaucoma stage.* The hallmark of this stage is *contracture* of the fibrovascular membrane.[51, 53] This tends to flatten the stroma of the iris, giving it a smooth, glistening appearance, and causes ectropion uvea and pupillary dilation. In the anterior chamber angle, the contracture leads to *peripheral anterior synechia* formation, with eventual total synechial closure of the angle. The glaucoma in this stage is typically severe and usually requires surgical intervention.

F. Management

The optimum approach to preventing blindness from neovascular glaucoma would be to treat the underlying disease before rubeosis iridis develops. Prophylactic measures are currently available with which rubeosis can be prevented in some eyes or arrested before the onset of neovascular glaucoma in other cases. When glaucoma is present, medical therapy and frequently surgical intervention are required.

1. *Prophylactic measures.* Although rubeosis iridis does not invariably lead to neovascular glaucoma, it does so with sufficient frequency that prophylactic measures to prevent the glaucoma appear to be warranted. Preliminary studies suggest that the following forms of treatment may provide such prophylaxis.

a. *Panretinal photocoagulation.* Ablation of peripheral retina with Xenon arc or Argon laser photocoagulation has been shown to significantly reduce or eliminate anterior segment neovascularization in many cases,[56-60] and to reduce the chances of developing rubeosis iridis in eyes with diabetic retinopathy or central retinal vein occlusion.[39, 46, 61] It has also been reported that carbon dioxide laser can be used for intraocular panretinal photocoagulation at the time of vitrectomy.[62] The mechanism by which panretinal photocoagulation influences neovascularization is uncertain, although it may be related to decreasing the retinal oxygen demand,[35] which is consistent with the reported observation that the photoreceptor-retinal pigment epithelial complex accounts for two-thirds of the total retinal oxygen consumption.[63]

Randomized, controlled studies show that treated eyes do better than untreated eyes in both diabetic[39] and central retinal vein occlusion cases.[58, 61] However, one study revealed that panretinal photocoagulation is more effective in controlling rubeosis in diabetics, than in patients with central retinal vein occlusion,[46] and the results of another investigation suggest that the treatment of retinal vascular occlusive cases should be limited to those eyes with retinal capillary nonperfusion.[58]

Panretinal photocoagulation appears to be most effective as prophylaxis against the development of rubeosis iridis or neovascular glaucoma. However, it is reported that the treatment may reverse intraocular pressure elevation in the open-angle glaucoma stage,[56, 57] and in some cases of early angle-closure neovascular glaucoma, provided the synechial closure has not exceeded 270°.[59] Even in the latter situation, panretinal photocoagulation may be useful in reducing anterior segment neovascularization prior to intraocular surgery.[5, 64] However, one study showed that panretinal photocoagulation prior to vitrectomy for diabetic retinopathy did not prevent postoperative rubeosis iridis.[65]

b. *Panretinal cryotherapy.* When cloudy media precludes panretinal photocoagulation, it has been reported that transscleral panretinal cryotherapy in eyes with neovascular glaucoma will control the intraocular pressure and reduce or abolish the neovascularization.[66] The preliminary results are difficult to interpret, however, since five of the six eyes also had cyclocryotherapy, and further study of this modality is needed.

c. *Goniophotocoagulation.* This technique involves the direct application of laser therapy to new vessels in the anterior chamber angle.[67] It is most effective when used in the early stages of the disease to prevent the progressive angle changes and eventual intractable neovascular glaucoma.[68] It may be used in conjunction with panretinal photocoagulation, and is primarily recommended for patients with a high risk of developing neovascular glaucoma, when panretinal photocoagulation has not been successful or is not possible or advisable, and prior to intraocular surgery.[64, 68]

2. *Medical management.* Once the intraocular pressure begins to rise, medical therapy is usually required and is frequently sufficient to control the pressure during the open-angle glaucoma stage. The mainstay of the therapy at this stage is drugs that reduce aqueous production, such as carbonic anhydrase inhibitors and timolol. Miotics and epinephrine are rarely helpful and should usually be avoided due to the complications with inflammation.[69] Topical corticosteroids may be useful in minimizing the inflammation and pain.[70] In addition, intravitreal triamcinolone has been shown to reduce retinal neovascularization in rabbit eyes,[71] raising the question of a possible direct benefit of topical steroids on rubeotic vessels. In far advanced or blind eyes, atropine is helpful for relief of pain. Hyperosmotic agents may also be required for temporary control of cases with marked intraocular pressure elevation.

3. *Surgical management.* If the disease follows its natural course to eventual angle-closure glaucoma, medical therapy nearly always becomes ineffective and surgical intervention is required. The many procedures that have been attempted for this condition bare witness to the difficulty of surgically treating neovascular glaucoma.

a. *Cyclocryotherapy.* Good results have been reported from some studies, and it has been suggested that cyclocryotherapy may be the procedure of choice for neovascular glaucoma.[72, 73] Other reports, however, have been less encouraging, such as one 2-year follow-up of 50 eyes in which one-third were uncontrolled and one-third developed phthisis.[74] Many surgeons consider this procedure to be preferable only to retrobulbar alcohol or enucleation.[74-76] In two cases of neovascular glaucoma associated with retinal detachment, intravitreal neovascularization developed from the ciliary body following cyclocryotherapy.[77]

b. *Filtering surgery.* It has been a general belief that standard filtering procedures in eyes with neovascular glaucoma are rarely successful, primarily due to the high risk of intraoperative bleeding and postoperative progression of the fibrovascular membrane. However, it has been emphasized that this is no longer true, if appropriate *pre-operative measures* are taken.[5, 64] A successful panretinal photocoagulation, possibly combined with goniophotocoagulation, will usually make it possible to perform a standard filtering operation, such as trabeculectomy, or a full-thickness filtering procedure.[5, 64] In addition, newer techniques of filtering surgery for neovascular glaucoma have been described, which include a modified trabeculectomy with intraocular bipolar cautery of peripheral iris and ciliary processes,[78] and creation of a limbal fistula with a carbon dioxide laser.[79] Preliminary experience has also been encouraging with the implantation of a tube[80, 81] or valve[82] into the anterior chamber in eyes with neovascular glaucoma. Details regarding the techniques and reported results of these procedures will be considered in Section Three.

c. *Hypophysectomy* is mentioned only out of historical interest. Its efficacy was never established with regard to rubeosis iridis and neovascular glaucoma. In one study, 62 patients were treated and compared to 73 untreated cases. Rubeosis iridis developed in 29% of the former group and 33% of the latter, while the incidence of neovascular glaucoma in eyes with rubeosis iridis was 27% and 33%, respectively.[38]

II. GLAUCOMA AND RETINAL DETACHMENT

The co-existence of glaucoma and retinal detachment in the same eye occurs under three circumstances: 1) glaucomas associated with retinal detachment, in which a cause-and-effect relationship is uncertain; 2) glaucoma secondary to retinal detachment; and 3) glaucomas secondary to treatment for retinal detachment. The first two situations will be discussed in this chapter, and the third will be considered in Chapter 18.

A. Glaucomas Associated with Retinal Detachment

1. *Primary open-angle glaucoma.*

a. *Epidemiology.* Primary open-angle glaucoma is more common in eyes with a *rhegmatogenous retinal detachment* than in the general population. In one study of 817 cases of retinal detachment, primary open-angle glaucoma was present in 4%, and an additional 6.5% had elevated intraocular pressure without glaucomatous damage.[83]

b. *Theories of mechanism.* It is not known why primary open-angle glaucoma and rhegmatogenous retinal detachment occur in the same eye more frequently than would be anticipated on the basis of chance occurrence. Myopia and the use of miotics have not been found to be the common denominator.[83] In 30 cases of spontaneous rhegmatogenous retinal detachment, 53% had a cup/disc ratio greater than 0.3 and 20% were high topical steroid responders.[84] These values are significantly higher than in the general population and resemble the findings in groups of patients with primary open-angle glaucoma, which led the authors to suggest that the two diseases may be related genetically by multifactorial inheritance.[84]

c. *Management.* When primary open-angle glaucoma and retinal detachment co-exist, one disorder may mask the presence of the other, necessitating careful attention to certain details during the management of either condition:[85]

(1). *Primary open-angle glaucoma.* When following a patient with primary open-angle glaucoma, the peripheral retina should be examined before initiating therapy and at least annually or whenever warning signs appear, such as floaters, flashing lights, loss of peripheral vision, or a sudden decrease in the intraocular pressure. Although the role of miotics in the pathogenesis of rhegmatogenous retinal detachment has not been clearly established, circumstantial evidence indicates that particular caution is warranted when these drugs are used.[86, 87]

(2). *Retinal detachment.* An eye with a rhegmatogenous retinal detachment typically has a reduced intraocular pressure, which may mask a pre-existing glaucoma. In addition, retinal detachment surgery lowers ocular rigidity, which will cause a Schiøtz tonometer to read falsely low.[88, 89] In one study of 115 eyes, the mean disparity between applanation and Schiøtz pressure measurements averaged 8.6 mmHg one month after retinal detachment surgery and 5.8 mm Hg 6 months postoperatively.[88] An applanation tonometer, therefore, should be used following retinal detachment surgery, and the optic nerve head should be carefully inspected during the fundus examination to avoid missing co-existing glaucoma.

The success of retinal detachment surgery is not adversely affected by the presence of glaucoma,[83] although the visual outcome may be worse due to the concomitant glaucomatous optic atrophy.[83, 90] Following retinal detachment surgery, special caution should be given to the use of topical steroids, due to the increased incidence of high topical steroid responders,[84] and miotics should be avoided in either eye if possible.

2. *Pigmentary glaucoma.* Patients with the pigment-dispersion syndrome, with or without glaucoma, may have an increased incidence of retinal detachment.[85] In addition, patients with retinal detachment are reported to have varying degrees of pigment dispersion in the anterior chamber angle in a significant number of cases.[85, 91] As in the case of primary open-angle glaucoma, no definite cause-and-effect

relationship has been established, but the same considerations as mentioned above must be employed in the management of these conditions.

B. Glaucoma Secondary to Retinal Detachment

As previously noted, a *rhegmatogenous retinal detachment* is commonly associated with a slight reduction in the intraocular pressure. However, the opposite occurs in a small number of cases, and the patient presents with unilateral pressure elevation, which may mask the underlying retinal detachment. The anterior chamber angle is typically open, and aqueous cells and flare are often seen.[92]

1. *Theories of mechanism.* The mechanism of the glaucoma is unclear, although many patients have a history of ocular trauma,[83, 92] and concomitant damage to the trabecular meshwork may be the cause of reduced aqueous outflow in some cases. Other suggested mechanisms include anterior uveitis secondary to the retinal detachment[92] and obstruction of the trabecular meshwork by pigment from the retinal pigment epithelium.[93]

2. *Management.* The treatment of both the rhegmatogenous retinal detachment and the secondary glaucoma is repair of the detachment, which typically results in resolution of the glaucoma within a few days.[92] In the differential diagnosis, it is important to remember that an eye with retinal detachment and glaucoma may harbor a *malignant melanoma*.[94]

III. GLAUCOMAS ASSOCIATED WITH OTHER DISORDERS OF THE RETINA, CHOROID, AND VITREOUS

A. Angle-closure Glaucomas

1. **Central retinal vein occlusion.** Neovascular glaucoma, which may follow retinal vascular occlusive disease, was discussed earlier in this chapter. In addition, a small number of cases have been described with shallowing of the anterior chamber after a central retinal vein occlusion, which can lead to transient angle-closure glaucoma.[95-97]

Examination typically reveals a forward shift of the lens-iris diaphragm in the involved eye and a normal anterior chamber depth in the fellow eye. The mechanism of the angle-closure is uncertain, although it has been postulated that transudation of fluid from the retinal vessels into the vitreous leads to forward displacement of the lens with a subsequent pupillary block.[95] The differential diagnosis should include primary angle-closure glaucoma, which may secondarily cause occlusion of the central retinal vein, and neovascular glaucoma, which can lead to synechial closure of the anterior chamber angle. The former situation might be recognized by a potentially occludable angle in the fellow eye, while the latter can usually be identified by the presence of rubeosis iridis.

Treatment should be medical, since the angle returns to normal depth over a several week period.[95-97] Acetazolamide and timolol may be helpful, and success has been reported with both pilocarpine[95, 96] and cycloplegics.[97]

2. **Nanophthalmos.** In this rare ocular anomaly, the eye is small but has a normal shape. The eyes are highly hyperopic due to the short axial length and frequently develop angle-closure glaucoma in the fourth to sixth decades of life.[98]

Uveal effusion and *non-rhegmatogenous retinal detachment* have been found following intraocular surgery in these cases.[98, 99] There is evidence that the uveal effusion may precede the surgery and actually cause the angle-closure glaucoma by causing a forward shift of the lens-iris diaphragm, leading to a pupillary block mechanism.[100] It has been proposed that the uveal effusion results from choroidal congestion due to impaired vortex venous drainage through the thick sclera, which is characteristic of nanophthalmos.[101]

This form of secondary glaucoma responds poorly to conventional medical or surgical therapy.[99] A suggested approach to managing the uveal effusion is vortex vein decompression and, in some cases, drainage of choroidal and/or subretinal fluid with air injection into the vitreous cavity.[101] Preliminary results suggest that laser iridoplasty may relieve the angle-closure glaucoma by causing contracture of the peripheral iris and pulling the anterior chamber angle open.[100]

3. **Retinal and vitreous abnormalities in the newborn.** Several developmental or acquired disorders of the retina and/or vitreous in the newborn can lead to forward displacement of the lens-iris diaphragm and eventual angle-closure glaucoma.

a. *Retrolental fibroplasia* (retinopathy of prematurity). Contracture of the retrolental mass can cause progressive shallowing of the anterior chamber with eventual angle-closure glaucoma. This complication coincides with the cicatricial phase of the disease, which usually has its onset at three to 6 months of age. However, the angle-closure glaucoma may occur later in childhood, and there is a need for continued observation. In one series of five patients with secondary angle-closure glaucoma, the glaucoma in each case occurred after age 2 years.[102] Lens aspiration, with anterior vitrectomy in some cases, has been successfully used to control the intraocular pressure, although the procedure is usually only to relieve pain and avoid enucleation, since vision is typically lost by this stage.[102–104]

b. *Retinal dysplasia.* This condition is usually bilateral and associated with multiple congenital anomalies, especially in trisomy 13-15.[105] The dysplastic retina may be pulled up behind the lens, and glaucoma may result from angle-closure or an associated mesodermal dysgenesis of the anterior chamber angle.

c. *Persistent hyperplastic primary vitreous.* Retention and hyperplasia of the primary vitreous is usually unilateral and often associated with microphthalmia and elongated ciliary processes.[106] Shallowing of the anterior chamber with subsequent angle-closure glaucoma may result from contracture of the fibrous retrolenticular mass and swelling of a cataractous lens. Small pupillary notches, due to anastomotic vessels between the anterior and posterior tunica vasculosa lentis, may be a helpful sign of persistent hyperplastic primary vitreous, especially when the diagnosis is obscured by an opaque lens.[107]

Aspiration of the lens and removal of the fibrovascular mass with scissors[108] or roto-extraction[109] may prevent or eliminate the angle-closure glaucoma. Postoperative visual rehabilitation, however, is difficult and treatment to avoid amblyopia is usually required.[108, 109]

B. Retinitis Pigmentosa

Retinitis pigmentosa has been described in association with primary glaucoma, which appears most often to be of the open-angle type.[110] However, the association is infrequent, and a true cause-and-effect relationship has not been established.[85]

References

1. Coats, G: Further cases of thrombosis of the central vein. Roy Land Ophthal Hosp Rep 16:516, 1906.
2. Weiss, DI, Shaffer, RN, Nehrenberg, TR: Neovascular glaucoma complicating carotid-cavernous fistula. Arch Ophthal 69:304, 1963.
3. Hoskins, HD Jr: Neovascular glaucoma: current concepts. Trans Am Acad Ophthal Otol 78:330, 1974.
4. Gartner, S, Henkind, P: Neovascularization of the iris (rubeosis iridis). Surv Ophthal 22:291, 1978.
5. Wand, M: Neovascular Glaucoma. In The Secondary Glaucomas, Ritch, R, Shields, MB, eds. CV Mosby Co, St Louis (in press).
6. Mandelcorn, MS, Blankenship, G, Machemer, R: Pars plana vitrectomy for the management of severe diabetic retinopathy. Am J Ophthal 81:561, 1976.
7. Aaberg, TM, Van Horn, DL: Late complications of pars plana vitreous surgery. Ophthalmology 85:126, 1978.
8. Michels, RG: Vitrectomy for complications of diabetic retinopathy. Arch Ophthal 96:237, 1978.
9. Miller, SA, Butler, JB, Myers, FL, Bresnick, GH: Pars plana vitrectomy. Treatment for tractional macula detachment secondary to proliferative diabetic retinopathy. Arch Ophthal 98:659, 1980.
10. Blankenship, G, Cortez, R, Machemer, R: The lens and pars plana vitrectomy for diabetic retinopathy complications. Arch Ophthal 97:1263, 1979.
11. Blankenship, GW: The lens influence on diabetic vitrectomy results. Report of a prospective randomized study. Arch Ophthal 98:2196, 1980.
12. Blankenship, G: Preoperative iris rubeosis and diabetic vitrectomy results. Ophthalmology 87:176, 1980.
13. Wolter, JR: Double embolism of the central retinal artery and one long posterior ciliary artery followed by secondary hemorrhagic glaucoma. Am J Ophthal 73:651, 1972.
14. Bresnick, GH, Gay, AJ: Rubeosis iridis associated with branch retinal arteriolar occlusions. Arch Ophthal 77:176, 1967.
15. Walton, DS, Grant, WM: Retinoblastoma and iris neovascularization. Am J Ophthal 65:598, 1968.
16. Goldberg, MF, Tso, MOM: Rubeosis iridis and glaucoma associated with sickle cell retinopathy: a light and electron microscopic study. Ophthalmology 85:1028, 1978.
17. Savir, H, Kurz, O: Fluorescein angiography in syphilitic retinal vasculitis. Ann Ophthal 8:713, 1976.
18. Hung, JY, Hilton, GF: Neovascular glaucoma in a patient with X-linked juvenile retinoschisis. Ann Ophthal 12:1054, 1980.

19. Young, NJA, Hitchings, RA, Sehmi, K, Bird, AC: Stickler's syndrome and neovascular glaucoma. Br J Ophthal 63:826, 1979.
20. Sugar, HS: Neovascular glaucoma after carotid-cavernous fistula formation. Ann Ophthal 11:1667, 1979.
21. Harris, GJ, Rice, PR: Angle closure in carotid-cavernous fistula. Ophthalmology 86:1521, 1979.
22. Huckman, MS, Haas, J: Reversed flow through the ophthalmic artery as a cause of rubeosis iridis. Am J Ophthal 74:1094, 1972.
23. Wise, GN: Retinal neovascularization. Trans Am Ophthal Soc 54:729, 1956.
24. Bresnick, GH, De Venecia, G, Myers, FL, Harris, JA, Davis, MD: Retinal ischemia in diabetic retinopathy. Arch Ophthal 93:1300, 1975.
25. Laatikainen, L, Kohner, EM: Fluorescein angiography and its prognostic significance in central retinal vein occlusion. Br J Ophthal 60:411, 1976.
26. Ernest, JT, Archer, DB: Vitreous body oxygen tension following experimental branch retinal vein obstruction. Invest Ophthal Vis Sci 18:1025, 1979.
27. Folkman, J, Merler, E, Abernathy, C, Williams, G: Isolation of a tumor factor responsible for angiogenesis. J Exp Med 133:275, 1971.
28. Glaser, BM, D'Amore, PA, Michels, RG, Brunson, SK, Fenselau, AH, Rice, T, Patz, A: The demonstration of angiogenic activity from ocular tissues. Preliminary report. Ophthalmology 87:440, 1980.
29. Federman, JL, Brown, GC, Felberg, NT, Felton, SM: Experimental ocular angiogenesis. Am J Ophthal 89:231, 1980.
30. Patz, A: Studies on retinal neovascularization. Invest Ophthal Vis Sci 19:1133, 1980.
31. Imre, G: Studies on the mechanism of retinal neovascularization. Role of lactic acid. Br J Ophthal 48:75, 1964.
32. Zauberman, H, Michaelson, IC, Bergmann, F, Maurice, DM: Stimulation of neovascularization of the cornea by biogenic amines. Exp Eye Res 8:77, 1969.
33. Ben Ezra, D: Neovasculogenesis. Triggering factors and possible mechanisms. Surv Ophthal 24:167, 1979.
34. Henkind, P: Ocular neovascularization. Am J Ophthal 85:287, 1978.
35. Wolbarsht, ML, Landers, MB III: The rationale of photocoagulation therapy for proliferative diabetic retinopathy: a review and a model. Ophthal Surg 11:235, 1980.
36. Ohrt, V: The frequency of rubeosis iridis in diabetic patients. Acta Ophthal 49:301, 1971.
37. Kluxen, G, Friedburg, D, Ruppert, A: Circular neovascularization of the circulus arteriosus iridis minor. Klin Monatsbl Augenheilkd 176:160, 1980.
38. Madsen, PH: Rubeosis of the iris and haemorrhagic glaucoma in patients with proliferative diabetic retinopathy. Br J Ophthal 55:368, 1971.
39. Wand, M, Dueker, DK, Aiello, LM, Grant, WM: Effects of panretinal photocoagulation on rubeosis iridis, angle neovascularization, and neovascular glaucoma. Am J Ophthal 86:332, 1978.
40. Madsen, PH: Haemorrhagic glaucoma. Comparative study in diabetic and nondiabetic patients. Br J Ophthal 55:444, 1971.
41. Pasco, M, Singer, L, Romem, M: Chronic simple glaucoma and thrombosis of the retinal vein. Eye Ear Nose Throat Monthly 52:47, 1973.
42. Ring, CP, Pearson, TC, Sanders, MD, Wetherley-Mein, G: Viscosity and retinal vein thrombosis. Br J Ophthal 60:397, 1976.
43. Cappin, JM, Whitelocke, R: The iris in central retinal vein thrombosis. Proc Roy Soc Med 67:16, 1974.
44. Hayreh, S, March, W, Phelps, CD: Ocular hypotony following retinal vein occlusion. Arch Ophthal 96:827, 1978.
45. Sinclair, SH, Gragoudas, ES: Prognosis for rubeosis iridis following central retinal vein occlusion. Br J Ophthal 63:735, 1979.
46. Tasman, W, Magargal, LE, Augsburger, JJ: Effects of argon laser photocoagulation on rubeosis iridis and angle neovascularization. Ophthalmology 87:400, 1980.

47. Priluck, IA, Robertson, DM, Hollenhorst, RW: Long-term follow-up of occlusion of the central retinal vein in young adults. Am J Ophthal 90:190, 1980.
48. Zegarra, H, Gutman, FA, Conforto, J: The natural course of central retinal vein occlusion. Ophthalmology 86:1931, 1979.
49. Laatikainen, L, Blach, RK: Behaviour of the iris vasculature in central retinal vein occlusion: a fluorescein angiographic study of the vascular response of the retina and the iris. Br J Ophthal 61:272, 1977.
50. Laatikainen, L: Development and classification of rubeosis iridis in diabetic eye disease. Br J Ophthal 63:150, 1979.
51. Schulze, RR: Rubeosis iridis. Am J Ophthal 63:487, 1967.
52. Jocson, VL: Microvascular injection studies in rubeosis iridis and neovascular glaucoma. Am J Ophthal 83:508, 1977.
53. Anderson, DM, Morin, JD, Hunter, WS: Rubeosis iridis. Can J Ophthal 6:183, 1971.
54. Goldberg, MF, Tso, MOM: Rubeosis iridis and glaucoma associated with sickle cell retinopathy: A light and electron microscopic study. Ophthalmology 85:1028, 1978.
55. Gartner, S, Taffet, S, Friedman, AH: The association of rubeosis iridis with endothelialisation of the anterior chamber: report of a clinical case with histopathological review of 16 additional cases. Br J Ophthal 61:267, 1977.
56. Little, HL, Rosenthal, AR, Dellaporta, A, Jacobson, DR: The effect of pan-retinal photocoagulation on rubeosis iridis. Am J Ophthal 81:804, 1976.
57. Laatikainen, L: Preliminary report on effect of retinal panphotocoagulation on rubeosis iridis and neovascular glaucoma. Br J Ophthal 61:278, 1977.
58. Laatikainen, L, Kohner, EM, Khoury, D, Blach, RK: Panretinal photocoagulation in central retinal vein occlusion: A randomised controlled clinical study. Br J Ophthal 61:741, 1977.
59. Jacobson, DR, Murphy, RP, Rosenthal, AR: The treatment of angle neovascularization with panretinal photocoagulation. Ophthalmology 86:1270, 1979.
60. Murphy, RP, Egbert, PR: Regression of iris neovascularization following panretinal photocoagulation. Arch Ophthal 97:700, 1979.
61. May, DR, Klein, ML, Peyman, GA: A prospective study of xenon arc photocoagulation for central retinal vein occlusion. Br J Ophthal 60:816, 1976.
62. Miller, JB, Smith, MR, Boyer, DS: Intraocular carbon dioxide laser photocautery. Indications and contraindications at vitrectomy. Ophthalmology 87:1112, 1980.
63. Weiter, JJ, Zuckerman, R: The influence of the photoreceptor-RPE complex on the inner retina. An explanation for the beneficial effects of photocoagulation. Ophthalmology 87:1133, 1980.
64. Wand, M, Hutchinson, BT: The surgical management of neovascular glaucoma. Pers Ophthal 4:147, 1980.
65. Goodart, R, Blankenship, G: Panretinal photocoagulation influence on vitrectomy results for complications of diabetic retinopathy. Ophthalmology 87:183, 1980.
66. May, DR, Bergstrom, TJ, Parmet, AJ, Schwartz, JG: Treatment of neovascular glaucoma with transscleral panretinal cryotherapy. Ophthalmology 87:1106, 1980.
67. Simmons, RJ, Dueker, DK, Kimbrough, RL, Aiello, LM: Goniophotocoagulation for neovascular glaucoma. Trans Am Acad Ophthal Otol 83:80, 1977.
68. Simmons, RJ, Deppermann, SR, Dueker, DK: The role of gonio-photocoagulation in neovascularization of the anterior chamber angle. Ophthalmology 87:79, 1980.
69. Grant, WM: Management of neovascular glaucoma in Symposium on Ocular Therapy, vol 7, Leopold, IH, ed. CV Mosby Co, St Louis, 1974, p 36.
70. Drews, RC: Corticosteroid management of hemorrhagic glaucoma. Trans Am Acad Ophthal Otol 78:334, 1974.
71. Tano, Y, Chandler, D, Machemer, R: Treatment of intraocular proliferation with intravitreal injection of triamcinolone acetonide. Am J Ophthal 90:810, 1980.

72. Feibel, RM, Bigger, JF: Rubeosis iridis and neovascular glaucoma. Evaluation of cyclocryotherapy. Am J Ophthal 74:862, 1972.
73. Boniuk, M: Cryotherapy in neovascular glaucoma. Trans Am Acad Ophthal Otol 78:337, 1974.
74. Krupin, T, Mitchell, KB, Becker, B: Cyclocryotherapy in neovascular glaucoma. Am J Ophthal 86:24, 1978.
75. Faulborn, J, Birnbaum, F: Cyclocryotherapy of haemorrhagic glaucoma: Clinical long time and histopathologic results. Klin Monatsbl Augenheilkd 170:651, 1977.
76. Faulborn, J, Hoster, K: Results of cyclocryotherapy in case of hemorrhagic glaucoma. Klin Monatsbl Augenheilkd 162:513, 1973.
77. Goldberg, MF, Ericson, ES: Intravitreal ciliary body neovascularization. Ophthal Surg 8:62, 1977.
78. Herschler, J, Agness, D: A modified filtering operation for neovascular glaucoma. Arch Ophthal 97:2339, 1979.
79. Ticho, U, Monselize, M, Levene, S, Kaye, R: Carbon dioxide laser filtering surgery in hemorrhagic glaucoma. Glaucoma 1:114, 1979.
80. Molteno, ACB, Van Rooyen, MMB, Bartholomew, RS: Implants for draining neovascular glaucoma. Br J Ophthal 61:120, 1977.
81. Egerer, I: Clinical experience in glaucoma surgery utilizing silicon catheters. Klin Monatsbl Augenheilk 174:434, 1979.
82. Krupin, R, Kaufman, P, Mandell, A, Ritch, R, Asseff, C, Podos, SM, Becker, B: Filtering valve implant surgery for eyes with neovascular glaucoma. Am J Ophthal 89:338, 1980.
83. Phelps, CD, Burton, TC: Glaucoma and retinal detachment. Arch Ophthal 95:418, 1977.
84. Shammas, HF, Halasa, AH, Faris, BM: Intraocular pressure, cup-disc ratio, and steroid responsiveness in retinal detachment. Arch Ophthal 94:1108, 1976.
85. Phelps, CD: Glaucomas Associated with Retinal Disorders. In The Secondary Glaucomas, Ritch, R, Shields, MB, eds. CV Mosby Co, St Louis (in press).
86. Pape, LG, Forbes, M: Retinal detachment and miotic therapy. Am J Ophthal 85:558, 1978.
87. Beasley, H, Fraunfelder, FT: Retinal detachments and topical ocular miotics. Ophthalmology 86:95, 1979.
88. Pemberton, JW: Schiøtz-applanation disparity following retinal detachment surgery. Arch Ophthal 81:534, 1969.
89. Syrdalen, P: Intraocular pressure and ocular rigidity in patients with retinal detachment. II. Postoperative study. Acta Ophthal 48:1036, 1970.
90. Burton, TC, Lambert, RW Jr: A predictive model for visual recovery following retinal detachment surgery. Ophthalmology 85:619, 1978.
91. Sebestyen, JG, Schepens, CL, Rosenthal, ML: Retinal detachment and glaucoma. I. Tonometric and gonioscopic study of 160 cases. Arch Ophthal 67:736, 1962.
92. Schwartz, A: Chronic open-angle glaucoma secondary to rhegmatogenous retinal detachment. Am J Ophthal 75:205, 1973.
93. Davidorf, FH: Retinal pigment epithelial glaucoma. Ophthal Dig 38:11, 1976.
94. Yanoff, M: Glaucoma mechanisms in ocular malignant melanoma. Am J Ophthal 70:898, 1970.
95. Hyams, SW, Neumann, E: Transient angle-closure glaucoma after retinal vein occlusion. Report of two cases. Br J Ophthal 56:353, 1972.
96. Grant, WM: Shallowing of the anterior chamber following occlusion of the central retinal vein. Am J Ophthal 75:384, 1973.
97. Bloome, MA: Transient angle-closure glaucoma in central retinal vein occlusion. Ann Ophthal 9:44, 1977.
98. Brockhurst, RJ: Nanophthalmos with uveal effusion. A new clinical entity. Arch Ophthal 93:1289, 1975.
99. Calhoun, FP Jr: The management of glaucoma in nanophthalmos. Tr Am Ophthal Soc 73:97, 1975.
100. Kimbrough, RL, Trempe, CS, Brockhurst, RJ, Simmons, RJ: Angle-closure

glaucoma in nanophthalmos. Am J Ophthal 88:572, 1979.
101. Brockhurst, RJ: Vortex vein decompression for nanophthalmic uveal effusion. Arch Ophthal 98:1987, 1980.
102. Pollard, ZF: Secondary angle-closure glaucoma in cicatricial retrolental fibroplasia. Am J Ophthal 89:651, 1980.
103. Hittner, HM, Rhodes, LM, McPherson, AR: Anterior segment abnormalities in cicatricial retinopathy of prematurity. Ophthalmology 86:803, 1979.
104. Layden, WE, Edwards, WC: Retinopathy of prematurity: The role of lens aspiration in management of angle closure glaucoma. Pers Ophthal 2:189, 1978.
105. Hoepner, J, Yanoff, M: Ocular anomalies in trisomy 13-15: An analysis of 13 eyes with two new findings. Am J Ophthal 74:729, 1972.
106. Reese, AB: Persistent hyperplastic primary vitreous. Am J Ophthal 40:317, 1955.
107. Meisels, HI, Goldberg, MF: Vascular anastomoses between the iris and persistent hyperplastic primary vitreous. Am J Ophthal 88:179, 1979.
108. Smith, RE, Maumenee, AE: Persistent hyperplastic primary vitreous: Results of surgery. Trans Am Acad Ophthal Otol 78:911, 1974.
109. Nankin, SJ, Scott, WE: Persistent hyperplastic primary vitreous. Rotoextraction and other surgical experience. Arch Ophthal 95:240, 1977.
110. Kogbe, OI, Follmann, P: Investigations into the aqueous humour dynamics in primary pigmentary degeneration of the retina. Ophthalmologica 171:165, 1975.

Chapter 16

GLAUCOMAS ASSOCIATED WITH OCULAR INFLAMMATION

GLAUCOMAS ASSOCIATED WITH OCULAR INFLAMMATION

The form of ocular inflammation which most frequently produces intraocular pressure elevation is primary iridocyclitis. In addition, when glaucoma is associated with other types of ocular inflammation, there is usually secondary involvement of the anterior uveal tract. We will, therefore, consider first the clinical forms of iridocyclitis and the mechanisms and management of the associated glaucomas, and then review the other forms of ocular inflammation that may lead to secondary glaucoma.

I. IRIDOCYCLITIS

A. Terminology

The general forms of iridocyclitis are classified primarily according to the clinical presentation and duration of active disease. A specific case of iridocyclitis, however, may manifest one or all of these clinical forms at different times during the course of the disease.

1. *Acute iridocyclitis.* The characteristic history for this type of iridocyclitis is the sudden onset of mild to moderate ocular pain, photophobia, and blurred vision. Physical examination typically reveals ciliary flush and a slight constriction of the pupil. Slit lamp biomicroscopy shows variable degrees of aqueous flare and cells, and usually fine inflammatory precipitates on the corneal endothelium (keratic precipitates). The intraocular pressure is often lower than in the fellow eye, although some patients will present with marked elevation of the pressure, which may be associated with severe pain and corneal edema.

2. *Subacute iridocyclitis.* Some cases of ocular inflammation produce few or no symptoms. The diagnosis may be made during a routine eye examination or as part of a work-up for a related systemic disease. This form of iridocyclitis can have serious consequences because complications, such as secondary glaucoma, may go undetected until advanced damage has occurred.

3. *Chronic iridocyclitis.* The clinical presentation in this form of iridocyclitis ranges from acute to subacute, but is characterized by a protracted course of months to years, often with remissions and exacerbations. It is this form of iridocyclitis that is particularly prone to cause secondary glaucoma.

B. Clinical Forms of Iridocyclitis and Glaucoma

1. In many cases, the iridocyclitis is non-specific and the underlying cause of the inflammation is never determined. This is seen more often with the acute form of iridocyclitis. These cases usually respond

to non-specific anti-inflammatory therapy, as discussed later in this chapter, although it is important to rule out related ocular or systemic disease.

2. **Sarcoidosis.** This is a multisystem inflammatory disorder of uncertain etiology, which has a predilection for young adults and black individuals. The typical histopathologic finding is non-caseating granulomas, and systemic involvement commonly includes pulmonary hilar lymphadenopathy, peripheral lymphadenopathy, and cutaneous lesions. In a review of 532 cases of sarcoidosis, 202 (38%) had ocular involvement, which included chorioretinitis, retinal periphlebitis, and occasional involvement of the optic nerve, orbit, or lacrimal glands.[1] By far the most common ocular abnormality, however, was anterior uveitis.

a. *Iridocyclitis. Acute iridocyclitis,* with the previously described features of ciliary flush, aqueous flare and cells, and occasional fine or large (mutton-fat) keratic precipitates, was noted in 30 (14.9%) of the 202 patients with ocular sarcoid.[1] In the acute phase, the inflammation was usually unilateral. A more frequent finding, indeed the most common ocular manifestation of sarcoidosis, was a *"chronic granulomatous uveitis,"* which was reported in 106 (52.5%) of the 202 cases.[1] This is more often bilateral, has a protracted course, and is typified by mutton-fat keratic precipitates, synechiae, and iris nodules. The nodules, which were seen in 23 (11.4%) of the 202 cases of ocular sarcoid,[1] characteristically involve the pupillary border (Koeppe nodules) and stroma of the iris (Busacca nodules), but may also be found in the anterior chamber angle and on the ciliary body.[2]

b. *Glaucoma.* This complication of the iridocyclitis occurred in 22 (10.9%) of the 202 patients with ocular sarcoid,[1] and was the most common cause of visual disturbance in another series.[3] The most common mechanism of secondary glaucoma in the latter study was obstruction of the trabecular meshwork by inflammatory debris or the nodules.[3] A more chronic form of glaucoma may also occur in association with iris bombe' or goniosynechiae,[3] and a subacute form with precipitates on the trabecular meshwork has been described,[4,5] and will be discussed later in this chapter.

3. **Iridocyclitis associated with arthritis.** The association of iridocyclitis with most forms of arthritis is the same as in the general population, with the following notable exceptions:

a. *Juvenile rheumatoid arthritis* (JRA). This is a spectrum of arthritic disorders in children. One form is characterized by *monoarticular,* or *pauciarticular* (involvement of four joints or less) onset, a predilection for girls, and minimal additional systemic manifestations. Other types of JRA have polyarticular onset or additional acute systemic involvement.

(1). *Iridocyclitis.* The reported prevalence of iridocyclitis in the monoarticular or pauciarticular form of JRA ranges from 19%[6] to 29%,[7] while the other types of JRA are rarely associated with this ocular finding.[6-10] The ocular inflammation may have an acute onset, with the typical features of acute iridocyclitis. However, many cases are asymptomatic, emphasizing the need for periodic ocular examinations of children with juvenile rheumatoid arthritis.[6, 7] The onset of the arthritis typically precedes that of the uveitis, and although the arthritis usually disappears in adult life, the iridocyclitis may persist.[8] Children with iridocyclitis rarely have a positive serology for rheumatoid factor, but they frequently have antinuclear antibody[8, 10] and HLA-B27 antigen,[10] and some eventually are found to have typical ankylosing spondylitis.[10]

(2). *Glaucoma.* Complications are more common when the ocular inflammatory course is protracted, and these include band keratopathy, cataracts, and secondary glaucoma. The reported prevalence of glaucoma in children with JRA and iridocyclitis ranges from 14 to 22%.[8-10] Glaucoma is a particularly serious complication, with half of the eyes in one study having a vision of 6/60 or less.[10] The glaucoma is usually of the pupillary block variety, but it may be related to alterations in the trabecular meshwork early in the course of the disease. Histologic studies of advanced cases revealed peripheral anterior synechiae and occlusion of the pupil.[11] Treatment is typically difficult, with many eyes responding only partially to corticosteroids. The addition of non-steroidal anti-inflammatory agents may be helpful in these cases.[9, 10] Anti-glaucoma drugs may be required to control intraocular pressure elevation, and glaucoma surgery is occasionally needed, although reported results in these cases are poor.[8]

b. *Ankylosing spondylitis* (Marie-Strumpell disease). This form of arthritis typically involves the cervical or lumbosacral spine and is associated with an intermittent acute iridocyclitis in 3.5 to 12.5% of reported cases.[12] A high percentage of these patients have the HLA-B27 antigen.[13] Recurrent uveitis may precede the arthritic symptoms, and there is evidence, based on HLA typing and sensitive bone scans, that the ocular inflammation may occur in the absence of overt symptoms or radiologic evidence of the spondilitis.[12] Glaucoma may result from trabecular damage or synechiae formation.

4. *Pars planitis* (chronic cyclitis). This protracted ocular inflammatory disorder primarily involves the ciliary body. A typical finding is a "snowbank" of the vitreous base overlying the pars plana inferiorly.[14] In a series of 100 cases with a 4 to 20 year follow-up, the incidence of glaucoma was 8%.[15] A clinicopathologic study of seven cases of pars planitis revealed glaucoma in five, and possible mechanisms of pressure elevation included peripheral anterior synechiae, iris bombé, and rubeosis iridis.[14] Steroid-induced glaucoma also may occur during the management of this chronic disorder, as with any inflammatory disease.

5. *Glaucomatocyclitic crises.* In 1948, Posner and Schlossman[16] described a uniocular disease in young to middle-aged adults, which was characterized by recurrent attacks of mild anterior uveitis with marked elevations of intraocular pressure. They called the syndrome

glaucomatocyclitic crises, although it is frequently referred to as the *Posner-Schlossman syndrome*.

a. *Clinical features.* The typical patient may experience slight ocular discomfort, blurred vision, and halos, which last for hours up to a few weeks or rarely more and tend to recur on a monthly or yearly basis.[16] Physical findings are minimal, with occasional mild ciliary flush, slight pupillary constriction, and corneal epithelial edema. Hypochromia of the iris is not a consistent finding, but has been reported in up to 40% of various series.[17] Early segmental iris ischemia with late congestion and leakage on fluorescein angiography has also been described.[18] Slit lamp biomicroscopy reveals occasional faint flare and a few fine, non-pigmented keratic precipitates, while gonioscopy shows a normal, open angle with characteristic absence of synechiae and occasional debris.[16, 17] The cause of the inflammation is unknown.

b. *Glaucoma.* The intraocular pressure is typically elevated in the range of 40 to 60 mmHg and coincides with the duration of the uveitis. Intraocular pressure and facility of aqueous outflow usually return to normal between attacks, although severe cases with optic nerve head and visual field damage have been reported.[19, 20] The glaucoma may be related to inflammatory changes in the trabecular meshwork, although other theories of mechanism include increased aqueous production, possibly due to elevated levels of aqueous prostaglandins,[21] and an association with primary open-angle glaucoma.[18, 19] Most cases can be controlled during attacks with corticosteroids and anti-glaucoma agents which reduce aqueous production,[17, 22] although rare, severe cases may require filtering surgery.[20, 23]

6. **Fuchs' heterochromic cyclitis.** In 1906, Fuchs[24] described a condition characterized by mild anterior uveitis, heterochromia, cataracts, and occasional glaucoma. The similarities and differences between this disease and glaucomatocyclitic crises should be noted to avoid confusing the two.

a. *Clinical features.* Fuchs' heterochromic cyclitis is usually unilateral, although bilateral involvement has been reported in up to 13% of the cases.[25] The typical age of onset is in the third or fourth decade,[26] and there is an equal incidence among men and women.[25] The uveitis in this disease is mild and tends to run a single, very protracted course. The patient is usually unaware of any difficulty until visual disturbance, primarily from cataract formation, becomes apparent. While *hypochromia* of the iris is more common than in glaucomatocyclitic crises, it is not a constant feature, and tends to develop gradually during the course of the disease.[25, 26] Gross signs of ocular inflammation are typically absent, although slit lamp biomicroscopy may reveal minimal aqueous flare and cells, with fine characteristic stellate keratic precipitates on the central cornea.[25] *Cataracts,* which usually first involve the posterior cortex, are common but typically develop late in the course of the disease.[26] In addition, white opacities may be seen in the anterior vitreous.[25] The iris frequently has extensive stromal atrophy, and transillumination of the iris is reported to demonstrate a characteristic light, even translucence.[27] Anterior segment fluorescein angiography shows delayed filling, sector ischemia, leakage, and neovascularization.[28, 29]

b. *Glaucoma.* Secondary intraocular pressure elevation is not a constant finding as in glaucomatocyclitic crises, but occurs as a late, serious complication in up to 13% of unilateral cases and 33% with bilateral involvement.[30] The glaucoma typically persists after the uveitis has subsided. The anterior chamber angle is open and characteristically free of synechiae, although *fine vessels*, which may hemorrhage, are often seen extending onto the trabecular meshwork.[30] The etiology of the uveitis and the precise mechanism of the glaucoma are both uncertain. Electron microscopic studies of the iris in two cases revealed abnormal melanocytes with scant, immature melanin granules, abundant plasma cells, and a membranous degeneration of nerve fibers, suggesting a primary or secondary abnormality of adrenergic innervation.[31] Based on fluorescein angiographic observations, a vascular pathogenesis has also been postulated.[28, 29] Histopathologic examination of the anterior chamber angle structures in one case revealed rubeosis, trabeculitis, and an inflammatory membrane over the angle,[32] while another study showed extensive atrophy of Schlemm's canal and the trabecular endothelium.[33] Whatever the cause, the glaucoma in this disease does not respond to steroid therapy, but requires standard medical or surgical management.[26]

7. *Glaucoma associated with precipitates on the trabecular meshwork.* Chandler and Grant[4] have described an uncommon form of secondary open-angle glaucoma in which the only evidence of ocular inflammation is precipitates on the trabecular meshwork. Since the condition is usually bilateral, it may be mistaken for primary open-angle glaucoma.[5] However, careful gonioscopy, which is essential in both the diagnosis and follow-up, reveals gray or slightly yellow precipitates on the meshwork and irregular peripheral anterior synechiae, which often attach to the trabecular precipitates.[5] The cause is unknown, although some cases subsequently demonstrate sarcoidosis, rheumatoid arthritis, ankylosing spondylitis, episcleritis, glaucomatocyclitic crisis, or chronic uveitis.[5] The glaucoma, which is presumed to be due to inflammatory changes in the trabecular meshwork, usually clears promptly with topical corticosteroid therapy, although anti-glaucoma drugs which reduce aqueous production may be temporarily required for pressure control. The condition often recurs, and the patients must be followed closely. Untreated cases may progress to synechial closure of the angle.

8. *Infectious diseases.* The following infectious processes may cause an iridocyclitis with the occasional association of glaucoma.

a. *Congenital rubella.* This disorder affects predominantly the heart, auditory apparatus, and eyes,[34] although virtually any organ may be involved.[35] Ocular defects occur in 30 to 60% of the cases and include cataracts, microphthalmia, retinopathy, and glaucoma.[36] The secondary glaucoma is reported to occur in 2 to 15% of children with congenital rubella.[37] Contrary to earlier reports, the cataracts and glaucoma occur together at a frequency that would be anticipated with each occurring independently.[38] The glaucoma is particularly severe, with blindness occurring in 8 of 15 children in one follow-up study.[38] Mechanisms of the glaucoma include iridocyclitis, angle anomalies resembling primary congenital glaucoma or mesodermal dysgenesis, and angle closure glaucoma due to a combination of microphthalmia and an intumescent lens or pupillary block after cataract extraction.[4] Although the ocular abnormalities are usually observed in the neonatal period, the glaucoma may also occur later in childhood or in young adults.[39] These cases are most often associated with microphthalmia and cataracts.[39]

b. *Syphilis. Congenital syphilis* may cause iridocyclitis with secondary glaucoma in either the early or late stages of the disease.[35] Glaucoma associated with the interstitial keratitis of congenital syphilis will be discussed later in this chapter. *Acquired syphilis* in adults may also cause iridocyclitis and intraocular pressure elevation.[40]

c. *Hansen's disease.* Uveitis is common in lepromatous leprosy and typically involves the iris and ciliary body, with four forms having been described: 1) chronic iridocyclitis, 2) acute plastic iridocyclitis, 3) iris pearls or miliary lepromata, which is pathognomonic of the disease, and 4) nodular lepromata, characterized by larger, less discrete masses on the iris.[41] Complications of keratitis and iridocyclitis are the main causes of blindness in this disease. In a study of 100 cases, 19 had acute or chronic iridocyclitis and 12 had evidence of glaucoma, which was usually secondary to chronic anterior uveitis.[42] Active iridocyclitis is reported to respond to treatment with dapsone, corticosteroids, and rifampin.[41]

d. *Metastatic endophthalmitis* arises from a primary extraocular infection and may be associated with obstruction of the anterior chamber angle by a blanket of cells. In one case report, bilateral meningococcal endophthalmitis led to acute glaucoma.[43]

e. *Cytomegalic inclusion retinitis* was described in two adult renal transplant patients, both of whom developed a secondary open-angle glaucoma presumably due to an associated anterior uveitis.[44]

f. *Adenovirus type 10* has been reported to cause keratoconjunctivouveitis with a transient increased intraocular pressure.[45]

g. *Hemorrhagic fever with renal syndrome* (nephropathia epidemica). This viral disease is characterized by fever, chills, malaise, nausea, vomiting, and headache, which progresses to back and abdominal pain, uremia, hematuria, oliguria, and proteinuria. Three patients have been described with associated transient angle-closure glaucoma, which was felt to be due to swelling of the ciliary body.[46]

h. *Herpetic kerato-uveitis* is commonly associated with secondary glaucoma. This condition will be discussed later under the heading of Keratitis.

C. Theories of Mechanisms for Associated Glaucoma

The possible mechanisms by which iridocyclitis may lead to an elevated intraocular pressure have already been mentioned with regard to certain specific forms of iridocyclitis, and will now be summarized. In general, iridocyclitis affects both aqueous production and resistance to aqueous outflow, with the subsequent change in intraocular pressure representing a balance between these two factors.

1. *Aqueous production.* Inflammation of the ciliary body usually leads to reduced aqueous production. If this outweighs a concomitant increased resistance to outflow, the intraocular pressure will be reduced, which is often the case with acute iridocyclitis.[47] However, prostaglandins, which have been demonstrated in the aqueous of eyes with uveitis,[48] are known to cause elevated intraocular pressure without a reduction in outflow facility,[49-52] suggesting that increased aqueous production may possibly occur in some cases of uveitis.

2. *Aqueous outflow.* When the aqueous outflow system is involved in an ocular inflammatory disease, increased resistance to outflow may result from a variety of acute and chronic mechanisms.

a. *Acute.* During the active phase of iridocyclitis, several mechanisms of obstruction to aqueous outflow may lead to a relatively sudden, but usually reversible, rise in intraocular pressure.

(1). *Open-angle mechanisms.* In the majority of cases, the anterior chamber angle is open, which is an important observation in ruling out primary angle-closure glaucoma. Obstruction of the trabecular meshwork may occur in several ways:

(a). A disruption in the blood-aqueous barrier allows *inflammatory cells* and *fibrin* to enter the aqueous and accumulate in the trabecular meshwork. Normal serum components have been shown to reduce outflow when perfused in enucleated human eyes.[53] Prostaglandins were demonstrated to increase aqueous protein content,[51, 52, 54] and it has been suggested that an accumulation of cyclic adenosine monophosphate (cAMP), due to prostaglandins or certain non-prostaglandin agents, causes the barrier damage.[55]

(b). In other cases, *swelling* or *dysfunction* of the *trabecular lamellae* or *endothelium* may lead to aqueous outflow obstruction.[47]

(c). *Precipitates* on the trabecular meshwork, as previously discussed, may also occur in eyes with ocular inflammation and elevated intraocular pressure.[4, 5]

(d). It must also be kept in mind that the use of corticosteroids in treating the inflammation may create yet another mechanism of intraocular pressure elevation (steroid-induced glaucoma), which will be discussed in Chapter 19.

(2). *Angle-closure mechanisms.* Much less commonly, an iridocyclitis, either of primary origin or secondary to other ocular inflammation, may lead to acute closure of the anterior chamber angle by a forward rotation of the ciliary body.[56] In addition, if a significant posterior uveitis is also present, angle-closure may result from displacement of the lens-iris diaphragm due to massive exudative retinal detachment.

b. *Chronic.* Several sequelae of active inflammation may lead to a chronic elevation of intraocular pressure.

(1). *Open-angle mechanisms.* Obstruction of aqueous outflow may result from *scarring* and obliteration of outflow channels, or from the overgrowth of an endothelial-cuticular or fibrovascular *membrane* in the open angle. The membranes, however, may contract, eventually leading to synechial closure of the angle.

(2). *Angle-closure mechanisms.* In addition to the influence of membrane contraction, *peripheral anterior synechiae* may result from the protein and inflammatory cells in the angle, which pull the iris toward the cornea. *Posterior synechiae* may also be a sequelae of anterior uveitis and can cause iris bombé.[47]

D. Management

In treating an eye with iridocyclitis and glaucoma, controlling the inflammatory component alone frequently leads to normalization of the intraocular pressure, and this is usually the first approach in the treatment plan. However, if the magnitude of the pressure elevation poses an immediate threat to vision or if the intraocular pressure does not respond adequately to anti-inflammatory therapy, medical and even surgical management of the glaucoma may also be indicated. The following basic principles of management apply to most cases of iridocyclitis, as well as other forms of ocular inflammation, with exceptions as noted in the discussions of the specific diseases.

1. *Management of the inflammation*

a. *Corticosteroids.* This group of drugs constitute the first line defense in most cases of ocular inflammation. Topical administration is preferred for anterior segment disease, and commonly used steroids include prednisolone 1.0% or dexamethasone 0.1%. In a rabbit model of anterior uveitis, frequent topical administration of prednisolone acetate 1.0% caused a significant decrease in protein levels and leukocytes in the anterior chamber.[57] Administration of the steroid every hour may be required initially, with gradual reduction in frequency as the inflammation subsides. In a rabbit model of keratitis, instillation every 15 min was even more effective than the hourly regimen, although five doses at 1-min intervals each hour was equivalent to the effect achieved by administration every 15 min.[58] When the response to topical administration is insufficient, periocular injections (*e.g.*, dexamethasone phosphate, prednisolone succinate, triamcinolone acetate, or methylprednisolone acetate) or a systemic corticosteroid (*e.g.*, prednisone) may be required.[47] With any form of administration, the many side effects of corticosteroids must be considered, including steroid-induced glaucoma.

b. *Non-steroidal anti-inflammatory agents.* When the use of corticosteroids are contraindicated or inadequate, other anti-inflammatory drugs may be helpful. *Prostaglandin synthetase inhibitors*, such as aspirin,[59] imidazole,[60] indoxole,[61] indomethacin,[61] and dipyridamole[62] have been effective in some cases of uveitis. With severe cases, *immunosuppressive agents*, such as methotrexate,[63] azathioprine,[64] or chlorambucil,[64] may be indicated. In a study of 25 patients with severe chronic uveitis who were poorly responsive or unresponsive to corticosteroid therapy, all responded to long-term daily administration of prednisone 10 to 15 mg combined with azathioprine 2.0 to 2.5 mg or chlorambucil 6 to 8 mg.[64] These patients must be monitored closely for hematologic reactions.

    c. In conjunction with anti-inflammatory agents, a *mydriatic-cycloplegic drug*, such as atropine 1%, homatropine 1 to 5%, or cyclopentolate 0.5 to 1%, is usually indicated to avoid posterior synechiae and to relieve the discomfort of ciliary muscle spasm.[65]

    2. *Management of the glaucoma*

    a. *Medical.* Since miotics are generally contraindicated in the inflamed eye, topical timolol or epinephrine is usually the first line anti-glaucoma drug in the treatment of glaucoma secondary to ocular inflammation. A carbonic anhydrase inhibitor may also be needed, and a hyperosmotic agent is occasionally required as a short-term emergency measure.

    b. *Surgical.* Intraocular surgery should be avoided whenever possible in eyes with active inflammation. However, when medical therapy is inadequate, surgery may be required. In these cases, it is best to do the least amount of surgery possible. A laser iridotomy may be safer than a surgical iridectomy, when an angle closure mechanism is present. Filtering surgery is indicated in open-angle cases that are uncontrolled on maximum tolerable medical therapy. A technique called trabeculodialysis, in which a goniotomy knife is used to incise above the trabecular meshwork and then peel the meshwork downward, was successful in a preliminary series of eyes with anterior uveitis and glaucoma.[66]

II. OTHER FORMS OF OCULAR INFLAMMATION

A. Choroiditis

    In the following conditions, a uveitis that is predominantly posterior may cause secondary glaucoma either by an associated anterior inflammatory component or by angle closure from a posterior mass effect.

    1. *Vogt-Koyanagi-Harada syndrome.* The systemic findings in this disorder include alopecia, poliosis, and meningeal signs. Ocular manifestations consist of anterior and posterior uveitis with exudative retinal detachment. In a review of 51 cases, secondary glaucoma was found in 20% of the patients.[67] Within the total group, a mild anterior uveitis was seen in all patients, posterior synechiae occurred in 36%, keratic precipitates in 30%, and nodules on the iris in 8.4%.[67]

    2. *Behcet's disease.* The cardinal features of this chronic systemic disease, in decreasing order of frequency, are oral ulcers, genital ulcers, uveitis, synovitis, cutaneous vasculitis, and meningoencephalitis.[68] The uveitis tends to occur later in the course of the disease and is eventually bilateral. In a study of 32 patients with Behcet's disease, 21 had uveitis.[68] Both the anterior and posterior uvea were involved

in all 21 cases, although the posterior uveitis appeared to be more significant, leading to a variety of retinal problems. The anterior uveitis may lead to secondary glaucoma.

3. *Sympathetic ophthalmia.* This form of ocular inflammation typically occurs weeks or months after traumatic or surgical penetration of the fellow eye. The severity of the inflammation is related to the degree of ocular pigmentation,[69] and the choroid is predominantly affected with frequent involvement of the overlying retina.[70] In a study of 17 cases with an average follow-up of 10.6 years, seven (43%) had secondary glaucoma.[70] The mechanism of the glaucoma is unknown, although in a histopathologic study of 105 cases, a high percentage had plasma cell infiltration of the iris and ciliary body,[70] suggesting an immune reaction near the area of aqueous outflow. Whatever the cause, the glaucoma is typically difficult to treat, requiring frequent adjustments of corticosteroids and occasional surgical intervention.[71]

B. Keratitis

1. *Interstitial keratitis.* As a feature of congenital syphilis, interstitial keratitis typically appears late in the course of the disease, between the ages of 5 and 16, although it may appear as early as birth or as late as 30 years of age.[72] The presenting symptoms of interstitial keratitis include marked ciliary flush, lacrimation, photophobia, and pain.[72] The mechanisms of glaucoma associated with interstitial keratitis, in addition to the previously noted concomitant iridocyclitis, include open-angle and angle-closure forms that usually appear later in life.[73, 74]

With *secondary open-angle glaucoma*, the eye may have irregular pigmentation of the anterior chamber angle, with occasional columnar peripheral anterior synechiae, and one histopathologic study revealed endothelium and a glassy membrane over the angle.[73] This condition responds poorly to medical therapy, but may be controlled by filtering surgery. Another form of secondary open-angle glaucoma in the adult is the recurrence of iridocyclitis in an eye that had interstitial keratitis in younger life.[73] The residual ghost vessels in the cornea may help in making this diagnosis.

Eyes with interstitial keratitis in infancy often have small anterior segments and narrow angles, which can lead to *angle-closure glaucoma* later in life. This is usually subacute and responds well to peripheral iridectomy.[73, 75] In some cases, multiple cysts of the iris may lead to angle-closure.

2. *Herpetic kerato-uveitis*

a. *Herpes simplex type 1 virus.* This viral infection may cause recurrent conjunctivitis, keratitis, and uveitis. In one study of patients with herpes simplex kerato-uveitis, 28% had intraocular pressure elevation, and 10% had glaucomatous damage.[76] The keratitis in cases with associated intraocular pressure elevation is typically disciform or stromal, rather than a superficial ulcer.[76] The pressure usually remains elevated for several weeks, and a rabbit model suggests a biphasic intraocular pressure response in which the uveitis during the first few days represents active infection, but subsequently is due to immune mechanisms.[77] An analysis of aqueous from 33 herpes patients revealed herpes simplex virus in eight cases, all of which had secondary glaucoma.[78] Histopathology of rabbit eyes with experimental herpetic kerato-uveitis showed mononuclear cells in the trabecular meshwork and peripheral anterior synechiae.[79]

Management of this condition requires attention to the infection, inflammation, and glaucoma, and one suggested regimen includes topical trifluorothymidine, corticosteroids, and cycloplegics along with anti-glaucoma agents that reduce aqueous production.[78] One study indicated that the severity of the uveitis and intraocular pressure rise in experimental secondary herpes simplex uveitis was lessened with dexamethasone 0.1% twice daily, but not with aspirin or cyclophosphamide.[80]

b. *Herpes zoster virus.* In addition to causing the characteristic cutaneous vesicular eruptions along the trigeminal distribution, this viral disease may produce a keratitis and uveitis. The anterior uveitis not uncommonly leads to a secondary glaucoma, which usually responds to topical corticosteroids.

C. Scleritis

This is an extremely painful, potentially disasterous form of ocular inflammation, which may primarily involve either the anterior or posterior segment of the eye.[81, 82] Anterior scleritis may present with diffuse or nodular edema of the deep scleral tissue with overlying episcleral congestion. Other anterior forms may have necrotizing granulomas surrounded by inflammation or without inflammation (scleromalacia perforans). Posterior scleritis, which is more difficult to diagnose, may present with pars planitis, exudative retinal detachment, optic nerve head edema, or proptosis.

In one study of 301 cases, glaucoma was present in 11.6%,[81] while in another series, the prevalence of elevated intraocular pressure was 18.7% with rheumatoid scleritis and 12% with non-rheumatoid scleritis.[83] In the vast majority of cases, the glaucoma is associated with anterior scleritis, and proposed mechanisms of pressure elevation in these patients include obstruction of the outflow channels by edema and long-standing uveitis with peripheral anterior synechiae.[81] Glaucoma associated with posterior scleritis is much less common, but may result from a forward shift of the lens-iris diaphragm or an anterior rotation of the ciliary body in association with choroidal effusion.[56] Treatment of scleritis and glaucoma generally consists of topical and systemic corticosteroids, with anti-glaucoma agents as needed, and surgical intervention for the glaucoma only when absolutely necessary.

D. Episcleritis

In contrast to scleritis, episcleritis produces only mild discomfort and does not typically lead to serious sequelae. The characteristic appearance is congestion of the episcleral vessels, which may be diffuse with chemosis and occasional lid edema (simple episcleritis) or localized with nodules in the episcleral tissue (nodular episcleritis).[81] Secondary glaucoma is uncommon in this condition,[81,83] but has been reported.[84] Presumed mechanisms of open-angle glaucoma include inflammation of the angle structures[84] and steroid-induced glaucoma.[81] Angle-closure glaucoma has also been observed in association with episcleritis.[83] In most cases, both the episcleritis and the secondary glaucoma respond to topical corticosteroids.

References

1. Obenauf, CD, Shaw, HE, Sydnor, CF, Klintworth, GK: Sarcoidosis and its ophthalmic manifestations. Am J Ophthal 86:648, 1978.
2. Mizuno, K, Watanabe, T: Sarcoid granulomatous cyclitis. Am J Ophthal 81:82, 1976.
3. Iwata, K, Nanba, K, Sobue, K, Abe, H: Ocular sarcoidosis: evaluation of intraocular findings. Ann NY Acad Sci 278:445, 1976.
4. Chandler, PA, Grant, WM: Lectures on Glaucoma. Lea & Febiger, Philadelphia, 1965, p 257.
5. Roth, M, Simmons, RJ: Glaucoma associated with precipitates on the trabecular meshwork. Ophthalmology 86:1613, 1979.
6. Calabro, JJ, Parrino, GR, Atchoo, PD, Marchesano, JM, Goldberg, LS: Chronic iridocyclitis in juvenile rheumatoid arthritis. Arth Rheum 13:406, 1970.
7. Schaller, J, Kupfer, C, Wedgwood, RJ: Iridocyclitis in juvenile rheumatoid arthritis. Pediatrics 44:92, 1969.
8. Key, SN III, Kimura, SJ: Iridocyclitis associated with juvenile rheumatoid arthritis. Am J Ophthal 80:425, 1975.
9. Chylack, LT Jr, Bienfang, DC, Bellows, R, Stillman, JS: Ocular manifestations of juvenile rheumatoid arthritis. Am J Ophthal 79:1026, 1975.
10. Kanski, JJ: Anterior uveitis in juvenile rheumatoid arthritis. Arch Ophthal 95:1794, 1977.
11. Sabates, R, Smith, T, Apple, D: Ocular histopathology in juvenile rheumatoid arthritis. Ann Ophthal 11:733, 1979.
12. Russell, AS, Lentle, BC, Percy, JS, Jackson, FI: Scintigraphy of sacroiliac joints in acute anterior uveitis. A study of thirty patients. Ann Intern Med 85:606, 1976.
13. Brewerton, DA, Hart, FD, Nicholls, A, Caffrey, M, James, DCO, Sturrock, RD: Ankylosing spondylitis and HL-A 27. Lancet 1:904, 1973.
14. Pederson, JE, Kenyon, KR, Green, WR, Maumenee, AE: Pathology of pars planitis. Am J Ophthal 86:762, 1978.
15. Smith, RE, Godfrey, WA, Kimura, SJ: Complications of chronic cyclitis. Am J Ophthal 82:277, 1976.
16. Posner, A, Schlossman, A: Syndrome of unilateral recurrent attacks of glaucoma with cyclitic symptoms. Arch Ophthal 39:517, 1948.
17. Hollwich, F: Clinical aspects and therapy of the Posner-Schlossmann-syndrom. Klin Monatsbl Augenheilkd 172:736, 1978.
18. Raitta, C, Vannas, A: Glaucomatocyclitic crisis. Arch Ophthal 95:608, 1977.
19. Kass, MA, Becker, B, Kolker, AE: Glaucomatocyclitic crisis and primary open-angle glaucoma. Am J Ophthal 75:668, 1973.
20. Hung, PT, Chang, JM: Treatment of glaucomatocyclitic crises. Am J Ophthal 77:169, 1974.

21. Nagataki, S, Mishima, S: Aqueous humor dynamics in glaucomato-cyclitic crisis. Invest Ophthal 15:365, 1976.
22. de Roetth, A Jr: Glaucomatocyclitic crisis. Am J Ophthal 69:370, 1970.
23. Sood, GC, Kapoor, S, Krishnamurthy, G, Reddy, S, Sood, M: Posner-Schlossman syndrome—surgical management. EENT Monthly 55:12, 1976.
24. Fuchs, E: uber Komplikationen der Heterochromie. Ztschr Augenh 15:191, 1906.
25. Franceschetti, A: Heterochromic cyclitis (Fuchs' syndrome). Am J Ophthal 39:50, 1955.
26. Kimura, SJ, Hogan, MJ, Thygeson, P: Fuchs' syndrome of heterochromic cyclitis. Arch Ophthal 54:179, 1955.
27. Saari, M, Vuorre, I, Nieminen, H: Infra-red transillumination stereophotography of the iris in Fuchs's heterochromic cyclitis. Br J Ophthal 62:110, 1978.
28. Saari, M, Vuorre, I, Nieminen, H: Fuchs's heterochromic cyclitis: a simultaneous bilateral fluorescein angiographic study of the iris. Br J Ophthal 62:715, 1978.
29. Berger, BB, Tessler, HH, Kottow, MH: Anterior segment ischemia in Fuchs' heterochromic cyclitis. Arch Ophthal 98:499, 1980.
30. Huber, VA: Das Glaukom bei komplizierter Heterochromie Fuchs. Ophthalmologica 142:66, 1961.
31. Melamed, S, Lahav, M, Sandbank, U, Yassur, Y, Ben-Sira, I: Fuch's heterochromic iridocyclitis: an electron microscopic study of the iris. Invest Ophthal Vis Sci 17:1193, 1978.
32. Perry, HD, Yanoff, M, Scheie, HG: Rubeosis in Fuchs heterochromic iridocyclitis. Arch Ophthal 93:337, 1975.
33. Benedikt, O, Roll, P, Zirm, M: The glaucoma in heterochromic cyclitis Fuchs. Gonioscopic studies and electron microscopic investigations of the trabecular meshwork. Klin Monatsbl Augenheilkd 173:523, 1978.
34. Cooper, LZ, Ziring, PR, Ockerse, AB, Fedun, BA, Kiely, B, Krugman, S: Rubella. Clinical manifestations and management. Am J Dis Child 118:18, 1969.
35. Chandler, SH: Ocular abnormalities associated with intrauterine infections. Pers Ophthal 3:249, 1979.
36. Rudolph, AJ, Desmond, MM: Clinical manifestations of the congenital rubella syndrome. Int Ophthal Clin 12:3, 1972.
37. Boniuk, M: Glaucoma in the congenital rubella syndrome. Int Ophthal Clin 12:121, 1972.
38. Wolff, SM: The ocular manifestations of congenital rubella. Tr Am Ophthal Soc 70:577, 1972.
39. Boger, WP III: Late ocular complications in congenital rubella syndrome. Ophthalmology 87:1244, 1980.
40. Schwartz, LK, O'Connor, GR: Secondary syphilis with iris papules. Am J Ophthal 90:380, 1980.
41. Michelson, JB, Roth, AM, Waring, GO III: Lepromatous iridocyclitis diagnosed by anterior chamber paracentesis. Am J Ophthal 88:674, 1979.
42. Shields, JA, Waring, GO III, Monte, LG: Ocular findings in leprosy. Am J Ophthal 77:880, 1974.
43. Jensen, AD, Naidoff, MA: Bilateral meningococcal endophthalmitis. Arch Ophthal 90:396, 1973.
44. Merritt, JC, Callender, CO: Adult cytomegalic inclusion retinitis. Ann Ophthal 10:1059, 1978.
45. Hara, J, Ishibashi, T, Fujimoto, F, Danjyo, S, Minekawa, Y, Maeda, A: Adenovirus type 10 keratoconjunctivitis with increased intraocular pressure. Am J Ophthal 90:481, 1980.
46. Saari, KM: Acute glaucoma in hemorrhagic fever with renal syndrome (nephropathia epidemica). Am J Ophthal 81:455, 1976.
47. Krupin, T: Glaucomas Associated with Uveitis. In The Secondary Glaucomas, Ritch, R, Shields, MB, eds. CV Mosby Co, St Louis (in press).
48. Leopold, IH: The therapeutic tumult and the ophthalmologist. Am J Ophthal 76:181, 1973.

49. Chiang, TS, Thomas, RP: Ocular hypertension following intravenous infusion of prostaglandin E_1. Arch Ophthal 88:418, 1972.
50. Chiang, TS, Thomas, RP: Consensual ocular hypertensive response to prostaglandin E_2. Invest Ophthal 11:845, 1972.
51. Kass, MA, Podos, SM, Moses, RA, Becker, B: Prostaglandin E_1 and aqueous humor dynamics. Invest Ophthal 11:1022, 1972.
52. Podos, SM, Becker, B, Kass, MA: Prostaglandin synthesis, inhibition, and intraocular pressure. Invest Ophthal 12:426, 1973.
53. Epstein, DL, Hashimoto, JM, Grant, WM: Serum obstruction of aqueous outflow in enucleated eyes. Am J Ophthal 86:101, 1978.
54. Neufeld, AH, Sears, ML: The site of action of prostaglandin E_2 on the disruption of the blood-aqueous barrier in the rabbit eye. Exp Eye Res 17:445, 1973.
55. Bengtsson, E: The effect of theophylline on the breakdown of the blood-aqueous barrier in the rabbit eye. Invest Ophthal Vis Sci 16:636, 1977.
56. Quinlan, MP, Hitchings, RA: Angle-closure glaucoma secondary to posterior scleritis. Br J Ophthal 62:330, 1978.
57. Bolliger, GA, Kupferman, A, Leibowitz, HM: Quantitation of anterior chamber inflammation and its response to therapy. Arch Ophthal 98:1110, 1980.
58. Leibowitz, HM, Kupferman, A: Optimal frequency of topical prednisolone administration. Arch Ophthal 97:2154, 1979.
59. Marsetio, M, Siverio, CE, Oh, JO: Effects of aspirin and dexamethasone on intraocular pressure in primary uveitis produced by herpes simplex virus. Am J Ophthal 81:636, 1976.
60. Kass, MA, Palmberg, P, Becker, B: The ocular anti-inflammatory action of imidazole. Invest Ophthal Vis Sci 16:66, 1977.
61. Spinelli, HM, Krohn, DL: Inhibition of prostaglandin-induced iritis. Topical indoxole vs indomethacin therapy. Arch Ophthal 98:1106, 1980.
62. Podos, SM: Effect of dipyridamole on prostaglandin-induced ocular hypertension in rabbits. Invest Ophthal Vis Sci 18:646, 1979.
63. Wong, VG, Hersh, EM: Methotrexate in the therapy of cyclitis. Trans Am Acad Ophthal Otol 69:279, 1965.
64. Andrasch, RH, Pirofsky, B, Burns, RP: Immunosuppressive therapy for severe chronic uveitis. Arch Ophthal 96:247, 1978.
65. Luntz, MH: A clinical approach to the medical treatment of uveitis. Adv Ophthal 36:187, 1978.
66. Hoskins, HD, Jr, Hetherington, J Jr, Shaffer, RN: Surgical management of the inflammatory glaucomas. Pers Ophthal 1:173, 1977.
67. Ohno, S, Char, DH, Kimura, SJ, O'Connor, GR: Vogt-Koyanagi-Harada syndrome. Am J Ophthal 83:735, 1977.
68. Colvard, DM, Robertson, DM, O'Duffy, JD: The ocular manifestations of Behcet's disease. Arch Ophthal 95:1813, 1977.
69. Marak, GE Jr, Ikui, H: Pigmentation associated histopathological variations in sympathetic ophthalmia. Br J Ophthal 64:220, 1980.
70. Lubin, JR, Albert, DM, Weinstein, M: Sixty-five years of sympathetic ophthalmia. A clinicopathologic review of 105 cases (1913–1978). Ophthalmology 87:109, 1980.
71. Makley, TA Jr, Azar, A: Sympathetic ophthalmia. A long-term follow-up. Arch Ophthal 96:257, 1978.
72. Tavs, LE: Syphilis. Maj Prob Clin Pediatr 19:222, 1978.
73. Grant, WM: Late glaucoma after interstitial keratitis. Am J Ophthal 79:87, 1975.
74. Tsukahara, S: Secondary glaucoma due to inactive congenital syphilitic interstitial keratitis. Ophthalmologica 174:188, 1977.
75. Sugar, HS: Late glaucoma associated with inactive syphilitic interstitial keratitis. Am J Ophthal 53:602, 1962.
76. Falcon, MG, Williams, HP: Herpes simplex kerato-uveitis and glaucoma. Trans Ophthal Soc UK 98:101, 1978.
77. Oh, JO: Effect of cyclophosphamide on primary herpes simplex uveitis in rabbits.

Invest Ophthal Vis Sci 17:769, 1978.

78. Sundmacher, R, Neumann-Haefelin, D: Herpes simplex virus isolations from the aqueous of patients suffering from focal iritis, endotheliitis, and prolonged disciform keratitis with glaucoma. Klin Monatsbl Augenheilkd 175:488, 1979.

79. Townsend, WM, Kaufman, HE: Pathogenesis of glaucoma and endothelial changes in herpetic kerato-uveitis in rabbits. Am J Ophthal 71:904, 1971.

80. Dennis, RF, Oh, JO: Aspirin, cyclophosphamide, and dexamethasone effects on experimental secondary herpes simplex uveitis. Arch Ophthal 97:2170, 1979.

81. Watson, PG, Hayreh, SS: Scleritis and episcleritis. Br J Ophthal 60:163, 1976.

82. Watson, P: Glaucoma Secondary to Keratitis, Episcleritis, and Scleritis. *In* The Secondary Glaucomas, Ritch, R, Shields, MB, eds. CV Mosby Co, St Louis (in press).

83. McGavin, DDM, Williamson, J, Forrester, JV, Foulds, WS, Buchanan, WW, Dick, WC, Lee, P, MacSween, RNM, Whaley, K: Episcleritis and scleritis. A study of their clinical manifestations and association with rheumatoid arthritis. Br J Ophthal 60:192, 1976.

84. Harbin, TS Jr, Pollack, IP: Glaucoma in episcleritis. Arch Ophthal 93:948, 1975.

Chapter 17

GLAUCOMAS ASSOCIATED WITH INTRAOCULAR HEMORRHAGE

GLAUCOMAS ASSOCIATED WITH INTRAOCULAR HEMORRHAGE

Intraocular hemorrhage is most commonly caused by trauma or surgery. In addition, hyphemas may occur spontaneously in association with several ocular disorders, most of which have been discussed in previous chapters. Whatever the initial cause of the intraocular hemorrhage may be, secondary intraocular pressure elevation frequently occurs when the aqueous outflow channels become obstructed by blood in various forms. In this chapter, we will consider the mechanisms and management of the blood-induced glaucomas, as well as some specific causes of intraocular hemorrhage that are not covered in other chapters.

I. GLAUCOMAS ASSOCIATED WITH FRESH HEMORRHAGE

A. Blunt Trauma

The most common source of intraocular hemorrhage is blunt trauma. This usually results from a tear in the ciliary body, causing small branches of the major arterial circle to bleed into the anterior chamber.

1. *General features.* Young people appear to be more prone to blunt ocular trauma, with 77% in one large series of patients with traumatic hyphemas being under 30 years of age.[1] The initial clinical finding may be a microscopic hyphema, which is characterized by red blood cells circulating in the aqueous. Other cases range from an inferior layered hyphema of variable size to a total hyphema, although the smaller hemorrhages are more common. In most cases, the blood clears within a few days, apparently primarily through the trabecular meshwork, and the prognosis is good unless the trauma caused other ocular injuries. However, complications may occur during the post-injury course which can have devastating results.

2. *Complications*

    a. Recurrent hemorrhage. Reports of the frequency with which eyes rebleed after a traumatic hyphema range from 4 to 35%.[2-16] Rebleeding usually occurs during the first week after the initial injury,[3] which is probably related to the normal lysis and retraction of the clot.[2, 10] Aspirin has been shown to have a detrimental effect on the frequency of rebleeding,[8, 13] and there is a suggestion that hypotony may also increase the chances of recurrent hemorrhage.[2, 4] Reports differ as to whether the size of the initial hyphema influences rebleeding.[3, 5, 14, 15]

    b. Secondary glaucoma. Although intraocular pressure elevation may occur following the initial bleed, it is more common after a recurrent hemorrhage, and constitutes the most serious complication of a traumatic hyphema.[1, 3, 6] The incidence of glaucoma associated with a traumatic hyphema is partially related to the size of the hemorrhage. In one study of 235 cases, glaucoma occurred in 13.5% of the eyes with a hyphema filling less than one-half of the anterior chamber, 27% of those with a bleed of greater than one-half, and 52% of the cases with a total hyphema.[16] It is important to distinguish between a total hyphema with bright red blood, and an "eight-ball" or "black-ball" hyphema, which is characterized by dark reddish-black blood, since the latter carries a more grave prognosis relative to secondary glaucoma.[3] In one series of 113 cases, elevated intraocular pressure occurred in one-third of those with a rebleed, but in all cases with eight-ball hyphemas.[3]

The *mechanism* of pressure elevation is related to *obstruction* of the *trabecular meshwork* in most cases of traumatic hyphema. Although fresh red blood cells are known to pass through the conventional aqueous outflow system with relative ease, it appears to be the overwhelming numbers of cells, combined with plasma, fibrin, and debris, that may lead to a transient obstruction of aqueous outflow.[17] In cases of *eight-ball hyphema*, it is presumably the formation of a clot, occasionally with degenerated red blood cells from an associated vitreous hemorrhage,[18] which further impedes outflow.[3] Another factor that increases the incidence of glaucoma in association with hyphema is *sickle cell hemaglobinopathies*, including sickle trait.[19-21] Erythrocytes have a greater tendency to sickle in the aqueous humor,[19, 20, 22] and the elongated, rigid cells pass more slowly through the trabecular meshwork,[23] leading to intraocular pressure elevation even with small amounts of intracameral blood.[19, 20] Furthermore, even moderate elevations of pressure may have a more deleterious effect on the optic nerve head in patients with a sickle cell hemoglobinopathy, possibly due to reduced vascular perfusion.[19, 20] Another mechanism of secondary open-angle glaucoma associated with sickle cell hemoglobinopathies is obstruction to aqueous outflow due to sickled erythrocytes in Schlemm's canal, which has been observed following blunt trauma and in one case with no antecedent trauma.[21]

c. *Corneal blood staining* is typically the result of a prolonged, total hyphema that is usually, but not always, associated with elevated intraocular pressure. This complication occurred in six of 289 patients (2%) with traumatic hyphema, all of whom has a secondary, total hyphema.[24] Histologically, the staining represents an infiltration of posterior stroma with red blood cell breakdown products.[24] This is seen clinically as a central or diffuse, rust-colored opacity, which begins to clear from the periphery, althouth total clearing may take up to two or three years.[24]

3. *Management* of a traumatic hyphema involves attempts to a) facilitate resorption of the blood, b) prevent secondary hemorrhage, and c) treat the complications when they occur.

a. *Conservative management.* Although there is general agreement that the uncomplicated hyphema should be managed nonsurgically, opinions vary as to the optimum conservative care plan. A commonly used protocol is to admit the patient for approximately 5 days of bed rest with elevation of the head of the bed and monocular or binocular patching.[3, 9, 25] However, one study showed no significant difference between patients treated with strict bed rest and patching as compared to a group that were allowed limited activity without patching.[26] A comparison of monocular and binocular patching also revealed no difference in outcome,[27] and it has been reported that over 90% of rebleeds occur at night, suggesting that rapid eye movements may be a factor.[28] Various drugs are also used by some physicians *to accelerate resorption* of the hyphema, but none of these have proven value in this regard. Rabbit studies have not supported the efficacy of atropine,[29] pilocarpine,[29] or acetazolamide[30] for this purpose, although there is a suggestion that hyperosmotics may accelerate resorption of a clotted hyphema.[31]

b. *Prevention of rebleed.* Numerous drugs have been evaluated regarding their ability to reduce the incidence of secondary hemorrhage, and the reported results are conflicting. Oral prednisone has been reported to significantly lower the rebleed rate,[7, 32] although other studies found neither steroids[14] nor estrogen[3] to be of value in this regard. *Antifibrinolytic agents* (including tranexamic acid[11, 12, 33] and aminocaproic acid[10]) have been used in an effort to minimize the natural lysis of the clot, and most reports indicate a significant reduction in rebleeds,[10, 12, 33] although one study found no significant difference from patients treated only with bed rest.[11] The influence of hydrostatic pressure on the damaged vessels has also been studied, and one report described fewer rebleeds with medical reduction of systemic blood pressure and elevation of the head of the bed.[34] As previously noted, a low intraocular pressure[2, 4] or the use of aspirin[8, 13] may increase the chances of secondary hemorrhage.

c. *Management of glaucoma.*

(1) *Medical* treatment of elevated intraocular pressure is occasionally needed to protect the optic nerve head and enhance the resorption of the hyphema, even though it may increase the risk of a rebleed. This pressure reduction is best accomplished with hyperosmotics and drugs which reduce aqueous production. However, caution should be given to the use of acetazolamide in patients with sickle cell hemoglobinopathies, since this increases the concentration of ascorbic acid in the aqueous humor, which leads to more sickling in the anterior chamber.[35]

(2) *Surgical* intervention has been advocated in the following situations: 1) corneal blood staining, 2) total hyphema with an intraocular pressure above 50 mmHg for more than 5 days, 3) a hyphema that was initially total and has not resolved below 50% after 6 days with the intraocular pressure above 25 mmHg, or 4) a hyphema that is unresolved after 9 days.[36] The fourth day after injury is said to be the optimum time for removal of the clot, because it has retracted from adjacent structures.[37, 38] The procedure most often advocated is

irrigation of the anterior chamber with saline,[39, 40] or a fibrinolytic agent (urokinase,[39-41] or fibrinolysin.[42-46]) The iris may prolapse into the incision due to pupillary block, necessitating a peripheral iridectomy,[47] and one report noted complete resorption of the hyphema following iridectomy alone.[48] In some cases, the clot cannot be removed by irrigation, and various suggestions for surgical removal of the clot include cryoextraction,[49] ultrasonic emulsification and extraction,[50] and removal with vitrectomy instruments.[51-53] Belcher and Simmons[54] have reported success with a technique, originally advocated by Chandler, in which the liquefied portion of a total hyphema is removed by paracentesis and the clot is allowed to resorb. When recurrent bleeding occurs during clot extraction, raising the intraocular pressure to 50 mmHg for 5 min has been used to stop the bleeding.[53] Cyclodiathemy has also been utilized to control intraocular bleeding.[55, 56]

B. Penetrating Injuries

Penetrating injuries are also frequently associated with intraocular hemorrhage, although secondary glaucoma is less common than with blunt trauma during the early post-injury period due to the open wound. However, intraocular pressure elevation may follow closure of the wound, especially if meticulous care is not given to reconstruction of the anterior chamber and treatment of the associated inflammation in the post-operative period.[57]

C. Hyphema Associated with Intraocular Surgery

Bleeding within the eye can be a serious complication of any intraocular procedure and may occur during the operation or in the early or even late postoperative period.

1. *During surgery.* As an intraoperative complication, bleeding is usually associated with damage to the ciliary body, as can occur when performing a cyclodialysis, filtering procedure, or iridectomy. This bleeding can usually be controlled by placing a large air bubble in the anterior chamber for a few minutes, which raises the intraocular pressure and acts as a tamponade. Direct, gentle pressure or the application of epinephrine 1:1000 to the ciliary body for 1 to 2 min can also be helpful in stopping ciliary body bleeding. Cautery is generally avoided in these cases, but may occasionally be necessary.

2. *Postoperatively.* Bleeding in the early postoperative period is usually not associated with serious sequelae and should be managed conservatively with limited activity and elevation of the head. Small hyphemas after intraocular surgery normally clear rapidly, although the time may be considerably longer in eyes with pre-existing glaucoma, due to delayed passage of red blood cells through the trabecular meshwork. When a postoperative hyphema is associated with elevated intraocular pressure, conservative medical management should be instituted as required, using drugs that lower aqueous production or hyperosmotics if necessary. Surgical intervention is reserved for

critical cases, although the indications may be somewhat more liberal than with a traumatic hyphema if there is danger of rupturing a corneoscleral wound or causing further atrophy to a nerve head that has previously been damaged by glaucoma.

Hemorrhage during the late postoperative period may result from reopening of a uveal wound or from disruption of new vessels growing across a corneoscleral incision. In a study of 58 eyes 5 to 10 years after cataract extraction, 12% had episcleral vessels in the inner aspects of the incision site and nearly half of these had evidence of mild intraocular hemorrhage.[58] Direct laser therapy may be used to treat such vessels, and preliminary experience suggests that limbal cryotherapy may also be useful in preventing intraocular hemorrhage in these cases.[58]

D. Spontaneous Hyphemas

Spontaneous hyphemas may occur in eyes with the following disorders, most of which were considered in previous chapters. In some cases, the hyphema may cause or contribute to an elevation of the intraocular pressure.

1. *Intraocular tumors.* As noted in Chapter 11, a spontaneous hyphema may occur in a child with juvenile xanthogranuloma, and intraocular hemorrhage may be a manifestation of an ocular malignant melanoma.

2. *Neovascularization* of the anterior ocular segment, which may lead to a spontaneous hyphema, is seen in the conditions referred to as rubeosis iridis and neovascular glaucoma (Chapter 15) and in Fuchs' heterochromic cyclitis (Chapter 16).

3. *Vascular tufts at the pupillary margin* (also referred to as iris neovascular tufts or iridic microhemangiomas) were first described in 1968,[59] and represent yet another source of spontaneous hyphema. They can be seen by slit lamp biomicroscopy as multiple vascular tufts along the pupillary margin, and fluorescein angiography of the iris is reported to demonstrate small areas of staining and leakage from the lesions.[59] A histopathologic examination revealed thin-walled new vessels at the pupillary margin of the iris with a mild inflammatory cell infiltration.[60] The condition is typically seen in elderly individuals, but may be found in young adults. Most of these patients have no systemic disease,[59] although associations with diabetes mellitus[59, 61] and myotonic dystrophy[61, 62] have been reported. Spontaneous hyphemas occur in a small number of these cases, occasionally causing transient intraocular pressure elevation.[63, 64] Laser photocoagulation was reported to successfully eradicate a vascular tuft that bled.[60] However, since it is rare to have recurrent hyphemas or permanent damage related to the transiently elevated intraocular pressure, Simmons (personal communication) advocates withholding treatment until one or more recurrences of bleeding are documented.

II. GLAUCOMAS ASSOCIATED WITH LONG-STANDING HEMORRHAGE

A. Glaucoma Due to Ghost Cells

In 1976, Campbell and co-workers[65] described a form of secondary glaucoma in which degenerated red blood cells (ghost cells) develop in the vitreous cavity and subsequently enter the anterior chamber where they temporarily obstruct aqueous outflow.

1. *Theories of mechanism.* [18, 65] Having entered the vitreous cavity by one of several mechanisms (trauma, surgery, or retinal disease), fresh erythrocytes are transformed from their typical bi-concave, pliable nature to tan or khaki-colored, spherical, less pliable structures, referred to as ghost cells. Histologically, these cells have thin walls and appear hollow except for clumps of denaturized hemoglobin, called Heinz bodies. Unlike fresh red blood cells, ghost cells do not pass readily through a 5 micron Millipore filter or human trabecular meshwork. The ghost cells develop within a matter of weeks and may then remain in the vitreous cavity for many months until a disruption of the anterior hyaloid allows them to enter the anterior chamber. Once in the anterior chamber, the abnormal cells accumulate in the trabecular meshwork where they may cause a temporary, but occasionally marked, elevation of intraocular pressure.

2. *Specific clinical settings.* Several situations have been described which may lead to ghost cell glaucoma:

a. *Cataract extraction* may be associated with glaucoma due to ghost cells in one of three ways[66]: 1) A large hyphema with vitreous hemorrhage occurs in the early post-operative period. As the hyphema clears, ghost cells, which developed in the vitreous, come forward and obstruct aqueous outflow. 2) A vitreous hemorrhage is present before cataract surgery, and disruption of the anterior hyaloid as a result of the operation allows the ghost cells to enter the anterior chamber. 3) A vitreous hemorrhage develops at some point after cataract extraction due to retinal disease, and the ghost cells develop and come forward through previously made defects in the anterior hyaloid.

b. *Vitrectomy* may lead to ghost cell glaucoma in eyes with pre-existing vitreous hemorrhage, if the anterior hyaloid is disrupted and the vitreous and cells are not completely removed.[67]

c. *Traumatic hyphemas*, including eight-ball hyphemas, may be associated with vitreous hemorrhage and subsequent glaucoma due to ghost cells. This may occur after the hyphema has cleared or may be masked by a persistent hyphema.[18]

3. *Clinical features.* [18, 65] Depending on the number of ghost cells in the anterior chamber, the intraocular pressure ranges from normal to marked elevation with pain and corneal edema. Slit lamp biomicroscopy reveals characteristic khaki-colored cells in the aqueous and on the corneal endothelium. If present in large quantities, the ghost cells may layer out inferiorly, creating a pseudohypopyon, which is occa-

sionally associated with a layer of fresher red blood cells (candy-stripe sign). The anterior chamber angle, on gonioscopy, is typically open and may appear normal or may be covered by scant to heavy amounts of khaki-colored cells.

4. *Differential diagnosis.*[18] Glaucoma due to ghost cells may be confused with the less common hemolytic and hemosiderotic glaucomas, which are discussed later in this chapter. In addition, neovascular glaucoma and glaucoma due to inflammation must be ruled out. Although the diagnosis is usually easily made on the basis of history and clinical features, it may be confirmed by examination of an aqueous aspirate, which reveals the typical ghost cells.

5. *Management.*[18, 65] Glaucoma due to ghost cells is not a permanent condition, but may last for months before the abnormal cells eventually clear from the anterior chamber angle. In the interim, it is often possible to control the intraocular pressure with standard antiglaucoma medication. Other cases, however, will require surgical intervention, which may consist of anterior chamber irrigation or vitrectomy.

B. Hemolytic Glaucoma

Fenton and Zimmerman[68] described a form of secondary glaucoma associated with intraocular hemorrhage in which macrophages ingest contents of the red blood cells and then accumulate in the trabecular meshwork where they temporarily obstruct aqueous outflow. Clinically, numerous red-tinted blood cells are seen floating in the aqueous, and the anterior chamber angle is typically open, with reddish brown pigment covering the trabecular meshwork.[69] Cytologic examination of the aqueous reveals macrophages containing golden-brown pigment,[69] and an ultrastructural study of seven eyes revealed red blood cells and macrophages with phagocytized blood and pigment in the trabecular spaces.[70] The endothelial cells of the trabecular meshwork were degenerated and also had phagocytized blood.[70] The condition is self-limiting and should be managed medically if possible. When surgical intervention is required, anterior chamber lavage has been recommended.[69]

C. Hemosiderotic Glaucoma

Hemosiderotic glaucoma is a rare condition in which hemoglobin from lysed red blood cells in the anterior chamber is phagocytized by endothelial cells of the trabecular meshwork. Iron in the hemoglobin subsequently causes *siderosis*, which is believed to produce tissue alterations in the trabecular meshwork, eventually resulting in obstruction to aqueous outflow.[71] However, an association between iron staining of the trabecular meshwork and impairment of aqueous outflow has yet to be clearly established.[72]

References

1. Pilger, IS: Medical treatment of traumatic hyphema. Surv Ophthal 20:28, 1975.
2. Howard, GM, Hutchinson, BT, Frederick, AR Jr: Hyphema resulting from blunt

trauma. Gonioscopic, tonographic, and ophthalmoscopic observations following resolution of the hemorrhage. Trans Am Acad Ophthal Otol 69:294, 1965.

3. Spaeth, GL, Levy, PM: Traumatic hyphema: Its clinical characteristics and failure of estrogens to alter its course. A double-blind study. Am J Ophthal 62:1098, 1966.
4. Milstein, BA: Traumatic hyphema: A study of 83 consecutive cases. South Med J 64:1081, 1971.
5. Giles, CL, Bromley, WG: Traumatic hyphema. A retrospective analysis from the University of Michigan Teaching Hospitals. J Pediatr Ophthal 9:90, 1972.
6. Edwards, WC, Layden, WE: Traumatic hyphema. A report of 184 consecutive cases. Am J Ophthal 75:110, 1973.
7. Yasuna, E: Management of traumatic hyphema. Arch Ophthal 91:190, 1974.
8. Crawford, JS, Lewandowski, RL, Chan, W: The effect of aspirin on rebleeding in traumatic hyphema. Am J Ophthal 80:543, 1975.
9. Fritch, CD: Traumatic hyphema. Ann Ophthal 8:1223, 1976.
10. Crouch, ER Jr, Frenkel, M: Aminocaproic acid in the treatment of traumatic hyphema. Am J Ophthal 81:355, 1976.
11. Mortensen, KK, Sjolie, AK: Secondary haemorrhage following traumatic hyphaema. A comparative study of conservative and tranexamic acid treatment. Acta Ophthal 56:763, 1978.
12. Bramsen, T: Fibrinolysis and traumatic hyphaema. Acta Ophthal 57:447, 1979.
13. Gorn, RA: The detrimental effect of aspirin on hyphema rebleed. Ann Ophthal 11:351, 1979.
14. Spoor, TC, Hammer, M, Belloso, H: Traumatic hyphema. Failure of steroids to alter its course: a double-blind prospective study. Arch Ophthal 98:116, 1980.
15. Rakusin, W: Traumatic hyphema. Am J Ophthal 74:284, 1972.
16. Coles, WH: Traumatic hyphema: An analysis of 235 cases. South Med J 61:813, 1968.
17. Sternberg, P Jr, Tripathi, RC, Tripathi, BJ, Chilcote, RR: Changes in outflow facility in experimental hyphema. Invest Ophthal Vis Sci 19:1388, 1980.
18. Campbell, DG: Ghost cell glaucoma. In The Secondary Glaucomas, Ritch, R, Shields, MB, eds. CV Mosby Co, St Louis (in press).
19. Goldberg, MF: The diagnosis and treatment of secondary glaucoma after hyphema in sickle cell patients. Am J Ophthal 87:43, 1979.
20. Goldberg, MF: Sickled erythrocytes, hyphema, and secondary glaucoma. I. The diagnosis and treatment of sickled erythrocytes in human hyphemas. Ophthal Surg 10:17, 1979.
21. Friedman, AH, Halpern, BL, Friedberg, DN, Wang, FM, Podos, SM: Transient open-angle glaucoma associated with sickle cell trait: report of 4 cases. Br J Ophthal 63:832, 1979.
22. Goldberg, MF: Sickled erythrocytes, hyphema, and secondary glaucoma. IV. The rate and percentage of sickling of erythrocytes in rabbit aqueous humor, in vitro and in vivo. Ophthal Surg 10:62, 1979.
23. Goldberg, MF, Tso, MOM: Sickled erythrocytes, hyphema, and secondary glaucoma: VII. The passage of sickled erythrocytes out of the anterior chamber of the human and monkey eye: light and electron microscopic studies. Ophthal Surg 10:89, 1979.
24. Brodrick, JD: Corneal blood staining after hyphaema. Br J Ophthal 56:589, 1972.
25. Edwards, WC, Layden, WE: Traumatic hyphema: Review of current medical and surgical therapy. Pers Ophthal 2:171, 1978.
26. Read, J, Goldberg, MF: Comparison of medical treatment for traumatic hyphema. Trans Am Acad Ophthal Otol 78:799, 1974.
27. Edwards, WC, Layden, WE: Monocular versus binocular patching in traumatic hyphema. Am J Ophthal 76:359, 1973.
28. Skalka, HW: Recurrent hemorrhage in traumatic hyphema. Ann Ophthal 10:1153, 1978.
29. Rose, SW, Coupal, JJ, Simmons, G, Kielar, RA: Experimental hyphema clearance in rabbits. Drug trials with 1% atropine and 2% and 4% pilocarpine. Arch Ophthal 95:1442, 1977.

30. Masket, S, Best, M: Therapy in experimental hyphema. II. Acetazolamide. Arch Ophthal 87:222, 1972.
31. Masket, S, Best, M, Fisher, LV, Kronenberg, SM, Galin, MA: Therapy in experimental hyphema. Arch Ophthal 85:329, 1971.
32. Rynne, MV, Romano, PE: Systemic corticosteroids in the treatment of traumatic hyphema. J Pediatr Ophthal Strabis 17:141, 1980.
33. Bramsen, T: Traumatic hyphaema treated with the antifibrinolytic drug tranexamic acid. Acta Ophthal 54:250, 1976.
34. Macdougald, TJ: The treatment of traumatic hyphaema. Trans Ophthal Soc UK 92:815, 1972.
35. Goldberg, MF: Sickled erythrocytes, hyphema, and secondary glaucoma: V. The effect of vitamin C on erythrocyte sickling in aqueous humor. Ophthal Surg 10:70, 1979.
36. Read, J: Traumatic hyphema: surgical vs medical management. Ann Ophthal 7:659, 1975.
37. Sears, ML: Surgical management of black ball hyphema. Trans Am Acad Ophthal Otol 74:820, 1970.
38. Wolter, JR, Henderson, JW, Talley, TW: Histopathology of a black ball blood clot removed four days after total traumatic hyphema. J Ped Ophthal 8:15, 1971.
39. Rakusin, W: Urokinase in the management of traumatic hyphaema. Br J Ophthal 55:826, 1971.
40. Rakusin, W: The role of urokinase in the management of traumatic hyphaema. Ophthalmologica 167:373, 1973.
41. Leet, DM: Treatment of total hyphema with urokinas. Am J Ophthal 84:79, 1977.
42. Oosterhuis, JA: Fibrinolysin irrigation in traumatic secondary hyphema. Ophthalmologica 155:357, 1968.
43. Podos, S, Liebman, S, Pollen, A: Treatment of experimental total hyphemas with intraocular fibrinolytic agents. II. Arch Ophthal 71:537, 1964.
44. Scheie, HG, Ashley, BJ, Burns, DT: Treatment of total hyphema with fibrinolysin. Arch Ophthal 69:147, 1963.
45. Polychronakos, D, Razoglou, C: Treatment of total hyphema with fibrinolysin. Ophthalmologica 154:31, 1967.
46. Horven, I: Fibrinolysis and hyphema. The effect of "thrombolysin" and "kabikanas" on clotted blood in camera anterior of the eye in rabbits. Acta Ophthal 46:320, 1962.
47. Heinze, J: The surgical management of total hyphaema. Austral J Ophthal 3:20, 1975.
48. Dizon, RV, Aquino, MV, Bernardino, VB Jr: Iridectomy for eight-ball hyphema. Philippine J Ophthal 6:37, 1974.
49. Hill, K: Cryoextraction of total hyphema. Arch Ophthal 80:368, 1968.
50. Kelman, CD, Brooks, DL: Ultrasonic emulsification and aspiration of traumatic hyphema. A preliminary report. Am J Ophthal 71:1289, 1971.
51. McCuen, BW, Fung, WE: The role of vitrectomy instrumentation in the treatment of severe traumatic hyphema. Am J Ophthal 88:930, 1979.
52. Diddie, KR, Ernest, JT: Rotoextractor evacuation of total hyphema. Ophthal Surg 7:49, 1976.
53. Stern, WH, Mondal, KM: Vitrectomy instrumentation for surgical evacuation of total anterior chamber hyphema and control of recurrent anterior chamber hemorrhage. Ophthal Surg 10:34, 1979.
54. Belcher, CD III, Simmons, RJ: Hyphema management by paracentesis, presented at Annual Meeting Am Acad Ophthal, San Francisco, 1979.
55. Glaser, B: Prophylaxis in traumatic hyphema. South Med J 57:195, 1964.
56. Gilbert, HD, Smith, RE: Traumatic hyphema: treatment of secondary hemorrhage with cyclodiathermy. Ophthal Surg 7:31, 1976.
57. Richardson, K: Acute glaucoma after trauma. In Ocular Trauma, Freeman, H MacK, ed. Appleton-Century-Crofts, New York, 1979, p 161.
58. Watzke, RC: Intraocular hemorrhage from vascularization of the cataract incision. Ophthalmology 87:19, 1980.

59. Cobb, B: Vascular tufts at the pupillary margin: a preliminary report on 44 patients. Trans Ophthal Soc UK 88:211, 1968.
60. Coleman, SL, Green, WR, Patz, A: Vascular tufts of pupillary margin of iris. Am J Ophthal 83:881, 1977.
61. Mason, GI: Iris neovascular tufts. Relationship to rubeosis, insulin, and hypotony. Arch Ophthal 97:2346, 1979.
62. Cobb, B, Shilling, JS, Chisholm, IH: Vascular tufts at the pupillary margin in myotonic dystrophy. Am J Ophthal 69:573, 1970.
63. Perry, HD, Mallen, FJ, Sussman, W: Microhaemangiomas of the iris with spontaneous hyphaema and acute glaucoma. Br J Ophthal 61:114, 1977.
64. Mason, GI, Ferry, AP: Bilateral spontaneous hyphema arising from iridic micro-hemangiomas. Ann Ophthal 11:87, 1979.
65. Campbell, DG, Simmons, RJ, Grant, WM: Ghost cells as a cause of glaucoma. Am J Ophthal 81:441, 1976.
66. Campbell, DG, Essigmann, EM: Hemolytic ghost cell glaucoma. Further studies. Arch Ophthal 97:2141, 1979.
67. Campbell, DG, Simmons, RJ, Tolentino, FI, McMeel, JW: Glaucoma occurring after closed vitrectomy. Am J Ophthal 83:63, 1977.
68. Fenton, RH, Zimmerman, LE: Hemolytic glaucoma. An unusual cause of acute open-angle secondary glaucoma. Arch Ophthal 70:236, 1963.
69. Phelps, CD, Watzke, RC: Hemolytic glaucoma. Am J Ophthal 80:690, 1975.
70. Grierson, I, Lee, WR: Further observations on the process of haemophagocytosis in the human outflow system. Albrecht v Graefes Arch klin exp Ophthal 208:49, 1978.
71. Vannas, S: Hemosiderosis in eyes with secondary glaucoma after delayed intra-ocular hemorrhages. Acta Ophthal 38:254, 1960.
72. Simmons, RJ, Kimbrough, RL: Late glaucoma after trauma. in Ocular Trauma, ed, Freeman, H MacK, Appleton-Century-Croft, New York, 1979, p 167.

Chapter 18

GLAUCOMAS ASSOCIATED WITH OCULAR TRAUMA

I. Blunt trauma
   A. Acute intraocular pressure elevation
   B. Iridocyclitis
   C. Intraocular hemorrhage
   D. Dislocation of the lens
   E. Trabecular damage

II. Penetrating injuries
   A. Tissue disruption
   B. Retained intraocular foreign bodies

III. Chemical burns
   A. Alkali burns
   B. Acid burns

GLAUCOMAS ASSOCIATED WITH OCULAR TRAUMA

A secondary elevation of the intraocular pressure may complicate several forms of ocular trauma, including blunt and penetrating injuries and chemical burns.

I. BLUNT TRAUMA

A blunt injury to the eye may lead to secondary glaucoma by several mechanisms, most of which have been discussed in previous chapters. In many cases, an injury may cause more than one of these mechanisms, and the clinician must be alert to the possibility of a second, delayed intraocular pressure elevation after the initial rise has subsided.

A. Acute Intraocular Pressure Elevation[1]

During the early postcontusion period, there may be a transient elevation of the intraocular pressure, which lasts for one to several weeks. This occurs in the absence of any other obvious damage to the eye. The anterior chamber angle is grossly normal by gonioscopy, and the mechanism of the pressure rise is unknown. It is best to treat such conditions medically, primarily with drugs that reduce aqueous production.

B. Iridocyclitis

Blunt trauma not uncommonly causes a transient anterior uveitis. This most often is associated with a reduction in intraocular pressure, although secondary glaucoma may occur by the mechanisms discussed in Chapter 16.

C. Intraocular Hemorrhage

As discussed in the previous chapter, blunt trauma often causes intraocular bleeding, and this may be associated with secondary intraocular pressure elevation of early or delayed onset.

D. Dislocation of the Lens

Trauma is the most common cause of a dislocated lens, which may lead to an early pupillary block form of glaucoma or a delayed intraocular pressure rise due to phacolysis. The diagnosis and management of these conditions were considered in Chapter 14.

E. Trabecular Damage

Trabecular damage is frequently associated with the above sequelae of blunt trauma and may lead to chronic intraocular pressure elevation.

1. *Associated injuries* (Fig. 18.1). The tissue alterations of the trabecular meshwork are subtle and often overshadowed by more obvious associated injuries. Although the latter are not directly responsible for the secondary glaucoma, it is important to recognize them as signs of previous trauma. A common finding following blunt ocular trauma is a condition referred to as *angle recession*. Histologically, this represents a tear between the longitudinal and circular muscles of the ciliary body, and gonioscopically, it is seen as an irregular widening of the ciliary band. An even more common gonioscopic finding is tears or detachments of uveal processes in the anterior chamber angle.[2] Other associated injuries include *iridodialysis*, or a tear in the root of the iris, and *cyclodialysis*, which is a separation of the ciliary body from the scleral spur. Trauma that is sufficient to cause an angle recession or other of these injuries is often also associated with a *hyphema*, which may be the initial finding when a patient presents for evaluation of a blunt eye injury. The reported prevalence of angle recession in eyes with traumatic hyphemas ranges from 60 to 94%.[2-6] The intraocular pressure during the early post-injury period may be lower than the fellow eye or, if elevated, it usually returns to normal as the initial effects of the injury subside. However, it is important to follow these patients indefinitely, since a reported 4 to 9% of those with angle recessions greater than 180° will eventually, often many years later, develop a chronic glaucoma.[3, 5, 7]

2. *Theories of mechanism.* The clinicopathologic correlation between blunt injury to the eye and the delayed development of glaucoma was noted by Wolff and Zimmerman,[8] who suggested that the angle recession provided evidence of past injury, but was not the actual cause of the glaucoma. They suggested that initial trauma to the trabecular meshwork stimulated proliferative and/or degenerative changes in the trabecular tissue, which led to obstruction of aqueous outflow. Herschler[9] supported this concept by human observations and animal studies which revealed *tears in the trabecular meshwork* just posterior to Schwalbe's line, during the early post-trauma period. This produced a flap of trabecular tissue, which was hinged at the scleral spur (Fig. 18.1). With time, scarring ensued, causing the initial trabecular injury to be less apparent, but also leading to chronic obstruction in portions of the aqueous outflow system. In addition to alterations within the trabecular meshwork, an *endothelial layer* with a Descemet's-like membrane may extend from the cornea over the anterior chamber angle.[8, 10, 11] It is important to understand this course of events, as well as the significance of associated injuries, since the diagnosis is difficult to make by the gonioscopic appearance of the trabecular meshwork alone. It is also important to note that the majority of eyes which eventually develop glaucoma after blunt injury appear to have an underlying predisposition to reduced aqueous outflow, as evidenced by frequent alterations of intraocular pressure in the fellow eye.[6, 9]

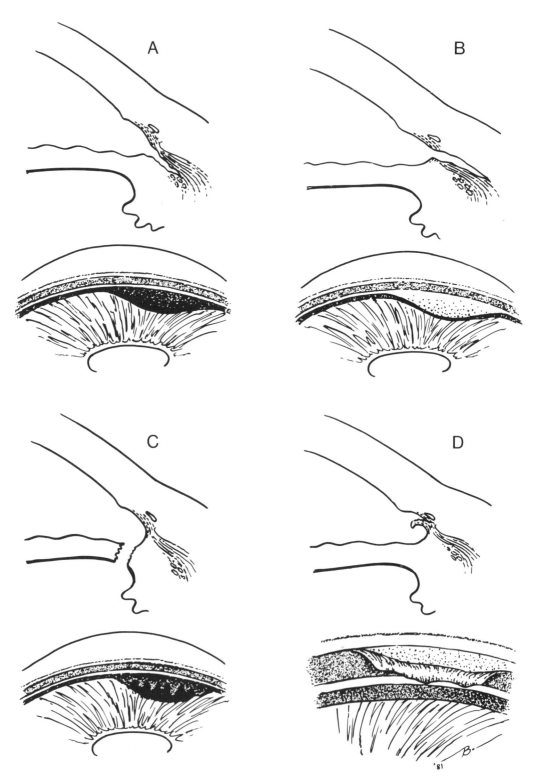

Figure 18.1. Forms of anterior chamber angle injury associated with blunt trauma, showing cross-sectional schematic and corresponding gonioscopic appearance. **A:** angle recession (tear between longitudinal

3.Management. Intraocular pressure elevation due to trabecular damage does not respond well to standard medical therapy. In one reported case with associated angle recession, pilocarpine caused a paradoxical pressure rise, while cycloplegics lowered the tension.[12] The authors theorized that the injured eye may have shifted to a predominantly uveoscleral mechanism of aqueous outflow, which is known to be impaired by miotics. They suggested that cycloplegics may have therapeutic value in these cases.[12] In addition, drugs which reduce aqueous production, such as carbonic anhydrase inhibitors and timolol maleate, may be more efficacious in eyes with scarring of the trabecular meshwork. Filtering surgery should be recommended only when the medical therapy is ineffective.

II. PENETRATING INJURIES

Penetrating injuries may lead to chronic intraocular pressure elevation either secondary to the gross disruption of ocular tissues or to retention of a foreign body, with subsequent tissue changes.

A. Tissue Disruption

During the early post-injury period, the intraocular pressure may be elevated due to inflammation, hyphema, or angle closure from a swollen, disrupted lens. In other cases, the eye may be hypotonous due to a large, open wound. In either situation, the initial management includes prompt and meticulous surgical reconstruction to minimize scarring and chronic glaucoma.[1] In some eyes, this may require removal of portions of incarcerated uveal tissue, aspiration of the lens if disrupted and swollen, or reformation of the anterior chamber. Postoperative management includes control of the inflammation and prophylactic antibiotic coverage. Failure to reform a flat anterior chamber or adequately treat the inflammation may lead to chronic pressure elevation due to peripheral anterior synechiae or posterior synechiae with iris bombe'. Additional, rare causes of delayed elevation of intraocular pressure include sympathetic ophthalmia and epithelial ingrowth, which are discussed in Chapters 16 and 19, respectively.

B. Retained Intraocular Foreign Bodies

Retained intraocular foreign bodies may be associated with the same tissue disruption and secondary glaucoma as noted above. In addition, prolonged intraocular retention of certain foreign materials, including the following metals, may lead to delayed tissue alterations.[13]

---

and circular muscles of ciliary body); **B:** cyclodialysis (separation of ciliary body from scleral spur, with widening of suprachoroidal space); **C:** iridodialysis (tear in root of iris); and **D:** trabecular damage[9] (tear in anterior portion of meshwork, creating a flap that is hinged at the scleral spur).

1. *Siderosis* results from the intraocular retention of *ferrous metal* (iron) but may also be due to intraocular *hemorrhage* (the ionized form of iron is indistinguishable from hemosiderin). This material can cause structural alterations in tissues throughout the eye. Glaucoma may be a complication of advanced cases, although there is no proof that trabecular outflow is impaired by iron staining of the trabecular structures.[14]

2. *Chalcosis. Copper* is also oxidized within the eye and can lead to tissue damage nearly as severe as that encountered with ferrous foreign bodies. Glaucoma appears to be less common in these patients, although retinal changes may lead to visual field defects that might be confused with those of glaucoma.[15]

III. CHEMICAL BURNS

A. Alkali Burns

Alkali burns produce a rapid initial rise in the intraocular pressure, reportedly due to shrinkage of the outer collagenous coats of the eye.[16] This is followed by a return to normal or subnormal pressure and then a slower, sustained elevation of tension, associated with release of prostaglandins.[16] A hypopyon may also develop and contribute to the pressure rise. In managing the secondary glaucoma associated with an alkali burn of the cornea, topical corticosteroids may be helpful if a significant inflammatory component is present. It has been shown in rabbits that topical steroids can be used for the first week without increasing the risk of corneal melting, but not thereafter.[17] In addition, the presence of prostaglandins during the delayed pressure rise suggests that the early use of drugs which inhibit prostaglandin synthesis, such as indomethacin and imidazole, may be beneficial. Anti-glaucoma agents, especially those that reduce aqueous production, are also frequently required in these cases. As with other forms of anterior uveitis, miotics should usually be avoided.

B. Acid Burns

Acid burns to the cornea have been shown to cause an intraocular pressure response in rabbits similar to that seen with alkali burns.[18] A rapid tension increase, lasting up to 3 hr, is felt to result from shrinkage of the outer ocular coats, while a subsequent sustained rise in considered to be mediated by prostaglandin release.[18] Treatment of secondary glaucoma in these cases is similar to that for alkali burns.

References

1. Richardson, K: Acute glaucoma after trauma. *In* Ocular Trauma, Freeman, H Mack, ed. Appleton-Century-Crofts, New York, 1979, p 161.
2. Howard, GM, Hutchinson, BT, Frederick, AR: Hyphema resulting from blunt trauma. Gonioscopic, tonographic, and ophthalmoscopic observations following resolution of the hemorrhage. Trans Am Acad Ophthal Otol 69:294, 1965.

3. Blanton, FM: Anterior chamber angle recession and secondary glaucoma. A study of the aftereffects of traumatic hyphemas. Arch Ophthal 72:39, 1964.
4. Tonjum, AM: Gonioscopy in traumatic hyphema. Acta Ophthal 44:650, 1966.
5. Mooney, D: Angle recession and secondary glaucoma. Br J Ophthal 57:608, 1973.
6. Spaeth, GL: Traumatic hyphema, angle recession, dexamethasone hypertension, and glaucoma. Arch Ophthal 78:714, 1967.
7. Kaufman, JH, Tolpin, DW: Glaucoma after traumatic angle recession. A ten-year prospective study. Am J Ophthal 79:648, 1974.
8. Wolff, SM, Zimmerman, LE: Chronic secondary glaucoma associated with retrodisplacement of iris root and deepening of the anterior chamber angle secondary to contusion. Am J Ophthal 54:547, 1962.
9. Herschler, J: Trabecular damage due to blunt anterior segment injury and its relationship to traumatic glaucoma. Trans Am Acad Ophthal Otol 83:239, 1977.
10. Lauring, L: Anterior chamber glass membranes. Am J Ophthal 68:308, 1969.
11. Iwamoto, T, Witmer, R, Landolt, E: Light and electron microscopy in absolute glaucoma with pigment dispersion phenomena and contusion angle deformity. Am J Ophthal 72:420, 1971.
12. Bleiman, BS, Schwartz, AL: Paradoxical intraocular pressure response to pilocarpine. A proposed mechanism and treatment. Arch Ophthal 97:1305, 1979.
13. Hogan, MJ, Zimmerman, LE: Ophthalmic Pathology. An Atlas and Textbook, 2nd ed. WB Saunders Co, Philadelphia, 1962, p 159.
14. Simmons, RJ, Kimbrough, RL: Late glaucoma after trauma. In Ocular Trauma, Freeman, H Mack, ed. Appleton-Century-Crofts, New York, 1979, p 167.
15. Rosenthal, AR, Marmor, MF, Leuenberger, P, Hopkins, JL: Chalcosis: a study of natural history. Ophthalmology 86:1956, 1979.
16. Paterson, CA, Pfister, RR: Intraocular pressure changes after alkali burns. Arch Ophthal 91:211, 1974.
17. Donshik, PC, Berman, MB, Dohlman, CH, Gage, J, Rose, J: Effect of topical corticosteroids on ulceration in alkali-burned corneas. Arch Ophthal 96:2117, 1978.
18. Paterson, CA, Eakins, KE, Paterson, E, Jenkins, RM II, Ishikawa, R: The ocular hypertensive response following experimental acid burns in the rabbit eye. Invest Ophthal Vis Sci 18:67, 1979.

Chapter 19

GLAUCOMAS FOLLOWING OCULAR SURGERY

GLAUCOMAS FOLLOWING OCULAR SURGERY

Secondary glaucoma may be a complication of any intraocular surgical procedure, as well as several extraocular procedures. The long list of these glaucomas that may follow ocular surgery is the subject of this chapter.

I. MALIGNANT (CILIARY BLOCK) GLAUCOMA
A. Terminology

In 1869, von Graefe[1] described a rare complication of certain ocular procedures, which was characterized by shallowing or flattening of the anterior chamber and an elevation of the intraocular pressure. He called the condition *"malignant glaucoma,"* because of the poor response to conventional therapy. Today, the concept of malignant glaucoma has been expanded to include a variety of clinical situations, which have the following common denominators: 1) shallowing or flattening of both the central and peripheral anterior chamber, 2) elevated intraocular pressure, and 3) unresponsiveness to, or even aggravation by, miotics but frequent relief with cycloplegic-mydriatic therapy.[2-4]

Studies regarding the mechanism of malignant glaucoma, which will be considered later in this chapter, have led some authors to recommend new terms for this group of diseases. Based on the theory that apposition of the ciliary processes against the equator of the lens, or the anterior hyaloid in aphakia, obstructs the normal forward flow of aqueous, the name, *"ciliary block glaucoma,"* has been proposed.[5, 6] To describe the concept that a forward shift of the lens pushes peripheral iris into the anterior chamber angle, the term, *"direct lens block angle closure,"* has also been suggested.[7] At the present time, there is no universal agreement regarding the terminology for this group of conditions, and the traditional term, malignant glaucoma, will be retained for purposes of discussion in this text.

B. Clinical Forms

It has yet to be established as to whether all clinical conditions that are called malignant glaucoma should actually be included within a single disease category. Nevertheless, the following disorders have been described under that name.

1. *Classic malignant glaucoma*[3, 4] is the prototype and most common form of this disease group. It follows surgical intervention for *angle-closure glaucoma*, and is reported to complicate 0.6 to 4% of these cases.[2-4, 8] Neither the type of surgery nor the level of intraocular pressure immediately prior to surgical intervention appear related to

the postoperative development of malignant glaucoma.[3, 4] However, partial or total closure of the anterior chamber angle at the time of surgery is associated with an increased incidence of this complication.[3, 4] Furthermore, the primary angle-closure attack itself may be a predisposing factor, since malignant glaucoma, when it occurs, nearly always does so in an eye that has had an attack of angle-closure glaucoma, even though the angle may be open pre-operatively.[8] However, the condition rarely if ever follows a prophylactic iridectomy, when the angle is open at the time of surgery.[8] The condition may occur immediately after surgery or months to years later, often corresponding to the cessation of cycloplegic therapy or the institution of miotic drops.[2-4]

2. *Malignant glaucoma in aphakia.* Although classic malignant glaucoma typically occurs in phakic eyes, it may persist after lens removal for treatment of the disease, demonstrating that the condition can exist in aphakia.[3, 4] Furthermore, malignant glaucoma has been reported following cataract extraction in eyes without pre-existing glaucoma.[4] The distinction between this condition and pupillary block glaucoma in aphakia will be considered later in this chapter.

3. *Miotic-induced malignant glaucoma.* As noted above, the onset of classic malignant glaucoma may correspond to the institution of miotic therapy, suggesting a causal relationship.[9] In addition, similar clinical pictures have been described in unoperated eyes on miotic therapy,[10] and in an eye treated with miotics after a filtering procedure for open-angle glaucoma.[11]

4. *Inflammation* and *trauma* have also been reported as precipitating factors of malignant glaucoma.[7] One report described a "fungal malignant glaucoma" in which a keratomycosis endophthalmitis led to a flat anterior chamber with marked intraocular pressure elevation.[12]

5. *Retinal detachment surgery* was said to cause the "malignant glaucoma syndrome" in a patient who developed choroidal detachments after a buckling procedure.[13]

6. *Spontaneous malignant glaucoma.* It has also been reported that malignant glaucoma may develop in eyes without previous surgery or miotic therapy.[4, 14]

C. Theories of Mechanism

There is a lack of general agreement regarding the sequence of events responsible for the development of malignant glaucoma, although the following are the more popular theories.

1. *Posterior pooling of aqueous.* Shaffer[15] hypothesized that an accumulation of aqueous behind a posterior vitreous detachment causes the forward displacement of the iris-lens or iris-vitreous diaphragm, and the concept was subsequently expanded to include the pooling of aqueous within vitreous pockets. This theory has been supported by an ultrasonographic study of eyes with malignant glaucoma in aphakia, demonstrating echo-free zones in the vitreous

from which aqueous was reportedly aspirated.[16] The mechanism(s) leading to the posterior diversion of aqueous is uncertain, although there is strong evidence to support the following possibilities.

(a). *Ciliolenticular (or ciliovitreal) block* (Figs. 19.1 and 19.2). It has been observed in cases of malignant glaucoma that the tips of the ciliary processes rotate forward and press against the lens equator in the phakic eye, or against the anterior hyaloid in aphakia, which might create the obstruction to forward flow of aqueous.[5, 17] As previously noted, it was this concept that led to the proposed term, "*ciliary block glaucoma,*" as a substitute for malignant glaucoma.[5]

(b). *Anterior hyaloid obstruction.* It has also been suggested that the anterior hyaloid may contribute to ciliolenticular block and that breaks in the hyaloid near the vitreous base possibly allow the posterior diversion of aqueous (Fig. 19.3).[6] The hyaloid breaks, however, have a one-way valve effect, since fluid coming anteriorly closes the vitreous face against the ciliary body, preventing forward flow.[6] Others who have observed the ciliolenticular contact note that the spaces between the ciliary processes seem to be open, with vitreous visible behind them.[3] These investigators report, however, that the anterior vitreous face is abnormally forward against the ciliary processes in both phakic and aphakic forms of malignant glaucoma.[3] Perfusion studies with both animal[18] and human[19, 20] eyes have shown that resistance to flow of a fluid through vitreous increases significantly with an elevation of pressure in the eye. It has been postulated

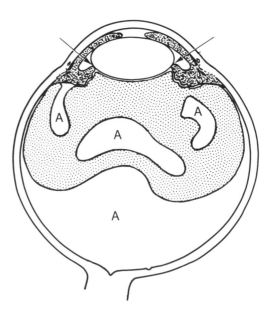

Figure 19.1. Concept of ciliolenticular block as the mehanism of malignant glaucoma. Apposition of ciliary processes to the lens equator (**arrows**) causes a posterior diversion of aqueous (**A**) which pools in and behind the vitreous with a forward shift of the lens-iris diaphragm.

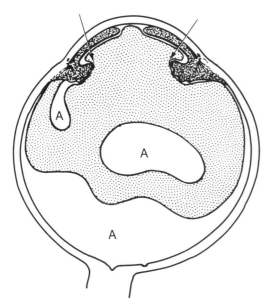

Figure 19.2. Concept of ciliovitreal block as the mechanism of malignant glaucoma in aphakia. Apposition of ciliary processes against the anterior hyaloid **(arrows)** leads to posterior diversion of aqueous **(A)**, which causes a forward shift of the vitreous.

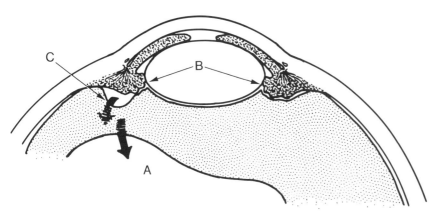

Figure 19.3. The anterior hyaloid may contribute to the ciliolenticular block **(B)**, and breaks in the hyaloid near the vitreous base **(C)** may allow the aqueous **(A)** to be diverted posteriorly **(arrows)**.

that the increased resistance might be due to compression of the vitreous as well as its displacement against the ciliary body, lens, and iris, thereby reducing the available area of anterior hyaloid through which fluid could flow.[19, 20] These clinical and laboratory observations support the concept that an intact anterior hyaloid may be important in preventing the forward movement of aqueous that has been trapped in or behind the vitreous.

2. *Slackness of lens zonules.* Chandler and Grant[21] have postulated that the forward movement of the lens-iris diaphragm in malignant glaucoma might be due to abnormal slackness or weakness of the zonules of the lens, as well as pressure from the vitreous. Others have also advocated this theory and suggested that the laxity of the zonules might be the result of severe, prolonged angle closure[8] or ciliary muscle spasm induced by surgery, miotics, inflammation, trauma, or unknown factors.[7] The concept that the lens subsequently pushes the peripheral iris into the anterior chamber angle, as noted earlier in this chapter, led to the proposed term, "*direct lens block angle closure.*"[7]

3. It seems very likely that malignant glaucoma is a multifactorial disease, in which elements of all the aforementioned mechanisms are involved to variable degrees.

D. Differential Diagnosis

The diagnosis of malignant glaucoma requires the exclusion of the following conditions, which can be facilitated by *surgical confirmation procedures*, when necessary.[4, 6]

1. *Pupillary block* is the most difficult entity to distinguish from malignant glaucoma, but must be ruled out before the latter diagnosis can be made. During slit lamp biomicroscopy, attention should be directed to two questions. First, is there moderate depth to the central anterior chamber with bowing of the peripheral iris into the chamber angle as with pupillary block, or is the entire lens-iris diaphragm shifted forward with marked shallowing or loss of the central anterior chamber as with malignant glaucoma? (Fig. 19.4) Second, and probably of more diagnostic value, is a patent iridectomy present? If the iridectomy is clearly patent, a pupillary block is unlikely. However, if patency cannot be confirmed, the diagnosis of pupillary block cannot be ruled out, and one should proceed with an iridectomy as a surgical confirmation procedure.

2. *Choroidal separation* is common after glaucoma filtering procedures and might be confused with malignant glaucoma due to the shallow or flat anterior chamber. However, these eyes are typically hypotonous and the light brown choroidal detachments are easily seen if there is adequate visibility of the posterior ocular segment. The surgical approach in this case is to make incisions through the scleral, usually in the inferior quadrants, to look for suprachoroidal fluid. If a characteristic straw-colored fluid is drained from the suprachoroidal space, the diagnosis of choroidal separation is made, and the procedure is completed by reforming the anterior chamber with air and/or saline.

3. *Suprachoroidal hemorrhage* may occur hours or days after ocular surgery and creates shallowing or loss of the anterior chamber associated with normal or elevated intraocular pressure. The eye is typically more inflamed than with choroidal detachment and the choroidal elevation is frequently dark reddish-brown. The surgical approach is the same as for choroidal detachments, except for the drainage of blood from the suprachoroidal space via the sclerotomies.

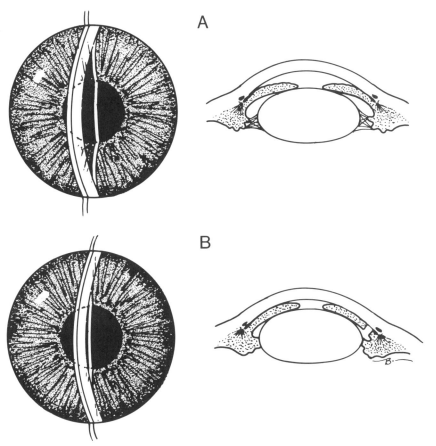

Figure 19.4. Slit-lamp biomicroscopic distinction between pupillary block glaucoma and malignant glaucoma. **A:** in pupillary block glaucoma, there is moderate depth to the central anterior chamber, with forward bowing of the peripheral iris and absence of a patent iridectomy; **B:** in malignant glaucoma, the entire lens-iris diaphragm is shifted forward with marked shallowing or loss of the central anterior chamber, and a patent peripheral iridectomy may be present.

E. Management

1. *Medical.* Chandler and Grant[21] reported in 1962 that mydriatic-cycloplegic treatment was effective in malignant glaucoma, and the following year, Weiss and co-workers[22] recommended the use of hyperosmotics to combat this condition. The value of a cycloplegic may be both to pull the lens back by tightening the zonules[21] and to break a ciliary block,[6] while the presumed benefit of a hyperosmotic is to reduce the pressure exerted by the vitreous.[22] These two measures, along with a carbonic anhydrase inhibitor to reduce the amount of aqueous that may be pooling posteriorly, constitute the standard medical approach to malignant glaucoma and may be used in the following manner[2-4]:

(a). Phenylephrine and atropine four times daily. (The patient is maintained on atropine indefinitely after the attack is broken to prevent recurrences.)

(b). Hyperosmotic agents (50% oral glycerol 1 ml/lb body weight or intravenous mannitol 2 g/kg body weight once to twice daily).

(c). Acetazolamide 250 mg orally four times daily.

2. *Surgical.* The above regimen is curative in approximately half of the cases within 5 days.[2-4] If the condition persists beyond this time, surgical intervention is usually indicated and consists of one or more of the following:

(a). *Posterior sclerotomy and air injection* (Fig. 19.5). A pars plana incision with aspiration of fluid from the vitreous and reformation of the anterior chamber with an air bubble has been advocated as the procedure of choice for classic malignant glaucoma.[2-4, 6] It has been suggested that the sclerotomy should be placed 3 mm posterior to the limbus to break the anterior hyaloid, thereby reducing its contribution to the blockade.[6] Postoperatively, the patients are generally maintained on atropine to avoid recurrence.

(b). *Lens extraction* is favored by some as the procedure of choice,[23] while others utilize this approach if the posterior sclerotomy and air injection fails. To be effective, lens extraction should be combined with an incision of the anterior hyaloid and possibly with deep incisions into fluid pockets in the vitreous.[2-4]

(c). *Vitrectomy* is the preferred procedure of some surgeons, especially in aphakic cases.[24, 25]

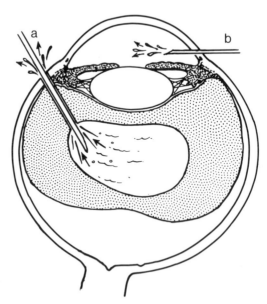

Figure 19.5. Posterior sclerotomy and air injection in the management of malignant glaucoma. Fluid is drained or aspirated from the vitreous via a pars plana incision **(a)**, and the anterior chamber is deepened with air **(b)**.

(d). *Laser photocoagulation* of ciliary processes as visualized through an iridectomy and followed by medical therapy is reported to have relieved cases of malignant glaucoma, possibly by breaking the ciliolenticular block.[26] Further evaluation of this therapeutic modality is needed to establish its efficacy and mechanism of action.[27]

(e). *Cyclocryotherapy* has also been advocated, with the presumed mechanism being alteration in the ciliary body or vitreous.[28]

(f). *Perilenticular incision* of the vitreous was described by Chandler,[29] but the procedure was generally abandoned due to the significant risks involved.

3. *Management of the fellow eye.*[2] When malignant glaucoma has occurred in one eye, there is a significant chance that it will develop in the fellow eye if surgery is performed following an acute angle closure attack. For this reason, it is best to do a prophylactic iridectomy early, and a laser iridectomy is probably the safest approach in these cases. However, if angle-closure glaucoma is present, every effort should be made to break the attack before surgery and, if the attack cannot be broken, mydriatic-cycloplegic therapy should be used vigorously post-iridectomy and continued indefinitely.

II. GLAUCOMAS IN APHAKIA

A. Terminology

Occasionally, the term "aphakic glaucoma" will be seen in the literature. It is mentioned in this text only to discourage its use, since it implies that a single form of glaucoma is associated with aphakia. As will be seen in the following discussion, there are many mechanisms by which cataract surgery can lead to glaucoma, and it is best to refer to these glaucomas in aphakia by terms which describe the particular events leading to the intraocular pressure elevation.

B. In Early Postoperative Period

1. *Transient intraocular pressure elevation with deep anterior chamber.*

(a). *General considerations.* A rise in intraocular pressure with a deep anterior chamber is not uncommon during the first several days after routine cataract extraction, although the frequency of this complication undoubtedly varies according to the surgical technique. Early studies in which the corneoscleral incision was approximated with various numbers of silk or gut sutures revealed no significant differences between pre- and postoperative pressures[30] and only occasional, minor fluctuations in tonographic facilities of outflow.[31] However, in a more recent series, in which a continuous fine perlon suture was used for wound closure, all eyes had a significant intraocular pressure rise within the first 24 hr after cataract extraction.[32]

The intraocular pressure has been noted to rise within 6 to 7 hr after routine cataract extraction,[32] and generally returns to normal within a week. A modest pressure rise is usually of no consequence, although high pressures may cause pain and occasional disruption of the corneoscleral wound. Furthermore, eyes with pre-existing glaucoma and advanced glaucomatous optic atrophy may not tolerate even short episodes of pressure elevation. In addition, anterior ischemic optic neuropathy has been reported to occur during these periods of elevated pressure in eyes with vulnerable optic nerve head circulation.[33]

(b). *Theories of mechanism.* The mechanism(s) responsible for the early, transient elevation of intraocular pressure following some cases of routine cataract extraction have not been fully established. There are most likely many factors involved, of which the following have been considered:

(1). *Distortion of the anterior chamber angle.* Kirsch and co-workers[34, 35] described the gonioscopic appearance of an *internal white ridge* resembling an inverted snow bank along the inner margins of the corneoscleral incision following routine cataract extraction. For about the first 2 weeks, the ridge typically obscures visualization of the trabecular meshwork and then gradually recedes over the next few months. There is some controversy regarding the pathogenesis of the internal ridge. Campbell and Grant[36] provided evidence that distortion of the anterior chamber angle might be induced by tight corneoscleral sutures. Kirsch and co-workers[35] could not confirm this, but suggested that edema of the deep corneal stroma was the mechanism. While the initiating factor(s) remain to be determined, the consequences of the ridge are known to include the formation of peripheral anterior synechiae, vitreous adhesions, and hyphema.[34] In addition, it is quite likely that the white ridge contributes, at least in some cases, to the early, transient pressure elevation after cataract surgery. In one study of 95 cataract extractions, early intraocular pressure rise occurred in 23% of the cases with limbal incisions, but in none with corneal incisions, suggesting that distortion produced by the corneoscleral wound temporarily influences the adjacent trabecular meshwork and aqueous outflow.[37]

(2). *Influence of α-chymotrypsin.* The enzyme, α-chymotrypsin, in dilutions of 1:5,000 to 1:10,000 rapidly produces a selective disintegration of lens zonules, which is characterized by fragmentation of the fibrils into uniform segments of approximately 1000 Å in length.[38] Barraquer,[39] in 1958, demonstrated the value of the enzymatic zonulolysis in facilitating cataract extraction, and the enzyme has since been commonly used for that purpose. In 1964, Kirsch[40] reported a study of 343 cataract extractions in which early, transient pressure rise occurred in 75% of the eyes in which 2 to 4 cc of a 1:5000 dilution of the enzyme was used, compared to a 24% incidence of high pressures in a group without enzyme. The complication was somewhat more common in patients with pre-existing open-angle glaucoma.[41] Tonographic studies showed a decrease in aqueous outflow facility,[42, 43] although no abnormal parameters were noted 2 to 4 months postoperatively.[44] The enzyme-induced pressure response has been produced experimentally in monkeys,[45-47] and histologic studies of these eyes suggested that the pressure rise was due to an accumulation of lens zonule fragments in the trabecular meshwork.[47, 48]

Based on the above clinical and laboratory observations, the term *"enzyme glaucoma"* is occasionally applied to those cases of early, transient intraocular pressure elevation with deep anterior chambers, in which the enzyme was used to facilitate lens extraction. However, it is still uncertain as to how important the enzyme is in causing this complication of cataract surgery. Several studies have noted no difference in the postoperative pressure course in groups with and without enzyme,[32, 37, 49, 50] even in eyes with pre-existing glaucoma.[51] It has been suggested that the volume or concentration of α-chymotrypsin might influence the enzyme-induced pressure response, in that eyes receiving 0.25 cc to 0.5 cc of 1:5000 to 1:10,000 dilution had pressure responses similar to cases without enzyme.[49, 50] Kirsch[52] also observed a dose relationship, but still found a 55% incidence of high pressures in the early postoperative period following the use of 0.25 cc of 1:5,000 α-chymotrypsin.

(2). *Inflammation and pigment dispersion.* Postoperative inflammation and dispersion of pigment from the iris occur to some degree after every cataract extraction. If either or both conditions are excessive, obstruction of the trabecular meshwork by inflammatory cells, fibrin, or pigment granules may lead to transient pressure elevations. The inflammatory response and secondary glaucoma may be particularly prominent when lens fragments are retained in the vitreous following extracapsular cataract extraction.[53]

(c). *Management.* If the early postoperative pressure rise is mild, anti-glaucoma medication may not be required. However, if there is pain or a threat to the optic nerve head, cornea, or cataract incision, temporary medical measures should be employed. Acetazolamide[54-56] and timolol[56-59] have been evaluated for efficacy in this specific clinical situation and, while the results are somewhat conflicting, both are generally felt to be useful in these cases. Pilocarpine was not felt to be of value in one study,[55] and epinephrine is generally avoided due to the danger of macular edema.[60] Steroids were reported to be ineffective in preventing "enzyme glaucoma,"[55] but may be helpful in controlling the pressure when inflammation is excessive. Indomethacin and aspirin have also been shown to reduce the postoperative pressure rise, presumably by inhibiting prostaglandin synthesis.[61] When uveitis and glaucoma are associated with retained lens fragments in the vitreous, pars plana vitrectomy is reported to yield good results.[53]

2. *Flat anterior chamber after cataract extraction.* Loss of the anterior chamber after cataract surgery may be associated with either hypotony or elevated intraocular pressure, both of which require prompt treatment to avoid permanent and serious sequelae.

(a). *Wound leak* is generally felt to be the most common cause of a flat anterior chamber after cataract extraction. It is often associated with *choroidal detachments*, which Chandler and Grant[62] have taught is due to hypotony from the wound leak. This leads to a vicious cycle, since the choroidal detachments cause decreased aqueous production with further hypotony and also contribute to the forward shift of the iris and vitreous. The mainstay of medical therapy is wide mydriasis to combat any pupillary block component, which may be present even in a hypotonous eye.[63] Topical steroids may help by minimizing synechiae formation, and hyperosmotics may lessen the forward bulge of vitreous by reducing vitreous volume. A flat anterior chamber should not be allowed to persist for more than 5 days due to the danger of peripheral anterior synechiae formation with subsequent chronic glaucoma.[62] If surgical intervention becomes necessary, the first step is to inspect the corneoscleral wound carefully for a leak, which may be easily overlooked. If a wound leak is present, it should be closed, and the anterior chamber reformed with air or saline. Drainage of choroidal detachments may also be required.

(b). *Glaucoma from pupillary block in aphakia* is a relatively rare complication of cataract extraction, but tends to occur more commonly with round pupil extractions.[64, 65] It is particularly likely to occur weeks after a transient flat anterior chamber secondary to the mechanisms noted above.[62] The condition is also more common following surgery for *congenital cataracts*, and a combination of sector and peripheral iridectomies with multiple sphincterotomies is reported to minimize this complication.[66]

The pathogenesis of pupillary block in aphakia is felt to be an adherence between the iris and anterior vitreous face, which prevents aqueous flow into the anterior chamber either through the pupil or iridectomy. The aqueous accumulates in pools behind the iris, causing a forward shift of the iris and closure of the anterior chamber angle (Fig. 19.6). The mechanism may be dependent on an intact anterior hyaloid, since fluorescein studies have shown that aqueous will flow through spontaneous openings in the vitreous face.[67] It may be possible to distinguish this condition from the much less common malignant glaucoma in aphakia by the deeper central anterior chamber and forward bowing of the peripheral iris in the former situation, although such a distinction is often difficult.

Treatment consists initially of mydriasis to relieve the pupillary block,[63-65] although an iridectomy or iridotomy is frequently required.[64, 65] To be effective, the iridectomy must be placed over a pocket of aqueous behind the iris, rather than an area in which the vitreous is in broad apposition to the posterior surface of the iris. The laser is particularly useful in these cases, since more than one iridectomy can be made until an aqueous pocket is found, as evidenced by a deepening of the peripheral anterior chamber. Suggested alternative surgical approaches include separating the iris from the vitreous adhesions with an iris repositor[68] and pars plana vitrectomy.[69]

3. *Vitreous filling the anterior chamber* was described by Grant[70] as a mechanism of acute open-angle glaucoma (Fig. 19.7). He reported

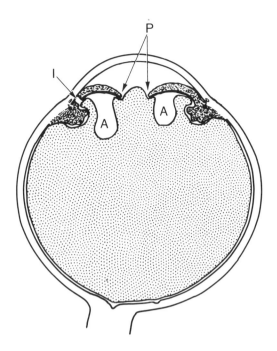

Figure 19.6. Pupillary block in aphakia. An adherence between the iris and anterior vitreous face blocks the flow of aqueous into the anterior chamber at both the pupil **(P)** and iridectomy site **(I)**. The posterior accumulation of aqueous **(A)** causes forward bowing of the peripheral iris with closure of the anterior chamber angle.

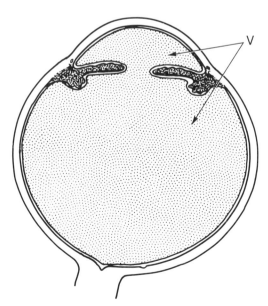

Figure 19.7. Vitreous **(V)** filling the anterior chamber as a mechanism of open-angle glaucoma in aphakia.

that this can be cured in some cases by mydriasis to minimize pupillary block, while other eyes require miosis to draw the vitreous from the angle. Simmons[71] noted that many cases will resolve spontaneously in several months. When surgical intervention is required, nearly all cases are relieved by iridectomy.

4. *Hemorrhage* as a mechanism of glaucoma following cataract surgery was discussed in Chapter 17. The bleeding may be seen immediately after surgery or may develop at a later date as new vessels begin to bridge the corneoscleral incision. When glaucoma secondary to blood in the anterior chamber is associated with vitreous hemorrhage, pars plana vitrectomy has been recommended.[72]

C. In Late Postoperative Period

Although most cases of intraocular pressure elevation after cataract surgery occur in the early postoperative period and are transient, a small number of eyes will retain a high pressure chronically after surgery despite a normal pre-operative tension, or will develop secondary glaucoma months or years after surgery.

1. *Peripheral anterior synechiae and/or trabecular damage.*

(a). *Clinical features and theories of mechanism.* In most cases of chronic glaucoma in aphakia, peripheral anterior synechiae are present, presumably due to a flat anterior chamber and/or excessive inflammation in the early postoperative period. In one series of 203 uncomplicated cataract extractions, 47% had some degree of peripheral anterior synechiae.[73] Secondary glaucoma occurred in 3% of the overall group, all of whom had goniosynechiae in more than one-fourth of the angle. However, in other cases of glaucoma in aphakia, the angle may be open in all quadrants and appear normal, except for variable degrees of increased pigmentation. This condition has also been described in patients years after surgery for congenital cataracts.[74] The mechanism of aqueous outflow obstruction in these cases is uncertain, but most likely relates to alterations within the trabecular meshwork as a result of the surgery, and possibly to a pre-existing reduction in outflow facility.

(b). *Management.* The majority of these cases can and should be managed medically. Miotic therapy is frequently effective, as is the use of drugs which reduce aqueous production, such as timolol and carbonic anhydrase inhibitors. Epinephrine is usually avoided due to the danger of macular edema.[60] Surgical intervention is reserved for cases that are uncontrolled on maximum tolerable medical therapy, since no procedure has been shown to be totally satisfactory in this situation. Filtering surgery often fails, presumably due to conjunctival scarring from the previous surgery and the influence of the vitreous. Operations that have been used for this form of chronic glaucoma in aphakia include cyclodialysis, cyclocryotherapy, and filtering surgery combined with partial or total vitrectomy.[75] In addition, favorable preliminary experience has been reported with transpupillary argon laser photocoagulation of the ciliary processes.[76]

2. *Epithelial ingrowth.* In this condition, an *epithelial membrane* grows into the eye through a penetrating wound. It extends over the posterior surface of the cornea, causing corneal edema, and also grows down across the anterior chamber angle and onto the iris, which may lead to secondary glaucoma. It is reported to occur in 0.09[77] to 0.11%[78] of eyes after cataract surgery, and has also been reported after penetrating trauma,[79, 80] penetrating keratoplasty,[81] and glaucoma surgery.[82]

(a). *Clinical features.* Early in the disease process, a wound leak may be demonstrated by the Seidel test. By slit-lamp biomicroscopy, the epithelial ingrowth on the cornea is seen as a thin gray translucent or transparent membrane with a scalloped, thickened leading edge.[79] Specular microscopy is reported to reveal a characteristic pattern of cell borders, which may have some diagnostic value.[82] The membrane on the iris is more difficult to see, but it typically causes a flattening of the stroma and can be delineated by the characteristic white burns that result from diagnostic laser photocoagulation.[83] Gonioscopy often reveals peripheral anterior synechiae, and glaucoma may be present. Cytologic evaluation of an aqueous aspirate has been described as a diagnostic aid,[84, 85] although the clinical features are usually sufficient to establish the diagnosis.

(b). *Theories of mechanism.* A wound leak is generally felt to be the initial factor leading to epithelial ingrowth, and is frequently seen at the time of diagnosis.[83, 86, 87] Reports differ as to whether the condition is more likely to occur with a fornix-based conjunctival flap during cataract surgery, as opposed to a limbus-based flap.[77, 78] Ultrastructural studies show well-developed epithelium, resembling that of the bulbar conjunctiva, growing over posterior cornea, anterior chamber angle, and the iris.[88–90] Several mechanisms have been proposed for the glaucoma secondary to epithelial ingrowth, including the growth of epithelium over the trabecular meshwork,[77, 91] areas of necrosis in the trabecular meshwork,[88] peripheral anterior synechiae,[77] pupillary block,[62] or desquamated epithelium in the aqueous outflow system.[91]

(c). *Management.* Epithelial ingrowth is generally a progressive and ultimately devastating condition, which usually requires radical surgical intervention. Maumenee[83] described a technique of excising the fistula and involved iris and destroying the epithelium on the posterior cornea with cryotherapy. Subsequent modifications have included *en bloc* excision of the involved chamber angle tissues,[92–94] excision of all involved tissue followed by keratoplasty,[93, 94] and the use of vitrectomy instruments to remove involved iris and vitreous.[87]

3. *Fibrous proliferation.* Two forms of this condition have been described[79]:

(a). *Fibrous ingrowth* is the result of inadequate wound closure after intraocular surgery or penetrating trauma. It has been reported to occur in approximately one-third of eyes enucleated after cataract extraction.[95–97] The hallmark of this form of fibrous proliferation is a break in the corneal endothelium and Descemet's membrane, which allows *fibroblasts* to enter the anterior chamber from subepithelial connective tissue[98] or from corneal or limbal stroma.[99, 100] The fibrous tissue, which is often vascularized, may grow over the corneal endothelium, the anterior chamber angle and iris, and into the vitreous cavity. Peripheral anterior synechiae are frequently seen in these cases.[100] Clinically, the condition may be difficult to distinguish from epithelial ingrowth, although it is usually less progressive and less destructive.[79] When glaucoma is present, it may either be the result of damage from the surgery or trauma or from the direct effect of the fibrous tissue in the anterior chamber angle. Treatment is generally confined to controlling the intraocular pressure, preferably with medications, although surgery, such as cyclocryotherapy, may be necessary.

(b). *Retrocorneal membranes* may result from a variety of inflammatory or traumatic insults to the cornea. Descemet's membrane is typically intact and the fibrous tissue is believed to represent metaplastic endothelial cells.[101] Glaucoma is not commonly associated, but may result from the initial insult.

4. *Proliferation of melanocytes* from the iris across the trabecular meshwork and posterior surface of the cornea has also been described as a mechanism of secondary glaucoma following cataract extraction.[102]

D. Glaucomas in Pseudophakia

The rapidly expanding use of intraocular lens implantation raises the following questions regarding glaucoma before and after cataract surgery: 1) Is it safe to implant a lens in an eye with pre-existing glaucoma? and 2) What additional forms of glaucoma after cataract extraction might be anticipated with lens implantation?

1. *Intraocular lens implantation in eyes with pre-existing glaucoma* is a controversial issue. Several investigators have concluded that it is a safe practice in well-controlled open-angle glaucoma.[103–107] Some even feel that the presence of chronic miosis is not a contraindication, since they perform a sector iridotomy to facilitate cataract delivery and then close the defect with polypropylene sutures before implanting the lens.[104] Herschler,[108] however, has provided several valid reasons for exercising extreme caution in these cases: 1) it is occasionally hard to anticipate the level of postoperative glaucoma control prior to cataract surgery, 2) the increased incidence of uveitis following some forms of lens implantation may be difficult to manage if the open-angle glaucoma patient is a steroid responder, 3) "non-absorbable" sutures in the iris may eventually absorb, and 4) glaucoma surgery in an eye with an intraocular lens may be more difficult. Drews[109] has also stated that "glaucoma remains a relative contraindication to lens implantation." More specifically, advanced glaucomas and most secondary forms of glaucoma are felt to be relative con-

traindications.[110] The presence of peripheral anterior synechiae is said to be a specific contraindication to lens implantation, since corneal endothelial loss, fibrous endothelial metaplasia, and angle cicatrization with glaucoma have been observed in such cases.[111]

2. *Glaucoma following lens implantation.* The reported incidence of secondary glaucoma after lens implantation is relatively low with the apparent exception of anterior chamber lenses.[112] In the interim Food and Drug Administration report, secondary glaucoma was reported in 6.3% of 6650 anterior chamber lenses, 3.9% of 14,360 with iris fixation, 2.1% of 5722 with iridocapsular fixation, and 3.5% of 1182 posterior chamber lens.[113] This is compared to a 3.6% incidence of glaucoma in 3132 cataract extractions without intraocular lens implantation.[113] The following specific forms of secondary glaucomas have been described in pseudophakic eyes:

(a). *Pupillary-block glaucoma* occurs primarily with anterior chamber or iris-supported intraocular lens.[114, 115] In a series of 106 eyes with iris-supported lens implants, four (3.8%) developed this form of secondary glaucoma.[114] The complication usually appears early in the postoperative course. The anterior chamber may be flat with an iris-supported lens, or the iris may be seen to bulge forward on either side of an anterior chamber lens. The condition may be aggravated by inflammation, hemorrhage, incarcerated vitreous, lens debris, and an incomplete or obstructed iridectomy.[114] Treatment should include mydriatic's to break the pupillary block, along with carbonic anhydrase inhibitors, hyperosmotic agents, and timolol. If medical therapy is inadequate, a laser or surgical iridectomy is usually effective. Success has also been reported with the use of laser to dilate the pupil in these cases.[116]

(b). *Uveitis, glaucoma, and hyphema* has been described as a syndrome in some cases of pseudophakia,[117] and has been called the "UGH" syndrome.[118] It is associated primarily with anterior chamber lens and appears to be related to the design and quality of specific lenses.[117, 118] The mechanism is felt to be contact of the rough posterior surface of the lens with the iris. Mild cases may be managed with mydriatics or miotic's to minimize iris movement against the lens. Steroids should be employed for the iritis and carbonic anhydrase inhibitors or timolol for the glaucoma. It has also been advised that bacteriologic studies should be obtained to rule out endophthalmitis when the inflammation is marked.[112] Recurrent hyphema and glaucoma is an indication to remove the lens.[118]

(c). *Steroid-induced glaucoma* is another mechanism that must be considered when prolonged treatment of postoperative uveitis is required.

(d). *Sodium hyaluronate* (Healon) is used by some surgeons to maintain a deep anterior chamber during implantation of the intraocular lens. This is reported to cause a marked elevation of the intraocular pressure during the first few postoperative days if it is not irrigated out before completion of the procedure.[119, 120]

III. GLAUCOMAS ASSOCIATED WITH PENETRATING KERATOPLASTY

A. Clinical Features

Penetrating keratoplasty, utilizing modern techniques of tight wound closure, is complicated by a significant incidence of intraocular pressure elevation in the early postoperative period.[121] In one series, the average maximum pressure in the first week was 24 mmHg in phakic eyes, 40 mmHg in aphakic cases, and 50 mmHg in those with combined keratoplasty and cataract extraction.[122] A significant number of patients will retain chronic pressure elevation after aphakic keratoplasty, especially if they had pre-existing glaucoma or an early postoperative pressure rise.[123] The incidence of secondary glaucoma is not only higher in aphakic eyes, but also following repeated penetrating keratoplasty.[124] Glaucoma after corneal grafting is dangerous not only from the standpoint of glaucomatous optic atrophy, but also from the high incidence of associated graft failures.[125, 126]

B. Theories of Mechanism

1. *In early postoperative period.* In some cases, the postoperative glaucoma after penetrating keratoplasty has the same pressure elevating mechanisms that are associated with other intraocular procedures, including uveitis, hemorrhage, pupillary block, and steroid-induced glaucoma.[127] However, additional mechanisms of secondary glaucoma occur early in the postoperative period, which are unique to eyes having undergone penetrating keratoplasty, especially when aphakia is also present. Two such mechanisms have been postulated.

(a). *Collapse of the trabecular meshwork* may result from the loss of anterior support, due to the incision in Descemet's membrane, which may be compounded in the aphakic eye by a reduction in posterior support from the loss of zonular tension.[128, 129] It was suggested that this hypothesis was supported by the observations that through-and-through suturing was associated with better facility of outflow in autopsy eyes[128] and lower early postoperative intraocular pressures as compared to eyes with conventional suturing.[129]

(b). *Compression of the anterior chamber angle* may be caused by the conventional techniques of penetrating keratoplasty, causing an early postoperative intraocular pressure rise as well as subsequent chronic glaucoma due to peripheral anterior synechiae.[130]

2. *In the late postoperative period.* Gradual flattening of the anterior chamber several months after aphakic keratoplasty has been described.[131] This phenomenon appeared to be related to an intact anterior vitreous face, and prophylactic vitrectomy has been suggested to avoid this complication. Another late-developing glaucoma occurs after keratoplasty for congenitally opaque corneas.[132] It is not associated with peripheral anterior synechiae, and the mechanism is unknown. Other forms of late-onset glaucoma may be due to peripheral anterior synechiae or steroid-induced glaucoma.[127]

C. Management

1. *Preventative measures.* Based on a mathematical model, it has been postulated that the following factors may minimize angle compression and also improve trabecular support: 1) a donor graft that is larger than the recipient trephine, 2) looser or shorter suture bites to minimize tissue compression, 3) smaller trephine size, 4) a thinner peripheral host cornea, and 5) a larger host corneal diameter.[130, 133] The concept that an oversized corneal donor graft improves outflow was not supported in a perfusion study with autopsy eyes.[134] However, one clinical study found that oversized grafts reduced the incidence of progressive angle closure,[135] while another investigation of aphakic eyes revealed significantly lower postoperative pressures with oversized grafts as compared to eyes with same sized grafts.[136] The use of through-and-through suturing and generous vitrectomy in aphakic eyes, as previously discussed, may also have value in preventing intraocular pressure elevation after penetrating keratoplasty. In addition, it has been emphasized that glaucoma following keratoplasty can be minimized by using meticulous wound closure, and extensive postoperative steroids.[137]

2. *Treatment of glaucoma.*

(a). *Medical therapy* should be tried first, unless a specific, treatable condition, such as pupillary block, is apparent.[121] However, attempts to alter the early postoperative pressure rise are frequently unsuccessful. Neither carbonic anhydrase inhibitors[138, 139] nor timolol[139] were significantly efficacious in this situation, although timolol was useful in controlling chronic glaucoma after keratoplasty, especially when used in combination with a miotic and a carbonic anhydrase inhibitor.[127] Hyperosmotic agents may be useful for the temporary control of extreme pressure elevation in the early postoperative period.[138] Miotics and epinephrine may also occasionally be of value.[121]

(b). *Surgical therapy* is indicated when either the optic nerve head or the graft is threatened by a persistent elevation of intraocular pressure. Cyclodialysis was successful in only 22 of 100 such cases in one study,[140] and another investigation found a 30% incidence of graft failure after any intraocular procedure.[141] *Cyclocryotherapy,* therefore, is the most commonly used surgical procedure for glaucoma following penetrating keratoplasty.[137, 142, 143]

IV. GLAUCOMAS ASSOCIATED WITH VITREOUS AND RETINAL PROCEDURES

A. Glaucomas Following Pars Plana Vitrectomy

1. *Incidence.* Intraocular pressure elevation is the most common major complication following pars plana vitreous surgery.[144-148] The reported incidence of postoperative glaucoma ranges from 20 to 26%.[146-148]

2. *Theories of mechanism.* Most of the factors that lead to intra-ocular pressure elevation after pars plana vitrectomy and the management of these conditions have been considered in other chapters. It may be helpful to review these various mechanisms according to the *time frame* in which they occur after vitreous surgery[147]:

(a). *First day*

(1). *Intraocular gas.* Air or sulfur hexafluoride, which occasionally is injected into the vitreous cavity to tamponade the retina, expands during the early postoperative period and not uncommonly leads to significant intraocular pressure elevation.[146, 147] Studies with living rabbit and enucleated human eyes indicate that the Schiøtz tonometer gives falsely low readings in this situation, and that applanation tonometry should be used to follow these cases.[149] Rarely, it is necessary to remove a portion of the gas to relieve extremely high intraocular pressures.[146]

(2). *Severe choroidal and ciliary body hemorrhage,* the equivalent of an expulsive hemorrhage in open-eye surgery, can cause angle closure glaucoma in the immediate postoperative period.[147]

(b). *First week.* Intraocular pressure elevation during this period is most likely due to one of the following, all of which are discussed in other chapters:

(1). Fresh hemorrhage, ghost cells, or hemolytic glaucoma (Chapter 17).

(2). Retained lens material with phacolytic glaucoma (Chapter 14).

(3). Uveitis (Chapter 16).

(4). Pre-existing glaucoma.

(c). *Two to four weeks* postoperatively, the cause of newly developed glaucoma is almost invariably *neovascular glaucoma,* which is discussed in Chapter 15.

B. Glaucoma Following Retinal Detachment Surgery

1. *Scleral buckling procedures* are reported to cause a transient shallowing of the anterior chamber and elevation of the intraocular pressure in 4 to 7% of the cases.[150-152] However, this is frequently asymptomatic and may go undetected unless slit lamp biomicroscopy and tonometry are performed in the early postoperative period. Experimental studies with monkeys suggest that occlusion of the vortex veins by an encircling band or sectorial scleral indentation causes congestion and forward rotation of the ciliary body with subsequent shallowing of the anterior segment.[153] The same study showed that occlusion of the vortex veins also caused the ciliary processes to produce a protein-rich aqueous, which might further reduce outflow.[153] Choroidal detachments are also commonly seen when the chamber is shallow and the pressure is elevated after retinal reattachment surgery.[151] These changes in the early postoperative period rarely lead to serious sequelae, although peripheral anterior synechiae may develop with subsequent chronic glaucoma. Suggested

treatment includes atropine to relieve ciliary muscle spasm and corticosteroids to reduce the inflammation and prevent synechia formation.[151] Carbonic anhydrase inhibitors, timolol, and epinephrine may be used when necessary for temporary pressure control. When surgical intervention is required, drainage of suprachoroidal fluid is said to be the procedure of choice.[152] A peripheral iridectomy is generally of no value in these cases.

2. *Other glaucoma mechanisms* include the use of *intraocular gas*, which was discussed earlier in this chapter, as well as the use of *silicone* as a retinal tamponade. In some eyes treated with intravitreal silicone, small bubbles of silicone will appear in the anterior chamber in either phakic or aphakic eyes.[154-156] In two series, this caused secondary glaucoma in a significant percentage of cases,[154, 155] although it had no influence on the intraocular pressure in another study.[156] *Steroid-induced glaucoma* is another mechanism that must be kept in mind if corticosteroid therapy is required for several weeks postoperatively.[151]

C. Glaucoma Following Retinal Photocoagulation

A transient shallowing of the anterior chamber, occasionally associated with elevated intraocular pressure, may follow extensive Xenon or laser photocoagulation of the retina.[157, 158] The mechanism is felt to be either swelling of the ciliary body[157] or an outpouring of fluid from the choroid to the vitreous with subsequent forward displacement of the lens-iris diaphragm.[158] The condition is temporary and should be managed medically in the same manner described for the early pressure rise and shallow anterior chamber after scleral buckling.

References

1. von Graefe, A: Beitrage zur pathologie und therapie des glaucoma. Archiv Fur Ophthal 15:108, 1869.
2. Chandler, PA, Simmons, RJ, Grant, WM: Malignant glaucoma. Medical and surgical treatment. Am J Ophthal 66:495, 1968.
3. Simmons, RJ: Malignant glaucoma. Br J Ophthal 56:263, 1972.
4. Simmons, RJ: Malignant glaucoma. In The Secondary Glaucomas, Ritch, R, Shields, MB, eds. CV Mosby Co, St Louis (in press).
5. Weiss, DI, Shaffer, RN: Ciliary block (malignant) glaucoma. Trans Am Acad Ophthal Otol 76:450, 1972.
6. Shaffer, RN, Hoskins, HD Jr: Ciliary block (malignant) glaucoma. Ophthalmology 85:215, 1978.
7. Levene, R: A new concept of malignant glaucoma. Arch Ophthal 87:497, 1972.
8. Lowe, RF: Malignant glaucoma related to primary angle closure glaucoma. Aust J Ophthal 7:11, 1979.
9. Pecora, JL: Malignant glaucoma worsened by miotics in a postoperative angle-closure glaucoma patient. Ann Ophthal 11:1412, 1979.
10. Rieser, JC, Schwartz, B: Miotic-induced malignant glaucoma. Arch Ophthal 87:706, 1972.
11. Merritt, JC: Malignant glaucoma induced by miotics postoperatively in open-angle glaucoma. Arch Ophthal 95:1988, 1977.
12. Jones, BR: Principles in the management of oculomycosis. Trans Am Acad Ophthal Otol 79:15, 1975.

13. Weiss, IS, Deiter, PD: Malignant glaucoma syndrome following retinal detachment surgery. Ann Ophthal 6:1099, 1974.
14. Schwartz, AL, Anderson, DR: "Malignant glaucoma" in an eye with no antecedent operation or miotics. Arch Ophthal 93:379, 1975.
15. Shaffer, RN: The role of vitreous detachment in aphakic and malignant glaucoma. Trans Am Acad Ophthal Otol 58:217, 1954.
16. Buschmann, W, Linnert, D: Echography of the vitreous body in case of aphakia and malignant aphakic glaucoma. Klin Monatsbl Augenheilkd 168:453, 1976.
17. Lippas, J: Mechanics and treatment of malignant glaucoma and the problem of a flat anterior chamber. Am J Ophthal 57:620, 1964.
18. Fatt, I: Hydraulic flow conductivity of the vitreous gel. Invest Ophthal Vis Sci 16:555, 1977.
19. Epstein, DL, Hashimoto, JM, Anderson, PF, Grant, WM: Experimental perfusions through the anterior and vitreous chambers with possible relationships to malignant glaucoma. Am J Ophthal 88:1078, 1979.
20. Quigley, HA: Malignant glaucoma and fluid flow rate (letter to editor). Am J Ophthal 89:879, 1980.
21. Chandler, PA, Grant, WM: Mydriatic-cycloplegic treatment in malignant glaucoma. Arch Ophthal 68:353, 1962.
22. Weiss, DI, Shaffer, RN, Harrington, DO: Treatment of malignant glaucoma with intravenous mannitol infusion. Medical reformation of the anterior chamber by means of an osmotic agent: a preliminary report. Arch Ophthal 69:154, 1963.
23. Bastian, A, Kohler, U: Therapy and functional results in malignant glaucoma. Klin Monatsbl Augenheilkd 161:316, 1972.
24. Sugar, HS: Bilateral aphakic malignant glaucoma. Arch Ophthal 87:347, 1972.
25. Koerner, FH: Anterior pars plana vitrectomy in ciliary and iris block glaucoma. Albrecht Graefes Arch Klin Exp Ophthal 214:119, 1980.
26. Herschler, J: Laser shrinkage of the ciliary processes. A treatment for malignant (ciliary block) glaucoma. Ophthalmology 87:1155, 1980.
27. Simmons, RJ: In Discussion of Herschler, J: Laser shrinkage of the ciliary processes. A treatment of malignant (ciliary block) glaucoma. Ophthalmology 87:1158, 1980.
28. Benedikt, O: A new operative method for the treatment of malignant glaucoma. Klin Monatsbl Augenheilkd 170:665, 1977.
29. Chandler, PA: A new operation for malignant glaucoma: A preliminary report. Tr Am Ophthal Soc 62:408, 1964.
30. Galin, MA, Baras, I, Perry, R: Intraocular pressure following cataract extraction. Arch Ophthal 66:80, 1961.
31. Lee, PF, Trotter, RR: Tonographic and gonioscopic studies before and after cataract extraction. Arch Ophthal 58:407, 1957.
32. Rich, WJ, Radtke, ND, Cohan, BE: Early ocular hypertension after cataract extraction. Br J Ophthal 58:725, 1974.
33. Hayreh, SS: Anterior ischemic optic neuropathy. IV. Occurrence after cataract extraction. Arch Ophthal 98:1410, 1980.
34. Kirsch, RE, Levine, O, Singer, JA: Ridge at internal edge of cataract incision. Arch Ophthal 94:2098, 1976.
35. Kirsch, RE, Levine, O, Singer, JA: Further studies on the ridge at the internal edge of the cataract incision. Trans Am Acad Ophthal Otol 83:224, 1977.
36. Campbell, DG, Grant, WM: Trabecular deformation and reduction of outflow facility due to cataract and penetrating keratoplasty sutures. Presented at Annual Meeting, Association for Research in Vision and Ophthalmology, Sarasota, Fla, April 25–29, 1977, abstract, p 126.
37. Rothkoff, L, Biedner, B, Blumenthal, M: The effect of corneal section on early increased intraocular pressure after cataract extraction. Am J Ophthal 85:337, 1978.
38. Ley, AP, Holmberg, AS, Yamashita, T: Histology of zonulolysis with alpha

chymotrypsin employing light and electron microscopy. Am J Ophthal 49:67, 1960.

39. Barraquer, J: Zonulolisis enzymatica. An Med Cirugia 34:148, 1958.
40. Kirsch, RE: Glaucoma following cataract extraction associated with use of alpha-chymotrypsin. Arch Ophthal 72:612, 1964.
41. Lantz, JM, Quigley, JH: Intraocular pressure after cataract extraction: Effects of alpha chymotrypsin. Can J Ophthal 8:339, 1973.
42. Kirsch, RE: Further studies on glaucoma following cataract extraction associated with the use of alpha-chymotrypsin. Trans Am Acad Ophthal Otol 69:1011, 1965.
43. Galin, MA, Barasch, KR, Harris, LS: Enzymatic zonulolysis and intraocular pressure. Am J Ophthal 61:690, 1966.
44. Jocson, VL: Tonography and gonioscopy: before and after cataract extraction with alpha chymotrypsin. Am J Ophthal 60:318, 1965.
45. Kalvin, NH, Hamasaki, DI, Gass, JDM: Experimental glaucoma in monkeys. I. Relationship between intraocular pressure and cupping of the optic disc and cavernous atrophy of the optic nerve. Arch Ophthal 76:82, 1966.
46. Lessell, S, Kuwabara, T: Experimental alpha-chymotrypsin glaucoma. Arch Ophthal 81:853, 1969.
47. Anderson, DR: Experimental alpha chymotrypsin glaucoma studied by scanning electron microscopy. Am J Ophthal 71:470, 1971.
48. Anderson, DR: Scanning electron microscopy of zonulolysis by alpha chymotrypsin. Am J Ophthal 71:619, 1971.
49. Barraquer, J, Rutllan, J: Enzymatic zonulolysis and postoperative ocular hypertension. Am J Ophthal 63:159, 1967.
50. Skalka, HW: Alpha-chymotrypsin glaucoma. Ann Ophthal 8:149, 1976.
51. Gombos, GM, Oliver, M: Cataract extraction with enzymatic zonulolysis in glaucomatous eyes. Am J Ophthal 64:68, 1968.
52. Kirsch, RE: Dose relationship of alpha chymotrypsin in production of glaucoma after cataract extraction. Arch Ophthal 75:774, 1966.
53. Hutton, WL, Snyder, WB, Vaiser, A: Management of surgically dislocated intravitreal lens fragments by pars plana vitrectomy. Ophthalmology 85:176, 1978.
54. Biedner, B, Rothkoff, L, Blumenthal, M: The effect of acetazolamide on early increased intraocular pressure after cataract extraction. Am J Ophthal 83:565, 1977.
55. Bloomfield, S: Failure to prevent enzyme glaucoma. A negative report. Am J Ophthal 64:405, 1968.
56. Packer, AJ, Fraioli, AJ, Epstein, DL: The effect of timolol and acetazolamide on transient intraocular pressure elevation following cataract extraction with alpha-chymotrypsin. Ophthalmology 88:239, 1981.
57. Obstbaum, SA, Galin, MA: The effects of timolol on cataract extraction and intraocular pressure. Am J Ophthal 88:1017, 1979.
58. Braverman, SD, Shields, MB: Efficacy of timolol in controlling intraocular pressure elevation after cataract extraction. Presented at Annual Meeting American Academy of Ophthalmology, San Francisco, Nov 5-9, 1979.
59. Haimann, MH, Phelps, CD: Prophylactic timolol for the prevention of high intraocular pressure after cataract extraction. A randomized, prospective, double-blind study. Ophthalmology 88:233, 1981.
60. Kolker, AE, Becker, B: Epinephrine maculopathy. Arch Ophthal 79:552, 1968.
61. Rich, WJCC: Prevention of postoperative ocular hypertension by prostaglandin inhibitors. Trans Ophthal Soc UK 97:268, 1977.
62. Chandler, PA, Grant, WM: Glaucoma, 2nd ed. Lea & Febiger, Philadelphia, 1979, p 224.
63. Weisel, J, Swan, KC: Mydriatic treatment of shallow chamber after cataract extraction. Arch Ophthal 58:126, 1957.
64. Chandler, PA: Glaucoma from pupillary block in aphakia. Arch Ophthal 67:14,

1962.

65. Chandler, PA: Glaucoma in aphakia. Trans Am Acad Ophthal Otol 67:483, 1963.
66. Chandler, PA: Surgery of congenital cataract. Trans Am Acad Ophthal Otol 72:341, 1968.
67. Zauberman, H, Yassur, Y, Sachs, U: Fluorescein pupillary flow in aphakics with intact and spontaneous openings of the vitreous face. Br J Ophthal 61:450, 1977.
68. Hitchings, RA: Acute aphakic pupil block glaucoma: an alternative surgical approach. Br J Ophthal 63:31, 1979.
69. Peyman, GA, Sanders, DR, Minatoya: Pars plana vitrectomy in the management of pupillary block glaucoma following irrigation and aspiration. Br J Ophthal 62:336, 1978.
70. Grant, WM: Open-angle glaucoma associated with vitreous filling the anterior chamber. Tr Am Ophthal Soc 61:196, 1963.
71. Simmons, RJ: The vitreous in glaucoma. Trans Ophthal Soc UK 95:422, 1975.
72. Brucker, AJ, Michels, RG, Green, WR: Pars plana vitrectomy in the management of blood-induced glaucoma with vitreous hemorrhage. Ann Ophthal 10:1427, 1978.
73. Racz, P, Szilvassy, I, Pinter, E: Findings in the anterior chamber angle after cataract extraction without complication. Klin Monatsbl Augenheilkd 164:218, 1974.
74. Phelps, CD, Arafat, NI: Open-angle glaucoma following surgery for congenital cataracts. Arch Ophthal 95:1985, 1977.
75. Herschler, J: The effect of total vitrectomy on filtration surgery in the aphakic eye. Ophthalmology 88:229, 1981.
76. Lee, PF: Argon laser photocoagulation of the ciliary processes in cases of aphakic glaucoma. Arch Ophthal 97:2135, 1979.
77. Bernardino, VB, Kim, JC, Smith, TR: Epithelialization of the anterior chamber after cataract extraction. Arch Ophthal 82:742, 1969.
78. Theobald, GD, Haas, JS: Epithelial invasion of the anterior chamber following cataract extraction. Trans Am Acad Ophthal Otol 52:470, 1948.
79. Stark, WJ, Bruner, W: Glaucoma Secondary to Epithelial Downgrowth and Fibrous Proliferation. In The Secondary Glaucomas, Ritch, R, Shields, MB, eds. CV Mosby Co, St Louis (in press).
80. Eldrup-Jorgensen, P: Epithelialization of the anterior chamber. A clinical and histopathological study of a Danish material. Acta Ophthal 47:328, 1969.
81. Sugar, A, Meyer, RF, Hood, CI: Epithelial downgrowth following penetrating keratoplasty in the aphake. Arch Ophthal 95:464, 1977.
82. Smith, RE, Parrett, C: Specular microscopy of epithelial downgrowth. Arch Ophthal 96:1222, 1978.
83. Maumenee, AE: Treatment of epithelial downgrowth and intraocular fistula following cataract extraction. Tr Am Ophthal Soc 62:153, 1964.
84. Calhoun, FP Jr: An aid to the clinical diagnosis of epithelial downgrowth into the anterior chamber following cataract extraction. Am J Ophthal 61:1055, 1966.
85. Verrey, F: Invasion epitheliale de la chambre anterieure: confirmation anatomique par l'examen cytologique de l'humeur aqueuse. Ophthalmologica 153:467, 1967.
86. Maumenee, AE, Paton, D, Morse, PH, Butner, R: Review of 40 histologically proven cases of epithelial downgrowth following cataract extraction and suggested surgical management. Am J Ophthal 69:598, 1970.
87. Stark, WJ, Michels, RG, Maumenee, AE, Cupples, H: Surgical management of epithelial ingrowth. Am J Ophthal 85:772, 1978.
88. Jensen, P, Minckler, DS, Chandler, JW: Epithelial ingrowth. Arch Ophthal 95:837, 1977.
89. Iwamoto, T, Srinivasan, BD, DeVoe, AG: Electron microscopy of epithelial downgrowth. Ann Ophthal 9:1095, 1977.
90. Zavala, EY, Binder, PS: The pathologic findings of epithelial ingrowth. Arch Ophthal 98:2007, 1980.

91. Terry, TL, Chisholm, JF Jr, Schonberg, AL: Studies on surface-epithelium invasion of the anterior segment of the eye. Am J Ophthal 22:1083, 1939.
92. Brown, SI: Treatment of advanced epithelial downgrowth. Trans Am Acad Ophthal Otol 77:618, 1973.
93. Brown, SI: Results of excision of advanced epithelial downgrowth. Ophthalmology 86:321, 1979.
94. Friedman, AH: Radical anterior segment surgery for epithelial invasion of the anterior chamber: report of three cases. Trans Am Acad Ophthal Otol 83:216, 1977.
95. Dunnington, JH: Wound rupture with tissue incarceration. In Symposium on Diseases and Surgery of the Lens. CV Mosby Co, St Louis, 1957, p 161.
96. Allen, JC: Epithelial and stromal ingrowths. Am J Ophthal 65:179, 1968.
97. Bettman, JW Jr: Pathology of complications of intraocular surgery. Am J Ophthal 68:1037, 1969.
98. Swan, KC: Fibroblastic ingrowth following cataract extraction. Arch Ophthal 89:445, 1973.
99. Sherrard, ES, Rycroft, PV: Retrocorneal membranes. II. Factors influencing their growth. Br J Ophthal 51:387, 1967.
100. Friedman, AH, Henkind, P: Corneal stromal overgrowth after cataract extraction. Br J Ophthal 54:528, 1970.
101. Michels, RG, Kenyon, KR, Maumenee, AE: Retrocorneal fibrous membrane. Invest Ophthal 11:822, 1972.
102. Ueno, H, Green, WR, Kenyon, KR, Hoover, RE: Trabecular and retrocorneal proliferation of melanocytes and secondary glaucoma. Am J Ophthal 88:592, 1979.
103. Smith, JA, Anderson, DR: Effect of the intraocular lens on intraocular pressure. Arch Ophthal 94:1291, 1976.
104. Clayman, HM, Jaffe, NS, Light, DS, Eichenbaum, DM: Lens implantation, miosis, and glaucoma. Am J Ophthal 87:121, 1979.
105. Taylor, DM, Stern, AL: Long-term follow-up of 43 intraocular lenses in eyes with primary glaucoma. AM Intra-ocular Implant Soc J 5:313, 1979.
106. Smith, JA: Glaucoma and the intraocular lens. Ann Ophthal 11:1853, 1979.
107. Taylor, DM, Dalburg, LA, Consentino, RT, Khaliq, A: Intraocular lenses: 500 consecutive intracapsular cataract extractions with lens implantation compared with 500 intracapsular extractions—observations and comments. Ophthal Surg 9:29, 1978.
108. Herschler, J: Glaucoma and the intraocular lens. Ann Ophthal 11:1057, 1979.
109. Drews, RC: Lens implantation in patients with glaucoma. Ophthalmology 87:665, 1980.
110. Layden, WE: Glaucomas following intraocular lens implantation. In The Secondary Glaucomas, Ritch, R, Shields, MB, eds. CV Mosby Co, St Louis (in press).
111. Rowsey, JJ, Gaylor, JR: Intraocular lens disasters. Peripheral anterior synechia. Ophthalmology 87:646, 1980.
112. Polack, FM: Management of anterior segment complications of intraocular lenses. Ophthalmology 87:881, 1980.
113. Worthen, DM, Boucher, JA, Buxton, JN, Hayreh, SS, Lowther, G, Reinecke, RD, Spencer, WH, Talbott, M, Weeks, DF: Interim FDA report on intraocular lenses. Ophthalmology 87:267, 1980.
114. Werner, D, Kaback, M: Pseudophakic pupillary-block glaucoma. Br J Ophthal 61:329, 1977.
115. Ferayorni, JJ: Intraocular lenses and secondary glaucoma: A retrospective study. Ann Ophthal 10:1447, 1978.
116. Obstbaum, SA, Galin, MA, Barasch, KR, Baras, I: Laser photomydriasis in pseudophakic pupillary block. AM Intra-ocular Implant Soc J 7:28, 1981.
117. Ellingson, FT: The uveitis-glaucoma-hyphema syndrome associated with the Mark-VII Choyce anterior chamber lens implant. AM Intra-ocular Implant Soc J 4:50, 1978.

118. Keates, RH, Ehrlich, DR: "Lenses of chance" complications of anterior chamber implants. Ophthalmology 85:408, 1978.
119. Binkhorst, CD: Inflammation and intraocular pressure after the use of Healon in intraocular lens surgery. AM Intra-ocular Implant Soc J 6:340, 1980.
120. Pape, LG: Intracapsular and extracapsular technique of lens implantation with Healon. Am Intra-ocular Implant Soc J 6:342, 1980.
121. Sugar, A: Glaucoma Following Penetrating Keratoplasty. In The Secondary Glaucomas, Ritch, R, Shields, MB, eds. The CV Mosby Co, St Louis (in press).
122. Irvine, AR, Kaufman, HE: Intraocular pressure following penetrating keratoplasty. Am J Ophthal 68:835, 1969.
123. Olson, RJ, Kaufman, HE: Prognostic factors of intraocular pressure after aphakic keratoplasty. Am J Ophthal 86:510, 1978.
124. Robinson, CH Jr: Indications, complications and prognosis for repeat penetrating keratoplasty. Ophthal Surg 10:27, 1979.
125. Heydenreich, A: Corneal regeneration and intraocular tension. Klin Monatsbl Augenheilkd 148:500, 1966.
126. Fine, M: Problems of keratoplasty in aphakic eyes. In Castroviejo, R, et al.: Symposium on the Cornea. CV Mosby Co, St Louis, 1972, p 144.
127. Lass, JH, Pavan-Langston, D: Timolol therapy in secondary angle-closure glaucoma post penetrating keratoplasty. Ophthalmology 86:51, 1979.
128. Zimmerman, TJ, Krupin, T, Grodzki, W, Waltman, SR: The effect of suture depth on outflow facility in penetrating keratoplasty. Arch Ophthal 96:505, 1978.
129. Zimmerman, TJ, Waltman, SR, Sachs, U, Kaufman, HE: Intraocular pressure after aphakic penetrating keratoplasty "through-and-through" suturing. Ophthal Surg 10:49, 1979.
130. Olson, RJ, Kaufman, HE: A mathematical description of causative factors and prevention of elevated intraocular pressure after keratoplasty. Invest Ophthal Vis Sci 16:1085, 1977.
131. Gnad, HD: Athalamia as a late complication after keratoplasty on aphakic eyes. Br J Ophthal 64:528, 1980.
132. Schanzlin, DJ, Goldberg, DB, Brown, SI: Transplantation of congenitally opaque corneas. Ophthalmology 87:1253, 1980.
133. Olson, RJ: Aphakic keratoplasty. Determining donor tissue size to avoid elevated intraocular pressure. Arch Ophthal 96:2274, 1978.
134. Zimmerman, TJ, Krupin, T, Grodzki, W, Waltman, SR, Kaufman, HE: Size of donor corneal button and outflow facility in aphakic eyes. Ann Ophthal 11:809, 1979.
135. Foulks, GN, Perry, HD, Dohlman, CH: Oversize corneal donor grafts in penetrating keratoplasty. Ophthalmology 86:490, 1979.
136. Zimmerman, T, Olson, R, Waltman, S, Kaufman, H: Transplant size and elevated intraocular pressure. Postkeratoplasty. Arch Ophthal 96:2231, 1978.
137. Thoft, RA, Gordon, JM, Dohlman, CH: Glaucoma following keratoplasty. Trans Am Acad Ophthal Otol 78:352, 1974.
138. Wood, TO, West, C, Kaufman, HE: Control of intraocular pressure in penetrating keratoplasty. Am J Ophthal 74:724, 1972.
139. Olson, RJ, Kaufman, HE, Zimmerman, TJ: Effects of timolol and Daranide on elevated intraocular pressure after aphakic keratoplasty. Ann Ophthal 11:1833, 1979.
140. Casey, TA, Gibbs, D: Complications in corneal grafting. Trans Ophth Soc UK 92:517, 1972.
141. Lemp, MA, Pfister, RR, Dohlman, CH: The effect of intraocular surgery on clear corneal grafts. Am J Ophthal 70:719, 1970.
142. Binder, PS, Abel, R Jr, Kaufman, HE: Cyclocryotherapy for glaucoma after penetrating keratoplasty. Am J Ophthal 79:489, 1975.
143. Maumenee, AE: Recent advances in corneal transplantation. Trans Ophthal Soc UK 96:462, 1976.

144. Wilensky, JT, Goldberg, MF, Alward, P: Glaucoma after pars plana vitrectomy. Trans Am Acad Ophthal Otol 83:114, 1977.
145. Huamonte, FU, Peyman, GA, Goldberg, MF: Complicated retinal detachment and its management with pars plana vitrectomy. Br J Ophthal 61:754, 1977.
146. Faulborn, J, Conway, BP, Machemer, R: Surgical complications of pars plana vitreous surgery. Ophthalmology 85:116, 1978.
147. Aaberg, TM, Van Horn, DL: Late complications of pars plana vitreous surgery. Ophthalmology 85:126, 1978.
148. Ghartey, KN, Tolentino, FI, Freeman, HM, McMeel, JW, Schepens, CL, Aiello, LM: Closed vitreous surgery. XVII. Results and complications of pars plana vitrectomy. Arch Ophthal 98:1248, 1980.
149. Aronowitz, JD, Brubaker, RF: Effect of intraocular gas on intraocular pressure. Arch Ophthal 94:1191, 1976.
150. Sebestyen, JG, Schepens, CL, Rosenthal, ML: Retinal detachment and glaucoma. I. Tonometric and gonioscopic study of 160 cases. Arch Ophthal 67:736, 1962.
151. Phelps, CD: Glaucomas associated with diseases of the retina. In The Secondary Glaucomas, Ritch, R, Shields, MB, eds. CV Mosby Co, St Louis (in press).
152. Simmons, RJ: Angle-closure glaucoma after scleral buckling operations for separated retina. In Glaucoma, 2nd ed, Chandler, PA, Grant, WM, eds. Lea & Febiger, Philadelphia, 1979, p 183.
153. Hayreh, SS, Baines, JAB: Occlusion of the vortex veins. An experimental study. Br J Ophthal 57:217, 1973.
154. Okun, E: Intravitreal surgery utilizing liquid silicone. A long term follow-up. Trans Pac Coast Oto-Ophthal Soc 49:141, 1968.
155. Grey, RHB, Leaver, PK: Results of silicone oil injection in massive preretinal retraction. Trans Ophthal Soc UK 97:238, 1977.
156. Watzke, RC: Silicone retinopiesis for retinal detachment. A long-term clinical evaluation. Arch Ophthal 77:185, 1967.
157. Mensher, JH: Anterior chamber depth alteration after retinal photocoagulation. Arch Ophthal 95:113, 1977.
158. Boulton, PE: A study of the mechanisms of transient myopia following extensive Xenon Arc photocoagulation. Trans Ophth Soc UK 93:287, 1973.

Chapter 20

STEROID-INDUCED GLAUCOMA

STEROID-INDUCED GLAUCOMA

In the discussion of primary open-angle glaucoma (Chapter 7), it was noted that a certain percentage of the general population will respond to repeated instillation of topical corticosteroids with a variable increase in the intraocular pressure. It was also pointed out that this occurs more commonly in individuals who have primary open-angle glaucoma or a family history of the disease. There are many unknown facets regarding the pressure response to steroids, such as the precise distribution of steroid responders in the general population, the reproducibility of these responses, and hereditary influence. Nevertheless, the critical fact is that certain people do manifest this response to chronic steroid therapy, and the intraocular pressure elevation can lead to glaucomatous optic atrophy and loss of vision. Such a condition is referred to as steroid-induced glaucoma.

I. HISTORICAL BACKGROUND

In 1950, McLean[1] reported intraocular pressure rise in response to the systemic administration of ACTH for the treatment of uveitis. Francois,[2] in 1954, noted that a similar elevation in tension could occur after local therapy with cortisone. Numerous reports followed these early observations, which confirmed that intraocular pressure rise may occur with topical, systemic, or periocular administration of corticosteroids, although more often after local therapy. This extensive literature has been well reviewed.[3]

II. CLINICAL FEATURES

A. Forms of Steroid-induced Glaucoma

Francois[4] has described two clinical forms of steroid-induced glaucoma:

1. *Chronic*. This is usually caused by topical steroid therapy and may develop within a few weeks with potent corticosteroids or in months with the weaker steroids. The clinical picture typically resembles that of primary open-angle glaucoma with an open, normal appearing anterior chamber angle and absence of symptoms.

2. *Acute*. Much less often, the condition may have the clinical presentation of acute angle-closure glaucoma except for an open angle. This has been seen with intensive systemic steroid therapy or the topical use of potent corticosteroids.

B. Variations

Variations of the above clinical forms depend on the patient's age and the condition of the eyes. Although children are reported to have a lower incidence of positive steroid responders than adults,[5] glaucoma has been precipitated or caused by treating external diseases in infants with corticosteroids.[6] It has also been reported that intraocular pressure elevation may occur in the first few weeks after a trabeculectomy despite a good filtering bleb.[7] Since the patients were receiving topical steroids, the authors suggested a steroid-induced mechanism of pressure elevation,[7] although further study is needed to establish such a cause-and-effect relationship.[8] In eyes with well-established filtering procedures, topical corticosteroids have been reported to increase the facility of aqueous outflow and reduce the intraocular pressure.[9] Another clinical variation of steroid-induced glaucoma is apparent low-tension glaucoma, which may result when the steroid-induced pressure elevation has damaged the optic nerve head and visual field and then returned to normal with cessation of the drug.[10]

III. THEORIES OF MECHANISM

It is generally agreed that the intraocular pressure elevation due to steroid administration results from reduction in facility of aqueous outflow.[11-14] In the rabbit eye, intravenously administered glucocorticoids are specifically bound in the nuclei of cells in the outflow pathway, suggesting that these may be target cells in the steroid-induced mediation of reduced outflow facility.[15] The precise mechanism responsible for the obstruction to outflow is unknown, but the following theories have been suggested:

A. Mucopolysaccharide Theory

Acid mucopolysaccharides (or glycosaminoglycans) are normally present in the aqueous outflow system. Francois[16-18] has postulated that mucopolysaccharides in the polymerized form become hydrated, producing a "biological edema" which may increase resistance to aqueous outflow. Catabolic enzymes, within lysosomes, depolymerize the mucopolysaccharides. Corticosteroids stabilize the lysosomal membrane, which leads to an accumulation of polymerized mucopolysaccharides in the trabecular meshwork. Francois has also suggested that the lysosomes reside primarily in fibroblasts in the meshwork, which he has called goniocytes. He feels that clones of goniocytes may have variable sensitivity to corticosteroids, accounting for the differences in individual pressure responses. Examinations of trabecular specimens from patients with steroid-induced glaucoma have been inconclusive, but there is some evidence, both in human eyes[19] as well as in experimental rabbit studies,[20] that an excess accumulation of mucopolysaccharides in the aqueous outflow system may be an important factor in steroid-induced glaucoma.

B. Suppressed Phagocytosis

Endothelial cells lining the trabecular meshwork have phagocytic properties, which may help to clean the aqueous of debris before it reaches the inner wall of Schlemm's canal. Corticosteroids are known to suppress phagocytic activity, and the possibility has been raised that suppressed phagocytosis by the trabecular endothelium may allow debris in the aqueous to accumulate in the meshwork and act as a barrier to outflow.[21] This theory is consistent with ultrastructural studies showing marked depositions of amorphous and fibrous or linear material in the juxtacanalicular meshwork of eyes with steroid-induced glaucoma.[22, 23]

C. Additional Observations

It has been observed in rabbits that long-term topical steroid administration is associated with a shift toward an alkaline aqueous and reduced ascorbic acid content.[24, 25] The authors suggest that these changes may be related to steroid-induced glaucoma, although more study is needed to establish this theory.

Additional ocular repsonses that may occur in some individuals on chronic topical corticosteroid therapy include a slight mydriasis and ptosis, and an increase in corneal thickness.[12] However, none of these changes appear to correlate with the intraocular pressure response.[12, 26]

IV. PREVENTION

To avoid loss of vision from steroid-induced glaucoma, the physician must know how to prevent or minimize the chances of its occurrence. This requires close attention to the patient's history and to the selection and use of steroids.

A. Patient Selection

As noted, individuals with primary open-angle glaucoma or a family history of the disease are more likely to respond to chronic steroid therapy with a significant rise in intraocular pressure. In addition, it has been noted that high myopes[27] and diabetics[28] have a similar predisposition. These patients, therefore, are at a somewhat higher risk of developing steroid-induced glaucoma. However, since it is not possible to predict which individuals without these predisposing factors will also have a pressure rise, all patients must be treated cautiously. This involves avoiding steroids when a safer drug will suffice, using the least amount of steroid necessary, establishing a baseline intraocular pressure before initiating therapy, and monitoring the tension closely for the duration of the corticosteroid therapy.

B. Drug Selection

When corticosteroid therapy is required for any disorder, the optimum drug is the one which will achieve the desired therapeutic response by the safest route of administration, in the lowest concentration, and with the fewest potential adverse reactions. With regard to the intraocular pressure response, the following facts should be considered:

1. *Routes of administration*

    a. *Topical* corticosteroid therapy is more often associated with an intraocular pressure rise than is the case with systemic administration. This may occur not only with drops or ointment applied directly to the eye, but also with steroid preparations used in treating the skin of the eyelids.[29, 30]

    b. *Periocular* injection is the most dangerous route of corticosteroid administration from the standpoint of steroid-induced glaucoma. Intraocular pressure elevation may occur in response to subconjunctival, sub-Tenons, or retrobulbar injections of steroids.[31-34] The patient's response to earlier topical steroid therapy does not always predict how he will respond to periocular corticosteroids.[34] Repository steroids are particularly dangerous because of their prolonged duration of action, and it may occasionally be necessary to surgically excise the remaining drug before the pressure can be brought under control.[33, 34] If repository steroids must be used, they should be injected in an inferior quadrant to avoid compromising the superior sites for possible future filtering surgery.

    c. *Systemic* administration of corticosteroids is least likely to induce glaucoma, although cases have been described.[35-38] It is reported that this response does not correlate with the dosage or duration of treatment, but is associated with the degree of pressure response to topical steroids.[37, 38] It has been noted that amounts of corticosteroids, sufficient to influence the intraocular pressure, can be absorbed from skin application in areas remote from the eyes.[19]

2. *Relative pressure-inducing effects of topical steroids.* Although topical corticosteroids are more likely to cause an elevation of the intraocular pressure than are systemic steroids, the topical route of administration is still generally preferred to avoid the additional dangers associated with systemic corticosteroid therapy. While no topical steroid is totally free of a pressure-inducing effect, the following observations have been reported regarding the relative tendencies of these drugs to induce an elevation in the intraocular pressure:

    a. *Potent corticosteroids.* In general, the anti-inflammatory potency of a topical steroid is proportional to its pressure-inducing effect. *Betamethasone, dexamethasone, prednisolone,* and *flurandrenolide*[39] represent the end of the spectrum with the highest of both properties. However, as might be anticipated, the pressure-inducing potency is related to the dosage of the drug. In a study of high topical steroid responders, betamethasone 0.01% caused significantly less pressure elevation than the 0.1% concentration.[40] In addition, the formulation may cause some dissociation of anti-inflammatory and pressure-inducing effects. In a rabbit study, dexamethasone acetate 0.1% had a better anti-inflammatory effect than dexamethasone alcohol 0.1% or dexamethasone sodium phosphate 0.1%, while the acetate and sodium phosphate preparations had the same effect on intraocular pressure elevation in humans.[41]

b. *Weaker corticosteroids.* A newer corticosteroid with high topical activity, *clobetasone butyrate 0.1%*, was found to be comparable to prednisolone phosphate 0.5% in both anti-inflammatory and pressure-inducing effects,[42] while it had significantly less of each property as compared to betamethasone phosphate 0.1%.[42, 43]

c. *Non-adrenal steroids.* A group of drugs, closely related to progesterone, have been shown to have useful anti-inflammatory properties with significantly less pressure-inducing effects than most corticosteroids. *Medrysone* is primarily of value in the treatment of extraocular disorders, since it has limited corneal penetration. However, it has been claimed to be effective in treating iritis.[44] Most reports describe little or no intraocular pressure elevation,[44–46] although a slight pressure response in some patients has been observed.[40, 47] *Fluorometholone* is more effacacious than medrysone in treating inflammation of the anterior ocular segment. Although the pressure-inducing effect of fluoromethalone is substantially less than that of the potent corticosteroids,[47, 48] significant pressure rises have been observed with the use of this drug,[49] and the same precautions must be taken with the non-adrenal steroids as with the corticosteroids.

V. MANAGEMENT

A. Discontinuation of the Corticosteroid

Discontinuation of the corticosteroid is the first line of defense and is often all that is required. The chronic form is said to normalize in 1 to 4 weeks, while the acute form typically resolves within days of stopping the steroid.[4] If continued corticosteroid therapy is essential, it may be possible to control the intraocular pressure with the additional use of anti-glaucoma medications or by changing to a steroid with less pressure-inducing potential.

B. Anti-glaucoma Medication

Anti-glaucoma medication is required when the return to normal intraocular pressure is slow or in the rare cases in which the glaucoma persists despite stopping all steroids. The latter situation occurred in 6 of 210 patients (2.8%) in one series, and all of these patients had a family history of glaucoma.[4] The medical management of these cases is essentially the same as for primary open-angle glaucoma.

C. Surgical Intervention

Surgical intervention is indicated when the glaucoma is uncontrolled on maximum tolerable medication. As previously noted, it may occasionally be necessary to exise a depot of periocular steroid if this appears to be responsible for the persistent pressure elevation.[33] In other cases of uncontrolled glaucomas, filtering surgery is usually the procedure of choice.

References

1. McLean, JM: Use of ACTH and cortisone. Discussion of paper by Woods, AC. Trans Am Ophthal Soc 48:293, 1950.
2. Francois, J: Cortisone et tension oculaire. Ann D'Oculist 187:805, 1954.
3. Hodapp, E, Kass, MA: Corticosteroid-induced glaucoma. *In* The Secondary Glaucomas, Ritch, R, Shields, MB, eds. CV Mosby Co, St Louis (in press).
4. Francois, J: Corticosteroid glaucoma. Ann Ophthal 9:1075, 1977.
5. Biedner, BZ, David, R, Grudsky, A, Sachs, U: Intraocular pressure response to corticosteroids in children. Br J Ophthal 64:430, 1980.
6. Gnad, HD, Martenet, AC: Kongenitales Glaukom and Cortison. Klin Monatsbl Augenheilkd 162:86, 1973.
7. Wilensky, JT, Snyder, D, Gieser, D: Steroid-induced ocular hypertension in patients with filtering blebs. Ophthalmology 87:240, 1980.
8. Kolker, AE: In discussion of Wilensky, JT, *et al*, Steroid-induced ocular hypertension in patients with filtering blebs. Ophthalmology 87:243, 1980.
9. Kronfeld, PC: The effect of topical steroid administration on intraocular pressure and aqueous outflow after fistulizing operations. Tr Am Ophthal Soc 62:375, 1964.
10. Sugar, HS: Low tension glaucoma: a practical approach. Ann Ophthal 11:1155, 1979.
11. Armaly, MF: Effect of corticosteroids on intraocular pressure and fluid dynamics. II. The effect of dexamethasone in the glaucomatous eye. Arch Ophthal 70:492, 1963.
12. Miller, D, Peczon, JD, Whitworth, CG: Corticosteroids and functions in the anterior segment of the eye. Am J Ophthal 59:31, 1965.
13. Weekers, R, Grieten, J, Collignon-Brach, J: Contribution a l'etude de l'hypertension oculaire provoquee par la dexamethasone dans le glaucome a angle ouvert. Ophthalmologica 152:81, 1966.
14. Kupfer, C, Ross, K: Studies of aqueous humor dynamics in man. I. Measurements in young normal subjects. Invest Ophthal 10:518, 1971.
15. Tchernitchin, A, Wenk, EJ, Hernandez, MR, Weinstein, BI, Dunn, MW, Gordon, GG, Southren, AL: Glucocorticoid localization by radioautography in the rabbit eye following systemic administration of ^{3}H-dexamethasone. Invest Ophthal Vis Sci 19:1231, 1980.
16. Francois, J, Victoria-Troncoso, V: Mucopolysaccharides and pathogenesis of cortisone glaucoma. Klin Monatsbl Augenheilkd 165:5, 1974.
17. Francois, J: The importance of the mucopolysaccharides in intraocular pressure regulation. Invest Ophthal 14:173, 1975.
18. Francois, J: Tissue culture of ocular fibroblasts. Ann Ophthal 11:1551, 1975.
19. Spaeth, GL, Rodrigues, MM, Weinreb, S: Steroid-induced glaucoma: A. Persistent elevation of intraocular pressure. B. Histopathological aspects. Tr Am Ophthal Soc 75:353, 1977.
20. Ticho, U, Lahav, M, Berkowitz, S, Yoffe, P: Ocular changes in rabbits with corticosteroid-induced ocular hypertension. Br J Ophthal 63:646, 1979.
21. Bill, A: The drainage of aqueous humor. Invest Ophthal 14:1, 1975.
22. Rohen, JW, Linner, E, Witmer, R: Electron microscopic studies on the trabecular meshwork in two cases of corticosteroid-glaucoma. Exp Eye Res 17:19, 1973.
23. Roll, P, Benedikt, O: Electronmicroscopic investigation of the trabecular meshwork in cortisonglaucoma. Klin Monatsbl Augenheilkd 174:421, 1979.
24. Schirru, A, Pecori-Giraldi, J, Pellegrino, N: Topical corticosteroids and vitreous dynamics in the rabbit. Acta Ophthal 51:811, 1973.
25. Virno, M, Schirru, A, Pecori-Giraldi, J, Pellegrino, N: Aqueous humor alkalosis and marked reduction in ocular ascorbic acid content following long-term topical cortisone (9_a-fluoro-16_a-methylprednisolone). Ann Ophthal 6:983, 1974.
26. Spaeth, GL: The effect of autonomic agents on the pupil and the intraocular pressure of eyes treated with dexamethasone. Br J Ophthal 64:426, 1980.

27. Podos, SM, Becker, B, Morton, WR: High myopia and primary open-angle glaucoma. Am J Ophthal 62:1039, 1966.
28. Becker, B: Diabetes mellitus and primary open-angle glaucoma. Am J Ophthal 71:1, 1971.
29. Cubey, RB: Glaucoma following the application of corticosteroid to the skin of the eyelids. Br J Dermatol 95:207, 1976.
30. Zugerman, C, Sauders, D, Levit, F: Glaucoma from topically applied steroids. Arch Dermatol 112:1326, 1976.
31. Kalina, RE: Increased intraocular pressure following subconjunctival corticosteroid administration. Arch Ophthal 81:788, 1969.
32. Nozik, RA: Periocular injection of steroids. Trans Am Acad Ophthal Otol 76:695, 1972.
33. Herschler, J: Intractable intraocular hypertension induced by repository triamcinolone acetonide. Am J Ophthal 74:501, 1972.
34. Herschler, J: Increased intraocular pressure induced by repository corticosteroids. Am J Ophthal 82:90, 1976.
35. Stern, JJ: Acute glaucoma during cortisone therapy. Am J Ophthal 36:389, 1953.
36. Covell, LL: Glaucoma induced by systemic steroid therapy. Am J Ophthal 45:108, 1958.
37. Godel, V, Feiler-Ofry, V, Stein, R: Systemic steroids and ocular fluid dynamics. I. Analysis of the sample as a whole. Influence of dosage and duration of therapy. Acta Ophthal 50:655, 1972.
38. Godel, V, Feiler-Ofry, V, Stein, R: Systemic steroids and ocular fluid dynamics. II. Systemic versus topical steroids. Acta Ophthal 50:664, 1972.
39. Brubaker, RF, Halpin, JA: Open-angle glaucoma associated with topical administration of flurandrenolide to the eye. Mayo Clinic Proc 50:322, 1975.
40. Kitazawa, Y: Increased intraocular pressure induced by corticosteroids. Am J Ophthal 82:492, 1976.
41. Leibowitz, HM, Kupperman, A, Stewart, RH, Kimbrough, RL: Evaluation of dexamethasone acetate as a topical ophthalmic formulation. Am J Ophthal 86:418, 1978.
42. Ramsell, TG, Bartholomew, RS, Walker, SR: Clinical evaluation of clobetasone butyrate: a comparative study of its effects in postoperative inflammation and on intraocular pressure. Br J Ophthal 64:43, 1980.
43. Dunne, JA, Travers, JP: Double-blind clinical trial of topical steroids in anterior uveitis. Br J Ophthal 63:762, 1979.
44. Bedrossian, RH, Eriksen, SP: The treatment of ocular inflammation with medrysone. Arch Ophthal 99:184, 1969.
45. Spaeth, GL: Hydroxymethylprogesterone. An anti-inflammatory steroid without apparent effect on intraocular pressure. Arch Ophthal 75:783, 1966.
46. Dorsch, W, Thygeson, P: The clinical efficacy of medrysone, a new ophthalmic steroid. Am J Ophthal 65:74, 1968.
47. Mindel, JS, Tavitian, HO, Smith, H Jr, Walker, EC: Comparative ocular pressure elevation by medrysone, fluorometholone, and dexamethasone phosphate. Arch Ophthal 98:1577, 1980.
48. Fairbairn, WD, Thorson, JC: Fluorometholone. Anti-inflammatory and intraocular pressure effects. Arch Ophthal 86:138, 1971.
49. Stewart, RH, Kimbrough, RL: Intraocular pressure response to topically administered fluorometholone. Arch Ophthal 97:2139, 1979.

Chapter 21

GLAUCOMAS ASSOCIATED WITH ELEVATED EPISCLERAL VENOUS PRESSURE

GLAUCOMAS ASSOCIATED WITH ELEVATED EPISCLERAL VENOUS PRESSURE

As discussed in Chapter 2, one factor contributing to the normal intraocular pressure is the episcleral venous pressure. This averages approximately 9 to 10 mmHg,[1-5] although values vary according to the measurement technique. Several instr ~ents have been devised for measuring episcleral venous pressure, all of which have the common principle of recording the pressure required to collapse or arrest blood flow in the vessel.[1-5] It is commonly felt that the introcular pressure rises mmHg for mmHg with an increase in the episcleral venous pressure, although it has been suggested that the magnitude of introcular pressure rise may be greater than the rise in venous pressure.[6] Studies of primary open-angle glaucoma have shown no abnormality of episcleral venous pressure.[2,7] However, there are a variety of conditions which can cause an elevation of the venous pressure and produce characteristic forms of secondary glaucoma.

I. GENERAL CLINICAL FEATURES

The following findings are common to most cases of glaucoma associated with elevated episcleral venous pressure[5]:

A. External Examination

The most consistent feature is variable degrees of dilation and tortuosity of the episcleral and bulbar conjunctival vessels. Additional findings may include chemosis, proptosis, and a bruit and pulsations over the orbit, although these are inconsistent findings that depend upon the underlying cause of the elevated episcleral venous pressure and will be discussed in more detail later.

B. Intraocular Pressure

As noted above, the rise in intraocular pressure is approximately equal to the rise in episcleral venous pressure. The resultant tension is typically in the mid-20s to mid-30s, and an increased ocular pulse is often present.[8]

C. Gonioscopy

The anterior chamber angle is typically open, and the only abnormality may be blood reflux into Schlemm's canal. However, the latter feature has limited diagnostic value, since it is an inconsistent finding in cases of elevated episcleral venous pressure and may be seen in normal eyes.

D. Tonography

The facility of aqueous outflow is characteristically normal. In fact, a study with monkeys revealed that elevated venous pressure was associated with increased outflow,[9] which may, at least in part, result from a widening of Schlemm's canal. However, prolonged elevation of episcleral venous pressure often leads to a reduction in outflow facility, which may persist after normalization of the venous pressure.[5,8]

II. SPECIFIC CLINICAL FEATURES

The forms of glaucoma associated with elevated episcleral venous pressure may be considered in three categories: 1) obstruction to venous flow, 2) arteriovenous fistulas, and 3) idiopathic episcleral venous pressure elevation.[5]

A. Venous Obstruction

1. *Thyrotropic ophthalmopathy*. This disorder is also referred to as endocrine exophthalmos or Graves' disease. The precise hormonal basis of the condition is uncertain, although the ocular pathology consists of orbital infiltration with lymphocytes, mast cells, and plasma cells. This is the most common cause of unilateral, as well as bilateral, proptosis and may lead to glaucoma by several mechanisms[10]:

a. *Elevated episcleral venous pressure* may occur in severe cases with marked proptosis and orbital congestion.

b. *The contracture of extraocular muscles*, which occurs in the later phases of this infiltrative ophthalmopathy, may influence the intraocular pressure in different fields of gaze. Typically, fibrosis of the inferior rectus muscle causes resistance to upgaze, which is associated with a rise in the intraocular pressure when the patient looks up. For this reason, the pressure should be measured in several fields of gaze.

c. Some patients may have a *reduced facility of aqueous outflow* of uncertain mechanism. It must be kept in mind, as discussed in Chapter 3, that thyroid dysfunction may be associated with abnormal scleral rigidity, and the intraocular pressure in these individuals should be measured by applanation tonometry.

d. *Corneal exposure*, due to proptosis and lid retraction, is another serious complication of thyrotropic ophthalmopathy. This can lead to a corneal ulcer, with anterior chamber inflammation and subsequent glaucoma.

2. *Superior vena cava syndrome*. Lesions of the upper thorax may obstruct venous return from the head, causing elevated episcleral venous pressure in association with exophthalmos, edema and cyanosis of the face and neck, and dilated veins of the head, neck, chest and upper extremities.[11]

3. Other conditions that may occasionally obstruct orbital venous drainage include *retrobulbar tumors* and *cavernous sinus thrombosis*.

B. Arteriovenous Fistulas

1. *Carotid-cavernous fistula.* The typical clinical appearance of this condition includes proptosis in nearly all patients with frequent ocular pulsations and bruits over the globe. There are several mechanisms by which a traumatic or spontaneous rupture of the intracavernous carotid artery or one of its branches into the surrounding venous sinus can lead to a rise in the intraocular pressure[12, 13]:

a. The mixing of arterial and venous blood leads to both a reduction in arterial pressure and an increase in orbital venous pressure. The venous back-pressure increases the *episcleral venous pressure*, which is the most common cause of an intraocular pressure rise with a carotid-cavernous fistula.

b. *Angle-closure glaucoma* has also been reported in association with a carotid-cavernous fistula.[14] The presumed mechanism was increased pressure in the vortex veins, which caused congestion of the uveal tract and subsequent angle closure with pupillary block.

c. The reduced arterial flow may also lead to ocular ischemia with rubeosis iridis and *neovascular glaucoma* (Chapter 15).[13, 15, 16]

2. *Orbital varices.* This condition is characterized by intermittent exophthalmos and elevated episcleral venous pressure, usually associated with stooping over or the Valsalva maneuver.[6, 17] Since venous pressure is typically normal between episodes, secondary glaucoma is not common. However, glaucomatous damage has been reported to occur, and it has been suggested that management with anti-glaucoma medications may be effective and should be tried before considering surgical intervention.[6]

3. *Sturge-Weber syndrome.* As discussed in Chapter 10, one mechanism of intraocular pressure elevation in this condition is believed to be elevated episcleral venous pressure due to the episcleral hemangiomas with arteriovenous fistulas.[18, 19]

C. Idiopathic Elevated Episcleral Venous Pressure

A familial form of glaucoma associated with elevated episcleral venous pressure has been described in a mother and daughter.[20] All the typical features of elevated episcleral venous pressure were present, but no cause could be found for the increased venous pressure. In another study, three patients had idiopathic, dilated episcleral vessels and open-angle glaucoma. The tonographic facilities of outflow were abnormal in these patients, and the episcleral venous pressures were not reported.[21] A case has also been reported of spontaneous hemorrhage into conjunctival lymphatic vessels, which might be considered in the differential diagnosis of dilated, tortuous, blood-filled conjunctival vessels.[22]

III. MANAGEMENT

In many cases, the initial therapy should be directed toward eliminating the cause of the elevated episcleral venous pressure. This is particularly true in patients with thyrotropic ophthalmopathy, superior vena cava syndrome, retrobulbar tumors, or cavernous sinus thrombosis. However, in cases of carotid-cavernous fistula and orbital varices, the risk of surgical intervention may be such that other measures of glaucoma control should be considered first.[6, 13] When treatment of the glaucoma is required, drugs which reduce aqueous production should be used, since those which improve outflow are rarely effective.[5] If surgical intervention becomes necessary, a filtering procedure should be employed. However, there is an increased risk of uveal effusion and expulsive hemorrhage when filtering eyes with elevated episcleral venous pressure, especially in the Sturge-Weber syndrome, and it has been recommended that drainage of the supra-choroid be routinely performed at the time of surgery.[23]

References

1. Brubaker, RF: Determination of episcleral venous pressure in the eye. A comparison of three methods. Arch Ophthal 77:110, 1967.
2. Podos, SM, Minas, TF, Macri, FJ: A new instrument to measure episcleral venous pressure. Comparison of normal eyes and eyes with primary open-angle glaucoma. Arch Ophthal 80:209, 1968.
3. Krakau, CET, Widakowich, J, Wilke, K: Measurements of the episcleral venous pressure by means of an air jet. Acta Ophthal 51:185, 1973.
4. Phelps, CD, Armaly, MF: Measurement of episcleral venous pressure. Am J Ophthal 85:38, 1978.
5. Yablonski, ME, Podos, SM: Glaucoma secondary to elevated episcleral venous pressure. In The Secondary Glaucomas, Ritch, R, Shields, MB, eds. CV Mosby Co, St Louis (in press).
6. Kollarits, CR, Gaasterland, D, Di Chiro, G, Christiansen, J, Yee, RD: Management of a patient with orbital varices, visual loss, and ipsilateral glaucoma. Ophthal Surg 8:54, 1977.
7. Linner, E: The outflow pressure in normal and glaucomatous eyes. Acta Ophthal 33:101, 1955.
8. Chandler, PA, Grant, WM: Glaucoma, 2nd ed. Lea & Febiger, Philadelphia, 1979, p 267.
9. Barany, EH: The influence of extraocular venous pressure on outflow facility in Cercopithecus ethiops and Macaca fascicularis. Invest Ophthal Vis Sci 17:711, 1978.
10. Kolker, AE, Hetherington, J, Jr: Becker-Shaffer's Diagnosis and Therapy of the Glaucomas, 4th ed. CV Mosby Co, St Louis, 1976, p256.
11. Alfano, JE, Alfano, PA: Glaucoma and the superior vena caval obstruction syndrome. Am J Ophthal 42:685, 1956.
12. Henderson, JW, Schneider, RC: The ocular findings in carotid cavernous fistula in a series of 17 cases. Am J Ophthal 48:585, 1959.
13. Sanders, MD, Hoyt, WF: Hypoxic ocular sequelae of carotid-cavernous fistulae. Study of the causes of visual failure before and after neurosurgical treatment in a series of 25 cases. Br J Ophthal 53:82, 1969.
14. Harris, GJ, Rice, PR: Angle closure in carotid-cavernous fistula. Ophthalmology 86:1521, 1979.
15. Spencer, WH, Thompson, HS, Hoyt, WF: Ischaemic ocular necrosis from carotid-cavernous fistula. Pathology of stagnant anoxic "inflammation" in orbital and ocular tissues. Br J Ophthal 57:145, 1973.
16. Weiss, DI, Shaffer, RN, Nehrenberg, TR: Neovascular glaucoma complicating carotid-cavernous fistula. Arch Ophthal 69:304, 1963.

17. Wright, JE: Orbital vascular anomalies. Trans Am Acad Ophthal Otol 78:606, 1974.
18. Weiss, DI: Dual origin of glaucoma in encephalotrigeminal hemangiomatosis. Trans Ophthal Soc UK 93:477, 1971.
19. Phelps, CD: The pathogenesis of glaucoma in Sturge-Weber syndrome. Ophthalmology 85:276, 1978.
20. Minas, TF, Podos, SM: Familial glaucoma associated with elevated episcleral venous pressure. Arch Ophthal 80:202, 1968.
21. Radius, RL, Maumenee, AE: Dilated episcleral vessels and open-angle glaucoma. Am J Ophthal 86:31, 1978.
22. Jampol, LM, Nagpal, KC: Hemorrhagic lymphangiectasia of the conjunctiva. Am J Ophthal 85:419, 1978.
23. Bellows, RA, Chylack, LT, Epstein, DL, Hutchinson, BT: Choroidal effusion during glaucoma surgery in patients with prominent episcleral vessels. Arch Ophthal 97:493, 1979.

Chapter 22

ANIMAL MODELS OF GLAUCOMA

To study the mechanisms of glaucoma and the efficacy of anti-glaucoma therapy, it would be useful to have animal models which resemble the human forms of glaucoma. To date, no animal model has proven to be totally satisfactory for these purposes, although the following spontaneous or induced forms of glaucoma in animals have been reported.

I. SPONTANEOUS GLAUCOMAS[1, 2]

A. Dogs

Of the few animals that have been reported to spontaneously develop glaucoma, dogs are the most common.

1. *Beagles* may inherit a form of glaucoma which typically begins at age 6 to 18 months with open anterior chamber angles.[3, 4] At this stage, the glaucoma may be a suitable model for drug studies.[4] Topical pilocarpine and epinephrine have been studied in normotensive and glaucomatous beagles, and dose-related pressure responses were found, with a greater percentage reduction in the glaucomatous animals.[5, 6] A late stage of the disease is characterized by a dislocated lens and angle closure with occasional phthisis.[3, 4]

2. *Basset hounds* have been reported to develop a familial, congenital glaucoma with goniodysgenesis, which may manifest one of two clinical forms. One type is described as acute congestive, while the other is an open-angle form similar to human primary open-angle glaucoma.[7]

3. *Cocker spaniels* may develop a primary angle-closure form of glaucoma.[1, 2]

B. Rabbits

Strains of rabbits have been observed with spontaneous buphthalmos, although this has not yet proven useful in studying glaucoma therapy.[1, 2]

C. Primates

No primate has yet been found to commonly manifest glaucoma, although a form of spontaneous buphthalmos has been observed in the *Lemur fulvus rufus*.[8] In addition, the intraocular pressures in two free-breeding colonies of *Rhesus monkeys* have been found to be remarkably similar to those of humans, which may provide a good model for studying intraocular pressure.[9]

II. INDUCED GLAUCOMA

In addition to the spontaneous forms, animal models of glaucoma have been induced by a variety of techniques.

A. Ocular Injections[1]

A wide variety of agents, including talc, cotton fibers, silicone, prostaglandins, alkali, alphachymotrypsin enzyme,[10] methylcellulose,[11] and autologous fixed red blood cells,[12] have been injected into the anterior chamber of animal eyes to produce elevated intraocular pressures. In addition, sclerosing agents have been injected subconjunctivally.[13] These are all generally successful in creating tension rises for variable periods of time, but have the disadvantage of inducing artificial circumstances that are not optimum for the study of glaucoma drugs.

B. Laser Applications

Applying laser burns to the trabecular meshwork of animal eyes can also cause a rise in intraocular pressure.[14]

C. Steroid-induced Glaucoma

Animal models of glaucoma have been created by the topical[15] or subconjunctival[16] administration of corticosteroids. Although reported to produce a satisfactory intraocular pressure elevation,[15, 16] others have found the response to be quite erratic.[1]

D. Reduced Serum Osmolarity

A temporary increase in the intraocular pressure can be accomplished by forced ingestion of water[17] or intravenous injections of 5% glucose solution.[18] In the latter situation, the glucose is rapidly removed from the circulation, leaving a lowered serum osmolarity. These techniques may be useful in drug studies because they do not directly alter the eye, although the drug effects must be considered against the backdrop of an altered physiological status of the eye.

E. Continuous Light Exposure

Continuous light exposure causes buphthalmos in domestic chicks, which is associated with an elevated intraocular pressure and reduced aqueous outflow.[19]

References

1. Podos, SM: Animal models of human glaucoma. Trans Am Acad Ophthal Otol 81:632, 1976.
2. Gelatt, KN: Animal models for glaucoma. Invest Ophthal 16:592, 1977.

3. Gelatt, KN. Peiffer, RL Jr, Gwin, RM, Sauk, JJ Jr: Glaucoma in the beagle. Trans Am Acad Ophthal Otol 81:636, 1976.
4. Gelatt, KN, Peiffer, RL Jr, Gwin,RM, Gum, GG, Williams, LW: Clinical manifestations of inherited glaucoma in the beagle. Invest Ophthal 16:1135, 1977.
5. Gwin, RM, Gelatt, KN, Gum, GG, Peiffer, RL Jr, Williams, LW: The effect of topical pilocarpine on intraocular pressure and pupil size in the normotensive and glaucomatous beagle. Invest Ophthal 16:1143, 1977.
6. Gwin, RM, Gelatt, KN, Gum, GG, Peiffer, RL Jr: Effects of topical *l*-epinephrine and dipivalyl epinephrine on intraocular pressure and pupil size in the normotensive and glaucomatous beagle. Am J Vet Res 39:83, 1978.
7. Wyman, M, Ketring, K: Congenital glaucoma in the basset hound: a biologic model. Trans Am Acad Ophthal Otol 81:645, 1976.
8. Ritch, R, Shields, MB, Pokorny, KS, Friedman, AH: Spontaneous buphthalmos in the lemur. Presented at annual Spring meeting, Association for Research in Vision and Ophthalmology, Sarasota, 1979, abstract p 242.
9. Bito, LZ, Merritt, SQ, DeRousseau, CJ: Intraocular pressure of rhesus monkeys (*Macaca mulatta*). I. An initial survey of two free-breeding colonies. Invest Ophthal Vis Sci 18:785, 1979.
10. Best, M, Rabinovitz, AZ, Masket, S: Experimental alphachymotrypsin glaucoma. Ann Ophthal 7:803, 1975.
11. Lorenzetti, OJ, Sancilio, LF: Procedure for evaluating drug effects on increased intraocular pressure. Arch Ophthal 78:624, 1967.
12. Quigley, HA, Addicks, EM: Chronic experimental glaucoma in primates. I. Production of elevated intraocular pressure by anterior chamber injection of autologous ghost red blood cells. Invest Ophthal Vis Sci 19:126, 1980.
13. Malik, SRK, Choudhry, S, Gupta, AK: Experimental production of glaucoma in rabbits. Am J Ophthal 69:1010, 1970.
14. Gaasterland, D, Kupfer, C: Experimental glaucoma in the rhesus monkey. Invest Ophthal 13:455, 1974.
15. Levene, RZ, Rothberger, M, Rosenberg, S: Corticosteroid glaucoma in the rabbit. Am J Ophthal 78:505, 1974.
16. Bonomi, L, Perfetti, S, Noya, E, Bellucci, R, Tomazzoli, L: Experimental corticosteroid ocular hypertension in the rabbit. Albrecht Graefes Arch Klin Exp Ophthal 209:73, 1978.
17. Thorpe, RM, Kolker, AE: A tonographic study of water loading in rabbits. Arch Ophthal 77:238, 1967.
18. Bonomi, L, Tomazzoli, L, Jaria, D: An improved model of experimentally induced ocular hypertension in the rabbit. Invest Ophthal 15:781, 1976.
19. Kinnear, A, Lauber, JK, Boyd, TAS: Genesis of light-induced avian glaucoma. Invest Ophthal 13:872, 1974.

Section Three

Pharmacology and Surgery for Glaucoma

Chapter 23

FUNDAMENTALS OF TOPICAL DRUGS

The majority of drugs used in the management of glaucoma are administered by topical instillation to the eye. Before studying these drugs individually, therefore, it is helpful to consider some of the general principles concerning topical medications.

For a drug to be effective as a topical agent, it must be able to 1) penetrate the cornea and 2) reach the appropriate intraocular structures in sufficient concentration.

I. CORNEAL PENETRATION

The ability of a drug to penetrate the cornea depends on 1) the nature of the cornea, 2) the nature of the drug, and 3) the formulation of the drug[1]:

A. The Cornea

It may be helpful to think of the cornea as a *lipid-water-lipid* sandwich, in that the lipid content of the epithelium and endothelium is approximately 100 times greater than that of the stroma.[2] As a result of this composition, the epithelium and endothelium are readily traversed by lipid-soluble substances (*i.e.*, compounds in a non-ionized or non-electrolyte form), but are impermeable to water-soluble agents (ionized compounds or electrolytes). The reverse is true for the corneal stroma, which is permeable to water-soluble compounds but impermeable to lipid-soluble substances. This difference in permeability characteristics creates a *selective barrier*, in that only drugs which can exist in both a water-soluble and lipid-soluble state are able to penetrate the intact cornea. This has been referred to as the differential solubility concept.[2] Although this barrier can be influenced by alterations in the cornea, such as damaging the epithelium, it is more practical to enhance penetration by altering the drug and its formulation.

B. Drug Properties

1. *Lipid-water solubility.* As noted above, for a drug to penetrate all layers of the cornea, it must have the potential to exist in both lipid-soluble and water-soluble forms. Such a substance is said to be

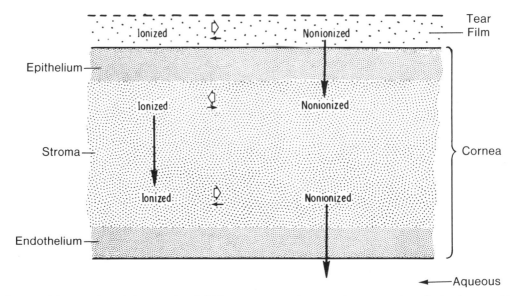

Figure 23.1. The differential solubility concept of corneal penetration. Only drugs with the potential to exist in both lipid-soluble (non-ionized) and water-soluble (ionized) forms are able to penetrate the intact cornea. The two forms are in equilibrium and, as one form penetrates a particular corneal layer, its concentration is replenished from the other form to maintain the equilibrium.

amphotheric. The two forms of the drug exist in equilibrium and, as one form penetrates a particular corneal layer, its concentration is replenished from the other form to maintain the equilibrium (Fig. 23.1).[2]

2. *Molecular weight* is not a major factor, since most topical ophthalmic drugs are less than 500 and will usually diffuse through biologic membranes.[1]

C. Formulation

1. *pH.* The lipid/water solubility ratio (partition coefficient) of a compound influences corneal penetration and is, in turn, influenced by the pH of the formulation. For example, pilocarpine penetration is better at pH 6.5 to 7.5 than at pH 4,[3,4] although no significant difference was noted between formulations at pH 4.1 and 5.8.[5] The pH is also important regarding stability and comfort to the eye, and each of these factors must be considered when formulating a drug.

2. *Concentration.* Corneal penetration is enhanced by increasing the concentration of a drug up to a point, beyond which the percentage of drug crossing the cornea decreases with increasing concentrations. In a monkey study, topical 1% pilocarpine had a greater percentage recovered in the aqueous than 4 or 8%.[6]

3. *Vehicle.* Corneal penetration is also influenced by the vehicle in which a drug is delivered. This relates primarily to the length of *time* that a vehicle allows the drug to remain in contact with the cornea.

a. *Ointments* provide longer corneal contact time[7, 8] and better corneal penetration[8, 9] than aqueous vehicles, but have the disadvantage of temporarily blurring vision.

b. *Water-soluble polymers* also improve corneal penetration by increasing viscosity, providing solution homogeneity (uniform suspension of drug particles in solution), and reducing surface tension.[10] The following polymers have been rated on the basis of corneal retention time or delivery rate of a marker compound, and are listed in decreasing order of effectiveness: hydroxypropylcellulose, hydroxyethylcellulose, hydroxypropylmethylcellulose, and polyvinyl alcohol.[11–13]

c. *Ocular insert devices* have been developed to provide *sustained release* of a drug. This has been shown to achieve the same therapeutic effect as frequent topical applications, but with significantly less medication.[14] Such devices include pre-soaked *hydrophilic contact lens*,[6, 15, 16] *polymers* of soluble[17, 18] or insoluble[19] material, and *polymeric membranes*.[20] Each of these devices offers promise as a drug delivery system, although only the polymeric membrane is commercially available for the treatment of glaucoma. This system will be discussed in Chapter 25.

4. *Additives.* Certain additives that are used in commercial formulations may also influence corneal penetration. The most notable of these is *benzalkonium chloride*, which is used in eye drops primarily as a "preservative" for its bacteriostatic property. It also acts as a wetting agent to enhance corneal penetration, which is necessary for some drugs, such as carbachol.[21]

II. INTRAOCULAR FACTORS INFLUENCING DRUG CONCENTRATIONS

Having penetrated the cornea, the drug must now pass through the aqueous to the appropriate structures in the anterior segment of the eye. Various factors influence the concentration of drug which finally reaches these sites:

A. Rate of Removal

The rate at which a drug is removed from the eye is influenced by diffusion into the vascular system and escape with the aqueous via the outflow system.

B. Binding to Melanin

Both cholinergic[22, 23] and adrenergic[23] drugs produce a greater response in eyes with less pigment. The explanation for this appears to be a binding of the drug to melanin in the anterior uveal tract, which prevents it from reaching the receptor site.[24–26] Histochemical studies show that adrenergic nerves are located close to melanocytes.[26] It has also been suggested, based on studies with pilocarpine in pigmented and albino rabbits, that a larger amount of the topically applied drug may be metabolized in the cornea of eyes with more pigment.[27]

C. Intraocular Metabolism

Some drugs are metabolized to inactive forms by enzymes in various ocular tissues.

References

1. Benson, H: Permeability of the cornea to topically applied drugs. Arch Ophthal 91:313, 1974.
2. Havener, WH: Ocular Pharmacology, 4th ed. CV Mosby Co, St Louis, 1978, pp 19, 429.
3. Anderson, RA, Cowle, JB: Influence of pH on the effect of pilocarpine on aqueous dynamics. Br J Ophthal 52:607, 1968.
4. Ramer, RM, Gasset, AR: Ocular penetration of pilocarpine: The effect of pH on the ocular penetration of pilocarpine. Ann Ophthal 7:293, 1975.
5. David, R, Goldberg, L, Luntz, MH: Influence of pH on the efficacy of pilocarpine. Br J Ophthal 62:318, 1978.
6. Asseff, CF, Weisman, RL, Podos, SM, Becker, B: Ocular penetration of pilocarpine in primates. Am J Ophthal 75:212, 1973.
7. Hardberger, R, Hanna, C, Boyd, CM: Effects of drug vehicles on ocular contact time. Arch Ophthal 93:42, 1975.
8. Hardberger, RE, Hanna, C, Goodart, R: Effects of drug vehicles on ocular uptake of tetracycline. Am J Ophthal 80:133, 1975.
9. Waltman, SR, Buerk, K, Foster, CS: Effects of ophthalmic ointments on intraocular penetration of topical fluorescein in rabbits and man. Am J Ophthal 78:262, 1974.
10. Lemp, MA, Holly, FJ: Ophthalmic polymers as ocular wetting agents. Ann Ophthal 4:15, 1972.
11. Bach, FC, Adam, JB, McWhirter, HC, Johnson, JE: Ocular retention of artificial tear solutions. Comparison of hydroxypropyl methylcellulose and polyvinyl alcohol vehicles using an argyrol marker. Ann Ophthal 4:116, 1972.
12. Capella, JA, Schaefer, IM: Comparison of ophthalmic vehicles using fluorescein uptake technique. Eye Ear Nose Throat Mthly 53:23, 1974.
13. Trueblood, JH, Rossomondo, RM, Carlton, WH, Wilson, LA: Corneal contact times of ophthalmic vehicles. Evaluation by microscintigraphy. Arch Ophthal 93:127, 1975.
14. Lerman, S, Reininger, B: Simulated sustained release pilocarpine therapy and aqueous humor dynamics. Can J Ophthal 6:14, 1971.
15. Maddox, YT, Bernstein, HN: An evaluation of the bionite hydrophilic contact lens for use in a drug delivery system. Ann Ophthal 4:789, 1972.
16. Hull, DS, Edelhauser, HF, Hyndiuk, RA: Ocular penetration of prednisolone and the hydrophilic contact lens. Arch Ophthal 92:413, 1974.
17. Maichuk, YF: Ophthalmic drug inserts. Invest Ophthal 14:87, 1975.
18. Katz, IM, Blackman, WM: A soluble sustained-release ophthalmic delivery unit. Am J Ophthal 83:72, 1977.
19. Leaders, FE, Hecht, G, VanHoose, M, Kellog, M: New polymers in drug delivery. Ann Ophthal 5:513, 1973.
20. Dohlman, CH, Pavan-Langston, D, Rose, J: A new ocular insert device for continuous constant-rate delivery of medication to the eye. Ann Ophthal 4:823, 1972.
21. Smolen, VF, Clevenger, JM, Williams, EJ, Bergdolt, MW: Biophasic availability of ophthalmic carbachol I: mechanisms of cationic polymer- and surfactant-promoted miotic activity. J Pharmaceut Sci 62:958, 1973.
22. Harris, LS, Galin, MA: Effect of ocular pigmentation on hypotensive response to pilocarpine. Am J Ophthal 72:923, 1971.

23. Melikian, HE, Lieberman, TW, Leopold, IH: Ocular pigmentation and pressure and outflow responses to pilocarpine and epinephrine. Am J Ophthal 72:70, 1971.
24. Lyons, JS, Krohn, DL: Pilocarpine uptake by pigmented uveal tissue. Am J Ophthal 75:885, 1973.
25. Newsome, DA, Stern, R: Pilocarpine adsorption by serum and ocular tissues. Am J Ophthal 77:918, 1974.
26. Path, PN, Jacobowitz, D: Unequal accumulation of adrenergic drugs by pigmented and nonpigmented iris. Am J Ophthal 78:470, 1974.
27. Lee, VHL, Hul, HW, Robinson, JR: Corneal metabolism of pilocarpine in pigmented rabbits. Invest Ophthal Vis Sci 19:210, 1980.

Chapter 24

BASIC PHARMACOLOGY OF THE AUTONOMIC NERVOUS SYSTEM

All topical drugs that are used to control the intraocular pressure in the management of glaucoma are thought to exert their pharmacologic effect by acting on the autonomic nervous system. The following review of that system will provide a framework on which to build an understanding of topical anti-glaucoma medications.

I. CELL MEMBRANE

The cell membrane is the site at which both physiologic mediators and most pharmacologic agents act to produce a particular cellular response. The cell membrane is composed of *lipid* and *protein*, although the actual arrangement of these components is uncertain. One theory, the "lipid-globular protein mosaic model," suggests that molecules of protein are imbedded in a layer of lipid, with protrusion of the globular protein on either side of the membrane.[1] Although this is an oversimplification of a highly complex and poorly understood subject, it provides a conceptual basis for a discussion of drug interactions. According to this hypothesis, the extracellular side of the protein globules contain *receptors*, with which physiologic mediators and some pharmacologic agents are believed to interact. *Catalysts* are felt to be located on the intracellular side of the protein and are involved in specific cellular functions in response to a physiologic mediator or drug.

II. AUTONOMIC NERVOUS SYSTEM

There are two main subdivisions of the autonomic nervous system. These subsystems differ on the basis of 1) receptors and 2) postganglionic physiologic mediators (Fig. 24.1)[1]:

A. Cholinergic (Parasympathetic) System

1. *Receptor.* It has traditionally been held that only one receptor type exists in the parasympathetic nervous system, although more

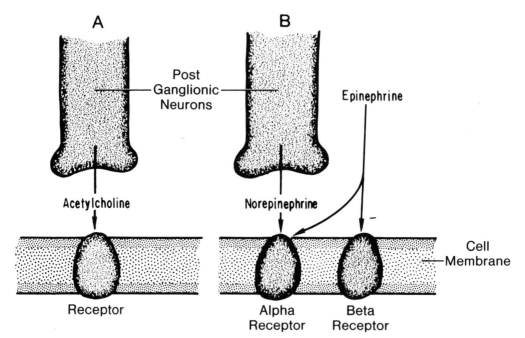

Figure 24.1. Main divisions of autonomic nervous system. **A:** cholinergic (parasympathetic) system is mediated by acetylcholine; **B:** adrenergic (sympathetic) system is mediated by norepinephrine and epinephrine.

recent studies have suggested the possibility of more than one cholinergic receptor.[2] Stimulation of the receptor(s) produces *miosis* and *increased aqueous outflow*. The mechanism of improved outflow facility appears to be related to contraction of the ciliary muscle.[3, 4] It has also been suggested that some cholinergic agents may reduce aqueous production,[5] although the mechanism of this effect, if it exists, is unknown.

2. *Physiologic mediator. Acetylcholine* is the post-ganglionic physiologic mediator of the cholinergic nervous system. It is produced in the post-ganglionic neuron, where it is stored and released when the membrane is polarized by increased Na^+ flux. After its release from the neuron, the mediator is rapidly inactivated by *acetylcholinesterase*.

B. Adrenergic (Sympathetic) System (Fig. 24.2)

1. *Receptors.* Two basic types of adrenergic receptors have been identified, although subdivisions are known to exist within these categories, and it is likely that there are additional receptors that have yet to be recognized.

a. *Alpha adrenergic receptor.* Stimulation of this receptor produces *mydriasis* and *vasoconstriction*. The effect of alpha adrenergic stimulation on aqueous humor dynamics is not fully understood. Current theories will be considered in Chapter 26.

b. *Beta adrenergic receptor.* The role of the beta adrenergic

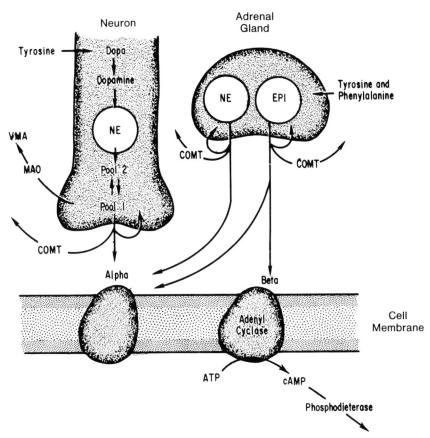

Figure 24.2. Adrenergic nervous system. Norepinephrine (**NE**) is produced in both post-ganglionic neurons and the adrenal glands and stimulates primarily alpha-adrenergic receptors; epinephrine (**E**) is produced in the adrenal glands and stimulates both alpha- and beta-adrenergic receptors. (See text for details).

system in aqueous humor dynamics is also a matter of controversy and speculation, although it is generally held that stimulation of the receptors increases aqueous outflow facility, while inhibition reduces aqueous production. The former mechanism appears to be related to the activation of *adenylate cyclase*, an enzyme at the catalyst site which catalyzes the conversion of ATP to *cyclic AMP*. Primate studies indicate that cyclic AMP in the anterior chamber mediates increased outflow facility.[6, 7] *Phosphodiesterase* inactivates cyclic AMP. The mechanism of reduced aqueous production by beta adrenergic inhibition is uncertain.

The beta system has been further subdivided into $beta_1$ and $beta_2$ types.[8] Stimulation of $beta_1$ receptors increases cardiac contractility and lypolysis, while the $beta_2$ subsystem is related to bronchodilation and vasodepression.

2. *Physiologic mediators.* There are two physiologic mediators in

the sympathetic nervous system. These are often referred to as *catecholamines:*

a. *Epinephrine* is secreted by the adrenal glands where it is produced from phenylalanine and tyrosine. It stimulates both *alpha* and *beta* receptors.

b. *Norepinephrine* is the post-ganglionic mediator and primarily stimulates the *alpha* receptor. It is also secreted by the adrenal glands where it is made from the same amino acids as epinephrine. In the post-ganglionic neuron, norepinephrine is produced from tyrosine alone and stored in two pools in the axon terminal. Slow release and re-uptake of the mediator constantly occur, and that which is not released is inactivated to *vanilmandelic acid* by *monoamine oxidase.* Following massive release of the mediator by nerve stimulation, 90% is recaptured by the nerve, a small amount is inactivated by *catechol-o-methyltransferase* and monoamine oxidase, and the remainder enters the circulation in active form.

III. AUTONOMIC DRUGS

Some of the physiologic mediators in the autonomic nervous system are used as pharmacologic agents. In addition, there are other compounds that act at some point within this nervous system to mimic or antagonize the action of the physiologic mediators. Drugs may mimic the effect of the physiologic mediator directly by stimulating the receptor or indirectly by enhancing the action of the physiologic mediator. Other compounds may compete with the physiologic mediator at the receptor site to inhibit the normal response of the particular autonomic system. Accordingly, the following scheme of autonomic drugs may be developed. Specific compounds within these categories will be considered in the next two chapters.

A. Cholinergic Drugs

1. *Parasympathomimetics* (stimulators or agonists)

a. *Direct stimulators.* This group of compounds, which includes the physiologic mediator, acetylcholine, directly stimulates the cholinergic receptors.

b. *Indirect stimulators.* These drugs enhance the action of acetylcholine by inhibiting the cholinesterases.

2. *Parasympatholytics.* These drugs, such as atropine, cyclopentolate, and tropicamide, block the response of acetylcholine at the receptor. This produces mydriasis and relaxation of the ciliary muscle and, as discussed in Section Two, these changes can lead to an elevation of intraocular pressure under certain circumstances.

B. Adrenergic Drugs

1. *Sympathomimetics* (stimulators or agonists)

a. *Alpha adrenergic agonists*

(1). *Direct alpha stimulators.* These compounds, including the physiologic mediators, epinephrine and norepinephrine, directly stimulate the alpha adrenergic receptors.

(2). *Indirect alpha stimulators.* Another group of drugs enhance the effect of norepinephrine by several mechanisms, which include stimulating its release from the axon terminal, increasing its release in response to nerve stimulation, decreasing its re-uptake, and inhibiting monoamine oxidase or catechol-o-methyltransferase.

b. *Beta adrenergic agonists*

(1). *Direct beta stimulators.* This group of drugs, including the physiologic mediator, epinephrine, directly stimulate the beta adrenergic receptors.

(2). *Indirect beta stimulators.* These pharmacologic agents mimic the effect of beta adrenergic stimulation by enhancing the effect of adenylate cyclase in various ways.

c. *Adrenergic potentiators.* There is another group of compounds which enhance the effect of epinephrine by producing adrenergic supersensitivity.

2. *Sympatholytics* (inhibitors, blockers, or antagonists)

a. *Alpha adrenergic antagonists.* These drugs compete with the catecholamines at the alpha receptors.

b. *Beta adrenergic antagonists.* This class of compounds compete with epinephrine for beta receptors.

References

1. Richardson, KT: Ocular microtherapy. Membrane-controlled drug delivery. Arch Ophthal 93:74, 1975.
2. Bito, LZ, Merritt, SQ: Paradoxical ocular hypertensive effect of pilocarpoine on echothiophate iodide-treated primate eyes. Invest Ophthal Vis Sci 19:371, 1980.
3. Kaufman, PL, Barany, EH: Loss of acute pilocarpine effect on outflow facility following surgical disinsertion and retrodisplacement of the ciliary muscle from the scleral spur in the cynomolgus monkey. Invest Ophthal 15:793, 1976.
4. Kaufman, PL, Barany, EH: Residual pilocarpine effects on outflow facility after ciliary muscle disinsertion in the cynomolgus monkey. Invest Ophthal 15:558, 1976.
5. Barsam, PC: Comparison of the effect of pilocarpine and echothiophate on intraocular pressure and outflow facility. Am J Ophthal 73:742, 1972.
6. Neufeld, AH, Dueker, DK, Vegge, T, Sears, ML: Adenosine 3',5'-monophosphate increases the outflow of aqueous humor from the rabbit eye. Invest Ophthal 14:40, 1975.
7. Neufeld, AH, Sears, ML: Adenosine 3',5'-monophosphate analogue increases the outflow facility of the primate eye. Invest Ophthal 14:688, 1975.
8. Lands, AM, Arnold, A, McAuliff, JP, Luduena, FP, Brown, TG: Differentiation of receptor systems activated by sympathomimetic amines. Nature 214:597, 1967.

Chapter 25

CHOLINERGIC DRUGS

I. **Pilocarpine**
   A. Mechanisms of action
   B. Administration
   C. Drug interactions
   D. Side effects

II. **Dual action parasympathomimetics**
   A. Carbachol
   B. Aceclidine

III. **Indirect Parasympathomimetics**
   A. Physostigmine
   B. Echothiophate iodide
   C. Other indirect parasympathomimetics

CHOLINERGIC DRUGS

The *parasympathomimetics*, often referred to as the *miotics* because of their common action on the pupil, were the first class of drugs to be used in the treatment of glaucoma, having been introduced in the 1870s. These compounds have the same basic effect on aqueous humor dynamics and differ primarily in duration of action and severity of side effects.

I. PILOCARPINE

This direct-acting parasympathomimetic is the most commonly used and the most extensively studied miotic.

A. Mechanisms of Action

1. *Increased facility of aqueous outflow.* The principle mode of intraocular pressure reduction by pilocarpine is enhanced aqueous outflow. In eyes with open anterior chamber angles, the mechanism of this action appears to be stimulation of *ciliary muscle contraction*. It has been demonstrated that aqueous outflow facility can be increased by accommodation,[1] a posterior depression of the lens,[2-4] tension on the choroid,[5] or a pull on the root of the iris.[6] In each of these situations, the common action appears to be traction on the scleral spur by virtue of its attachment to the ciliary musculature. The displacement of the scleral spur leads to an increased facility of aqueous outflow presumably by altering the configuration of the trabecular meshwork, Schlemm's canal, or both. Pilocarpine, and the other miotics, exert a similar traction on the scleral spur by causing contraction of the ciliary muscle.

More direct evidence for the influence of pilocarpine-induced cyclotonia on outflow facility is that disinsertion of the ciliary muscle from the scleral spur in monkeys, eliminates the effect of pilocarpine on intraocular pressure and facility of outflow.[7, 8] To rule out other possible mechanisms, it was shown that the disinsertion did not alter conventional outflow[9] nor cause histologic changes in the ciliary muscle, trabecular meshwork, or Schlemm's canal.[10] Histologic studies of human eyes treated with pilocarpine prior to enucleation for malignant melanoma demonstrated a posterior, internal pull on the scleral spur, with widening of the trabecular spaces, distention of the endothelial meshwork, an increase in the number of giant vacuoles, and larger, more frequent pores in the inner endothelium of Schlemm's canal.[11, 12] Primate studies suggested that the greater number of giant vacuoles was a result of increased aqueous flow through the outflow system, rather than a direct action of pilocarpine on the endothelium of Schlemm's canal.[13]

2. *Miosis.* The *miotic* effect of pilocarpine is useful in the short-term management of certain angle-closure glaucomas. However, this

does not appear to be related to the improvement of aqueous outflow facility in open-angle glaucomas, since total iridectomies in monkeys did not alter the facility response to intravenous pilocarpine.[14]

3. *Decreased aqueous production.* It may be that part of the intraocular pressure lowering effect of pilocarpine is related to decreased aqueous inflow, since the reduction in pressure has been reported to exceed[15] and outlast[16] the improvement in outflow facility. Barany[17] has suggested that prolonged treatment with pilocarpine may result in subsensitivity of the ciliary muscle, with a shift in emphasis to inhibition of aqueous secretion by an unknown mechanism.

4. Episcleral venous pressure does not appear to be altered by pilocarpine.[15]

5. It should also be noted that pilocarpine decreases extracanalicular (uveoscleral) outflow.[18] This may have clinical significance in eyes with markedly reduced conventional outflow. As these eyes become increasingly dependent on extracanalicular drainage, pilocarpine may cause a paradoxical rise in intraocular pressure.[19]

B. Administration

1. *Ocular penetration.* Although the cornea is the main route by which topical pilocarpine enters the eye,[20] this tissue may also impede ocular penetration. It has been shown that pilocarpine concentrates in the corneal stroma,[21, 22] where it is largely complexed or degraded,[23, 24] with only a small percentage entering the anterior chamber.[23-26] Selecting the optimum drug concentration, frequency of administration, and delivery system may improve the efficiency of ocular penetration.

2. *Drug concentration.* The intraocular pressure-lowering effect of pilocarpine is dose-related up to a concentration of 4%.[27-30] Studies differ, however, as to whether there is a significant dose-response curve with single dose instillations.[27, 28] Furthermore, higher concentrations of pilocarpine, such as 6 to 8%, may cause additional pressure reduction in darkly pigmented eyes.[31]

3. *Frequency of administration.* Following topical instillation in animals, the maximum concentrations of pilocarpine in the aqueous and iris were reached in approximately 20 min,[22] and aqueous levels were gone in 4 hr.[25] In studies of ocular hypertensive individuals, the maximum effect on intraocular pressure occurred within 2 hr and lasted for at least 8 hr, with a reduction in intraocular pressure of approximately 20%.[28] The pressure response began to decline by the 9th hr, although there was still a 14 to 15% reduction at 12 to 15 hr after instillation.[29] To insure adequate pressure control, standard pilocarpine drops are generally given four times daily. Efficiency may be improved by frequent, repeated instillations[32] or by continuous infusion[33, 34] of dilute solutions. Since these methods have obvious practical limitations for long-term therapy, efforts are being made to achieve similar results with newer drug delivery systems.

4. *Delivery systems.* A goal of any drug therapy is to achieve the

desired pharmacologic effect with the least amount of medicine. Animal and human studies suggest that the volume of pilocarpine delivered by commercial droppers may be significantly in excess of that needed to produce the desired response.[35, 36] It is also possible that the required dosage of a drug can be further reduced by utilizing vehicles which prolong corneal contact time[37]:

a. *Oily solutions.* Pilocarpine has a greater degree and duration of effect on the pupil when delivered in an oily vehicle than the same drug in an aqueous solution.[38]

b. *Polymer vehicles.* As discussed in Chapter 23, various polymers may increase corneal retention time. However, the results of clinical studies with pilocarpine in such vehicles have been conflicting. Pilocarpine in 1.6% polyvinylpyrrolidone and other water-soluble polymers (Adsorbocarpine) was reported to have a prolonged duration of action and improved pressure control,[39-41] allowing twice daily administration.[39] However, this was not confirmed by subsequent studies.[42-44] Preliminary experience with pilocarpine in another new polymer (Piloplex), given twice daily, suggests that it may be more effective than pilocarpine hydrochloride, four times a day.[45-48]

c. *Gels.* A *pilocarpine gel* applied once daily at bedtime was equivalent to pilocarpine hydrochloride drops instilled four times daily up to the 4 PM pressure measurement.[49]

d. *Soft contact lenses.* A soft contact lens that has been soaked in pilocarpine is reported to give longer corneal contact time,[50, 51] greater aqueous drug levels,[25, 52] and longer intraocular pressure control[53] than topically applied pilocarpine. This mode of drug delivery, however, has not yet been recommended for general clinical use.

e. *Membrane-controlled delivery system.*[54] Pilocarpine between two polymeric membranes provides a constant drug release of 20 μg/ hr (Ocusert P-20) or 40 μg/hr (Ocusert P-40), which is roughly comparable to 1 to 2% and 4% pilocarpine, respectively.[55-60] The insert device is retained in the cul-de-sac and is effective for up to 7 days,[57, 61] although both relative effectiveness[62] and duration of action[58, 59] must be established for each patient by therapeutic trial.

This therapeutic delivery system is commercially available and offers distinct advantages over topical instillation of pilocarpine. The constant rate of release (zero order delivery) provides comparable pressure control with one-fifth the amount of medicine delivered by drops,[55, 63] which reduces side effects.[55, 64, 65] Two exceptions to this steady delivery rate is an initial period of increased drug release following insertion of the device and occasional subsequent episodes of transient increased release, which has been called the sudden leakage phenomenon.[56] Another advantage of this delivery system is that it partially levels out the diurnal curve.[66] The primary disadvantages are occasional discomfort and retention problems[67, 68]

f. *Synthetic biosoluble matrix.* Preliminary experience with pilocarpine in a synthetic biosoluble matrix has shown that this system can provide constant drug release for up to 24 hr when placed in the cul-de-sac.[69] With further study of new designs, the ocular insert devices may become an increasingly useful form of drug delivery in the treatment of glaucoma.

g. It has also been reported that *subconjunctival* injection of 0.15 to 0.2 ml of 4% pilocarpine achieves a more rapid and sustained miosis than with instillation of pilocarpine drops.[70] Intraocular injection of pilocarpine should be avoided, since it has been shown to cause corneal edema, presumably due to the osmotic effect of the solution.[71]

C. Drug Interactions

1. *Other miotics.* When other miotics are administered in combination with pilocarpine, they not only fail to increase the pressure lowering effect, but may interfere with the action of pilocarpine. *Echothiophate iodide*, a potent indirect-acting parasympathomimetic, is as effective alone as in combination with pilocarpine.[72] Furthermore, pre-treating monkeys with echothiophate iodide or *diisopropyl fluorophosphate*, another potent indirect-acting parasympathomimetic, produced a reversible subsensitivity or insensitivity to pilocarpine.[73-76] One such study showed that pilocarpine paradoxically increased the intraocular pressure after pre-treatment with echothiophate iodide, while the miotic effect of pilocarpine was only partially abolished.[77] This was felt to suggest the presence of two cholinergic receptor populations. *Physostigmine* (eserine), a slightly weaker indirect-acting parasympathomimetic, had no additive effect on tonographic values when added to pilocarpine therapy.[78]

2. *Additional anti-glaucoma medications. Epinephrine*[78, 79] or *timolol*,[80] a beta adrenergic antagonist, will produce additional intraocular pressure reduction when combined with pilocarpine. However, the effect of either combination is less than the additive effect of the two drugs. Pilocarpine may also be used effectively in combination with *carbonic anhydrase inhibitors* or *hyperosmotic agents*.

D. Side Effects

1. *Systemic toxicity.* Pilocarpine can produce systemic effects similar to those of *muscarine* [81, 82]:

a. Diaphoresis (perspiration).

b. Stimulation of glands, including salivary, lacrimal, gastric, pancreatic, intestinal, and mucosa of the respiratory tract. Pulmonary edema resulting from the latter may be fatal.

c. Contraction of smooth muscle, involving the gastrointestinal system (causing nausea, vomiting, and diarrhea), bronchi (the resulting bronchospasm can be fatal), ureters, urinary bladder, gall bladder, and capsular muscle of spleen (causing leukocytosis).

d. Blood pressure and pulse may rise or fall, depending on the degree of autonomic stimulation.

e. High concentrations of pilocarpine may weaken myocardial contractility.

Systemic toxicity is rare with the usual doses of pilocarpine used in the chronic management of glaucoma. The danger comes when large doses are given within a short period of time, as was once the practice for angle-closure glaucoma.[82] The problem is compounded by the fact that pilocarpine-induced toxicity may be confused with that of concomitant hyperosmotic therapy or of the disease itself. The antidote of systemic pilocarpine toxicity is *atropine*.

2. *Ocular side effects* are common with pilocarpine and can interfere with the patient's compliance to therapy.

a. *Ciliary muscle spasm* may lead to a browache, which usually subsides with continued therapy. A more debilitating effect is *induced myopia*, which is due to shallowing of the anterior chamber, axial thickening of the lens, and forward shift in the lens position.[83-87] This is more marked in young individuals, but also occurs in presbyopes.[88] Following instillation of 2% pilocarpine, the induced myopia begins in approximately 15 min, peaks in 45 to 60 min, and lasts for 1½ to 2 hr.[83, 88] A statistically significant dose-related response was found for the duration, but not the magnitude, of the effects on anterior chamber depth and lens thickness.[84]

b. *Miosis* may cause dimness of vision and alterations in the visual fields as discussed in Chapter 5, especially if cataracts are present.

c. *Retinal detachment* due to the use of miotics has been suspected on the basis of circumstantial evidence, although a definite cause-and-effect relationship has not been established.[89-91] These are typically rhegmatogenous detachments, and it is presumed that ciliary body contraction exerts vitreoretinal traction, which causes the retinal tears. The degree of risk appears to be related to pre-existing retinal pathology,[89-91] and possibly to the potency of the miotic. A *macular hole* was also reported to develop in a patient within weeks after starting therapy with 2% pilocarpine.[92]

d. A *cataractogenic* effect of pilocarpine has been suggested from observing patients on long-term uniocular miotic therapy.[93]

e. *Corneal endothelial toxicity* was dose related in *in vitro* rabbit studies.[94] As previously noted, corneal edema may occur with intracameral injection of pilocarpine, although this is more likely related to the osmotic effect of the solution.[71]

f. An *atypical band keratopathy* was once observed in patients on long-term pilocarpine therapy,[95] but this was found to result from the preservative, *phenylmercuric nitrate*,[96] which is no longer used.

II. DUAL ACTION PARASYMPATHOMIMETICS

The following two drugs have both a direct and indirect action on the parasympathetic nervous system:

A. Carbachol

Carbachol produces direct motor end plate stimulation as well as an indirect parasympathomimetic effect by inhibition of acetylcholinesterase. A concentration of 1.5%, instilled three times daily, has a more potent and prolonged pressure effect than 2% pilocarpine, four times a day.[97] However, carbachol causes more accommodative spasm and pain than pilocarpine.[87] Furthermore, as noted in Chapter 23, carbachol has poor corneal penetration and requires an adjuvant such as benzalkonium chloride to achieve effective aqueous levels.[98]

B. Aceclidine

Aceclidine (available in Europe as Glaucostat) is a synthetic ester with direct motor end plate action and weak anticholinesterase activity.[99, 100] The intraocular pressure lowering[100, 101] and miotic[87, 101] effects are comparable to those of pilocarpine, while aceclidine has the advantage of less accommodative spasm.[87, 99, 102, 103]

III. INDIRECT PARASYMPATHOMIMETICS

The pure inhibitors of acetylcholinesterase have been divided, somewhat arbitrarily, into two groups, designated "reversible" and "irreversible." Actually, none of these drugs are totally irreversible, and more precise definitions might be relatively "weaker" and "stronger" cholinesterase inhibitors, respectively.

A. Physostigmine

Physostigmine (eserine) is a "weaker" cholinesterase inhibitor. It is administered as a 0.5% ointment, usually twice daily. As previously noted, it is not additive with pilocarpine.[78] Furthermore, as is true of all the cholinesterase inhibitors, it causes vascular congestion, which may be a disadvantage in eyes with angle-closure glaucoma.

B. Echothiophate Iodide

Echothiophate iodide is a strong, relatively irreversible cholinesterase inhibitor.

1. *Mechanism of action.* Human ocular tissue contains true cholinesterase,[104] while pseudocholinesterase is found in human plasma.[105] *In vitro* and *in vivo* studies of cat irides indicate that *true cholinesterase* is the enzyme portion related to the drug-induced alteration of the iris sphincter and is the portion primarily inhibited by echothiophate iodide.[106, 107]

2. *Administration.* *In vitro* studies indicate that echothiophate iodide has the same efficacy (maximum effect produced by a drug regardless of dose) as most of the other miotics.[108] Clinical trials have shown that a concentration of 0.03% echothiophate iodide has a potency (effect produced by a particular concentration) equivalent to 1 to 2% pilocarpine,[16] while 0.06% echothiophate iodide is comparable to 4% pilocarpine.[30] No additional intraocular pressure reduction is normally achieved with concentrations of echothiophate iodide above 0.06%.[30, 109] However, echothiophate has the advantage of a *prolonged duration* of action, with the maximum effect occurring in 4 to 6 hr

and a substantial residual present after 24 hr.[16] The usual dosage of echothiophate iodide is 0.03 to 0.06%, twice daily.

3. *Side effects* significantly limit the usefulness of echothiophate iodide.

a. *Systemic toxicity* is related to *cholinesterase depletion*. Echothiophate iodide depletes both true cholinesterase in red blood cells and pseudocholinesterase in the plasma. This depletion begins in the first 2 weeks of chronic therapy, peaks in 5 to 7 weeks, and requires several weeks to recover after discontinuing the drug.[110] Pseudocholinesterase may also be depleted in newborns whose mothers received echothiophate in late pregnancy.[111]

Pseudocholinesterase hydrolyzes *succinylcholine*, and general anesthesia can be complicated by prolonged respiratory paralysis if this muscle relaxant is used in a patient depleted of cholinesterase.[110] *Local anesthetics* of the ester linkage group, such as procaine and tetracaine, are also hydrolyzed by pseudocholinesterase, and depletion of the enzyme may lead to toxic reactions to the anesthetic.[112]

In addition, topical echothiophate iodide may rarely cause the parasympathomimetic reactions of diarrhea, nausea, abdominal cramps, and malaise. A case was reported in which these symptoms developed following bilateral conjunctivodacryocystorhinostomies with Jones' tubes in a patient on long-term treatment with echothiophate iodide.[113] The danger of increased systemic absorption after this operation should be considered with all topical medications.

The antidote for echothiophate iodide toxicity is *pralidoxime chloride* (Protopam). This frees cholinesterase from the complex and prevents further inhibition, but does not alter the intraocular pressure lowering effect.[114]

b. A *cataractogenic effect* has been observed with the chronic use of echothiophate for the management of glaucoma.[115, 116] The cataracts have been described as initially having fine anterior subcapsular vacuoles,[115] although nuclear and posterior subcapsular changes have also been observed.[116] The side effect appears to be dose-related[116] and has not been observed in patients receiving cholinesterase inhibitor therapy for accommodative esotropia or in pesticide workers who are chronically exposed to cholinesterase inhibiting organophosphates.[117]

Experimental models of echothiophate-induced cataracts have been produced in monkeys,[118-121] which reveal swollen lens fibers, reduced protein concentration, and abnormal material in the intercellular spaces.[121] The mechanism is unclear, although alterations in cation and water balance due to increased lens permeability have been proposed.[122] It has also been suggested that mannitol, which is used as a vehicle, may contribute to the cataract formation.[123] Glutathione was not significantly decreased in rabbit eyes with echothiophate-induced cataracts.[124] One study suggested that atropine inhibited the cataractogenic effect in monkeys.[125]

Whatever the mechanism and frequency of this side effect may be, most physicians feel that it is of sufficient danger that the drug should be reserved primarily for aphakic eyes.

c. *Other ocular side effects*

(1). A *disruption of the blood-aqueous barrier* may cause increased inflammation following intraocular surgery, and it is usually advisable to discontinue the drug several weeks before surgery.

(2). *Retinal detachments* may be associated with miotic therapy, as discussed previously in this chapter.

(3). *Iris cysts* near the pupillary margin are not uncommon in children receiving echothiophate iodide for the treatment of accommodative esotropia. Structural alterations have been observed in the iris, ciliary muscle, ciliary processes, and trabecular meshwork of monkey eyes receiving chronic topical applications of echothiophate iodide.[126]

(4). *Ocular pseudopemphigoid*[127] and periorbital *allergic contact dermatitis*[128] have both been associated with the use of echothiophate iodide.

(5). *Corneal epithelial toxicity* with echothiophate iodide is reported to be greater than with pilocarpine, but less than with carbachol.[129]

C. Other Indirect Parasympathomimetics

Other strong, relatively irreversible cholinesterase inhibitors include:

1. *Diisopropyl fluorophosphate.* This drug is similar in action and side effects to echothiophate iodide, but produces more intense ciliary spasm and is susceptible to contamination with water.

2. *Demecarium.* This compound is also similar to the other indirect parasympathomimetics, but may be effective when echothiophate iodide has failed.

3. *Tetraethyl pyrophosphate* was found to be comparable to other strong miotics, but had the disadvantage of a considerable tendency to induce local sensitization.[130, 131]

References

1. Armaly, MF, Jepson, NC: Accommodation and the dynamics of the steady-state intraocular pressure. Invest Ophthal 1:480, 1962.
2. Van Buskirk, EM, Grant, WM: Lens depression and aqueous outflow in enucleated primate eyes. Am J Ophthal 76:632, 1973.
3. Van Buskirk, EM: Changes in the facility of aqueous outflow induced by lens depression and intraocular pressure in excised human eyes. Am J Ophthal 82:736, 1978.
4. Van Buskirk, EM: The canine eye: lens depression and aqueous outflow. Invest Ophthal Vis Sci 19:789, 1980.
5. Moses, RA, Grodzki, WJ Jr: Choroid tension and facility of aqueous outflow. Invest Ophthal Vis Sci 16:1062, 1977.
6. Cairns, JE: Goniospasis: A method designed to relieve canalicular blockade in primary open-angle glaucoma. Ann Ophthal 8:1417, 1976.
7. Kaufman, PL, Barany, EH: Residual pilocarpine effects on outflow facility after ciliary muscle disinsertion in the cynomolgus monkey. Invest Ophthal 15:558, 1976.

8. Kaufman, PL, Barany, EH: Loss of acute pilocarpine effect on outflow facility following surgical disinsertion and retrodisplacement of the ciliary muscle from the scleral spur in the cynomolgus monkey. Invest Ophthal 15:793, 1976.

9. Kaufman, PL, Bill, A, Barany, EH: Formation and drainage of aqueous humor following total iris removal and ciliary muscle disinsertion in the cynomolgus monkey. Invest Ophthal Vis Sci 16:226, 1977.

10. Lutjen-Drecoll, E, Kaufman, PL, Barany, EH: Light and electron microscopy of the anterior chamber angle structures following surgical disinsertion of the ciliary muscle in the cynomolgus monkey. Invest Ophthal Vis Sci 16:218, 1977.

11. Grierson, I, Lee, WR, Abraham, S: Effects of pilocarpine on the morphology of the human outflow apparatus. Br J Ophthal 62:302, 1978.

12. Grierson, I, Lee, WR, Moseley, H, Abraham, S: The trabecular wall of Schlemm's canal: a study of the effects of pilocarpine by scanning electron microscopy. Br J Ophthal 63:9, 1979.

13. Grierson, I, Lee, WR, Abraham, S: The effects of topical pilocarpine on the morphology of the outflow apparatus of the baboon (*Papio cynocephalus*). Invest Ophthal Vis Sci 18:346, 1979.

14. Kaufman, PL: Aqueous humor dynamics following total iridectomy in the cynomolgus monkey. Invest Ophthal Vis Sci 18:870, 1979.

15. Gaasterland, D, Kupfer, C, Ross, K: Studies of aqueous humor dynamics in man. IV. Effects of pilocarpine upon measurements in young normal volunteers. Invest Ophthal 14:848, 1975.

16. Barsam, PC: Comparison of the effect of pilocarpine and echothiophate on intraocular pressure and outflow facility. Am J Ophthal 73:742, 1972.

17. Barany, EH: A pharmacologist looks at medical treatment in glaucoma—in retrospect and in prospect. Ophthalmology 86:80, 1979.

18. Bill, A, Phillips, CI: Uveoscleral drainage of aqueous humour in human eyes. Exp Eye Res 12:275, 1971.

19. Bleiman, BS, Schwartz, AL: Paradoxical intraocular pressure response to pilocarpine. A proposed mechanism and treatment. Arch Ophthal 97:1305, 1979.

20. Doane, MG, Jensen, AD, Dohlman, CH: Penetration routes of topically applied eye medications. Am J Ophthal 85:383, 1978.

21. Van Hoose, MC, Leaders, FE: The role of the cornea in the biologic response to pilocarpine. Invest Ophthal 13:377, 1974.

22. Lazare, R, Horlington, M: Pilocarpine levels in the eyes of rabbits following topical application. Exp Eye Res 21:281, 1975.

23. Krohn, DL: Flux of topical pilocarpine to the human aqueous. Trans Am Ophthal Soc 76:502, 1978.

24. Krohn, DL, Breitfeller, JM: Transcorneal flux of topical pilocarpine to the human aqueous. Am J Ophthal 87:50, 1979.

25. Asseff, CF, Weisman, RL, Podos, SM, Becker, B: Ocular penetration of pilocarpine in primates. Am J Ophthal 75:212, 1973.

26. Chrai, SS, Robinson, JR: Corneal permeation of topical pilocarpine nitrate in the rabbit. Am J Ophthal 77:735, 1974.

27. Harris, LS, Galin, MA: Dose response analysis of pilocarpine-induced ocular hypotension. Arch Ophthal 84:605, 1970.

28. Drance, SM, Nash, PA: The dose response of human intraocular pressure to pilocarpine. Canad J Ophthal 6:9, 1971.

29. Drance, SM, Bensted, M, Schulzer, M: Pilocarpine and intraocular pressure. Duration of effectiveness of 4% and 8% pilocarpine instillation. Arch Ophthal 91:104, 1974.

30. Harris, LS: Comparison of pilocarpine and echothiophate iodide in open-angle glaucoma. Ann Ophthal 4:736, 1972.

31. Harris, LS, Galin, MA: Effect of ocular pigmentation of hypotensive response to pilocarpine. Am J Ophthal 72:923, 1971.

32. Lerman, S, Reininger, B: Simulated sustained release pilocarpine therapy and aqueous humor dynamics. Can J Ophthal 6:14, 1971.

33. Birmingham, AT, Galloway, NR, Spencer, SA: A comparison of the pupillocon-

strictor effect of pilocarpine solution administered to the conjunctival sac as a single drop or as a continuous infusion in normal subjects. Br J Ophthal 60:568, 1976.

34. Birmingham, AT, Galloway, NR, Walker, DA: Intraocular pressure reduction in chronic simple glaucoma by continuous infusion of dilute pilocarpine solution. Br J Ophthal 63:808, 1979.

35. Patton, TF, Francoeur, M: Ocular bioavailability and systemic loss of topically applied ophthalmic drugs. Am J Ophthal 85:225, 1978.

36. File, RR, Patton, TF: Topically applied pilocarpine. Human pupillary response as a function of drop size. Arch Ophthal 98:112, 1980.

37. Fraunfelder, FT, Hanna, C: Ophthalmic drug delivery systems. Surv Ophthal 18:292, 1974.

38. Smith, SA, Smith, SE, Lazare, R: An increased effect of pilocarpine on the pupil by application of the drug in oil. Br J Ophthal 62:314, 1978.

39. Barsam, PC: The most commonly used miotic—now longer acting. Ann Ophthal 6:809, 1974.

40. Magder, H, Boyaner, D: The use of a longer acting pilocarpine in the management of chronic simple glaucoma. Can J Ophthal 9:285, 1974.

41. Sherman, SE: Clinical comparison of pilocarpine preparations in heavily pigmented eyes: an evaluation of the influence of polymer vehicles on corneal penetration, drug availability, and duration of hypotensive activity. Ann Ophthal 9:1231, 1977.

42. Quigley, HA, Pollack, IP: Intraocular pressure control with twice-daily pilocarpine in two vehicle solutions. Ann Ophthal 9:427, 1977.

43. Green, K, Downs, SJ: Ocular penetration of pilocarpine in rabbits. Arch Ophthal 93:1165, 1975.

44. Harbin, TS Jr, Kaback, MB, Podos, SM, Becker, B: Comparative intraocular pressure effects of Adsorbocarpine and Isopto Carpine. Ann Ophthal 10:59, 1978.

45. Ticho, U, Blumenthal, M, Zonis, S, Gal, A, Blank, I, Mazor, ZW: Piloplex, a new long-acting pilocarpine polymer salt. A: long-term study. Br J Ophthal 63:45, 1979.

46. Mazor, Z, Ticho, U, Rehany, U, Rose, L: Piloplex, a new long-acting pilocarpine polymer salt. B: comparative study of the visual effects of pilocarpine and Piloplex eye drops. Br J Ophthal 63:48, 1979.

47. Ticho, U, Blumenthal, M, Zonis, S, Gal, A, Blank, I, Mazor, ZW: A clinical trial with Piloplex—a new long-acting pilocarpine compound: preliminary report. Ann Ophthal 11:555, 1979.

48. Blumenthal, M, Ticho, U, Zonis, S, Gal, A, Blank, I, Mazor, Z: Further clinical trial with Piloplex—a new long-acting pilocarpine salt. Glaucoma 1:145, 1979.

49. Goldberg, I, Ashburn, FS Jr, Kass, MA, Becker, B: Efficacy and patient acceptance of pilocarpine gel. Am J Ophthal 88:843, 1979.

50. Krohn, DL, Breitfeller, JM: Quantitation of pilocarpine flux enhancement across isolated rabbit cornea by hydrogel polymer lenses. Invest Ophthal 14:152, 1975.

51. Ruben, M, Watkins, R: Pilocarpine dispensation for the soft hydrophilic contact lens. Br J Ophthal 59:455, 1975.

52. Ramer, RM, Gasset, AR: Ocular penetration of pilocarpine: The effect of hydrophilic soft contact lenses on the ocular penetration of pilocarpine. Ann Ophthal 6:1325, 1974.

53. Podos, SM, Becker, B, Asseff, C, Hartstein, J: Pilocarpine therapy with soft contact lenses. Am J Ophthal 73:336, 1972.

54. Shell, JW, Baker, RW: Diffusional systems for controlled release of drugs to the eye. Ann Ophthal 6:1037, 1974.

55. Place, VA, Fisher, M, Herbst, S, Gordon, L, Merrill, RC: Comparative pharmacologic effects of pilocarpine administered to normal subjects by eyedrops or by ocular therapeutic systems. Am J Ophthal 80:706, 1975.

56. Lee, P, Shen, Y, Eberle, M: The long-acting Ocusert-pilocarpine system in the management of glaucoma. Invest Ophthal 14:43, 1975.

57. Quigley, HA, Pollack, IP, Harbin, RS Jr: Pilocarpine Ocuserts. Long-term

clinical trials and selected pharmacodynamics. Arch Ophthal 93:771, 1975.

58. Friederich, RL: The pilocarpine Ocusert: A new drug delivery system. Ann Ophthal 6:1279, 1974.
59. Armaly, MF, Rao, KR: The effect of pilocarpine Ocusert with different release rates on ocular pressure. Invest Ophthal 12:491, 1973.
60. Worthen, DM, Zimmerman, TJ, Wind, CA: An evaluation of the pilocarpine Ocusert. Invest Ophthal 13:296, 1974.
61. Drance, SM, Mitchell, DWA, Schultzer, M: The duration of action of pilocarpine Ocusert on intraocular pressure in man. Can J Ophthal 10:450, 1975.
62. Macoul, KL, Pavan-Langston, D: Pilocarpine Ocusert system for sustained control of ocular hypertension. Arch Ophthal 93:587, 1975.
63. Sendelbeck, L, Moore, D, Urquhart, J: Comparative distribution of pilocarpine in ocular tissues of the rabbit during adminstration by eyedrop or by membrane-controlled delivery systems. Am J Ophthal 80:274, 1975.
64. Brown, HS, Meltzer, G, Merrill, RC, Fisher, M, Ferre, C, Place, VA: Visual effects of pilocarpine in glaucoma. Comparative study of administration by eyedrops or by ocular therapeutic systems. Arch Ophthal 94:1716, 1976.
65. Francois, J, Goes, F, Zagorski, Z: Comparative ultrasonographic study of the effect of pilocarpine 2% and Ocusert P 20 on the eye components. Am J Ophthal 86:233, 1978.
66. Fraunfelder, FT, Shell, JW, Herbst, SF: Effect of pilocarpine ocular therapeutic systems on diurnal control of intraocular pressure. Ann Ophthal 8:1031, 1976.
67. Smith, SE, Smith, SA, Friedman, AI, Chaston, JM: Comparison of the pupillary, refractive, and hypotensive effects of Ocusert-40 and pilocarpine eyedrops in the treatment of chronic simple glaucoma. Br J Ophthal 63:228, 1979.
68. Stewart, RH, Novak, S: Introduction of the Ocusert ocular system to an ophthalmic practice. Ann Ophthal 10:325, 1978.
69. Bensinger, R, Shin, DH, Kass, MA, Podos, SM, Becker, B: Pilocarpine ocular inserts. Invest Ophthal 15:1008, 1976.
70. Mehta, HK: Subconjunctival injection of pilocarpine. Trans Ophthal Soc UK 96:184, 1976.
71. Jay, JL, MacDonald, M: Effects of intraocular miotics on cultured bovine corneal endothelium. Br J Ophthal 62:815, 1978.
72. Kini, MM, Dahl, AA, Roberts, CR, Lehwalder, LW, Grant, WM: Echothiophate, pilocarpine, and open-angle glaucoma. Arch Ophthal 89:190, 1973.
73. Kaufman, PL, Barany, EH: Subsensitivity to pilocarpine in primate ciliary muscle following topical anticholinesterase treatment. Invest Ophthal 14:302, 1975.
74. Kaufman, PL, Barany, EH: Subsensitivity to pilocarpine of the aqueous outflow system in monkey eyes after topical anticholinesterase treatment. Am J Ophthal 82:883, 1976.
75. Kaufman, PL: Anticholinesterase-induced cholinergic subsensitivity in primate accommodative mechanism. Am J Ophthal 85:622, 1978.
76. Bito, LZ, Baroody, RA: Gradual changes in the sensitivity of rhesus monkey eyes to miotics and the dependence of these changes on the regimen of topical cholinesterase inhibitor treatment. Invest Ophthal Vis Sci 18:794, 1979.
77. Bito, LZ, Merritt, SQ: Paradoxical ocular hypertensive effect of pilocarpine on echothiophate iodide-treated primate eyes. Invest Ophthal Vis Sci 19:371, 1980.
78. Kronfeld, PC: The efficacy of combinations of ocular hypotensive drugs. A tonographic approach. Arch Ophthal 78:140, 1967.
79. Harris, LS, Mittag, TW, Galin, MA: Aqueous dynamics of pilocarpine-treated eyes. The influence of topically applied epinephrine. Arch Ophthal 86:1, 1971.
80. Knupp, JA, Mandell, AI, Hurvitz, LM, Spaeth, GL, Shields, MB: Comparison of dipivefrin and pilocarpine used concomitantly with timolol in the management of open-angle glaucoma. Presented at annual meeting American Academy of Ophthalmology, Chicago, Nov 2-7, 1980, abstract, p 129.
81. Havener, WH: Ocular Pharmacology, 4th ed. CV Mosby Co, St. Louis, 1978, p 286.

82. Greco, JJ, Kelman, CD: Systemic pilocarpine toxicity in the treatment of angle closure glaucoma. Ann Ophthal 5:57, 1973.
83. Abramson, DH, Coleman, DJ, Forbes, M, Franzen, LA: Pilocarpine. Effect on the anterior chamber and lens thickness. Arch Ophthal 87:615, 1972.
84. Abranson, DH, Chang, S, Coleman, DJ, Smith, ME: Pilocarpine-induced lens changes. An ultrasonic biometric evaluation of dose response. Arch Ophthal 92:464, 1974.
85. Abranson, DH, Chang, S, Coleman, DJ: Pilocarpine therapy in glaucoma. Effects on anterior chamber depth and lens thickness in patients receiving long-term therapy. Arch Ophthal 94:914, 1976.
86. Poinoosawmy, D, Nagasubramanian, S, Brown, NAP: Effect of pilocarpine on visual acuity and on the dimensions of the cornea and anterior chamber. Br J Ophthal 60:676, 1976.
87. Francois, J, Goes, F: Ultrasonographic study of the effect of different miotics on the eye components. Ophthalmologica 175:328, 1977.
88. Abramson, DH, Franzen, LA, Coleman, DJ: Pilocarpine in the presbyope. Demonstration of an effect on the anterior chamber and lens thickness. Arch Ophthal 89:100, 1973.
89. Pape, LG, Forbes, M: Retinal detachment and miotic therapy. Am J Ophthal 85:558, 1978.
90. Beasley, H, Fraunfelder, FT: Retinal detachments and topical ocular miotics. Ophthalmology 86:95, 1979.
91. Alpar, JJ: Miotics and retinal detachment: a survey and case report. Ann Ophthal 11:395, 1979.
92. Garlikov, RS, Chenoweth, RG: Macular hole following topical pilocarpine. Ann Ophthal 7:1313, 1975.
93. Levene, RZ: Uniocular miotic therapy. Trans Am Acad Ophthal Otol 79:376, 1975.
94. Coles, WH: Pilocarpine toxicity. Effects on the rabbit corneal endothelium. Arch Ophthal 93:36, 1975.
95. Kennedy, RE, Roca, PD, Landers, PH: Atypical band keratopathy in glaucomatous patients. Am J Ophthal 72:917, 1971.
96. Kennedy, RE, Roca, PD, Platt, DS: Further observations on atypical band keratopathy in glaucoma patients. Trans Am Ophthal Soc 72:107, 1974.
97. O'Brien, CS, Swan, KC: Carbaminoylcholine chloride in the treatment of glaucoma simplex. Arch Ophthal 27:253, 1942.
98. Smolen, VF, Clevenger, JM, Williams, EJ, Bergdolt, MW: Biophasic availability of ophthalmic carbachol I: mechanisms of cationic polymer- and surfactant-promoted miotic activity. J Pharm Sci 62:958, 1973.
99. Fechner, PU, Teichmann, KD, Weyrauch, W: Accommodative effects of aceclidine in the treatment of glaucoma. Am J Ophthal 79:104, 1975.
100. Drance, SM, Fairclough, M, Schulzer, M: Dose response of human intraocular pressure to aceclidine. Arch Ophthal 88:394, 1972.
101. Riegel, D, Leydhecker, W: Experiences with aceclidine in the treatment of simple glaucoma. Klin Monatsbl Augenheilkd 151:882, 1967.
102. Fechner, PU: Avoiding spasm of accommodation in the treatment of young glaucoma patients. Klin Monatsbl Augenhielkd 158:112, 1971.
103. Pilz, A, Lommatzsch, P, Ulrich, WD: Experimentelle und klinsche Untersuchungen mit Aceclidin (Glaucostat). Ophthalmologica 168:376, 1974.
104. Leopold, IH, Furman, M: Cholinesterase isoenzymes in human ocular tissue homogenates. Am J Ophthal 72:460, 1971.
105. Juul P: Human plasma cholinesterase isoenzymes. Clin Chim Acta 19:205, 1968.
106. Harris, LS, Shimmyo, M, Mittag, TW: Cholinesterases and contractility of cat irides. Effect of echothiophate iodide. Arch Ophthal 89:49, 1973.
107. Harris, LS, Shimmyo, M, Mittag, TW: Effects of echothiophate on cholinesterases in cat irides. Arch Ophthal 91:57, 1974.
108. Harris, LS, Shimmyo, M, Hughes, J: Dose-response of cholinergic agonists on cat irides. Arch Ophthal 91:299, 1974.

109. Harris, LS: Dose-response analysis of echothiophate iodide. Arch Ophthal 86:502, 1971.
110. Ellis, PP, Esterdahl, M: Echothiophate iodide therapy in children. Effect upon blood cholinesterase levels. Arch Ophthal 77:598, 1967.
111. Birks, DA, Prior, VJ, Silk, E, Whittaker, M: Echothiophate iodide treatment of glaucoma in pregnancy. Arch Ophthal 79:283, 1968.
112. Ellis, PP, Littlejohn, K: Effects of topical anticholinesterases on procaine hydrolysis. Am J Ophthal 77:71, 1974.
113. Wood, JR, Anderson, RL, Edwards, JJ: Phospholine iodide toxicity and Jones' tubes. Ophthalmology 87:346, 1980.
114. Lipson, ML, Holmes, JH, Ellis, PP: Oral administration of pralidoxime chloride in echothiophate iodide therapy. Arch Ophthal 82:830, 1969.
115. Axelsson, U, Holmberg, A: The frequency of cataract after miotic therapy. Acta Ophthal 44:421, 1966.
116. Thoft, RA: Incidence of lens changes in patients treated with echothiophate iodide. Arch Ophthal 80:317, 1968.
117. Pietsch, RL, Bobo, CB, Finklea, JF, Vallotton, WW: Lens opacities and organophosphate cholinesterase-inhibiting agents. Am J Ophthal 73:236, 1973.
118. Kaufman, PL, Axelsson, U: Induction of subcapsular cataracts in aniridic vervet monkeys by echothiophate. Invest Ophthal 14:863, 1975.
119. Kaufman, PL, Axelsson, U, Barany, EH: Induction of subcapsular cataracts in cynomolgus monkeys by echothiophate. Arch Ophthal 95:499, 1977.
120. Albrecht, M, Barany, E: Early lens changes in Macaca fascicularis monkeys under topical treatment with echothiophate or carbachol studied by slit-image photography. Invest Ophthal Vis Sci 18:179, 1979.
121. Philipson, B, Kaufman, PL, Fagerholm, P, Axelsson, U, Barany, EH: Echothiophate cataracts in monkeys. Electron microscopy and microradiography. Arch Ophthal 97:340, 1979.
122. Michon, J Jr, Kinoshita, JH: Experimental miotic cataract. II. Permeability, cation transport, and intermediary metabolism. Arch Ophthal 79:611, 1968.
123. Lazar, M, Nowakowski, J, Furman, M, Shore, B: Ocular penetration of topically applied mannitol. Am J Ophthal 70:849, 1970.
124. Firth, JM, Vucicevic, ZM, Tsou, KC: The influence of miotics on the lens. Ann Ophthal 5:685, 1973.
125. Kaufman, PL, Axelsson, U, Barany, EH: Atropine inhibition of echothiophate cataractogenesis in monkeys. Arch Ophthal 95:1262, 1977.
126. Lutjen-Drecoll, E, Kaufman, PL: Echothiophate-induced structural alterations in the anterior chamber angle of the cynomolgus monkey. Invest Ophthal Vis Sci 18:918, 1979.
127. Patten, JT, Cavanagh, HD, Allansmith, MR: Induced ocular pseudopemphigoid. Am J Ophthal 82:272, 1976.
128. Mathias, CGT, Maibach, HI, Irvine, A, Adler, W: Allergic contact dermatitis to echothiophate iodide and phenylephrine. Arch Ophthal 97:286, 1979.
129. Krejci, L, Harrison, R: Antiglaucoma drug effects on corneal epithelium. A comparative study in tissue culture. Arch Ophthal 84:766, 1970.
130. Grant, WM: Miotic and antiglaucomatous activity of tetraethyl pyrophosphate in human eyes. Arch Ophthal 39:579, 1948.
131. Grant, WM: Additional experiences with tetraethyl pyrophosphate in treatment of glaucoma. Arch Ophthal 44:362, 1950.

Chapter 26

ADRENERGIC DRUGS

ADRENERGIC DRUGS

I. EPINEPHRINE

This direct-acting sympathomimetic stimulates both *alpha* and *beta* adrenergic receptors and is a standard topical drug for the chronic management of open-angle forms of glaucoma.

A. Mechanisms of Action

Reports have been conflicting regarding the mechanism of intraocular pressure reduction by epinephrine. Early observations suggested that the primary action was decreased aqueous production.[1-4] It was subsequently noted, however, that an improvement in aqueous outflow facility occurs after prolonged use of epinephrine.[5, 6] Still more recent studies have indicated that increased outflow also occurs early and is the predominant feature of the pressure-lowering effect.[7-13] Rabbit[14] and human[15] studies indicate that the early effect on outflow is greatest with epinephrine concentrations of 1% or more and the response is larger in ocular hypertensives or open-angle glaucoma patients.[8, 10] The precise mechanisms by which epinephrine influences aqueous inflow and outflow are not fully understood, although the following observations and theories have been reported.

1. *Unified concept.* Sears and Neufeld[16, 17] have proposed a *three phase* mechanism for the action of epinephrine on aqueous humor dynamics.

a. *Decreased aqueous production* is the earliest effect, occurring within minutes of instillation. It is postulated that this may be due to vasoconstriction, an alpha adrenergic effect, which reduces the ultrafiltration of plasma into the stroma of the ciliary processes. This is consistent with observations in monkeys that topical epinephrine reduces blood flow by 59% in the iris and 20% in the ciliary processes for at least 6 hr.[18]

b. An *early increase in outflow facility* overlaps with phase one and has two components. The first portion is actually a part of phase one and is believed to be an alpha adrenergic effect. The second component occurs hours after administration, when the vasoconstrictor and mydriatic effects are gone. Fluorophotometric studies in normal human eyes show that intraocular pressure reduction for at least the first 7 hr after topical instillation of epinephrine is associated with improved facility of outflow and an actual increase in the rate of aqueous production.[19] Concomitant tonographic studies suggest that epinephrine may increase the rate of outflow via the extracanalicular (uveoscleral) pathway.[19] The receptor site in the outflow system is uncertain, but the mechanism is probably a beta adrenergic response, stimulating the synthesis of cyclic adenosine monophosphate (AMP), since the latter has been shown to mediate increased outflow facility in primates.[20-22] This portion of phase two lasts for several hours.

c. A *late increase in outflow facility* occurs weeks to months after continued administration of epinephrine. The mechanism is uncertain, but may be related to decreased mucinous material in the trabecular meshwork. This is consistent with the observation that epinephrine activates lysosomal hyaluronidase in the rabbit iris.[23] It has also been noted that long-term epinephrine therapy causes a supersensitivity to topical epinephrine,[24] which might relate to the increased effectiveness of the drug with continued use.

2. A modified concept of the adrenergic influence on aqueous humor dynamics has been postulated by Thomas and Epstein,[25] based primarily on observed interactions between epinephrine and the beta adrenergic antagonist, timolol. The hypothetical model may be considered to have three components. (The application of this model to the intraocular pressure-lowering mechanism of beta adrenergic antagonists and the clinical implications regarding combined therapy with beta adrenergic agonists and antagonists will be discussed later in this chapter.)

a. *Alpha adrenergic effect on aqueous inflow.* This is the same as for the unified concept of Sears and Neufeld,[16, 17] *i.e., reduced aqueous production*, probably due to vasoconstriction.

b. *Beta adrenergic effect on aqueous inflow.* The model postulates that stimulation of beta adrenergic receptors in the inflow system *increases* aqueous production. This is consistent with the previously noted fluorophotometric observations on inflow in response to epinephrine.[19] However, when epinephrine is applied to eyes pretreated with timolol, fluorophotometric studies reveal a slight decrease in aqueous production,[26] suggesting that the beta adrenergic antagonist blocks the beta-mediated effect of epinephrine on inflow.

c. *Beta adrenergic effect on aqueous outflow.* Stimulation of beta adrenergic receptors in the outflow system is believed to *increase* aqueous outflow, which is supported by tonographic studies. Timolol also blocks this effect of epinephrine, which is consistent with the observation that the beta adrenergic antagonist blocks catecholamine-stimulated increase in cyclic AMP.[27]

B. Administration

1. *Concentrations.* Studies have shown that the pressure-lowering effect of epinephrine is proportional to the concentration of *free base* (or active form of the drug) within the range of 0.25 to 1%,[16] and that 2% may have some additional efficacy over the 1% concentration.[4] It has also been shown that topical epinephrine may be an effective ocular hypotensive drug in concentrations as low as 0.06%.[28] Standard commercial preparations are available in concentrations of 0.5, 1, and 2%.

2. *Frequency of administration.* Twice daily instillation provides a continuous pressure lowering effect in most cases. However, a ques-

tion which needs further study is whether more frequent administration, *e.g.*, four times daily, might maximize the early effect of decreased aqueous production.

3. *Formulations.* Standard commercial preparations are available in three salt forms: hydrochloride, borate, and bitartrate. No significant difference has been found in the pressure lowering efficacy of these three preparations.[9]

a. *Epinephrine hydrochloride* has the advantage of stability and is available in all three concentrations (0.5, 1, and 2%) of the free base. It has the disadvantage of irritation upon instillation because of a low pH of approximately 3.5.

b. *Epinephryl borate* is a complex of boric acid and epinephrine and causes less irritation due to a higher pH of 7.4.[29] It is only available in the 0.5% of 1% concentrations of free base.

c. *Epinephrine bitartrate* also has the disadvantage of irritation with instillation due to a low pH. In addition, the stated concentration of commercial preparations may be less than the free base of epinephrine. This salt form has been tested in rabbits in a *polymeric matrix*, which releases the drug osmotically at a rate of 1 to 4 µg of free base per hour over a 12-hr period.[30] This form of drug delivery provided intraocular pressure control equivalent to that of the drug in drop form, but with considerably less total medication and without reducing the tear film pH.

C. Methods to Enhance Epinephrine Effect

1. *Adrenergic supersensitivity.* One method for enhancing the effect of epinephrine is to increase the sensitivity of ocular tissues to the drug.

a. *6-hydroxydopamine.* This compound produces a "chemical sympathectomy" by causing temporary degeneration of axon terminals.[31–35] The result is a transient increase in outflow facility due to an initial release of norepinephrine, and a more sustained effect on intraocular pressure reduction by enhancing the action of exogenous epinephrine. A similar effect has been demonstrated in rabbits with *alpha-methyl-para-tyrosine*, an inhibitor of norepinephrine synthesis.[36, 37] These drugs produce both an alpha and beta adrenergic supersensitivity, although the latter appears to be the predominant effect with 6-hydroxydopamine.[31–34] A practical disadvantage of 6-hydroxydopamine is that it must be administered subconjunctivally or by iontophoresis at weekly to monthly intervals.[38, 39] Furthermore, both 6-hydroxydopamine and alpha-methyl-para-tyrosine cause a subsensitivity to cholinergic drugs in rabbits.[36, 37]

b. *Guanethidine.* This drug is a post-ganglionic adrenergic antagonist which creates an adrenergic supersensitivity by depleting stores of catecholamines.[40] It may lower the intraocular pressure when given alone, presumably by an effect on both aqueous production and outflow,[41] but is particularly effective when used in combination with epinephrine.[42, 43] Clinical trials with such a combined drop have revealed significant, sustained reductions in intraocular pressure.[44–50]

However, one study revealed a biphasic response in which a phase of elevated intraocular pressure occurred due to increased aqueous production.[51] Although guanethidine is reported to cause soreness, conjunctival hyperemia, corneal epithelial changes, lid edema and ptosis in some patients,[52] the combination drops are said to be generally well tolerated.[44-50] The effect of ptosis by topical guanethidine, however, has actually been used to treat thyrotoxic lid retraction.[40, 53, 54]

2. *Dipivefrin.* Another way to enhance the effect of epinephrine is to modify the parent compound. Dipivefrin, or dipivalyl epinephrine, is created by the addition of two pivalic acid groups to epinephrine.[55-56] The new compound is significantly more lipophilic than epinephrine, which increases the corneal penetration by 17-fold.[57] In addition, dipivefrin is a *prodrug*, which is a drug that undergoes biotransformation before exhibiting its pharmacologic effect. The compound is hydrolyzed to epinephrine after absorption into the eye,[58] with the majority of the hydrolysis occurring in the cornea.[59] Clinical trials indicate that the pressure-lowering effect of 0.1% dipivefrin is somewhere between that of 1 and 2% epinephrine,[60-63] while the side effects of burning and irritation with instillation are significantly reduced.[64] Additional benefits may be less systemic toxicity and lack of hydrophilic contact lens discoloration,[65] as occurs with topical epinephrine. However, external ocular toxicity may occur with prolonged use of dipivefrin.[66] Rabbit studies suggest that cholinesterase inhibitors inactivate the esterase which converts dipivefrin to epinephrine,[67] although further study is needed before the clinical implications of this observation are known.

D. Side Effects

Side effects are common with the topical administration of standard epinephrine preparations. It is helpful to think of these in three categories: systemic, extraocular, and intraocular.

1. *Systemic toxicity* includes elevated blood pressure, tachycardia, arrhythmias, headaches, tremor, nervousness, and anxiety. Since dipivefrin is administered in the lower concentration of 0.1% and is not converted to active epinephrine until it enters the eye, fewer systemic effects might be anticipated with this form of epinephrine.

2. *Local extraocular reactions* constitute the most common side effects encountered with topical epinephrine therapy.

    a. *Burning* on instillation is practically universal with the hydrochloride and bitartrate preparations, but may be minimized with the use of epinephryl borate or dipivefrin.

    b. *Reactive hyperemia* occurs with all forms of epinephrine. The patient often fails to associate this with use of the drug, since the initial vasoconstrictive effect of epinephrine tends to whiten the conjunctiva, and the hyperemia appears later.

    c. *Adrenochrome pigmentation.* Oxidation and polymerization of epinephrine converts the drug to adrenochrome, a pigment of the melanin family, which may be deposited in several ocular structures.

In the lower *conjunctiva*, it forms small, round deposits, which are usually asymptomatic,[68] while deposits in the upper conjunctiva tend to be branching or "staghorn" in shape and may abrade the cornea.[69-71] When intraocular pressure elevation and bullous keratopathy are present, adrenochrome may deposit in the superficial cornea, producing a so-called *"black cornea."*[72-79] Adrenochrome may also deposit in the lacrimal sac[80] or nasolacrimal duct.[81] It may also discolor soft contact lenses,[82, 83] which, as previously noted, is reported not to occur with dipivefrin.[65]

    d. Other less common extraocular reactions include tearing, photophobia, blurred vision, epidermalization of the lacrimal punctum,[84] and madarosis (loss of eyelashes).[85] An association with ocular pemphigoid has been suggested,[86] although a clear cause-and-effect relationship has not been established, and true allergic reactions with topical epinephrine are not common.

    3. *Intraocular reactions*, while less common than the extraocular side effects, generally have more serious consequences. With regard to dipivefrin, it should be anticipated that the intraocular reactions will be the same as with other forms of epinephrine, since it becomes the active drug after entering the eye.

    a. *Mydriasis* is a standard, although somewhat variable, response to epinephrine. It is usually of no consequence, but may precipitate *angle-closure glaucoma* in the predisposed eye, and is clearly contraindicated in such cases.

    b. *Epinephrine maculopathy* is a form of cystoid macular edema, which occurs in some aphakic eyes receiving topical epinephrine.[87-89] A fluorescein angiographic study of 128 consecutive eyes revealed macular edema in 28% of those receiving epinephrine and in 13% of those not on the drug.[90] The mechanism is uncertain, but the condition is usually reversible and probably dose related.

    c. *Corneal endothelial damage* has been observed with intracameral injection of epinephrine 1:1000 in rabbit and monkey eyes, but not with a 1:5000 concentration.[91] Decreased endothelial cell counts have been reported in glaucoma patients after prolonged use of topical epinephrine.[92]

    d. It has also been suggested that epinephrine might reduce optic nerve head perfusion by causing vasoconstriction of the adrenergically-innervated vessels behind the lamina cribrosa, and that this might particularly be a problem in the unprotected fellow eye during uniocular treatment with epinephrine.[93]

II. OTHER ADRENERGIC STIMULATORS (AGONISTS)

A. Direct Alpha-adrenergic Stimulators

    1. *Norepinephrine*, the post-ganglionic physiologic mediator of the adrenergic nervous system, has had limited clinical usefulness because of instability. However, newer more stable preparations have led to a re-evaluation of the drug. Concentrations of 2 to 4%, given twice daily, significantly lowered the intraocular pressure, presum-

ably by an alpha-induced increase in outflow facility, without causing beta-induced side effects, such as tachycardia.[94-96] Rabbit studies reveal an early mydriasis and rise in intraocular pressure[97, 98] before the pressure reduction occurs.[97] The ocular effects of norepinephrine can be potentiated by bilateral cervical ganglionectomy,[98] monoamine oxidase inhibitors (pargyline or pheniprazone),[99] or protriptyline,[100] which potentiates adrenergic activity by blocking catecholamine uptake into postganglionic neurons.

2. *Clonidine hydrochloride* is a centrally acting systemic anti-hypertensive agent, which has been shown to lower the intraocular pressure and produce mydriasis.[101, 102] Concentrations of 0.125 and 0.25% have been shown to lower the pressure, although neither was as effective as 2% pilocarpine.[101] The drug binds to alpha-adrenergic receptors in homogenized rabbit iris-ciliary body preparations,[103] and studies with cat eyes suggest that it decreases aqueous humor formation by causing constriction of afferent vessels in the ciliary processes.[104] Clonidine requires an intact adrenergic nervous system to be effective.[105]

B. Indirect Alpha-adrenergic Stimulator

Pargyline, a monoamine oxidase inhibitor, is an indirect alpha-adrenergic stimulator, used in the treatment of systemic hypertension.[106] It has been shown to lower the intraocular pressure in rabbits by decreasing aqueous production,[106, 107] provided the adrenergic nervous system is intact.[108] Pargyline 0.5% significantly lowered the pressure in open-angle glaucoma patients, without effecting the pupil.[109]

C. Beta-adrenergic Stimulator

Isoproterenol is a direct beta-adrenergic stimulator. The racemic form, *dl*-isoproterenol, reduces intraocular pressure in man,[110, 111] but causes tachycardia with palpitation and weakness,[111] which is an *l*-isomer effect.[111, 112] *d*-Isoproterenol also reduces the intraocular pressure in rabbits,[112, 113] without causing tachycardia, vasoconstriction, or mydriasis.[112] However, *d*-isoproterenol does not appear to have the same pressure effect in human eyes.[113]

III. ALPHA-ADRENERGIC BLOCKING AGENTS (ANTAGONISTS)

A. Thymoxamine

This drug competes with norepinephrine for alpha-adrenergic receptors. As a result, it produces *miosis* by inhibiting the dilator muscle of the iris, without influencing the ciliary muscle-induced facility of aqueous outflow.[114] This provides several potential clinical applications for the drug, most of which have been considered in previous chapters. (At the present time, however, the drug is not commercially available in the United States.)

1. *Reversal of mydriasis.* 0.1% thymoxamine can reverse the mydriatic effect of 0.5% ephedrine, but not when the latter is combined with 0.5% homotropine.[115]

2. *Management of angle-closure glaucoma.* Thymoxamine has the advantages of 1) causing miosis despite pressure-induced ischemia of the iris sphincter and 2) not increasing the posterior vector force of the iris, which might aggravate the pupillary block.[116, 117] In a study of patients with acute angle-closure glaucoma, 0.5% thymoxamine was administered every minute for five times and then every 15 min for 2 to 3 hr. The attacks were broken in all cases, except those with peripheral arterior synechiae or prolonged angle closure.[116, 117]

3. *Differentiating angle-closure glaucoma from open-angle glaucoma with narrow angles.* Since thymoxamine produces miosis without affecting the ciliary muscle-controlled facility of outflow, it will break an angle-closure attack, but have no effect on open-angle glaucoma.[118] It has been demonstrated that this property of thymoxamine can be used as a diagnostic adjunct to gonioscopy in distinguishing between angle-closure glaucoma and open-angle glaucoma with narrow angles.[119]

4. *Management of pigmentary glaucoma.* One theory for the mechanism of pigment dispersion in pigmentary glaucoma, as discussed in Chapter 13, is contact between the iris pigment epithelium and packets of lens zonules.[120] It has been suggested that miosis without cyclotonia, as produced by thymoxamine, theoretically provides the optimum means of minimizing this effect.[120]

5. *Management of eyelid retraction.* 0.5% thymoxamine was found to cause a substantial narrowing of the palpebral fissure in many patients with eyelid retraction, especially cases secondary to thyroid disease.[121] It has been suggested that this may have value in the diagnosis of thyroid eye disease and possibly in the medical treatment of eyelid retraction.[121]

B. Prazosin

Prazosin is a post-synaptic alpha-adrenergic antagonist, which is used as an oral medication to lower blood pressure and produce peripheral vasodilation.[122, 123] Rabbit studies have shown that topical administration of 0.001 to 0.1% prazosin causes a dose-related lowering of intraocular pressure[122, 123] by reducing aqueous humor formation.[123]

IV. BETA-ADRENERGIC BLOCKING AGENTS (ANTAGONISTS)

A. Early Experience

Propranolol hydrochloride was the first commercially available beta-adrenergic antagonist in the United States, having been introduced in 1967 for the treatment of cardiac arrhythmias, angina pectoris, and systemic hypertension. The drug was also found to reduce the intraocular pressure when given orally,[124–128] topically,[129–130] or intravenously.[131]

B. Limiting factors

Numerous *side effects* of many beta blockers limit their usefulness as topical anti-glaucoma agents:

1. *Corneal anesthesia*, due to membrane stabilizing activity, occurs when propranolol is given topically.[129]

2. *Reduced tear production* is also a problem with propranolol[132] and certain other beta blockers. This is particularly true of practolol, which causes a severe dry eye syndrome in some patients, occasionally associated with subconjunctival fibrosis, corneal ulcers, and a skin rash.[133-135] The practolol-induced ocular toxicity may have an immunologic pathogenesis.[134]

3. An *intrinsic sympathomimetic effect* causing an early, transient adrenergic agonist action, occurs with some beta blockers. An example is *pindolol*, which is reported to have a good ocular hypotensive effect without altering corneal sensitivity.[136]

4. *Carcinogenicity* in test animals has also been observed with the beta blockers, *pamatolol* and *tolamolol*.[137]

C. Timolol Maleate

This beta$_1$ and beta$_2$ adrenergic antagonist was found in preliminary trials to have none of the adverse reactions noted above.[138, 139] In 1978, the topical agent was approved by the Food and Drug Administration for the treatment of open-angle glaucoma.

1. *Preliminary trials*. Rabbit studies revealed an intraocular pressure-lowering effect in both the treated[140, 141] and untreated eye.[141] Single doses in human volunteers were effective in normotensive individuals[138] as well as those with primary open-angle glaucoma,[142, 143] and short-term multiple-dose trials in open-angle glaucoma patients demonstrated a sustained ocular hypotensive effect.[144-147] Comparative studies showed the intraocular pressure-lowering efficacy of timolol to be greater than that of epinephrine[148] and equivalent to or slightly more than that of pilocarpine.[149-152] In all of these trials, ocular and systemic side effects were minimal.

2. *Mechanism of action*. Tonographic[153, 154] and fluorophotometric[155, 156] studies in humans indicate that the pressure-lowering effect of timolol is primarily due to *reduced aqueous production*. Some reports of tonographic studies have also suggested a slight improvement in outflow facility.[144, 157] Experiments with cat eyes also indicate that timolol-induced intraocular pressure reduction is related to inhibition of aqueous humor formation with no significant change in outflow.[158] The hypothetical model of adrenergic receptors, discussed earlier in this chapter, assumes that the beta-adrenergic receptors related to aqueous inflow have a resting "tone," while those associated with outflow have no tone.[25] Consequently, blocking both sets of receptors reduces aqueous production, but does not affect the facility of aqueous outflow.

The precise mechanism by which timolol reduces aqueous production is unknown. It has been suggested that timolol may act directly on the ciliary epithelia to block active transport or ultrafiltration.[159]

The possibility of direct action by beta-adrenergic agents on the formation of aqueous humor is supported by the reported observation of beta-adrenergic receptors in rabbit ciliary processes.[160] As previously noted, timolol has been shown to block the catecholamine-stimulated synthesis of cyclic AMP,[27] although the duration of this effect is shorter than the length of the intraocular pressure reduction.[27, 159] The drug has also been demonstrated to block catecholamine stimulation of chloride transport in isolated frog and rabbit corneas.[161]

3. *Concentrations and frequency of administration.* Rabbit studies demonstrated good corneal penetration of timolol.[162] Experience with open-angle glaucoma patients indicated that a 0.5% concentration gave the maximum intraocular pressure-reducing effect, which peaked in 2 hr[138, 142] and lasted for at least 24 hr.[143] The drug is commercially available in 0.25 and 0.5% concentrations, and the optimum frequency of administration in most cases is twice daily, although once-a-day treatment has been shown to be effective in many cases.[163] One study indicated that the ocular hypotensive effect of 0.5% timolol is longer but not stronger than that of 0.25%.[164] Individuals with darker irides appear to require higher concentrations.[165]

4. *Drug interactions.* Long-term, multiple-drug studies have shown that timolol will cause additional lowering of intraocular pressure in many cases when added to maximum tolerable anti-glaucoma therapy.[166–169] More specifically, it is reported to impart significant additional pressure reduction when added to miotics[170–174] or carbonic anhydrase inhibitors.[170, 171, 173, 175] However, the reports regarding an interaction between timolol and epinephrine have been conflicting. While some studies suggested that the combined pressure-lowering effect of the two drugs was significantly greater than that of either drug alone,[157, 171–173] other investigations have shown that this may not be the case. When epinephrine or dipivefrin is given to eyes pretreated with timolol, there is little or no additional pressure reduction.[25, 174, 176–178] However, when timolol is given to eyes pretreated with an epinephrine compound, there is a significant additional pressure reduction at first,[25, 176, 177] but this only lasts for a few weeks.[25, 177] Thomas and Epstein[25] have shown that timolol blocks the beta-adrenergic effect of epinephrine on aqueous outflow, which may explain the failure of epinephrine to produce added pressure reduction when administered to eyes pretreated with timolol. When timolol is added to eyes already receiving epinephrine, it may be that time is required before timolol blocks the effect of epinephrine on outflow, and this may explain the period of added pressure reduction.[25] Topical and oral timolol did not produce an additive effect on intraocular pressure, pulse, or blood pressure.[179]

5. *Clinical indications.* Although timolol was originally evaluated and approved for the treatment of primary open-angle glaucoma, it has subsequently been found to control the intraocular pressure in nearly all forms of glaucoma.[180, 181] Since it lowers the intraocular

pressure by reducing aqueous production and does not alter the pupil, it is helpful in situations in which conventional aqueous outflow cannot be improved medically and in which miosis or mydriasis are not desirable. Timolol is reported to help control glaucoma in aphakia during the early postoperative period[182–184] as well as in chronic cases.[157, 181] The drug has also been found to control secondary angle-closure glaucoma after penetrating keratoplasty,[185] but was not effective in a series of aphakic keratoplasties.[186] Timolol has been used successfully following an iridectomy for angle-closure glaucoma when the pressure elevation persisted postoperatively.[187] Limited experience in children suggests timolol may be of value in some cases.[188, 189]

6. *Continued efficacy.* It has been observed that the intraocular pressure-responsiveness to timolol will decrease with continued administration in some patients. This occurs in two phases, which Boger[190] has called the "short term 'escape' and long term 'drift.'"

a. *Early "escape."* Many patients will experience a dramatic reduction in intraocular pressure with the initiation of timolol therapy. However, the pressure nearly always rises during the next few days to finally plateau at a maintenance level.[149, 170, 191] It has been demonstrated that the number of beta receptors in ocular tissues increases during the first few days of timolol therapy,[192] which may explain this "escape" phenomenon.[190]

b. *Late "drift."* Once the intraocular pressure has leveled off following the initiation of timolol therapy, control will be maintained in most cases. Some patients, however, will have a slow decline in pressure response to timolol, usually beginning 3 months to a year after starting treatment.[157, 169, 193–195] No physiologic explanation has yet been provided for this phenomenon.

7. *Side effects.* As previously noted, early clinical experience suggested that adverse ocular and systemic reactions are unusually low with timolol therapy. Specifically, the drug does not affect the pupillary size,[196] accommodation, or corneal endothelial permeability,[197] and rarely causes burning or conjunctival hyperemia. However, continued experience has disclosed side effects, some of which can have serious consequences.

a. *Ocular toxicity* is uncommon with timolol therapy, but the following observations have been reported. Burning and conjunctival hyperemia may occasionally occur and are frequently associated with *superficial punctate keratopathy* and *corneal anesthesia.*[198–201] In a series of 25 patients, four had markedly diminished corneal sensitivity.[201] *Reduced central visual acuity* has also been noted.[198–200] In some cases this is due to a change in the refractive error associated with discontinuation of miotic therapy, although the cause in other patients is not clear. *Tear production* may be reduced, although this is usually of no consequence unless the patient has low baseline tear flow.[202] A fluorescein angiographic study revealed dye leakage from vessels of the peripupillary iris after topical instillation of timolol.[203]

b. *Systemic toxicity* has been reported more often than ocular reactions and constitutes the more significant adverse effects of topical timolol therapy:

(1). *Cardiovascular.* Blockade of beta$_1$ adrenergic receptors slows the pulse rate and weakens myocardial contractility, which may lead to bradycardia, arrhythmias, heart failure, and syncope.[198–200, 204, 205]

(2). *Respiratory.* Blockade of beta$_2$ adrenergic receptors produces contraction of bronchial smooth muscle, which may cause bronchospasm and airway obstruction, especially in asthmatics.[198, 200, 204, 206] Dyspnea[204] and apneic spells in a neonate[207] have also been reported.

(3). *Central nervous system* effects may be the most common class of systemic reactions to timolol therapy and include depression, anxiety, confusion, dysarthria, hallucinations, lightheadedness, drowsiness, weakness, fatique, tranquilization, dissociative behavior, disorientation, and emotional lability.[198–200, 204]

(4). *Other systemic reactions* include gastrointestinal distress (nausea, diarrhea, and cramping),[198, 200, 204] dermatological disorders (maculopapular rash, alopecia, and hives),[200, 204] sexual impotence,[198, 199] and exacerbation of myasthenia gravis.[208]

D. Other Beta-adrenergic Blockers

Other beta adrenergic blockers that have been evaluated for the treatment of glaucoma include the following:

1. *Atenolol* is a selective beta$_1$-adrenergic antagonist with no intrinsic sympathomimetic or membrane-stabilizing properties.[209, 210] An oral dose of 50 mg had a better intraocular pressure-lowering effect than 40 mg of propranolol[211] or 500 mg of acetozolamide.[212] Topical administrations of 2% atenolol were comparable to 2% pilocarpine,[213] and 4% atenolol was more effective than 1% epinephrine.[214] However, a long-term study showed that the initial pressure control gradually wore off in some patients.[215]

2. Other beta-adrenergic antagonists that have been encouraging in preliminary studies include pindolol[136] and metoprolol.[216]

3. *Labetalol* is a combined alpha- and beta-adrenergic blocking agent which has been shown to produce a significant, dose-related intraocular pressure reduction in rabbits.[217, 218]

References

1. Weekers, R, Prijot, E, Gustin, J: Recent advances and future prospects in the medical treatment of ocular hypertension. Br J Ophthal 38:742, 1954.
2. Weekers, R, Delmarcelle, Y, Gustin, J: Treatment of ocular hypertension by adrenalin and diverse sympathomimetic amines. Am J Ophthal 40:666, 1955.
3. Becker, B, Ley, AP: Epinephrine and acetazolamide in the therapy of the chronic glaucomas. Am J Ophthal 45:639, 1958.
4. Garner, LL, Johnston, WW, Ballintine, EJ, Carroll, ME: Effect of 2% levo-rotary epinephrine on the intraocular pressure of the glaucomatous eye. Arch Ophthal 62:230, 1959.
5. Becker, B, Pettit, TH, Gay, AJ: Topical epinephrine therapy of open-angle glaucoma. Arch Ophthal 66:219, 1961.

6. Ballintine, EJ, Garner, LL: Improvement of the coefficient of outflow in glaucomatous eyes. Prolonged local treatment with epinephrine. Arch Ophthal 66:314, 1961.

7. Kronfeld, PC: Dose-effect relationships as an aid in the evaluation of ocular hypotensive drugs. Invest Ophthal 3:258, 1964.

8. Krill, AE, Newell, FW, Novak, M: Early and long-term effects of levoepinephrine on ocular tension and outflow. Am J Ophthal 59:833, 1965.

9. Criswick, VG, Drance, SM: Comparative study of four different epinephrine salts on intraocular pressure. Arch Ophthal 75:768, 1966.

10. Richards, JSF, Drance, SM: The effect of 2% epinephrine on aqueous dynamics in the human eye. Can J Ophthal 2:259, 1967.

11. Kronfeld, PC: Early effects of single and repeated doses of L-epinephrine in man. Am J Ophthal 72:1058, 1971.

12. Vannas, S, Linkova, M: Adrenalin therapy in glaucoma. Acta Ophthalmologica XX Meeting of Nordic Ophthalmologists 1971, p 39.

13. Green, K, Padgett, D: Effect of various drugs on pseudofacility and aqueous humor formation in the rabbit eye. Exp Eye Res 28:239, 1979.

14. Lorenzetti, OJ: Dose-dependent influence of topically instilled adrenergic agents on intraocular pressure and outflow facility in the rabbit. Exp Eye Res 12:80, 1971.

15. Obstbaum, SA, Kolker, AE, Phelps, CD: Low-dose epinephrine effect on intraocular pressure. Arch Ophthal 92:118, 1974.

16. Sears, ML: The mechanism of action of adrenergic drugs in glaucoma. Invest Ophthal 5:115, 1966.

17. Sears, ML, Neufeld, AH: Adrenergic modulation of the outflow of aqueous humor. Invest Ophthal 14:83, 1975.

18. Alm, A: The effect of topical l-epinephrine on regional ocular blood flow in monkeys. Invest Ophthal Vis Sci 19:487, 1980.

19. Townsend, DJ, Brubaker, RF: Immediate effect of epinephrine on aqueous formation in the normal human eye as measured by fluorophotometry. Invest Ophthal Vis Sci 19:256, 1980.

20. Neufeld, AH, Jampol, LM, Sears, ML: Cyclic-AMP in the aqueous humor: The effects of adrenergic agents. Exp Eye Res 14:242, 1972.

21. Neufeld, AH, Dueker, DK, Vegge, T, et al: Adenosine 3^1, 5^1-monophosphate increases the outflow of aqueous humor from the rabbit eye. Invest Ophthal 14:40, 1975.

22. Neufeld, AH, Sears, ML: Adenosine $3^1,5^1$-monophosphate analogue increases the outflow facility of the primate eye. Invest Ophthal 14:688, 1975.

23. Hayasaka, S, Sears, M: Effects of epinephrine, indomethacin, acetylsalicylic acid, dexamethasone, and cyclic AMP on the in vitro activity of lysosomal hyaluronidase from the rabbit iris. Invest Ophthal Vis Sci 17:1109, 1978.

24. Flach, AJ, Kramer, SG: Supersensitivity to topical epinephrine after long-term epinephrine therapy. Arch Ophthal 98:482, 1980.

25. Thomas, JV, Epstein, DL: Timolol and epinephrine in primary open angle glaucoma. Transient additive effect. Arch Ophthal 99:91, 1981.

26. Higgins, RG, Brubaker, RF: Acute effect of epinephrine on aqueous humor formation in the timolol-treated normal eye as measured by fluorophotometry. Invest Ophthal Vis Sci 19:420, 1980.

27. Bartels, SP, Roth, O, Jumblatt, MM, Neufeld, AH: Pharmacological effects of topical timolol in the rabbit eye. Invest Ophthal Vis Sci 19:1189, 1980.

28. Harris, LS, Galin, MA, Lerner, R: The influence of low dose L-epinephrine on intraocular pressure. Ann Ophthal 2:253, 1970.

29. Vaughan, D, Shaffer, R, Riegelman, S: A new stabilized form of epinephrine for the treatment of open-angle glaucoma. Arch Ophthal 66:108, 1961.

30. Birss, SA, Longwell, A, Heckbert, S, Keller, N: Ocular hypotensive efficacy of topical epinephrine in normotensive and hypertensive rabbits: continuous drug delivery vs eyedrops. Ann Ophthal 10:1045, 1978.

31. Holland, MG: Treatment of glaucoma by chemical sympathectomy with 6-

hydroxydopamine. Trans Am Acad Ophthal Otol 76:437, 1972.

32. Holland, MG, Wei, CP, Gupta, S: Review and evaluation of 6-hydroxydopamine (6-HD): chemical sympathectomy for the treatment of glaucoma. Ann Ophthal 5:539, 1973.
33. Holland, MG, Wei, CP: Epinephrine dose-response characteristics of glaucomatous human eyes following chemical sympathectomy with 6-hydroxydopamine. Ann Ophthal 5:633, 1973.
34. Holland, MG, Wei, CP: Chemical sympathectomy in glaucoma therapy: An investigation of alpha and beta adrenergic supersensitivity. Ann Ophthal 5:783, 1973.
35. Diamond, JG: 6-hydroxydopamine in treatment of open-angle glaucoma. Arch Ophthal 94:41, 1976.
36. Colasanti, BK, Kosa, JE, Trotter, RR: Responsiveness of the rabbit eye to adrenergic and cholinergic agonists after treatment with 6-hydroxydopamine or alpha-methyl-para-tyrosine. I. Pupillary changes. Ann Ophthal 10:1067, 1978.
37. Colasanti, BK, Trotter, RR: Responsiveness of the rabbit eye to adrenergic and cholinergic agonists after treatment with 6-hydroxydopamine or alpha-methyl-para-tyrosine. II. Intraocular pressure changes. Ann Ophthal 10:1209, 1978.
38. Kitazawa, Y, Nose, H, Horie, T: Chemical sympathectomy with 6-hydroxydopamine in the treatment of primary open-angle glaucoma. Am J Ophthal 79:98, 1975.
39. Watanabe, H, Levene, RZ, Bernstein, MR: 6-hydroxydopamine therapy in glaucoma. Trans Am Acad Ophthal Otol 83:69, 1977.
40. Sneddon, JM, Turner, P: The interactions of local guanethidine and sympathomimetic amines in the human eye. Arch Ophthal 81:622, 1969.
41. Bonomi, L, Di Comite, P: Outflow facility after guanethidine sulfate administration. Arch Ophthal 78:337, 1967.
42. Crombie, AL: Adrenergic supersensitization as a therapeutic tool in glaucoma. Trans Ophthal Soc UK 94:570, 1974.
43. Jones, DEP, Norton, DA, Harvey, J, Davies, DJG: Effect of adrenaline and guanethidine in reducing intraocular pressure in rabbits' eyes. Br J Ophthal 59:304, 1975.
44. Nagasubramanian, S, Tripathi, RC, Poinoosawmy, D, Gloster, J: Low concentration guanethidine and adrenaline therapy of glaucoma. A preliminary report. Trans Ophthal Soc UK 96:179, 1976.
45. Mills, KB, Ridgway, AEA: A double blind comparison of guanethidine-and-adrenaline drops with 1% adrenaline alone in chronic simple glaucoma. Br J Ophthal 62:320, 1978.
46. Hoyng, FJ, Dake, CL: The combination of guanethidine 3% and adrenaline 0.5% in 1 eyedrop (GA) in glaucoma treatment. Br J Ophthal 63:56, 1979.
47. Romano, J, Patterson, G: Evaluation of a 5% guanethidine and 0·5% adrenaline mixture (Ganda 5·05) and of a 3% guanethidine and 0·5% adrenaline mixture (Ganda 3·05) in the treatment of open-angle glaucoma. Br J Ophthal 63:52, 1979.
48. Jones, DEP, Norton, DA, Davies, DJG: Control of glaucoma by reduced dosage guanethidine-adrenaline formulation. Br J Ophthal 63:813, 1979.
49. Hoyng, FJ, Dake, CL: Maintenance therapy of glaucoma patients with guanethidine (3%) and adrenaline (0.5%) once daily. Albrecht Graefes Arch Klin Exp Ophthal 214:269, 1980.
50. Van Husen, H: A combination of 1% guanethidine and 0.2% epinephrine in drop form to lower IOP in open angle glaucoma (Germ). Klin Monatsbl Augenheilkd 177:622, 1980.
51. Hoyng, FJ, Dake, CL: The aqueous humor dynamics and the biphasic response in intraocular pressure induced by guanethidine and adrenaline in the glaucomatous eye. Albrecht Graefes Arch Klin Exp Ophthal 214:263, 1980.
52. Gloster, J: Guanethidine and glaucoma. Trans Ophthal Soc UK 94:573, 1974.
53. Asregadoo, ER: Guanethidine ophthalmic solution 5%. Use in the treatment of endocrine exophthalmos. Arch Ophthal 84:21, 1970.

54. Riley, FC, Moyer, NJ: Experimental Horner's syndrome: A pupillographic evaluation of guanethidine-induced adrenergic blockade in humans. Am J Ophthal 69:442, 1970.
55. Kaback, MB, Podos, SM, Harbin, TS Jr, Mandell, A, Becker, B: The effects of dipivalyl epinephrine on the eye. Am J Ophthal 81:768, 1976.
56. Bigger, JF: Dipivefrin and glaucoma. Pers Ophthal 4:87, 1980.
57. Mandell, AI, Stentz, F, Kitabchi, AE: Dipivalyl epinephrine: A new pro-drug in the treatment of glaucoma. Ophthalmology 85:268, 1978.
58. Wei, CP, Anderson, JA, Leopold, I: Ocular absorption and metabolism of topically applied epinephrine and a dipivalyl ester of epinephrine. Invest Ophthal Vis Sci 17:315, 1978.
59. Anderson, JA, Davis, WL, Wei, CP: Site of ocular hydrolysis of a prodrug, dipivefrin, and a comparison of its ocular metabolism with that of the parent compound, epinephrine. Invest Ophthal Vis Sci 19:817, 1980.
60. Kass, MA, Mandell, AI, Goldberg, I, Paine, M, Becker, B: Dipivefrin and epinephrine treatment of elevated intraocular pressure. A comparative study. Arch Ophthal 97:1865, 1979.
61. Kohn, AN, Moss, AP, Hargett, NA, Ritch, R, Smith, H Jr, Podos, SM: Clinical comparison of dipivalyl epinephrine and epinephrine in the treatment of glaucoma. Am J Ophthal 87:196, 1979.
62. Bischoff, P: Clinical studies conducted with a new epinephrine derivative for the treatment of glaucoma (dipivalyl epinephrine). Klin Monatsbl Augenheilkd 172:565, 1978.
63. Krieglstein, GK, Leydhecker, W: The dose-response relationships of dipivalyl epinephrine in open-angle glaucoma. Albrecht Graefes Arch Klin Exp Ophthal 205:141, 1978.
64. Yablonski, ME, Shin, DH, Kolker, AE, Kass, M, Becker, B: Dipivefrin use in patients with intolerance to topically applied epinephrine. Arch Ophthal 95:2157, 1977.
65. Newton, MJ, Nesburn, AB: Lack of hydrophilic lens discoloration in patients using dipivalyl epinephrine for glaucoma. Am J Ophthal 87:193, 1979.
66. Theodore, JA, Leibowitz, HM: External ocular toxicity of dipivalyl epinephrine. Am J Ophthal 88:1013, 1979.
67. Abramovsky, I, Mindel, JS: Dipivefrin and echothiophate contraindications to combined use. Arch Ophthal 97:1937, 1979.
68. Corwin, ME, Spencer, WH: Conjunctival melanin depositions. A sideeffect of topical epinephrine therapy. Arch Ophthal 69:73, 1963.
69. Veirs, ER, McGrew, JC: Ocular complications from topical epinephrine therapy of glaucoma. EENT Mthly 42:46, 1963.
70. Cashwell, LF, Shields, MB, Reed, JW: Adrenochrome pigmentation. Arch Ophthal 95:514, 1977.
71. Pardos, GJ, Krachmer, JH, Mannis, MJ: Persistent corneal erosion secondary to tarsal adrenochrome deposit. Am J Ophthal 90:870, 1980.
72. Reinecke, RD, Kuwabara, T: Corneal deposits secondary to topical epinephrine. Arch Ophthal 70:170, 1963.
73. Krejci, L, Harrison, R: Corneal pigment deposits from topically administered epinephrine. Experimental production. Arch Ophthal 82:836, 1969.
74. Krejci, L, Harrison, R: Epinephrine effects on corneal cells in tissue culture. Arch Ophthal 83:451, 1970.
75. Green, WR, Kaufer, GJ, Dubroff, S: Black cornea. A complication of topical use of epinephrine. Ophthalmologica 154:88, 1967.
76. Cleasby, G, Donaldson, DD: Epinephrine pigmentation of the cornea. Arch Ophthal 78:74, 1967.
77. Madge, GE, Geeraets, WJ, Guerry, DP III: Black cornea secondary to topical epinephrine. Am J Ophthal 71:402, 1971.
78. Levine, RA: Ocular pigmentation due to topical epinephrine: Review and case report. Ophthal Dig, Feb 1973, p 34.
79. McCarthy, RW, LeBlanc, R: A 'black cornea' secondary to topical epinephrine. Can J Ophthal 11:336, 1976.

80. Barishak, R, Romano, A, Stein, R: Obstruction of lacrimal sac caused by topical epinephrine. Ophthalmologica 159:373, 1969.

81. Spaeth, GL: Nasolacrimal duct obstruction caused by topical epinephrine. Arch Ophthal 77:355, 1967.

82. Sugar, J: Adrenochrome pigmentation of hydrophilic lenses. Arch Ophthal 91:11, 1974.

83. Miller, D, Brooks, SM, Mobilia, E: Adrenochrome staining of soft contact lenses. Ann Ophthal 8:65, 1976.

84. Romano, A, Barishak, R, Stein, R: Obstruction of lacrimal puncta caused by topical epinephrine. Ophthalmologica 166:301, 1973.

85. Kass, MA, Stamper, RL, Becker, B: Madarosis in chronic epinephrine therapy. Arch Ophthal 88:429, 1972.

86. Kristensen, EB, Norn, MS: Benign mucous membrane pemphigoid. I. Secretion of mucus and tears. Acta Ophthal 52:266, 1974.

87. Kolker, AE, Becker, B: Epinephrine maculopathy. Arch Ophthal 79:552, 1968.

88. Michels, RG, Maumenee, AE: Cystoid macular edema associated with topically applied epinephrine in aphakic eyes. Am J Ophthal 80:379, 1975.

89. Obstbaum, SA, Galin, MA, Poole, TA: Topical epinephrine and cystoid macular edema. Ann Ophthal 8:455, 1976.

90. Thomas, JV, Gragoudas, ES, Blair, NP, Lapus, JV: Correlation of epinephrine use and macular edema in aphakic glaucomatous eyes. Arch Ophthal 96:625, 1978.

91. Hull, DS, Chemotti, T, Edelhauser, HF, Van Horn, DL, Hyndiuk, RA: Effect of epinephrine on the corneal endothelium. Am J Ophthal 79:245, 1975.

92. Waltman, SR, Yarian, D, Hart, W Jr, Becker, B: Corneal endothelial changes with long-term topical epinephrine therapy. Arch Ophthal 95:1357, 1977.

93. Kramer, SG: Considerations on epinephrine therapy in glaucoma. Ann Ophthal 10:1077, 1978.

94. Pollack, IP, Rossi, H: Norepinephrine in treatment of ocular hypertension and glaucoma. Arch Ophthal 93:173, 1975.

95. Pollack, IP: Effect of l-norepinephrine and adrenergic potentiators on the aqueous humor dynamics of man. Am J Ophthal 76:641, 1973.

96. Bigger, JF: Norepinephrine therapy in patients allergic to or intolerant of epinephrine. Ann Ophthal 11:183, 1979.

97. Potter, DE, Rowland, JM: Adrenergic drugs and intraocular pressure: Effects of selective beta-adrenergic agonists. Exp Eye Res 27:615, 1978.

98. Waitzman, MB, Woods, WD, Cheek, WV: Effects of prostaglandins and norepinephrine on ocular pressure and pupil size in rabbits following bilateral cervical ganglionectomy. Invest Ophthal Vis Sci 18:52, 1979.

99. Colasanti, BK, Barany, EH: Potentiation of the mydriatic effect of norepinephrine in the rabbit after monoamine oxidase inhibition. Invest Ophthal Vis Sci 18:200, 1979.

100. Kitazawa, Y: Topical adrenergic potentiators in primary open-angle glaucoma. Am J Ophthal 74:588, 1972.

101. Harrison, R, Kaufmann, CS: Clonidine. Effects of a topically administered solution on intraocular pressure and blood pressure in open-angle glaucoma. Arch Ophthal 95:1368, 1977.

102. Koss, MC, San, LC: Analysis of clonidine-induced mydriasis. Invest Ophthal 15:566, 1976.

103. Neufeld, AH, Page, ED: In vitro determination of the ability of drugs to bind to adrenergic receptors. Invest Ophthal Vis Sci 16:1118, 1977.

104. Macri, FJ, Cevario, SJ: Clonidine. Effects on aqueous humor formation and intraocular pressure. Arch Ophthal 96:2111, 1978.

105. Allen, RC, Langham, ME: The intraocular pressure response of conscious rabbits to clonidine. Invest Ophthal 15:815, 1976.

106. Zeller, EA, Shoch, D, Cooperman, SG, Schnipper, RI: Enzymology of the refractory media of the eye. IX. On the role of monoamine oxidase in the regulation of aqueous humor dynamics of the rabbit eye. Invest Ophthal 6:618, 1967.

107. Zeller, EA, Shoch, D, Czerner, TB, Hsu, MY, Knepper, PA: Enzymology of the refractory media of the eye. X. Effects of topically administered bradykinin, amine releasers, and pargyline on aqueous humor dynamics. Invest Ophthal 10:274, 1971.

108. Bausher, LP: Identification of A and B forms of monoamine oxidase in the iris-ciliary body, superior cervical ganglion, and pineal gland of albino rabbits. Invest Ophthal 15:529, 1976.

109. Mehra, KS, Roy, PN, Singh, R: Pargyline drops in glaucoma. Arch Ophthal 92:453, 1974.

110. Bietti, G, Virno, M, Pecori-Giraldi, J, Pellegrino, N, Motolese, E: Possibility of isoproterenol therapy with soft contact lenses: ocular hypotension without systemic effects. Ann Ophthal 8:819, 1976.

111. Ross, RA, Drance, SM: Effects of topically applied isoproterenol on aqueous dynamics in man. Arch Ophthal 83:39, 1970.

112. Seidehamel, RJ, Dungan, KW, Hickey, TE: Specific hypotensive and antihypertensive ocular effects of d-isoproterenol in rabbits. Am J Ophthal 79:1018, 1975.

113. Kass, MA, Reid, TW, Neufeld, AH, Bausher, LP, Sears, ML: The effect of d-isoproterenol on intraocular pressure of the rabbit, monkey, and man. Invest Ophthal 15:113, 1976.

114. Wand, M, Grant, WM: Thymoxamine hydrochloride: an alpha-adrenergic blocker. Surv Ophthal 25:75, 1980.

115. Small, S, Stewart-Jones, JH, Turner, P: Influence of thymoxamine on changes in pupil diameter and accommodation produced by homatropine and ephedrine. Br J Ophthal 60:132, 1976.

116. Rutkowski, PC, Fernandez, JL, Galin, MA, Halasa, AH: Alpha-adrenergic receptor blockade in the treatment of angle-closure glaucoma. Trans Am Acad Ophthal Otol 77:137, 1973.

117. Halasa, AH, Rutkowski, PC: Thymoxamine therapy for angle-closure glaucoma. Arch Ophthal 90:177, 1973.

118. Wand, M, Grant, WM: Thymoxamine hydrochloride: Effects on the facility of outflow and intraocular pressure. Invest Ophthal 15:400, 1976.

119. Wand, M, Grant, WM: Thymoxamine test: differentiating angle-closure glaucoma from open-angle glaucoma with narrow angles. Arch Ophthal 96:1009, 1978.

120. Campbell, DG: Pigmentary dispersion and glaucoma. A new theory. Arch Ophthal 97:1667, 1979.

121. Dixon, RS, Anderson, RL, Hatt, MU: The use of thymoxamine in eyelid retraction. Arch Ophthal 97:2147, 1979.

122. Smith, BR, Murray, DL, Leopold, IH: Influence of topically applied prazosin on the intraocular pressure of experimental animals. Arch Ophthal 97:1933, 1979.

123. Krupin, T, Feitl, M, Becker, B: Effect of Prazosin on aqueous humor dynamics in rabbits. Arch Ophthal 98:1639, 1980.

124. Wettrell, K, Pandolfi, M: Effect of oral administration of various beta-blocking agents on the intraocular pressure in healthy volunteers. Exp Eye Res 21:451, 1975.

125. Pandolfi, M, Ohrstrom, A: Treatment of ocular hypertension with oral beta-adrenergic blocking agents. Acta Ophthal 52:464, 1974.

126. Wettrell, K, Pandolfi, M: Early dose response analysis of ocular hypotensive effects of propranolol in patients with ocular hypertension. Br J Ophthal 60:680, 1976.

127. Wettrell, K, Pandolfi, M: Propranolol vs acetazolamide. A long-term double-masked study of the effect on intraocular pressure and blood pressure. Arch Ophthal 97:280, 1979.

128. Ohrstrom, A, Pandolfi, M: Long-term treatment of glaucoma with systemic propranolol. Am J Ophthal 86:340, 1978.

129. Musini, A, Fabbri, B, Bergamaschi, M, Mandelli, V, Shanks, RG: Comparison of the effect of propranolol, lignocaine, and other drugs on normal and raised intraocular pressure in man. Am J Ophthal 72:773, 1971.

130. Maerte, HF, Merkle, W: Long-term treatment of glaucoma with propranolol ophthalmic solution. Klin Monatsbl Augenheilkd 177:437, 1980.
131. Takats, I, Szilvassy, I, Kerek, A: Intraocular pressure and circulation of aqueous humour in rabbit eyes following intravenous administration of propranolol (Inderal). Albrecht Graefes Arch Klin Exp Ophthal 185:331, 1972.
132. Cubey, RB, Taylor, SH: Ocular reaction to propranolol and resolution on continued treatment with a different beta-blocking drug. Br Med J 4:327, 1975.
133. Rahi, AHS, Chapman, CM, Garner, A, Wright, P: Pathology of practololinduced ocular toxicity. Br J Ophthal 60:312, 1976.
134. Garner, A, Rahi, AHS: Practolol and ocular toxicity. Antibodies in serum and tears. Br J Ophthal 60:684, 1976.
135. Skegg, DCG, Doll, R: Frequency of eye complaints and rashes among patients receiving practolol and propranolol. Lancet 2:475, 1977.
136. Bonomi, L, Steindler, P: Effect of pindolol on intraocular pressure. Br J Ophthal 59:301, 1975.
137. Status report on beta-blockers. FDA Drug Bulletin 8:13, 1978.
138. Katz, IM, Hubbard, WA, Getson, AJ, Gould, AL: Intraocular pressure decrease in normal volunteers following timolol ophthalmic solution. Invest Ophthal 15:489, 1976.
139. Zimmerman, TJ: Timolol maleate—a new glaucoma medication? Invest Ophthal Vis Sci 16:687, 1977.
140. Vareilles, P, Silverstone, D, Plazonnet, B, Le Douarec, JC, Sears, ML, Stone, CA: Comparison of the effects of timolol and other adrenergic agents on intraocular pressure in the rabbit. Invest Ophthal Vis Sci 16:987, 1977.
141. Radius, RL, Diamond, GR, Pollack, IP, Langham, ME: Timolol. A new drug for management of chronic simple glaucoma. Arch Ophthal 96:1003, 1978.
142. Zimmerman, TJ, Kaufman, HE: Timolol. A beta-adrenergic blocking agent for the treatment of glaucoma. Arch Ophthal 95:601, 1977.
143. Zimmerman, TJ, Kaufman, HE: Timolol: dose response and duration of action. Arch Ophthal 95:605, 1977.
144. Obstbaum, SA, Galin, MA, Katz, IM: Timolol: Effect on intraocular pressure in chronic open-angle glaucoma. Ann Ophthal 10:1347, 1978.
145. Ritch, R, Hargett, NA, Podos, SM: The effect of 1.5% timolol maleate on intraocular pressure. Acta Ophthal 56:6, 1978.
146. Moss, AP, Ritch, R, Hargett, NA, Kohn, AN, Smith, H Jr, Podos, SM: A comparison of the effects of timolol and epinephrine on intraocular pressure. Am J Ophthal 86:489, 1978.
147. Zimmerman, TJ, Kass, MA, Yablonski, ME, Becker, B: Timolol maleate. Efficacy and safety. Arch Ophthal 97:656, 1979.
148. Sonntag, JR, Brindley, GO, Shields, MB, Arafat, NIT, Phelps, CD: Timolol and epinephrine. Comparison of efficacy and side effects. Arch Ophthal 97:273, 1979.
149. Boger, WP III, Steinert, RF, Puliafito, CA, Pavan-Langston, D: Clinical trial comparing timolol ophthalmic solution to pilocarpine in open-angle glaucoma. Am J Ophthal 86:8, 1978.
150. Diamond, GR, Werblin, TP, Richter, R, Radius, R, Pollack, IP, Maumenee, AE: Extended clinical studies using timolol in patients with ocular hypertension and chronic open-angle glaucoma. Glaucoma 1:63, 1979.
151. Hass, I, Drance, SM: Comparison between pilocarpine and timolol on diurnal pressures in open-angle glaucoma. Arch Ophthal 98:480, 1980.
152. Merte, HJ, Merkle, W: Experiences in a double-blind study with different concentrations of timolol and pilocarpine. Klin Monatsbl Augenheilkd 177:443, 1980.
153. Zimmerman, TJ, Harbin, R, Pett, M, Kaufman, HE: Timolol and facility of outflow. Invest Ophthal Vis Sci 16:623, 1977.
154. Sonntag, JR, Brindley, GO, Shields, MB: Effect of timolol therapy on outflow facility. Invest Ophthal Vis Sci 17:293, 1978.
155. Coakes, RL, Brubaker, RF: The mechanism of timolol in lowering intraocular pressure in the normal eye. Arch Ophthal 96:2045, 1978.

156. Yablonski, ME, Zimmerman, TJ, Waltman, SR, Becker, B: A fluorophotometric study of the effect of topical timolol on aqueous humor dynamics. Exp Eye Res 27:135, 1978.

157. Lin, LL, Galin, MA, Obstbaum, SA, Katz, I: Long-term timolol therapy. Surv Ophthal 23:377, 1979.

158. Liu, HK, Chiou, GCY, Garg, LC: Ocular hypotensive effects of timolol in cat eyes. Arch Ophthal 98:1467, 1980.

159. Neufeld, AH: Experimental studies on the mechanism of action of timolol. Surv Ophthal 23:363, 1979.

160. Bromberg, BB, Gregory, DS, Sears, ML: Beta-adrenergic receptors in ciliary processes of the rabbit. Invest Ophthal Vis Sci 19:203, 1980.

161. Candia, OA, Podos, SM, Neufeld, AH: Modification by timolol of catechol-amine stimulation of chloride transport in isolated corneas. Invest Ophthal Vis Sci 18:691, 1979.

162. Schmitt, CJ, Lotti, VJ, LeDouarec, JC: Penetration of timolol into the rabbit eye. Measurements after ocular instillation and intravenous injection. Arch Ophthal 98:547, 1980.

163. Soll, DB: Evaluation of timolol in chronic open-angle glaucoma. Once a day vs twice a day. Arch Ophthal 98:2178, 1980.

164. Collignon-Brach, J, Weekers, R: Timolol. Etude clinique. J Fr Ophtalmol 2:603, 1979.

165. Katz, IM, Berger, ET: Effects of iris pigmentation on response of ocular pressure to timolol. Surg Ophthal 23:395, 1979.

166. Ashburn, FS Jr, Gillespie, JE, Kass, MA, Becker, B: Timolol plus maximum tolerated antiglaucoma therapy: A one-year follow-up study. Surv Ophthal 23:389, 1979.

167. Sonty, S, Schwartz, B: The additive effect of timolol on open angle glaucoma patients on maximal medical therapy. Surv Ophthal 23:381, 1979.

168. Zimmerman, TJ, Gillespie, JE, Kass, MA, Yablonski, ME, Becker, B: Timolol plus maximum-tolerated antiglaucoma therapy. Arch Ophthal 97:278, 1979.

169. Brindley, GO, Sonntag, JR, Shields, MB: Timolol: After the first year. Pers Ophthal 4:97, 1980.

170. Boger, WP III, Puliafito, CA, Steinert, RF, Langston, DP: Long-term experience with timolol ophthalmic solution in patients with open-angle glaucoma. Ophthalmology 85:259, 1978.

171. Keates, EU: Evaluation of timolol maleate combination therapy in chronic open-angle glaucoma. Am J Ophthal 88:565, 1979.

172. Smith, RJ, Nagasubramanian, S, Watkins, R, Poinoosawmy, D: Addition of timolol maleate to routine medical therapy: a clinical trial. Br J Ophthal 64:779, 1980.

173. Nielsen, NV, Eriksen, JS: Timolol in maintenance treatment of ocular hyperten-sion and glaucoma. Acta Ophthal 57:1070, 1979.

174. Knupp, JA, Mandell, A, Hurvitz, L, Spaeth, GL, Shields, MB: Comparison of dipivefrin and pilocarpine used concomitantly with timolol in the management of open-angle glaucoma. Presented at Annual Meeting American Academy Ophthalmology, Chicago, Nov 2-7, 1980.

175. Scharrer, A, Ober, M: Timolol and acetazolamide in the treatment of increased intraocular pressure. Albrecht Graefes Arch Klin Exp Ophthal 212:129, 1979.

176. Goldberg, I, Ashburn, FS Jr, Palmberg, PF, Kass, MA, Becker, B: Timolol and epinephrine. A clinical study of ocular interactions. Arch Ophthal 98:484, 1980.

177. Keates, EC, Stone, RA: Safety and effectiveness of concomitant administration of dipivefrin and timolol maleate. Am J Ophthal 91:243, 1981.

178. Ohrstrom, A, Pandolfi, M: Regulation of intraocular pressure and pupil size by beta-blockers and epinephrine. Arch Ophthal 98:2182, 1980.

179. Batchelor, ED, O'Day, DM, Shand, DG, Wood, AJ: Interaction of topical and oral timolol in glaucoma. Ophthalmology 86:60, 1979.

180. Wilson, RP, Kanal, N, Spaeth, GL: Timolol: its effectiveness in different types of glaucoma. Ophthalmology 86:43, 1979.

181. Zimmerman, TJ, Canale, P: Timolol—further observations. Ophthalmology

86:166, 1979.

182. Obstbaum, SA, Galin, MA: The effects of timolol on cataract extraction and intraocular pressure. Am J Ophthal 88:1017, 1979.

183. Braverman, SD, Shields, MB: Efficacy of timolol in controlling intraocular pressure elevation after cataract extraction. Presented at Annual Meeting American Academy Ophthalmology, San Francisco, Nov 5-9, 1979.

184. Haimann, MH, Phelps, CD: Prophylactic timolol for the prevention of high intraocular pressure after cataract extraction. A randomized, prospective, double-blind trial. Ophthalmology 88:233, 1981.

185. Lass, JH, Pavan-Langston, D: Timolol therapy in secondary angle-closure glaucoma post penetrating keratoplasty. Ophthalmology 86:51, 1979.

186. Olson, RJ, Kaufman, HE, Zimmerman, TJ: Effects of timolol and daranide on elevated intraocular pressure after aphakic keratoplasty. Ann Ophthal 11:1833, 1979.

187. Phillips, CI: Timolol in operated closed-angle glaucoma. Br J Ophthal 64:240, 1980.

188. McMahon, CD, Hetherington, J Jr, Hoskins, HD Jr, Shaffer, RN: Timolol and pediatric glaucomas. Ophthalmology 88:249, 1981.

189. Boger, WP III, Walton, DS: Timolol in uncontrolled childhood glaucomas. Ophthalmology 88:253, 1981.

190. Boger, WP III: Timolol: Short term "escape" and long term "drift." Ann Ophthal 11:1239, 1979.

191. Oksala, A, Salminen, L: Tachyphylaxis in tomolol therapy for chronic glaucoma. Klin Monatsbl Augenheilkd 177:451, 1980.

192. Neufeld, AH, Zawistowski, KA, Page, ED, Bromberg, BB: Influences on the density of beta-adrenergic receptors in the cornea and iris-ciliary body of the rabbit. Invest Ophthal Vis Sci 17:1069, 1978.

193. Krieglstein, GK: A follow-up study on the intraocular pressure response of timolol eye drops. Klin Monatsbl Augenheilkd 175:627, 1979.

194. Merte, HJ, Merkle, W: Results of long-term treatment of glaucoma with timolol ophthalmic solution. Klin Monatsbl Augenheilkd 177:562, 1980.

195. Steinert, RF, Thomas, JV, Boger, WP III: Long-term drift and continued efficacy after multiyear timolol therapy. Arch Ophthal 99:100, 1981.

196. Johnson, SH, Brubaker, RF, Trautman, JC: Absence of an effect of timolol on the pupil. Invest Ophthal Vis Sci 17:924, 1978.

197. Brubaker, RF, Coakes, RL, Bourne, WM: Effect of timolol on the permeability of corneal endothelium. Ophthalmology 86:108, 1979.

198. McMahon, CD, Shaffer, RN, Hoskins, HD Jr, Hetherington, J Jr: Adverse effects experienced by patients taking timolol. Am J Ophthal 88:736, 1979.

199. Wilson, RP, Spaeth, GL, Poryzees, E: The place of timolol in the practice of ophthalmology. Ophthalmology 87:451, 1980.

200. Van Buskirk, EM: Adverse reactions from timolol administration. Ophthalmology 87:447, 1980.

201. Van Buskirk, EM: Corneal anesthesia after timolol maleate therapy. Am J Ophthal 88:739, 1979.

202. Bonomi, L, Zavarise, G, Noya, E, Michieletto, S: Effects of timolol maleate on tear flow in human eyes. Albrecht Graefes Arch Klin Exp Ophthal 213:19, 1980.

203. Kottow, MH: Effects of topical timolol on iris vessels. Glaucoma 2:383, 1980.

204. Fraunfelder, FT: Interim report: national Registry of possible drug-induced ocular side effects. Ophthalmology 87:87, 1980.

205. Britman, NA: Cardiac effects of topical timolol. N Engl J Med 300:566, 1979.

206. Jones, FL Jr, Ekberg, NL: Exacerbation of asthma by timolol. N Engl J Med 301:270, 1979.

207. Olson, RJ, Bromberg, BB, Zimmerman, TJ: Apneic spells associated with timolol therapy in a neonate. Am J Ophthal 88:120, 1979.

208. Shaivitz, SA: Timolol and myasthenia gravis. JAMA 252:1611, 1979.

209. Wettrell, K, Pandolfi, M: Effect of topical atenolol on intraocular pressure. Br J Ophthal 61:334, 1977.

210. Elliot, MJ, Cullen, PM, Phillips, CI: Ocular hypotensive effect of atenolol (Tenormin, I.C.I.). A new beta-adrenergic blocker. Br J Ophthal 59:296, 1975.
211. MacDonald, MJ, Cullen, PM, Phillips, CI: Atenolol versus propranolol. A comparison of ocular hypotensive effect of an oral dose. Br J Ophthal 60:789, 1976.
212. MacDonald, MJ, Gore, SM, Cullen, PM, Phillips, CI: Comparison of ocular hypotensive effects of acetazolamide and atenolol. Br J Ophthal 61:345, 1977.
213. Wettrell, K, Wilke, K, Pandolfi, M: Topical atenolol versus pilocarpine: a double-blind study of the effect on ocular tension. Br J Ophthal 62:292, 1978.
214. Phillips, CI, Gore, SM, Gunn, PM: Atenolol versus adrenaline eye drops and an evaluation of these two combined. Br J Ophthal 62:296, 1978.
215. Brenkman, RF: Long-term hypotensive effect of atenolol 4% eyedrops. Br J Ophthal 62:287, 1978.
216. Alm, A, Wickstrom, CP: Effects of systemic and topical administration of metoprolol on intraocular pressure in healthy subjects. Acta Ophthal 58:740, 1980.
217. Leopold, IH, Murray, DL: Ocular hypotensive action of labetalol. Am J Ophthal 88:427, 1979.
218. Murray, DL, Podos, SM, Wei, CP, Leopold, IH: Ocular effects in normal rabbits of topically applied labetalol. A combined alpha- and beta-adrenergic antagonist. Arch Ophthal 97:723, 1979.

Chapter 27

CARBONIC ANHYDRASE INHIBITORS

CARBONIC ANHYDRASE INHIBITORS

The carbonic anhydrase inhibitors are presently the only drugs that are commonly used as systemically administered agents in the long-term management of glaucoma. The prototype, *acetazolamide*, was introduced as an ocular hypotensive drug in 1954,[1] and most of our understanding of the carbonic anhydrase inhibitors comes from experience with this compound. Other members of the drug class include methazolamide, dichlorphenamide, and ethoxzolamide. The carbonic anhydrase inhibitors all share the same basic mechanisms of action and have side effects which differ primarily only in degree. Therefore, these aspects will first be considered collectively before discussing unique features of the individual compounds.

I. MECHANISM OF ACTION

A. Carbonic Anhydrase

Carbonic anhydrase (CA) is an enzyme that catalyzes the conversions (in both directions) between carbon dioxide and bicarbonate[2, 3]:

$$\overset{\text{CA}}{CO_2 + H_2O \leftrightarrows H_2CO_3 \leftrightarrows HCO_3^- + H^+}$$

Theories as to how this enzyme relates to aqueous production were discussed in Chapter 2. The most likely explanation is that carbonic anhydrase helps to maintain a pH that is optimum for the enzymes involved in ion transport. Carbonic anhydrase exists in many forms throughout the body, but in the *ciliary processes* of human eyes it is almost purely *isoenzyme C*.[4, 5] The enzyme activity is found in several sites in the ciliary processes, and the exact location of critical inhibition by clinical doses of carbonic anhydrase inhibitors is unknown.[6]

B. Carbonic Anhydrase Inhibitors

Carbonic anhydrase inhibitors belong to the *sulfonamide* class of compounds. They have an active moiety, which is identical to carbonic acid and complimentary to carbonic anhydrase, that interferes with the function of the enzyme.[2, 3] The carbonic anhydrase inhibitors lower intraocular pressure by a 50 to 60% *reduction of aqueous humor formation.*[7] The mechanism by which this is accomplished is uncertain, but the following theories have been considered:

1. *Ion transport* associated with secretion of aqueous humor may be altered, possibly by creation of a local acid environment.[8] The principal ion that appears to be affected by carbonic anhydrase inhibitors differs according to the animal model being studied,[8-10] and has not been established in human eyes.

2. *Metabolic acidosis* is known to reduce intraocular pressure and has been proposed as the mechanism of action for carbonic anhydrase

inhibitors.[11] However, studies have shown that the ocular hypotensive effect of these drugs is neither time-related to the metabolic acidosis[12] nor is it dependent upon alterations of pH in the blood[13, 14] or aqueous.[14] Nevertheless, strong carbonic anhydrase inhibitors, which do create a metabolic acidosis, may exert an additional pressure-lowering effect by this mechanism.

3. An adrenergic effect of carbonic anhydrase inhibitors has also been considered, since the action of acetazolamide in dogs was found to be altered by adrenalectomy or adrenergic blocking agents.[15]

4. The diuretic effect of the carbonic anhydrase inhibitors is not a factor in the reduction of intraocular pressure.[16, 17] Furthermore, although acetazolamide was shown to reduce the venous pressure of the cat eye, which paralleled the intraocular pressure fall,[18] ocular blood flow does not appear to be involved in the pressure-lowering action of this drug.[19]

II. ADMINISTRATION

A. Routes of Delivery

Carbonic anhydrase inhibitors are effective when given orally, intramuscularly, or intravenously, but do not exert their ocular hypotensive effect when given topically[17] or subconjunctivally.[17] These observations suggest that an effect on carbonic anhydrase in the blood may be necessary for the action of carbonic anhydrase inhibitors on aqueous humor formation.

B. Dose-response Curve

The *dose-response curve* for carbonic anhydrase inhibitors is very restricted, in that aqueous production is not significantly reduced until more than 90% of the carbonic anhydrase activity is inhibited.[20] For this reason, it is important that the drug not be used in inadequate doses.[21] However, it may be that some of the dosages in common use exceed that required for maximum benefit, which will be considered in the discussion of the individual carbonic anhydrase inhibitors.

C. Distribution and Metabolism

Carbonic anhydrase inhibitors are not distributed randomly throughout the body fluids, but have a preferential affinity for certain tissues, including the iris and ciliary processes.[22] The drugs are not metabolized, but are excreted unchanged in the urine.

III. SIDE EFFECTS

Side effects are common with carbonic anhydrase inhibitor therapy and frequently necessitate discontinuation of the drugs.

A. Common, Transient Effects

Paresthesias of the fingers, toes, and around the mouth, as well as *urinary frequency* from the diuretic action, are experienced by nearly all patients initially. However, both of these effects are usually transient and of no consequence.

B. Serum Electrolyte Imbalances

Serum electrolyte imbalances may create more debilitating problems.

1. *Metabolic acidosis,* associated with bicarbonate depletion, occurs with the higher dosages of carbonic anhydrase inhibitors and should be avoided in patients with hepatic insufficiency, renal failure, adrenocortical insufficiency, hyperchloremic acidosis, depressed sodium or potassium levels, or severe pulmonary obstruction.[23] In addition, a common *symptom-complex*[24] of malaise, fatigue, weight loss, anorexia, depression and decreased libido[25] was correlated with the degree of metabolic acidosis, and preliminary experience suggests that treatment with sodium bicarbonate might help to minimize this situation.[24] It has also been reported that combined therapy with a carbonic anhydrase inhibitor and aspirin may cause serious acid-base imbalance and salicylate intoxication.[26]

2. *Potassium depletion* may occur during the initial phase of carbonic anhydrase inhibitor therapy, due to increased urinary excretion, especially if diuresis is brisk. However, this is normally transient[27] and does not lead to significant hypokalemia unless it is given concomitantly with chlorothiazide diuretics,[24] digitalis, corticosteroids, or ACTH, or in patients with hepatic cirrhosis. Potassium supplement is only indicated when significant hypokalemia is documented.

3. Serum sodium and chloride may also be transiently reduced, although the latter occurs primarily with dichlorphenamide.[3]

C. Gastrointestinal Symptoms

Gastrointestinal symptoms are also very common and include vague abdominal discomfort, a peculiar metallic taste, nausea, and diarrhea. These symptoms do not appear to be related to any serum chemical change, and the cause is unknown, although taking the medication with meals may help to reduce the symptoms in some cases.[24]

D. Sulfonamide-related Reactions

The following side effects are common to the sulfonamide group of drugs, of which the carbonic anhydrase inhibitors are members.

1. *Renal calculi* formation is probably the most common serious adverse reaction associated with carbonic anhydrase inhibitor therapy. The precise mechanism is unknown, but there may be an association with reduced excretion of urinary citrate[28, 29] or magnesium,[29] since both are believed to help keep calcium salts in solution. An alkaline urine is also known to predispose to precipitation of calcium salts, and this has been proposed as the mechanism of urolithiasis associated with carbonic anhydrase inhibitor therapy.[30, 31]

However, it has been shown that the urinary pH returns to pretreatment levels once the initial acetazolamide-induced bicarbonate diuresis subsides,[32] and some patients with renal stones during acetazolamide therapy may actually have an acidic urine.[33] *Renal colic* may also be associated with carbonic anhydrase inhibitor therapy and may rarely cause hematuria or anuria.[34]

2. *Blood dyscrasias* are rare, but thrombocytopenia, agranulocytosis, aplastic anemia, and neutropenia have been reported with acetazolamide or methazolamide therapy.[29, 35–37]

3. Other sulfonamide-related side effects include exfoliative dermatitis, hypersensitive nephropathy, and acute myopia.[29] The latter is the only ocular reaction commonly associated with carbonic anhydrase inhibitor therapy, and it is idiosyncratic and transient.

E. Other Adverse Reactions

Other adverse reactions that have been reported in association with carbonic anhydrase inhibitor therapy include elevated blood uric acid,[29] hirsutism,[38] and a transient (30 min) elevation of cerebral blood flow and cerebrospinal fluid pressure.[29] Teratogenic effects have been observed in rats, but not in humans, although caution during pregnancy is advised.[39] It has also been noted that an oral hypoglycemic agent, acetohexamide, was inadvertently substituted for acetazolamide because of the similar names.[40]

IV. SPECIFIC CARBONIC ANHYDRASE INHIBITORS

A. Acetazolamide (Diamox)

As previously noted, acetazolamide is the prototype of the carbonic anhydrase inhibitors, and most of the preceding information in this chapter is based on experience with this drug.

1. *Administration.* The traditional oral dosage for long-term therapy in adults is 250 mg tablets every 6 hr or 500 mg sustained release capsules twice a day. However, a single dose study showed that 63 mg gave the maximum effect on the intraocular pressure.[41] In the same study, 250 mg gave a slightly longer duration of action, but 500 mg had no advantage. In addition, it has been shown that a daily 500 mg sustained-release capsule provided a substantial pressure-lowering effect for at least 23 hr.[42] However, one capsule twice a day was more effective than the daily dose in controlling the pressure, and was as effective as one 250-mg tablet every 6 hr.[42] The recommended dose for children is 5 to 10 mg/kg of body weight every 4 to 6 hr.[3]

In tablet form, the ocular hypotensive effect peaks in 2 hr and lasts up to 6 hr, while that of the capsule peaks in 8 hr and persists beyond 12 hr. For more rapid action, the drug may be given intravenously, which provides a peak effect in 15 min and a duration of 4 hr. A useful routine for emergency situations, such as acute angle-closure glaucoma, is to give 250 mg intramuscularly and 250 mg intravenously. Metabolic acidosis is greater with intravenous injections of acetazolamide than with oral adminstration.[12] An oral drug delivery system has been investigated, which releases acetazolamide at a rate of 15 mg/hr and is reported to cause fewer side effects.[43]

2. *Advantages.* The main advantage of acetazolamide over the other carbonic anhydrase inibitors is that more is known about the drug, by virtue of larger laboratory and clinical experience. In addition, acetazolamide sustained release capsules, given twice daily, were found in a cross-over, randomized study to be better tolerated than four time a day dosages of methazolamide 50 mg (which was the next best tolerated), ethoxzolamide 125 mg, acetazolamide 250 mg, or dichlorphenamide 50 mg.[44]

B. Methazolamide (Neptazane)

1. *Administration.* Although methazolamide has been recommended in dosages of up to 100 mg three times daily,[3] studies suggest that considerably less is needed in most cases to provide the desired therapeutic effect.[45-48] A dose of 25 mg twice daily was found to produce significant intraocular pressure reduction without metabolic acidosis.[45, 46] Studies differ as to whether higher doses of methazolamide produce additional pressure reduction,[46, 47] but a 500 mg sustained release capsule of acetazolamide was shown to have a greater ocular hypotensive effect than either 25 or 50 mg of methazolamide.[46] A suggested regimen for the titrated use of carbonic anhydrase inhibitor therapy is to begin with methazolamide 25 mg twice a day, advancing to 50 mg of methazolamide twice daily if necessary, and finally to the acetazolamide 500 mg sustained release capsule twice a day as required to achieve the desired effect.[49]

2. *Advantages.* The main advantage of methazolamide, as seen from the above discussion, is that the drug can be used in smaller dosages, which causes fewer side effects. This is due to low protein binding, which allows the drug to diffuse more readily into tissue and thereby be more active on a weight basis in reducing aqueous production.[45, 46] It also has a significantly longer plasma half-life than acetazolamide. In addition, there is evidence that methazolamide causes significantly less renal side effects,[28, 50] although renal stone formation during methazolamide therapy has been reported.[51, 52]

C. Dichlorphenamide

Dichlorphenamide (Daranide, Oratrol) is recommended in doses of 25 to 100 mg three times a day. Its greater potency is probably due to a double molecular configuration resembling carbonic acid. The drug causes less metabolic acidosis, due to increased chloride excretion, but often has sustained diuresis with chronic use.[3]

D. Ethoxzolamide

Ethoxzolamide (Cardrase, Ethamide) is given in a dosage of 125 mg every 6 hr and is similar in action and side effects to acetazolamide.[3]

References

1. Becker, B: Decrease in intraocular pressure in man by a carbonic anhydrase inhibitor, Diamox. Am J Ophthal 37:13, 1954.
2. Becker, B: Chronic anhydrase and the formation of aqueous humor. Am J Ophthal 47:342, 1959.
3. Havener, WH: Ocular Pharmacology, 4th ed. CV Mosby Co, St Louis, 1978, p 475.
4. Dobbs, PC, Epstein, DL, Anderson, PJ: Identification of isoenzyme C as the principal carbonic anhydrase in human ciliary processes. Invest Ophthal Vis Sci 18:867, 1979.
5. Wistrand, PJ, Garg, LC: Evidence of a high-activity C type of carbonic anhydrase in human ciliary processes. Invest Ophthal Vis Sci 18:802, 1979.
6. Bárány, EH: A pharmacologist looks at medical treatment in glaucoma—in retrospect and in prospect. Ophthalmology 86:80, 1979.
7. Becker, B, Constant, MA: Experimental tonography. The effect of the carbonic anhydrase inhibitor acetazolamide on aqueous flow. Arch Ophthal 54:321, 1955.
8. Berggren, L: Direct observation of secretory pumping in vitro of the rabbit eye ciliary processes. Influence of ion milieu and carbonic anhydrase inhibition. Invest Ophthal 3:266, 1964.
9. Maren, TH: The rates of movement of Na^+, Cl^-, and HCO_3^- from plasma to posterior chamber: effect of acetazolamide and relation to the treatment of glaucoma. Invest Ophthal 15:356, 1976.
10. Holland, MG, Gipson, CC: Chloride ion transport in the isolated ciliary body. Invest Ophthal 9:20, 1970.
11. Bietti, G, Virno, M, Pecori-Giraldi, J, Pellegrino, N: Acetazolamide, metabolic acidosis, and intraocular pressure. Am J Ophthal 80:360, 1975.
12. Soser, M, Ogriseg, M, Kessler, B, Zirm, H: New findings concerning changes in intraocular pressure and blood acidosis after peroral application of acetazolamide. Klin Monatsbl Augenheilkd 176:88, 1980.
13. Benedikt, O, Zirm, M, Harnoncourt, K: Relations between metabolic acidosis and intraocular pressure after inhibition of carboanhydrase with acetazolamide. Albrecht Graefes Arch Klin Exp Ophthal 190:247, 1974.
14. Mehra, KS: Relationship of pH of aqueous and blood with acetazolamide. Ann Ophthal 11:63, 1979.
15. Thomas, RP, Riley, MW: Acetazolamide and ocular tension. Notes concerning the mechanism of action. Am J Ophthal 60:241, 1965.
16. Peczon, JD, Grant, WM: Diuretic drugs in glaucoma. Am J Ophthal 66:680, 1968.
17. Becker, B: The mechanism of the fall in intraocular pressure induced by the carbonic anhydrase inhibitor, Diamox. Am J Ophthal 39:177, 1955.
18. Macri, FJ: Acetazolamide and the venous pressure of the eye. Arch Ophthal 63:953, 1960.
19. Bill, A: Effects of acetazolamide and carotid occlusion on the ocular blood flow in unanesthetized rabbits. Invest Ophthal 13:954, 1974.
20. Friedenwald, JS: Current studies on acetazolamide (Diamox) and aqueous humor flow. Am J Ophthal 40:139, 1955.
21. Becker, B: Misuse of acetazolamide. Am J Ophthal 43:799, 1957.
22. Goren, SB, Newell, FW, O'Toole, JJ: The localization of Diamox-S^{35} in the rabbit eye. Am J Ophthal 51:87, 1961.
23. Block, ER, Rostand, RA: Carbonic anhydrase inhibition in glaucoma: hazard or benefit for the chronic lunger? Surv Ophthal 23:169, 1978.
24. Epstein, DL, Grant, WM: Carbonic anhydrase inhibitor side effects. Serum chemical analysis. Arch Ophthal 95:1378, 1977.
25. Wallace, TR, Fraunfelder, FT, Petursson, GJ, Epstein, DL: Decreased libido—a side effect of carbonic anhydrase inhibitor. Ann Ophthal 11: 1563, 1979.
26. Anderson, CJ, Kaufman, PL, Sturm, RJ: Toxicity of combined therapy with carbonic anhydrase inhibitors and aspirin. Am J Ophthal 86:516, 1978.
27. Spaeth, GL: Potassium, acetazolamide, and intraocular pressure. Arch Ophthal

78:578, 1967.

28. Constant, MA, Becker, B: The effect of carbonic anhydrase inhibitors on urinary excretion of citrate by humans. Am J Ophthal 49:929, 1960.
29. Grant, WM: Antiglaucoma drugs: problems with carbonic anhydrase inhibitors. In Symposium on Ocular Therapy, vol 6, Leopold, IH, ed. CV Mosby Co, St Louis, 1972, p 19.
30. Simpson, DP: Effect of acetazolamide on citrate excretion in the dog. Am J Physiol 206:883, 1964.
31. Kondo, T, Sakaue, E, Koyama, S, Matsuo, M, Takahashi, Y: Urolithiasis during treatment of carbonic anhydrase inhibitors. Folia Ophthal Jap 19:576, 1968.
32. Parfitt, AM: Acetazolamide and renal stone formation. Lancet 2:153, 1970.
33. Persky, L, Chambers, D, Potts, A: Calculus formation and ureteral colic following acetazolamide (Diamox) therapy. JAMA 161:1625, 1956.
34. Charron, RC, Feldman, F: Acetazolamide therapy with renal complications. Can J Ophthal 9:282, 1974.
35. Wisch, N, Fischbein, FI, Siegel, R, Glass, JL, Leopold, I: Aplastic anemia resulting from the use of carbonic anhydrase inhibitors. Am J Ophthal 75:130, 1973.
36. Gangitano, JL, Foster, SH, Contro, RM: Nonfatal methazolamide-induced aplastic anemia. Am J Ophthal 86:138, 1978.
37. Werblin, TP, Pollack, IP, Liss, RA: Blood dyscrasias in patients using methazolamide (Neptazane) for glaucoma. Ophthalmology 87:350, 1980.
38. Weiss, IS: Hirsutism after chronic administration of acetazolamide. Am J Ophthal 78:327, 1974.
39. Maren, TH: Teratology and carbonic anhydrase inhibition. Arch Ophthal 85:1, 1971.
40. Hargett, NA, Ritch, R, Mardirossian, J, Kass, MA, Podos, SM: Inadvertent substitution of acetohexamide for acetazolamide. Am J Ophthal 84:580, 1977.
41. Friedland, BR, Mallonee, J, Anderson, DR: Short-term dose response characteristics of acetazolamide in man. Arch Ophthal 95:1809, 1977.
42. Berson, FG, Epstein, DL, Grant, WM, Hutchinson, BT, Dobbs, PC: Acetazolamide dosage forms in the treatment of glaucoma. Arch Ophthal 98:1051, 1980.
43. Theeuwes, F, Bayne, W, McGuire, J: Gastrointestinal therapeutic system for acetazolamide. Efficacy and side effects. Arch Ophthal 96:2219, 1978.
44. Lichter, PR, Newman, LP, Wheeler, NC, Beall, OV: Patient tolerance to carbonic anhydrase inhibitors. Am J Ophthal 85:495, 1978.
45. Maren, TH, Haywood, JR, Chapman, SK, Zimmerman, TJ: The pharmacology of methazolamide in relation to the treatment of glaucoma. Invest Ophthal Vis Sci 16:730, 1977.
46. Stone, RA, Zimmerman, TJ, Shin, DH, Becker, B, Kass, MA: Low-dose methazolamide and intraocular pressure. Am J Ophthal 83:674, 1977.
47. Dahlen, K, Epstein, DL, Grant, WM, Hutchinson, BT, Prien, EL, Krall, JM: A repeated dose-response study of methazolamide in glaucoma. Arch Ophthal 96:2214, 1978.
48. Merkle, W: Effect of methazolamide on the intraocular pressure of patients with open-angle glaucoma. Klin Monatsbl Augenheilkd 176:181, 1980.
49. Zimmerman, TJ: Acetazolamide and methazolamide. Ann Ophthal 10:509, 1978.
50. Becker, B: Use of methazolamide (Neptazane) in the therapy of glaucoma. Comparison with acetazolamide (Diamox). Am J Ophthal 49:1307, 1960.
51. Ellis, PP: Urinary calculi with methazolamide therapy. Documenta Ophthalmologica 34:137, 1973.
52. Shields, MB, Simmons, RJ: Urinary calculus during methazolamide therapy. Am J Ophthal 81:622, 1976.

Chapter 28

HYPEROSMOTIC AGENTS

HYPEROSMOTIC AGENTS

The drugs discussed in this chapter represent a second class of compounds that may be administered systemically (orally or intravenously) for the control of elevated intraocular pressure. Unlike the carbonic anhydrase inhibitors, however, the use of these medications is generally limited to short-term, emergency situations, such as acute angle-closure glaucoma or secondary glaucomas with dangerously high pressures. Another clinical use for hyperosmotic agents is the reduction of vitreous volume, which is frequently employed as a prophylactic measure prior to intraocular surgery. The mechanisms of action and the side effects of the drugs within this class of compounds are similar, with some notable exceptions, and these features will be discussed collectively before considering specific aspects of the individual agents.

I. MECHANISMS OF ACTION

A. Reduced Vitreous Volume

As noted above, one action of hyperosmotic agents is reduction of vitreous volume. It is this effect which is generally believed to be responsible for lowering the intraocular pressure. This concept is supported by rabbit studies, which demonstrated a reduction in vitreous body weight of approximately 3 to 4% with various hyperosmotic agents.[1] The mechanism of vitreous shrinkage is commonly considered to result from an *osmotic gradient* between the blood and ocular tissues, which initially pulls fluids from the eye.

With time, a variable amount of the hyperosmotic agent may enter the eye, depending upon the permeability of the blood-ocular barriers and the size of the drug molecules. As the compound is cleared from the systemic circulation, there may be a reversal of the osmotic gradient resulting, in some cases, in a transient rise in intraocular pressure.

B. Hypothalamic-neural Theory

Some studies have shown that changes in intraocular pressure and serum osmolarity do not always correlate,[2, 3] and it may be that additional factors are involved in the ocular hypotensive effect of hyperosmotics. One alternative theory is that osmotic agents (both hyperosmotics and hypo-osmotics) influence the intraocular pressure through the central nervous system.

It has been observed that human eyes with *optic nerve* lesions do not manifest the usual reduction in intraocular pressure after water drinking.[4] Unilateral optic nerve transection in rabbits and monkeys also was associated with a reduced ocular hypertensive response to hypo-osmotics, as well as a diminished intraocular pressure lowering effect with hyperosmotic agents.[2, 5 6] These observations raised the possibility that the influence of osmotic agents on the intraocular pressure is mediated by the optic nerve.[2, 4-6]

Additional studies suggested that the central nervous system effect of osmotic agents on intraocular pressure might originate in the *hypothalamus.* Phenobarbital is known to have a depressant effect on the hypothalamus. The drug lowers the intraocular pressure in rabbits, presumably by inhibition of aqueous humor formation, and this action was shown to be reduced by optic nerve transection.[7] Furthermore, pretreatment with phenobarbital prevented the ocular hypotensive response to hyperosmotic agents in rabbits with intact optic nerves.[8] In addition, the injection of osmotic agents into the third ventricle of rabbits altered the intraocular pressure without affecting serum osmolarity, and this effect was eliminated by optic nerve transection.[9] Bilateral lesions in the supraoptic nuclei (an area of the hypothalamus near the optic tracts which is known to be related to water balance) abolished the intraocular pressure response to hypo-osmotics in rabbits.[10]

The above observations are felt to support the theory that osmotic agents exert their influence on intraocular pressure through the central nervous system, possibly originating in the hypothalamus and mediated by efferent fibers in the optic nerve.[2, 4-6, 8] The exact mechanism of pressure reduction is uncertain, although preliminary evidence suggests a decrease in aqueous production.[8]

Other reported studies have not confirmed the observation that unilateral optic nerve transection in rabbits alters the intraocular pressure response to osmotic agents.[11, 12] An alternative explanation that has been proposed for the diminished intraocular pressure response to osmotic agents in eyes with optic atrophy is that an associated reduction in the retinal vasculature decreases the available route of fluid movement from the eye.[11] Another study, however, indicated that optic atrophy is not invariably associated with reduced vasculature of the retina,[13] and there is clearly a need for further investigation of this question.

C. Altered Ciliary Epithelium

It has been observed in monkey studies that intra-arterial injections of hyperosmotic agents cause a breakdown of the blood-aqueous barrier associated with destruction of the non-pigmented ciliary epithelium.[14-16] However, similar changes do not occur following intravenous administration,[14, 15] and it is unlikely that this is part of the ocular hypotensive effect associated with clinical hyperosmotic therapy.

II. SIDE EFFECTS

Side effects with hyperosmotic therapy are common and can be serious,[17] or even fatal,[18, 19] although the magnitude of these adverse reactions varies with the specific agent and mode of administration:

A. Nausea and Vomiting

Nausea and *vomiting* are frequently encountered, especially with the oral (liquid) agents, presumably due to the heavy sweet taste. This is transient and usually of no consequence, but can be a problem if the vomiting occurs during surgery or leads to loss of the medication. The nausea can be minimized by serving the medication with ice and a tart flavoring.

B. Diuresis

Diuresis is a standard response to hyperosmotic therapy and is particularly a problem with the use of intravenous agents. In some cases, massive diuresis during surgery may necessitate the use of an indwelling catheter.

C. Other Reactions

Other reactions that may occur with all hyperosmotics, but which are worse with intravenous agents, include headache, backache, giddiness, diarrhea, confusion and disorientation,[17] chills and fever, cardiovascular overload, intracranial hemorrhage,[18] pulmonary edema, acidemia, and renal insufficiency.[19]

III. SPECIFIC HYPEROSMOTIC AGENTS

A. Oral Agents

1. **Glycerol** is administered as a liquid in a dosage of 1 to 1.5 g/kg body weight of a 50% solution.[20, 21] The ocular hypotensive effect occurs within 10 min of administration, peaks in 30 min, and lasts for approximately 5 hr.[20, 21] Glycerol is distributed throughout the extracellular body fluids and has poor ocular penetration, which enhances the osmotic gradient effect and allows effective repeated administrations.[20] In addition, the drug is metabolized, which causes less diuresis and increased safety. However, the *caloric content* of 4.32 kcal/g[21] and the osmotic diuresis with resultant dehydration can cause problems with repeated administration in diabetics.[22]

2. **Isosorbide** is a newer oral hyperosmotic agent, which became commercially available in 1980. Numerous studies have confirmed the ocular hypotensive efficacy of this agent.[23-29] The drug has an advantage over glycerol in that 95% is excreted unchanged in the urine,[23] which eliminates the caloric problem.[25] Other side effects are also reported to be less with isosorbide than with other hyperosmotics.[23-28] The recommended dosage is 1.5 g/kg body weight of a 50% solution, which produces a peak ocular hypotensive effect in 1 to 3 hr and lasts for 3 to 5 hr.[28] As in the case of glycerol, it may also be given in repeated doses. It should be noted that *isosorbide dinitrate* (Isordil), an organic nitrate used in the treatment of angina

pectoris, has a similar name, and care must be taken to avoid confusing these two drugs.[30]

3. *Other oral drugs* that have been found to be effective as hyperosmotic agents in lowering the intraocular pressure include glycine,[31] sodium lactate,[32] propylene glycol,[33] and ethyl alcohol, although the latter is only effective in large doses.[34]

B. Intravenous Agents

Intravenous agents generally produce a greater ocular hypotensive effect than oral hyperosmotics. They may be indicated when the oral agents are felt to be insufficient or when they cannot be taken for reasons such as nausea.

1. **Mannitol** is reported to have an equivalent[35] or greater[36] ocular hypotensive effect than urea, and is said to be more efficacious than glycerol.[36] In one study, intravenous mannitol and oral isosorbide produced equivalent pressure reduction at 30 and 60 min, although mannitol was more effective in maintaining the reduction.[24] The drug is distributed in the extracellular fluid compartments and has poor ocular penetration.[20] Although it is rapidly excreted unmetabolized in the urine, the transient rise in blood volume requires caution in patients with poor cardiac output. In general, side effects are infrequent, but may include headache, angina-like chest pains[35] and an anaphylactic reaction.[37] Death has been reported in a patient who developed pulmonary edema, acidemia, an anuria following mannitol therapy, and special caution is advised in patients with compromised renal function.[19]

The standard dose is 2 g/kg body weight of a 20% solution, given intravenously in 30 min,[20] although preliminary evidence suggests that significantly lower doses may be equally effective.[38] The onset of action is in 30 to 60 min, and the duration is approximately 6 hr.[20, 35]

2. **Urea** may be slightly less effective than mannitol, because it diffuses more freely throughout the body water and eventually penetrates into the eye.[20] In addition, urea has the significant disadvantage of causing tissue necrosis if it extravasates during intravenous administration.[17] Death from a subdural hematoma has occurred following urea administration for the diagnosis of systemic hypertension.[18]

3. *Glycerol*[39–41] and glycerol with sorbital[40, 41] have also been given intravenously, and preliminary experience suggests that these may prove to have value as intravenous hyperosomtic agents.

References

1. Robbins, R, Galin, MA: Effect of osmotic agents on the vitreous body. Arch Ophthal 82:694, 1969.
2. Podos, SM, Kruptin, T, Becker, B: Effect of small-dose hyperosmotic injections on intraocular pressure of small animals and man when optic nerves are transected and intact. Am J Ophthal 71:898, 1971.
3. Ramsell, JT, Ellis, PP, Paterson, CA: Intraocular pressure changes during hemodialysis. Am J Ophthal 72:926, 1971.

4. Riise, D, Simonsen, SE: Intraocular pressure in unilateral optic nerve lesion. Acta Ophthal 47:750, 1969.
5. Krupin, T, Podos, SM, Becker, B: Effect of optic nerve transection on osmotic alterations of intraocular pressure. Am J Ophthal 70:214, 1970.
6. Krupin, T, Podos, SM, Lehman, RAW, Becker, B: Effects of optic nerve transection on intraocular pressure in monkeys. Arch Ophthal 84:668, 1970.
7. Becker, B, Krupin, T, Podos, SM: Phenobarbital and aqueous humor dynamics: effect in rabbits with intact and transected optic nerves. Am J Ophthal 70:686, 1970.
8. Podos, SM, Krupin, T, Becker, B: Mechanism of intraocular pressure response after optic nerve transection. Am J Ophthal 72:79, 1971.
9. Krupin, T, Podos, SM, Becker, B: Alteration of intraocular pressure after third ventricle injections of osmotic agents. Am J Ophthal 76:948, 1973.
10. Cox, CE, Fitzgerald, CR, King, RL: A preliminary report on the supraoptic nucleus and control of intraocular pressure. Invest Ophthal 14:26, 1975.
11. Serafano, DM, Brubaker, RF: Intraocular pressure after optic nerve transection. Invest Ophthal Vis Sci 17:68, 1978.
12. Lam, KW, Shihab, Z, Fu, YA, Lee, PF: The effect of optic nerve transection upon the hypotensive action of ascorbate and mannitol. Ann Ophthal 12:1102, 1980.
13. Landers, MB III, Bradbury, MJ, Sydnor, CF: Retinal vascular changes in retrograde optic atrophy. Am J Ophthal 86:177, 1978.
14. Laties, AM, Rapoport, S: The blood-ocular barriers under osmotic stress. Studies on the freeze-dried eye. Arch Ophthal 94:1086, 1976.
15. Shabo, AL, Maxwell, DS, Kreiger, AE: Structural alterations in the ciliary process and the blood-aqueous barrier of the monkey after systemic urea injections. Am J Ophthal 81:162, 1976.
16. Okisaka, S , Kuwabara, T, Rapoport, SI: Effect of hyperosmotic agents on the ciliary epithelium and trabecular meshwork. Invest Ophthal 15:617, 1976.
17. Tarter, RC, Linn, JG Jr: A clinical study of the use of intravenous urea in glaucoma. Am J Ophthal 52:323, 1961.
18. Marshall, S, Hinman, F Jr: Subdural hematoma following administration of urea for diagnosis of hypertension. JAMA 182:813, 1962.
19. Grabie, MT, Gipstein, RM, Adams, DA, Hepner, GW: Contraindications for mannitol in aphakic glaucoma. Am J Ophthal 91:265, 1981.
20. Havener, WH: Ocular Pharmacology, 4th ed. CV Mosby Co, St Louis, 1978, p 440.
21. Virno, M, Cantore, P, Bietti, C, Bucci, MG: Oral glycerol in ophthalmology. A valuable new method for the reduction of intraocular pressure. Am J Ophthal 55:1133, 1963.
22. Oakley, DE, Ellis, PP: Glycerol and hyperosmolar nonketotic coma. Am J Ophthal 81:469, 1976.
23. Becker, B, Kolker, AE, Krupin, T: Isosorbide. An oral hyperosmotic agent. Arch Ophthal 78:147, 1967.
24. Barry, KG, Khoury, AH, Brooks, MH: Mannitol and isosorbide. Sequential effects on intraocular pressure, serum osmolality, sodium, and solids in normal subjects. Arch Ophthal 81:695, 1969.
25. Krupin, T, Kolker, AE, Becker, B: A comparison of isosorbide and glycerol for cataract surgery. Am J Ophthal 69:737, 1970.
26. Wisznia, KI, Lazar, M, Leopold, IH: Oral isosorbide and intraocular pressure. Am J Ophthal 70:630, 1970.
27. Mehra, KS, Singh, R, Char, JN, Rajyashree, K: Lowering of intraocular tension. Effects of isosorbide and glycerin. Arch Ophthal 85:167, 1971.
28. Mehra, KS, Singh, R: Lowering of intraocular pressure by isosorbide. Effects of different doses of drugs. Arch Ophthal 86:623, 1971.
29. Wood, TO, Waltman, SR, West, C, Kaufman, HE: Effect of isosorbide on intraocular pressure after penetrating keratoplasty. Am J Ophthal 75:221, 1973.
30. Buckley, EG, Shields, MB: Isosorbide and isorbide dinitrate. Am J Ophthal 89:457, 1980.

31. Fox, SL, Krantz, JC Jr: The use of glycine in the reduction of intraocular pressure. EENT Mthly 51:469, 1972.
32. Chiang, TS, Stocks, SA, Jones, C, Thomas, RP: The ocular hypotensive effect of sodium lactate in rabbits. Arch Ophthal 86:566, 1971.
33. Bietti, G: Recent experimental, clinical, and therapeutic research on the problems of intraocular pressure and glaucoma. Am J Ophthal 73:475, 1972.
34. Obstbaum, SA, Podos, SM, Kolker, AE: Low-dose oral alcohol and intraocular pressure. Am J Ophthal 76:926, 1973.
35. Smith, EW, Drance, SM: Reduction of human intraocular pressure with intravenous mannitol. Arch Opthal 68:734, 1962.
36. Vucicevic, ZM, Tark, E III, Ahmad, S: Echographic studies of osmotic agents. Ann Ophthal 11:1331, 1979.
37. Spaeth, GL, Spaeth, EB, Spaeth, PG, Lucier, AC: Anaphylactic reaction to mannitol. Arch Ophthal 78:583, 1967.
38. Worthen, DM, Quon, D: Dose response of intravenous mannitol on the human eye. Presented at Annual Meeting of Association for Research in Vision and Ophthalmology, Orlando, Fla, May 4–9, 1980, abstract, p 140.
39. Holtmann, HW: Experiences with glycerin infusions for intra-ocular pressure-lowering. Klin Monatsbl Augenheilkd 161:322, 1972.
40. Masiakowski, J, Warchalowska, D, Orlowski, WJ: Effect of osmotic agents on intraocular pressure. I. Survey of pharmacological possibilities. Klin Oczna 43:365, 1973.
41. Barkowska-Orlowska, M, Orlowski, WJ, Warchalowska, D, Masiakowski, J: Effect of osmotic agents on intraocular pressure. II. Intravenous administration of glycerol and glycerol with sorbitol under experimental conditions. Klin Oczna 43:371, 1973.

Chapter 29

INVESTIGATIONAL ANTI-GLAUCOMA DRUGS

INVESTIGATIONAL ANTI-GLAUCOMA DRUGS

Several of the drugs that have been discussed in the preceding chapters, specifically miotics, epinephrine compounds, and the carbonic anhydrase inhibitors, have time-proven value in the long-term management of glaucoma. In addition, early experience with β-adrenergic blockers suggests that these drugs will one day achieve similar status. However, because of intolerable side effects and lack of efficacy in some cases, these drugs are not always able to prevent progressive glaucomatous damage. There is a need, therefore, to continue the search for new and better anti-glaucoma medications. Much of this work is presently being done with new forms of drugs from the classes that were discussed in previous chapters. In addition, research is also being conducted with the following groups of drugs.

I. CANNABINOIDS

In 1971, Hepler and Frank[1] reported that smoking a marihuana cigarette caused a significant reduction in the intraocular pressure. It has subsequently been shown in animal and human studies that several derivatives of *tetrahydrocannabinol* (THC), the primary class of active ingredients in marihuana, effectively lower the intraocular pressure when given orally,[2-5] intravenously,[6-9] or topically.[2, 10-13] Such observations have stimulated the search for cannabinoids that would be suitable for the long-term management of glaucoma. To date, these studies have yielded the following data.

A. Mechanism of action

It was once thought that smoking marihuana might lower the intraocular pressure indirectly by the drug-induced relaxation effect.[14] Extensive animal studies, however, have confirmed a direct ocular hypotensive effect, which appears to have two components: local sympathomimetic activity and a central nervous system action.[8, 15, 16] The local effect is primarily due to vasodilation of the efferent vessels in the anterior uvea, which reduces the ultrafiltration pressure for aqueous humor formation.[9, 17, 18] This action is inhibited by ganglionectomy,[8, 15] beta-adrenergic blockers,[15] or vasodilators.[16] The intraocular pressure reduction is also associated with increased facility of outflow,[8, 9, 17] which is blocked by ganglionectomy[8, 15] or α-adrenergic antagonists.[15, 18] The cannabinoids have also been shown to increase aqueous protein,[9] and to antagonize the *in vivo* ocular production of prostaglandin from arachidonic acid.[19]

B. Clinical efficacy

Although marihuana and many of the cannabinoids are known to be highly effective in lowering the intraocular pressure, the numerous *side effects* of all the compounds thus far tested in humans seriously limits their general usefulness in the long-term management of glaucoma.[4, 20, 21] The best known of these is the *altered mental status*, which has been observed during trial therapy with inhalation of marihuana[22] and oral administration of tetrahydrocannabinol derivatives.[4, 5] Ocular side effects associated with marihuana inhalation include conjunctival hyperemia, a slight miosis, and reduced tear production.[20, 21, 23, 24] Individuals who had used marihuana chronically for 10 years or more, but had abstained for at least 3 hr prior to testing, had increased basal lacrimation, decreased dark adaptation, decreased color-match limits, decreased Snellen acuity, and slightly increased intraocular pressure as compared to matched non-user controls.[25]

From the standpoint of controlling glaucoma, the most disturbing adverse reaction is *systemic hypotension*, which has been observed with oral[4, 5] and intravenous[7] cannabinoids as well as marihuana inhalation.[22] If the drop in blood pressure is found to be associated with reduced perfusion of the optic nerve head, the cannabinoids could be lowering the intraocular pressure without protecting against progressive glaucomatous optic atrophy.[4, 26] Even with topical administration, animal studies suggest that cannibinoids reduce the intraocular pressure by a systemic mechanism,[12] and this has been found in trials with glaucoma patients to occasionally be associated with systemic hypotension.[13] It is clear that considerably more study is needed before any derivative of marihuana can be recommended for the management of glaucoma.

II. PROSTAGLANDINS

Large doses of topical prostaglandins or prostaglandin precursors, such as arachidonic acid, normally cause an initial rise in intraocular pressure, probably due to an inflammatory action. However, it has been shown in rabbits that 25 to 200 μg will produce a pressure reduction for 15 to 20 hr after the initial rise.[27] Furthermore, 5 μg will cause the reduction with no initial rise.[27] The ocular hypotensive phase is associated with a reduction in aqueous outflow resistance,[27] and adrenergic antagonists are reported to block the prostaglandin-induced increase in total outflow facility.[18] Neither indomethacin nor sympathectomy altered the ocular hypotensive effect, suggesting that the mechanism does not involve *de novo* synthesis of prostanglandin or release of endogenous norepinephrine.[27]

III. VANADATE

Vanadate is a potent inhibitor of sodium-potassium-activated adenosine triphosphatase (Na^+K^+ ATPase) that has been shown to lower the intraocular pressure when administered topically to rabbits and monkeys.[28, 29] The mechanism of action appears to be reduced aqueous production, presumably due to inhibition of the enzyme,

Na^+K^+ ATPase, or activation of adenyl cyclase in the ciliary epithelial membrane.[28, 29]

IV. VALINOMYCIN

Valinomycin is a cyclic peptide which increases the permeability of the mitochondrial membrane to potassium. Subconjunctival or topical administration in rabbits and monkeys caused a significant intraocular pressure reduction, although side effects include transient corneal edema and increased aqueous protein.[30]

V. ANTAZOLINE

Antazoline, an antihistamine in the ethylenediamine class, reduced the intraocular pressure when given topically to rabbits.[31] The mechanism of action appered to be decreased aqueous production, which was blocked by an α-adrenergic antagonist, but not by an anti-cholinergic or β-adrenergic blocking agent.

VI. DIRECT OPTIC NERVE HEAD PROTECTORS

All of the drugs previously discussed indirectly protect the optic nerve head from progressive glaucomatous atrophy by lowering the intraocular pressure. An alternative approach would be to give a medication that directly protects the nerve head from the effects of the elevated pressure. This might be particularly desirable in cases of low-tension glaucoma, where maximum medical therapy and even surgery are often unable to lower the intraocular pressure sufficiently to stop the progressive glaucomatous damage.

This concept should be credited to McGuire[32] who, in 1948, reported the use of bishydroxycoumarin (Dicumarol) to protect the optic nerve head by improving vascular perfusion. However, other investigators could not confirm his findings.[33] Subsequently, diphenylhydantoin (Dilantin)[34] and phosphatide complexes[35] were also reported to directly protect the optic nerve head from progressive glaucomatous damage in preliminary studies. Although none of these observations have been confirmed, they do represent an important potential approach to glaucoma therapy which clearly deserves further investigation

References

1. Hepler, RS, Frank, IR: Marihuana smoking and intraocular pressure. JAMA 217:1392, 1972.
2. Green, K, Kim, K: Acute dose response of intraocular pressure to topical and oral cannabinoids. Proc Soc Exp Biol Med 154:228, 1977.
3. Newell, FW, Stark, P, Jay, WM, Schanzlin, DJ: Nabilone: A pressure-reducing synthetic benzopyran in open-angle glaucoma. Ophthalmology 86:156, 1979.
4. Tiedeman, JS, Shields, MB, Weber, PA, Crow, JW, Cocchetto, DM, Harris, WA, Howes, JF: Effect of synthetic cannabinoids on elevated intraocular pressure. Ophthalmology 88:270, 1981.
5. Merritt, JC, McKinnon, S, Armstrong, JR, Hatem, G, Reid, LA: Oral Δ^9-tetrahy-

drocannabinol in heterogeneous glaucomas. Ann Ophthal 12:947, 1980.

6. Purnell, WD, Gregg, JM: Δ^9-tetrahydrocannabinol, euphoria and intraocular pressure in man. Ann Ophthal 7:921, 1975.

7. Cooler, P, Gregg, JM: Effect of delta-9-tetrahydrocannabinol on intraocular pressure in humans. So Med J 70:951, 1977.

8. Green, K, Kim, K: Mediation of ocular tetrahydrocannabinol effects by adrenergic nervous system. Exp Eye Res 23:443, 1976.

9. Green, K, Pederson, JE: Effect of Δ^1-tetrahydrocannabinol on aqueous dynamics and ciliary body permeability in the rabbit. Exp Eye Res 15:499, 1973.

10. Green, K, Kim, K, Wynn, H, Shimp, RG: Intraocular pressure, organ weights and the chronic use of cannabinoid derivatives in rabbits for one year. Exp Eye Res 25:465, 1977.

11. Green, K, Bigger, JF, Kim, K, Bowman, K: Cannabinoid penetration and chronic effects in the eye. Exp Eye Res 24:197, 1977.

12. Merritt, JC, Peiffer, RL, McKinnon, SM, Stapleton, SS, Goodwin, T, Risco, JM: Topical Δ^9-tetrahydrocannabinol on intraocular pressure in dogs. Glaucoma 3:13, 1981.

13. Merritt, JC, Olsen, JL, Armstrong, JR, McKinnon, SM: Topical Δ^9-tetrahydrocannabinol in hypertensive glaucomas. J Pharm Pharmacol 33:40, 1981.

14. Flom, MC, Adams, AJ, Jones, RT: Marijuana smoking and reduced pressure in human eyes: drug action or epiphenomenon? Invest Opthal 14:52, 1975.

15. Green, K, Bigger, JF, Kim, K, Bowman, K: Cannabinoid action on the eye as mediated through the central nervous system and local adrenergic activity. Exp Eye Res 24:189, 1977.

16. Green, K, Kim, K: Papaverine and verapamil interaction with prostaglandin E_2 and Δ^9-tetrahydrocannabinol in the eye. Exp Eye Res 24:207, 1977.

17. Green, Wynn, H, Padgett, D: Effects of Δ^9-tetrahydrocannabinol on ocular blood flow and aqueous humor formation.Exp Eye Res 26:65, 1978.

18. Green, K, Kim, K: Interaction of adrenergic antagonists with prostaglandin E_2 and tetrahydrocannabinol in the eye. Invest Ophthal 15:102, 1976.

19. Green, K, Podos, SM: Antagonism of arachidonic acid-induced ocular effects by Δ^1-tetrahydrocannabinol. Invest Ophthal 13:422, 1974.

20. Green, K: Marihuana and the eye. Invest Ophthal 14:261, 1975.

21. Green, K, Roth, M: Marijuana in the medical management of glaucoma. Pers Ophthal 4:101, 1980.

22. Merritt, JC, Crawford, WJ, Alexander, PC, Anduze, AL, Gelbart, SS: Effect of marihuana on intraocular and blood pressure in glaucoma. Ophthalmology 87:222, 1980.

23. Hepler, RS, Frank, IM, Ungerleider, JT: Pupillary constriction after marijuana smoking. Am J Ophthal 74:1185, 1972.

24. Brown, B, Adams, AJ, Haegerstrom-Portnoy, G, Jones, RT, Flom, MC: Pupil size after use of marijuana and alcohol. Am J Ophthal 83:350, 1977.

25. Dawson, WW, Jimenez-Antillon, CF, Perez, JM, Zeskind, JA: Marijuana and vision—after ten years' use in Costa Rica. Invest Ophthal Vis Sci 16:689, 1977.

26. Gaasterland, DE: Efficacy in glaucoma treatment—the potential of marijuana. Ann Ophthal 12:448, 1980.

27. Camras, CB, Bito, LZ, Eakins, KE: Reduction of intraocular pressure by prostaglandins applied topically to the eyes of conscious rabbits. Invest Ophthal Vis Sci 16:1125, 1977.

28. Becker, B: Vanadate and aqueous humor dynamics. Invest Ophthal Vis Sci 19:1156, 1980..

29. Krupin, T, Becker, B, Podos, SM: Topical vanadate lowers intraocular pressure in rabbits. Invest Ophthal Vis Sci 19:1360, 1980.

30. Lee, PF, Lam, KW: The effect of valinomycin on intraocular pressure. Ann Ophthal 5:33, 1973.

31. Krupin, T, Silverstein, B, Feitl, M, Roshe, R, Becker, B: The effect of H_1-blocking antihistamines on intraocular pressure in rabbits. Ophthalmology 87:1167, 1980.

32. McGuire, WP: The effect of dicumarol on the visual fields in glaucoma. A

preliminary report. Trans Am Ophthal Soc 84:96, 1948.

33. Shields, MB, Wadsworth, JAC: An evaluation of anticoagulation in glaucoma therapy. Ann Ophthal 9:1115, 1977.
34. Becker, B, Stamper, RL, Asseff, C, Podos, SM: Effect of diphenylhydantoin on glaucomatous field loss. A preliminary report. Trans Am Acad Ophthal Otol 76:412, 1972.
35. Hruby, K, Weiss, H: Therapeutic utilization of phosphatide complexes in ophthalmology. Ophthal Digest June 1976, p 9.

Chapter 30

SURGICAL ANATOMY OF GLAUCOMA

All standard surgical procedures for the treatment of glaucoma are performed on the anterior segment of the eye. A thorough understanding of and familiarity with the anatomy in this area is essential for the successful execution of these operations. In this chapter, we will briefly consider these anatomical structures as they relate to glaucoma surgery (Fig. 30.1).

I. LIMBUS

The limbus is a translucent zone between sclera and cornea and is the site of most glaucoma procedures. Knowledge of the relationship between the internal and external landmarks and structures in this region is critical in achieving the desired surgical result and in avoiding serious complications.

A. Internal Boundaries

The *internal boundaries* are the scleral spur with the insertion of the ciliary muscle, posteriorly, and Schwalbe's line, anteriorly. Between these structures is the trabecular meshwork, measuring 0.6 to 0.9 mm.

B. External Boundaries

1. The *sclerolimbal junction*, also referred to as the surgical or posterior limbus, is the junction of the opaque, white sclera and the translucent, bluish-gray limbus. The latter zone is visible only when conjunctiva and Tenon's capsule have been reflected. The sclerolimbal junction is the only consistent landmark of the limbus that can be used in surgery. An incision, perpendicular to the surface at this point, would pass through trabecular meshwork anterior to Schlemm's canal. Therefore, surgical incisions at the sclerolimbal junction are usually slanted toward the anterior chamber to avoid the trabecular meshwork.

2. The *corneolimbal junction*, also called the apparent or anterior limbus, has been defined as the termination of Bowman's membrane, which is approximately 0.5 mm anterior to the insertion of the

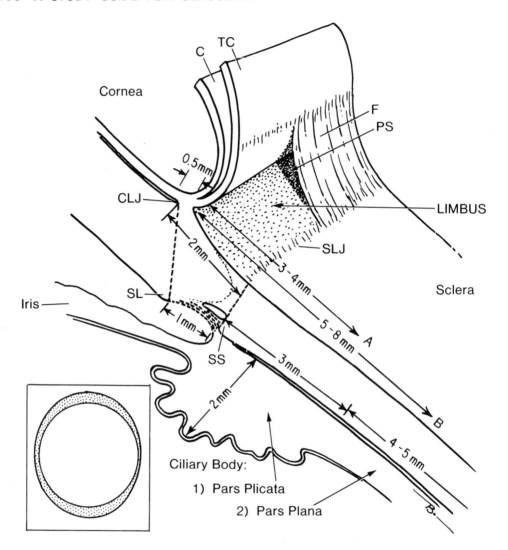

Figure 30.1. Surgical anatomy of glaucoma. The limbus is bounded internally by the scleral spur **(SS)** and Schwalbe's line **(SL)** and externally by the sclerolimbal junction **(SLJ)** and corneolimbal junction **(CLJ)**. Inset shows that the width of the limbus varies from a maximum superiorly to a minimum on the sides. The conjunctiva **(C)** and Tenon's capsule **(TC)** fuse before inserting approximately 0.5 mm behind the corneolimbal junction. A potential space **(PS)** is created by a fusion **(F)** between Tenon's capsule and episclera near the sclerolimbal junction. The ciliary body is divided into the pars plicata and pars plana. Destructive procedures of the ciliary body should be placed over the pars plicata **(point A)**, while a posterior sclerotomy should be made through the pars plana **(point B)**.

conjunctiva and Tenon's capsule. This anatomical landmark is less useful in surgery, due to the inconsistent insertion of the conjunctiva. This results in a variable external width of the limbus, ranging from a maximum of 1 to 1.5 mm above, to slightly less below, to a minimum of 0.3 to 0.5 mm on the sides.

II. CONJUNCTIVA-TENON'S CAPSULE

Tenon's capsule is loosely attached by weak connective tissue strands to the overlying conjunctiva and the underlying episclera. Near the corneolimbal junction, however, conjunctiva and Tenon's capsule fuse to form a single layer. In addition, the capsule is more firmly attached to the episclera along a line just behind the sclerolimbal junction. Anterior to this attachment the capsule splits into two layers forming a potential space. It is important to dissect this adherence between capsule and episclera in order to adequately expose the limbus. It is also helpful to note that the variable insertion of the conjunctiva, as previously described, provides the widest exposure of the limbus at the 12 o'clock position, which may be important in selecting the site for a filtering procedure. The thickness of Tenon's capsule differs considerably among individuals, with children and young adults generally having thicker tissue. The possible significance of this with regard to glaucoma filtering surgery will be considered in Chapter 31.

III. IRIS

The root of the iris inserts into the ciliary body just posterior and internal to the scleral spur, which places it approximately 2 mm posterior to the corneolimbal junction. This is a consideration when performing a peripheral iridectomy, since an incision slanted too far anteriorly will result in a less basal iridectomy, while one slanted too far posteriorly may involve the ciliary body and cause serious bleeding.

IV. CILIARY BODY

The *ciliary body* attaches to the sclera at the scleral spur. The anterior ciliary arteries enter the ciliary body behind the scleral spur in locations corresponding to the positions of the rectus muscle tendons. These vessels must be avoided when performing a cyclodialysis to prevent excessive bleeding. The size and location of the two divisions of the ciliary body are also important surgical landmarks:

A. Pars Plicata

The *pars plicata*, or corona ciliaris, is approximately 3 mm wide and 2 mm thick. In performing destructive procedures of the ciliary body, the lesions should be placed over this tissue, *i.e.*, 3 to 4 mm behind the corneolimbal junction, allowing for the previously discussed variation in this landmark.

B. Pars Plana

The *pars plana* is approximately 4 mm wide and located just behind the pars plicata. Posterior sclerotomies made through this zone should be placed 5 to 8 mm behind the corneolimbal junction.

Reference

 1. Sugar, HS: Surgical anatomy of glaucoma. Surv Ophthal 13:143, 1968.

Chapter 31

GLAUCOMA FILTERING PROCEDURES

GLAUCOMA FILTERING PROCEDURES

The operation most frequently used for open-angle forms of glaucoma, especially in adults, is commonly referred to as a filtering procedure. Although a number of variations for this procedure have been described, all filtering operations share the same basic mechanism of action and general surgical principles. We will first consider these aspects and then discuss specific filtration techniques and potential complications.

I. MECHANISM OF ACTION

A. Drainage Fistula

The basic mechanism of all filtering procedures is the creation of an opening, or fistula, at the limbus, which allows aqueous humor to drain from the anterior chamber, thereby circumventing the pathologic obstruction to outflow. The aqueous flows directly or indirectly into subconjunctival spaces and is then removed by one or more routes.

B. Transconjunctival Route

Studies have shown that aqueous in the subconjunctival spaces usually filters through the conjunctiva[1] and mixes with the tear film,[2,3] or is absorbed by degenerated vascular[1] or perivascular[4] conjunctival tissue. The conjunctiva in the area of filtration becomes elevated, avascular, and thin-walled to variable degrees, and is referred to as a *filtering bleb.* The histology of a successfully functioning filtering bleb reveals degenerative changes in the collagen.[4] It has been shown that aqueous humor inhibits the growth of fibroblasts in tissue culture,[5-7] suggesting that something in the aqueous may alter the conjunctiva and Tenon's capsule in a way that promotes filtration. However, aqueous humor that is obtained shortly after intraocular surgery[7] or is mixed with 20% desiccated embryo extract[8] actually supports fibroblast growth. In addition, aqueous humor obtained from glaucoma patients before surgery does not always inhibit fibroblast growth,[6] and it may be that alterations in aqueous humor content lead to failure of adequate filtering bleb formation in some cases.[6,7]

C. Other Routes

Less commonly a filtering procedure may control the intraocular pressure in the absence of an apparent filtering bleb. This is more common when the fistula is covered by a partial-thickness scleral flap, and reported mechanisms of possible aqueous drainage include flow through 1) lymphatic vessels near the scarred margins of the surgical area, 2) atypical, newly incorporated aqueous veins, and 3) normal aqueous veins.[1,4]

II. GENERAL SURGICAL PRINCIPLES

The various types of filtering surgery differ primarily according to the method used to create the drainage fistula. The other aspects of the operation, as well as the postoperative care, are basically the same for all filtering procedures and will be discussed first before considering specific fistulizing techniques.

A. Anesthesia

Most surgeons prefer local lid akinesia and retrobulbar injection for adults. General anesthesia is used for children and uncooperative patients, or when a retrobulbar injection is felt to be contraindicated. These principles apply, in general, to all forms of glaucoma surgery.

B. Limbal Stab Incision (Fig. 31.1)

Some surgeons first make a beveled incision into the anterior chamber at the limbus, usually in an inferior quadrant, as a route for injecting fluid at the end of the procedure. This can be done with a Wheeler knife, with the cutting edge facing the anterior chamber angle. The tip of the blade is rotated toward the angle during the withdrawal, to widen the inner portion of the incision.

C. The Conjunctival Flap (Fig. 31.2)

The preparation of the conjunctival flap is a critical step in all filtering procedures, since the most common cause of failure is scarring of the filtering bleb.[9] While techniques differ among surgeons, all agree that meticulous detail with minimal tissue damage and bleeding is essential.

1. *Preparation of the flap.* Some surgeons elect to make the flap at the 12 o'clock position to take advantage of the wider limbus in this area. Others prefer one of the superior quadrants, leaving the adjacent quadrant available for future surgery if required. Although a limbus-

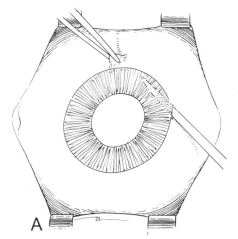
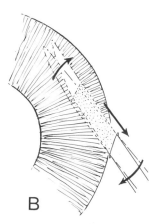

Figure 31.1. Limbal stab incision. **A:** entry at limbus with cutting edge of blade facing the anterior chamber angle; **B:** rotation of knife tip toward the angle during withdrawal.

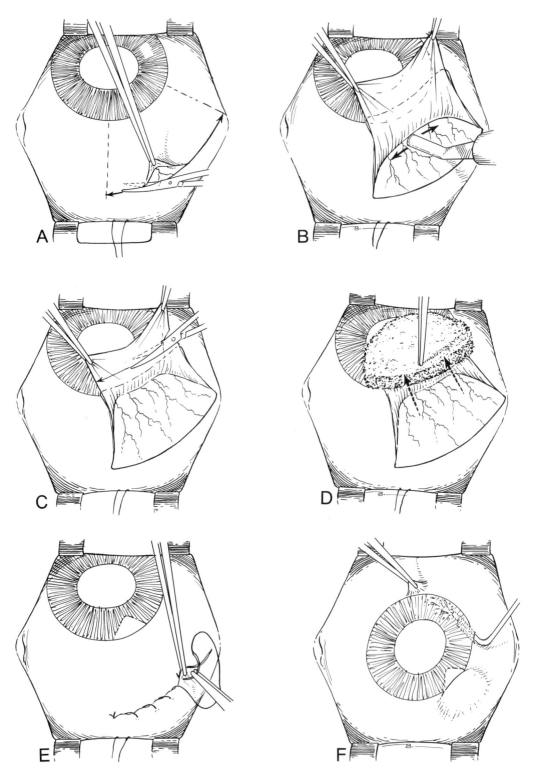

Figure 31.2. Preparation of a limbus-based conjunctival flap. **A:** incision through conjunctiva and Tenon's capsule; **B:** blunt dissection of Tenon's capsule from underlying episclera; **C:** partial excision of Tenon's capsule; **D:** retraction of conjunctival flap over cornea with moist Gelfoam sponge; **E:** closure of conjunctival flap; **F:** injection of balanced salt solution into anterior chamber, with elevation of conjunctival flap. (Portions reprinted with permission from Ophthal. Surg. 11:498, 1980.[12])

based flap is most commonly employed, some surgeons advocate a fornix-based flap, particularly in association with a trabeculectomy.[10, 11] Blunt dissection is desirable when possible. An instrument for this purpose has been fashioned from a #64 Beaver blade by blunting the cutting edge and bending it at a 45° angle.[12]

2. *Management of Tenon's capsule.* There is some controversy regarding the value of removing all or a portion of Tenon's capsule in the area of the conjunctival flap. In one study of similar filtering procedures, no difference in postoperative intraocular pressure control was noted between eyes with subtotal excision of the capsular tissue as compared to those in which it was left intact.[13] However, Tenon's capsule is typically thicker in children and young adults,[14] which may contribute to the poorer success rate of filtering surgery in these groups.[15] For this reason, many surgeons will excise variable portions of Tenon's capsule when it appears to be unusually thick. This can be accomplished by dissecting between the conjunctiva and Tenon's capsule and then excising the capsule from the episclera. An alternative approach is to dissect Tenon's capsule from underlying episclera, strip a portion of the capsule from the conjunctiva with gentle traction, and then excise that portion of the capsular tissue.

3. *During the fistulizing procedure*, it is important to keep the conjunctival flap moist and to minimize handling of the tissue. This can be conveniently accomplished by reflecting the flap over the cornea with a moist Gelfoam sponge.[12] A Weck-Cel surgical spear with the tip cut off may also be used to gently retract the flap.[16]

D. Peripheral Iridectomy

A *peripheral iridectomy* is a routine part of all standard filtering procedures, and is usually made after the fistula has been prepared. However, if the iris prolapses into the limbal wound, it is generally best to make the iridectomy and then complete the fistula. A large iridectomy is desirable to prevent adherence of the iris to the edges of the fistula.[17]

E. Closure of the Conjunctival Flap (Fig. 31.2)

This is also a critical aspect of any filtering procedure, since a leaking wound may lead to a persistently flat anterior chamber and failure of the filtering bleb to develop properly. Opinions vary widely as to the optimum suture for closure, but it is generally agreed that a running suture with close bites provides the tightest closure. Some surgeons prefer to further enhance the integrity of the wound closure by suturing Tenon's capsule and conjunctiva separately.[14]

F. Injection of Fluid (Fig. 31.2)

If a limbal stab incision was made at the outset, as previously described, the final step in the filtering operation is to inject a balanced salt solution into the anterior chamber via that incision. This deepens the anterior chamber and elevates the conjunctival flap, thereby demonstrating patency of the fistula and water-tight closure of the flap. Sodium hyaluronate (Healon) is a viscous substance, which may be used instead of a balanced salt solution and is reported to maintain a deep anterior chamber and promote superior bleb formation.[18]

G. Postoperative Management

Topical mydriatic-cycloplegic and antibiotic therapy should be used routinely for the first 2 to 3 weeks. In addition, most surgeons prefer to use a topical corticosteroid to reduce scar formation of the filtering bleb. One study suggested that chronic steroid therapy following filtering surgery may lead to intraocular pressure elevation despite a good filtering bleb,[19] although this has yet to be substantiated.

III. FISTULIZING TECHNIQUES

The two basic types of fistulas differ according to whether they extend through the full thickness of the limbal tissue or are covered by a partial-thickness scleral flap. In addition, efforts have been made to maintain patency of the fistula by implanting various materials in the opening.

A. Full-thickness Fistulas

The original type of limbal fistula, and one which is still in common use, involves creation of a direct opening through the full thickness of the limbal tissue. The fistula may be created by a variety of techniques.

1. *Sclerectomy.* In 1906, LaGrange[20] described a technique in which a full-thickness limbal incision was made, and a piece of tissue was then excised from the anterior lip of the wound to create a limbal fistula. Holth[21] modified this procedure 3 years later by performing the sclerectomy with a *punch*. A variety of sclerectomy punches have subsequently been developed, and surgical variations have included excision of tissue from the anterior lip of the wound,[22, 23] the anterior and posterior lips[24, 25] or the lateral lip of a radial incision.[26] However, the sclerectomy technique most often discussed in recent literature is the *posterior lip sclerectomy*, described by Iliff and Haas (Fig. 31.3).[27]

a. A scratch incision is begun just behind the insertion of the conjunctival flap in an area of sclera that has been lightly cauterized. The incision is beveled inward at an angle of approximately 75° to the limbal surface and is continued until the anterior chamber is entered. Scissors are then used to widen the incision to about five mm.

b. A 1.5-mm Holth punch is used to excise full-thickness limbal tissue from the posterior lip of the incision, creating a fistula of approximately 1 × 3 mm. Care must be taken to avoid cutting into the ciliary body, which can lead to significant bleeding.

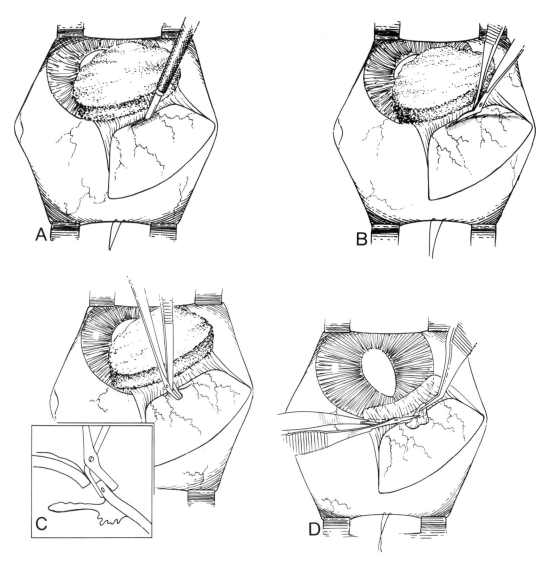

Figure 31.3. Posterior lip sclerectomy. **A:** beveled incision into anterior chamber; **B:** enlargement of limbal incision with scissors; **C:** excision of full-thickness tissue from posterior lip of incision with sclerectomy punch; **D:** peripheral iridectomy created, as for all standard filtering procedures. (Portions reprinted with permission from Ophthal. Surg. 11:498, 1980.[12])

    c. This technique may be modified slightly by applying light cautery to the posterior margins of the sclerectomy.[12, 23] This further enlarges the fistula and may help to inhibit postoperative scarring.[23, 28]

    d. As with all routine filtering procedures, a peripheral iridectomy is made after the fistula has been completed, or sooner if the iris prolapses during preparation of the fistula.

    2. *Trephination.* In 1909, Elliot[29] and Fergus[30] both described a

glaucoma filtering procedure in which the fistula was created with a small *trephine* placed just behind the corneolimbal junction. Elliot[31] later modified the technique by splitting the peripheral cornea and placing the trephine more anteriorly (sclero-corneal trephining). However, because this modification produced a thinner filtering bleb and a greater chance of late infection, Sugar[32] advocated a return to the original, more posterior trephining, which he called *limboscleral trephination* (or trepanation). The subsequent experience of Sugar[15, 33, 34] and others has supported the merit of this technique (Fig. 31.4).

a. A 1.5 or 2.0 mm trephine blade is placed over the limbus just behind the corneolimbal junction. The trephine is tilted forward so that the anterior edge of the blade enters the anterior chamber first. Entry into the anterior chamber is usually indicated by a movement of the upper pupillary margin toward the trephine.

b. The trephine button, which is hinged on the scleral side and may rotate forward due to prolapse of the iris, is excised by cutting across the hinge with scissors. As with other filtering procedures, care must be taken to avoid cutting into the ciliary body.

3. **Thermal sclerostomy.** Preziosi,[35] in 1924, described a filtering technique in which a limbal fistula was created by entering the anterior chamber angle with electro-cautery. Scheie[36] later described a procedure, which also utilized *cautery* but differed significantly from the Preziosi operation in that a limbal scratch incision was first made, and the cautery was then used to retract the wound edges, thereby creating the fistula. Various modifications have subsequently

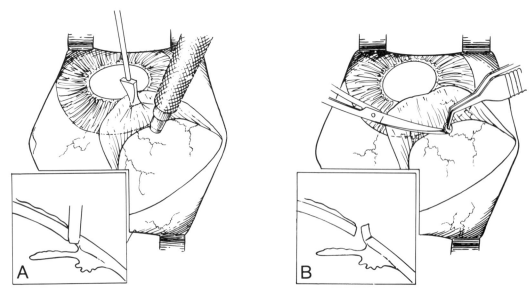

Figure 31.4. Limboscleral trephination. **A:** trephine button partially excised by tilting the trephine anteriorly; **B:** completion of excision by cutting posterior attachment with scissors.

been described,[37-40] although the basic technique of Scheie[36] remains a popular approach to this glaucoma filtering procedure (Fig. 31.5).

a. Light cautery is applied to the sclera in a 1 × 5 mm area behind the corneolimbal junction. A 5-mm limbal scratch incision is then made through the cauterized area, perpendicular to the scleral surface, and cautery is applied to the lips of the incision until the wound edges separate by at least one mm.

b. The escape of aqueous from the limbal incision may interfere with the application of cautery, and this can be partially avoided by stopping the initial scratch incision just before it enters the anterior chamber, applying cautery, and then completing the incision.[40] In addition, bipolar cautery can be effectively used in a wet field.

4. *Iridencleisis* differs from the other forms of full-thickness filtering surgery in that a wedge of iris is incarcerated into the limbal incision in an effort to maintain a patent channel for aqueous outflow.[41] This was once a popular procedure, but it lost favor partly due to the suspicion that the associated incidence of sympathetic ophthalmia was higher than with other filtering procedures. Although this fear has not been substantiated, the operation never regained popularity.

5. The use of *argon laser* to create a full-thickness glaucoma fistula has also been described.[42]

B. Partial-thickness Fistulas (Trabeculectomy)

Full-thickness filtering procedures may be complicated by excessive aqueous filtration, which can lead to a prolonged flat anterior

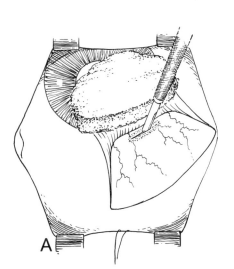
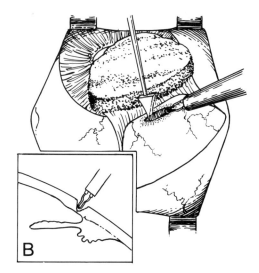

Figure 31.5. Thermal sclerostomy. **A:** limbal incision created (may initially be partial or full-thickness); **B:** application of cautery to the lips of the incision to separate the wound edges. A partial-thickness incision is then extended into the anterior chamber and cautery is applied to the depths of the wound, while a dry field is maintained with a sponge.

chamber, associated with corneal decompensation, synechiae formation, and cataracts. In addition, the filtering blebs often become very
thin and may rupture, creating the danger of endophthalmitis. (Surgical complications will be considered in more detail later in this
chapter.) One attempt to minimize these complications has been to
place a partial-thickness scleral flap over the fistula. This concept was
suggested by Sugar[43] in 1961, but was popularized by the 1968 report
of Cairns.[44] Both authors referred to the technique as a *trabeculectomy*.

1. *Theories of mechanism* (Fig. 31.6). It was originally thought that
aqueous might flow into the cut ends of Schlemm's canal.[44] Subsequent studies, however, showed fibrotic closure of the canal at its cut
ends in monkey[45] and human[46] eyes, and the presence of Schlemm's
canal in the "trabeculectomy" specimen did not correlate with the
outcome of the procedure.[47,48] Furthermore, the majority of successful
cases have a filtering bleb,[49] indicating that *external filtration* is the
principal mode of intraocular pressure reduction.

Whether the route of external filtration is primarily through or
around the partial-thickness scleral flap remains a matter of contro-

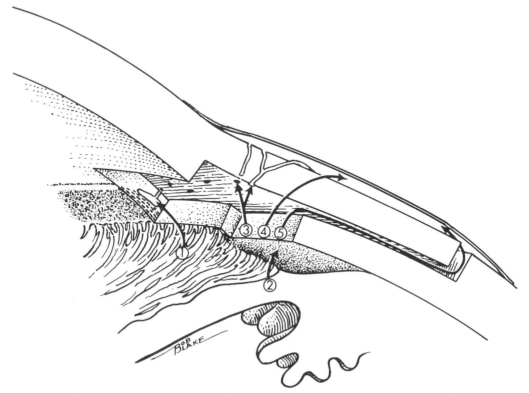

Figure 31.6.   Trabeculectomy, possible mechanisms of action. **1:** aqueous flow into cut
ends of Schlemm's canal (rare); **2:** cyclodialysis (if tissue is dissected posterior to scleral
spur); **3:** Filtration through outlet channels in scleral flap; **4:** filtration through connective
tissue substance of scleral flap; **5:** filtration around the margins of the scleral flap.

versy. Although the outer layers of limbus and anterior sclera do not differ ultrastructurally from the inner layers in any way that might predispose to increased passage of aqueous,[50] perfusion studies showed that flow through this tissue in enucleated eyes with a trabeculectomy (margins sealed with adhesive) can significantly increase the rate of outflow.[51] However, fluorescein angiographic studies of eyes with successful trabeculectomies suggested that the primary route of external filtration, in these cases, was around the margins of the scleral flap.[12] It may be that external filtration occurs by either route, depending on how tightly the scleral flap is sutured.

Other possible mechanisms of intraocular pressure reduction by trabeculectomy include cyclodialysis[45] or aqueous outflow through newly developed aqueous veins, lymphatic vessels, or normal aqueous veins.[52, 53]

2. *Basic trabeculectomy technique* (Fig. 31.7):

a. The margins of a 5 × 5 mm scleral flap, adjacent to the corneolimbal junction, are outlined with half-thickness scleral incisions. It is helpful to apply light cautery before making the incisions to minimize bleeding. A half-thickness lamellar flap, hinged at the cornea, is then raised until at least one mm of the bluish-gray limbus is exposed.

b. The anterior chamber is entered with a knife in front of Schwalbe's line just behind the hinge of the scleral flap. The incision is widened with scissors to approximately 4 mm and is extended posteriorly on either end for 1 mm. The 1 × 4 mm block of tissue is then reflected until the pigmented trabecular meshwork can be visualized, and the tissue is excised with scissors along the scleral spur.

c. After making the iridectomy, the scleral flap is then approximated with a variable number of sutures.

3. *Modifications.* The numerous variations of the guarded filtering procedure that have been reported primarily involve modifications in the scleral flap or in the fistulizing technique.

a. *Variations in the scleral flap.* Rather than making a square flap, some surgeons prefer a triangular[54] or semicircular[55] shape. With regard to suturing the flap, some like a tight closure with multiple sutures, while other surgeons not only prefer few[12] or no[56] sutures, but take steps to enhance filtration around the flap by lightly cauterizing the margins[12] or excising the distal two mm of the flap.[56]

b. *Variations in the fistulizing technique.* Watson[57–59] modified Cairn's basic technique by starting the dissection of the tissue block posteriorly over ciliary body, separating it from the underlying structure, and excising it at Schwalbe's line. Other techniques that have been used to create the subscleral fistula include trephination,[55, 60–63] posterior lip sclerectomy,[64, 65] thermal sclerostomy,[66–69] and a carbon dioxide laser.[70, 71] Another reported variation is to leave the trabecular tissue flap attached at its nasal end and suture it diagonally across the scleral bed to keep the flap from scarring down.[72]

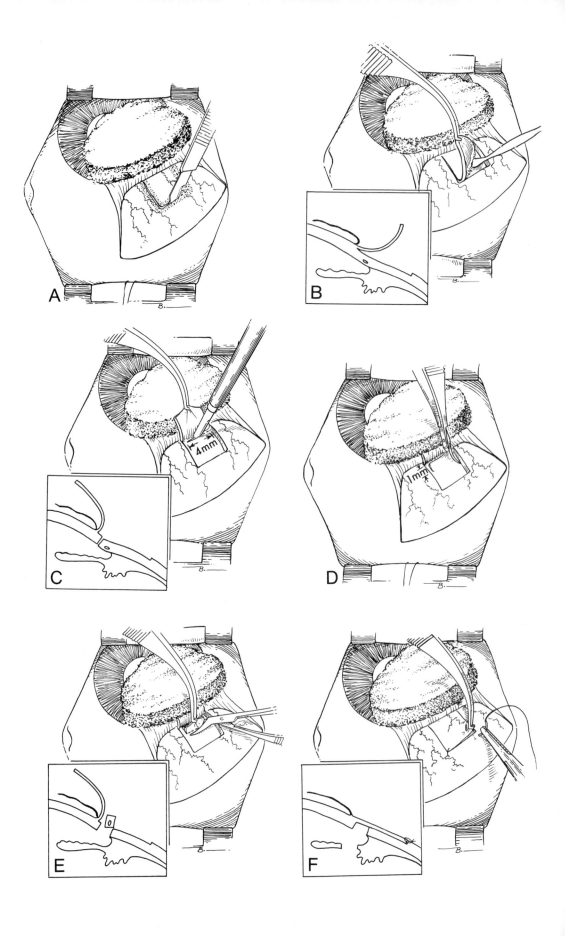

c. The trabeculectomy procedure has also been modified for *neovascular glaucoma.* One variation includes excision of a large trabecular segment, partial nonpenetrating cyclodiathermy in the scleral bed, and partial ablation of abnormal iris vessels with a wide sector iridectomy.[73] Another technique utilizes bipolar cautery to directly treat vessels in the anterior chamber angle and the ciliary processes in the area of the filtering surgery.[74]

C. Implant (Seton) Procedures

In an attempt to maintain patency of the drainage fistula in either full-thickness or guarded filtering operations, a wide variety of foreign materials have been placed in the fistula. Although these have been almost uniformly unsuccessful over the years, continued research with newer designs is beginning to show promise.

1. *Tubes.* The success of newer implant operations appears to be due, at least in part, to the concept of aqueous drainage through patent translimbal tubes. Animal studies have shown that catheters can maintain flow from the anterior chamber to a subconjunctival space for at least 6 months after implantation.[75] Devices that have been successfully used in humans include a stripe of hydrogel with parallel capillary channels,[76] and a silicone tube attached to a thin acrylic plate on the sclera.[77] The latter is reported to be particularly useful in eyes with neovascular glaucoma,[78] and chronic glaucoma in aphakia.[79]

2. *Valves* (Fig. 31.8). One step beyond the concept of tube implants is the creation of a valve which allows one-way flow from the anterior chamber and which opens at a pre-determined intraocular pressure level. Krupin and co-workers[80] developed such a valve, composed of an internal Supramid tube cemented to an external (subconjunctival) Silastic tube. The valve-effect is created by making slits in the closed external end of the Silastic tube. Preliminary experience, especially with neovascular glaucoma, has been encouraging.[81]

IV. PREVENTION AND MANAGEMENT OF COMPLICATIONS

The following complications may occur with any filtering procedure, although some operations and techniques appear to provide certain advantages over others. We will first consider the complications in general and then compare the merits of the various filtering procedures. It is helpful to think of these complications in three phases: operative, early postoperative, and late postoperative.

Figure 31.7. Trabeculectomy, basic technique. **A:** Margins of scleral flap are outlined by partial-thickness incisions; **B:** dissection of scleral flap; **C:** anterior chamber is entered with a knife just behind the hinge of the scleral flap; **D:** completion of anterior and lateral margins of deep limbal incision with scissors; **E:** flap of deep limbal tissue is excised by cutting along scleral spur; **F:** approximation of scleral flap. (Portions reprinted with permission from Ophthal. Surg. 11:498, 1980.[12])

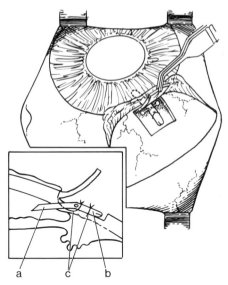

Figure 31.8. Glaucoma valve implant. An internal Supramid tube **(a)**, cemented to an external Silastic tube with a slit valve **(b)**, is inserted through a limbal incision into the anterior chamber and sutured **(c)** beneath a partial-thickness scleral flap.

A. Operative Complications

1. *Tearing or buttonholing the conjunctival flap* during various steps of the operation can be minimized by gentle handling of the tissues as outlined earlier in this chapter. When it does occur, it may be possible to close the defect using fine nylon suture on a round, tapered needle[82] or by applying tissue adhesive.[83] For very small holes, light bipolar cautery may effectively seal the defect. However, if the hole is large or directly over the fistula site, it may be best to shift to another quadrant of the eye to complete the procedure.

2. *Hemorrhage.* Episcleral bleeding is particularly common in glaucoma patients who have been on long-term anti-glaucoma medication. It can be managed with irrigation or light cautery, and should be under control before the anterior chamber is entered. As previously noted, inadvertent cutting of the *ciliary body* may cause brisk bleeding. Cautery is difficult and frequently counterproductive in these cases, and gentle, sustained pressure over the fistula with a sponge or a large air bubble in the anterior chamber will usually eventually control the bleeding. A *choroidal*, or expulsive, hemorrhage is a particularly devastating complication that usually results from sudden reduction in the intraocular pressure with rupture of a large choroidal vessel. It is managed by immediately closing the fistula, placing a scleral incision in the inferior temporal quadrant, and allowing the blood to drain from this site until it stops spontaneously.[41] Hemorrhage into the lens has also been reported as a rare complication of glaucoma surgery.[84]

3. *Choroidal effusion* may occur during glaucoma filtering surgery, especially in eyes with prominent episcleral vessels, as in cases of

Sturge-Weber syndrome.[85] This is usually recognized by a sudden shallowing of the anterior chamber during the operation and can be managed by making a scleral incision to release the suprachoroidal fluid.[85]

4. *Vitreous loss* may occur during creation of the fistula or iridectomy, due to rupture of the lens zonules and hyaloid membrane, which usually results from excessive manipulation. The vitreous should be removed from the surgical site with sponges and scissors or a vitrectomy instrument.

B. Early Postoperative Complications

During the first several days after a filtering procedure, the complications most often facing the surgeon are related either to an eye that is filtering too well or to one that is not filtering adequately.

1. *Hypotony* is common during the first few postoperative days, especially with full-thickness filtering procedures, and is typically associated with a very shallow anterior chamber, which usually deepens gradually with conservative management. However, if the chamber is flat, and especially if there is corneal decompensation, attention must be given to the cause and correction of the problem:

a. *Conjunctival defect.* If there is an obvious hole in the conjunctival flap, it may be possible to achieve spontaneous closure with a pressure patch. If this is not successful, tissue adhesive[83] or suturing of the defect[82] may be effective. However, when the defect is large, it may be necessary to develop a new conjunctival flap from tissue posterior to the defect.[86]

b. *Choroidal detachments* with decreased aqueous production are frequently found in hypotonous eyes with flat anterior chambers. It is occasionally necessary in these cases to drain the suprachoroidal fluid through scleral incisions in the inferior quadrants and then to deepen the chamber with a balanced salt solution.[87] An analysis of the suprachoroidal fluid suggests that it is derived from blood, and it is postulated that hypotony allows increased flow across the walls of the choriocapillaris, leading to the accumulation of the suprachoroidal fluid.[88] Less commonly, *serous retinal detachment* may occur after filtering surgery, presumably by a similar mechanism. These usually resolve spontaneously.

c. *Excessive filtration* may result from a large fistula or an exceptionally large filtering bleb. It is in this regard that *trabeculectomies* are felt to offer one of their advantages, since the protective scleral flap minimizes excessive filtration. Another technique that has been developed to prevent the early flat anterior chamber after filtering surgery is the *shell tamponade*, in which a plastic shell is temporarily sutured over the filtering bleb.[89, 90] In addition, a *guarded thermal sclerostomy* has been described, in which a suture is placed across the fistula to temporarily regulate the rate of filtration.[38]

Management of excessive filtration usually first involves firm patching of the eye. A small cotton ball may be placed over the lid in the area of the fistula to act as a tamponade. If this step is used, the patient should be kept awake, with his eyes open and looking straight ahead, since the Bell's phenomenon of sleep may place the tamponade over the center of the cornea. If the chamber cannot be reformed after several days, and especially if corneal decompensation is present, surgical intervention is usually indicated.[87] If choroidal detachments are large, these should be drained as previously noted. Otherwise it may be sufficient to deepen the anterior chamber with a large air bubble.[91]

2. *Elevated intraocular pressure* during the early postoperative period may be associated with either a flat or deep anterior chamber.

a. A *flat anterior chamber* suggests malignant (ciliary block) glaucoma or a pupillary block mechanism, both of which were discussed in Section Two.

b. A *deep anterior chamber* indicates inadequate filtration due to 1) obstruction of the fistula by iris, ciliary processes, lens, or vitreous, or 2) an absent or poorly functioning filtering bleb. The former category can be largely avoided by making an adequate fistula and iridectomy and by minimizing excessive surgical manipulation. However, once the complication occurs, there is frequently no recourse but to resume antiglaucoma medication and usually to repeat the procedure at a later date.

Management of a failing filtering bleb consists primarily of the copious use of steroids to minimize scarring and the intermittent application of digital pressure to expand the subconjunctival space by forcing aqueous into it.[90] The use of an ophthalmodynamometer has been suggested as an alternative to digital pressure, since it allows visualization of the bleb during pressure application as well as monitoring of the force being applied.[92] A perilimbal suction cup placed over the surgical site has also been used in an attempt to salvage a failing filtering bleb,[93] although reports of the benefit of this technique are conflicting.[94, 95]

It has also been reported that approximately one-third of the eyes treated by *trabeculectomy* have an intraocular pressure rise on the second postoperative day, which becomes normal within a week and does not influence the final result.[96]

3. *Uveitis* and *hyphema* may also occur during the early postoperative period. The former is treated with topical corticosteroids and mydriatics and the latter is managed conservatively with elevation of the head and limited activity.

4. *Loss of a small central island* of vision after glaucoma filtering surgery is rare, but has been reported.[97] Nevertheless, the incidence of this complication is so low that such a preoperative visual field is not considered to be a contraindication to surgery.[98, 99]

C. Late Postoperative Complications

1. *Late failure of filtration* may result from a filtering bleb that becomes cystic and scarred down[100] or from closure of the fistula by a proliferation of episcleral[101] or endothelial[102] tissue. Various surgical[100, 101] and laser [103] techniques have been described to re-establish

filtration in these cases, although most eventually require a repeat filtering procedure.

2. A *ruptured filtering bleb* may occur when the bleb wall has become too thin, and this may lead to loss of the anterior chamber and endophthalmitis. In some cases, the defect can be closed with tissue adhesive, although most require creation of a new conjunctival flap from tissue posterior to the defect.[86] A histologic examination of 10 leaking filtering blebs revealed an epithelial tract running from the surface of the bleb to the episclera in eight cases, and it was suggested that the bleb should be excised before bringing down the new flap to prevent epithelial downgrowth.[104]

3. *Overhanging filtering blebs.* In some cases, a large bleb may be gradually massaged downward over the cornea by the lid movements.[105] These can be surgically removed by lifting the bleb from the cornea with an iris spatula, excising it near the limbus, and suturing the free edges.[105]

4. *Endophthalmitis* associated with a ruptured filtering bleb may be somewhat less severe in a phakic eye than following cataract surgery, although both demand prompt, aggressive management.[106-109] For bacterial postoperative endophthalmitis in general, a recommended approach is to establish the diagnosis with aqueous and vitreous aspirates,[110] and then treat with high-dose parenteral and periocular antibiotics and systemic and periocular corticosteroids.[111] Endophthalmitis is generally more common with a thin-walled filtering bleb,[112] as following trephinations.[113] However, one study found the incidence of endophthalmitis to be the same between thermal sclerostomy and trabeculectomy.[114]

5. *Sympathetic ophthalmia* following glaucoma surgery is a rare complication. Studies suggest that this is not related to the type of operation, but rather to the pre-operative condition of the eye, in that it occurs more commonly when operating on a blind, painful eye.[115]

6. *Cataracts* are reported to occur in 30 to 40% of eyes after filtering surgery.[97, 116-120] The mechanism of this complication is uncertain, but possible factors include[116] 1) patient age, 2) duration of miotic therapy, 3) surgical manipulation, 4) postoperative iritis,[121] 5) prolonged flat anterior chamber, and 6) nutritional changes.

7. *Spontaneous hyphema* may occur weeks to years after filtering surgery.[122] Bimanual bipolar diathermy has been recommended to treat bleeding from the anterior chamber angle.[123] Laser photocoagulation may also be effective in these cases.

8. A *staphyloma* has been reported as a late complication of trabeculectomy.[124]

9. *Upper eyelid retraction* after glaucoma filtering surgery was described in two patients, and was thought to result from the adrenergic effect of aqueous humor on Mueller's muscle.[125]

V. COMPARISON OF FILTERING PROCEDURES

There is no universal agreement among surgeons regarding the filtering procedure of choice. Favorable results have been reported by proponents of each basic technique, and many of these are referenced in the discussion below. In comparing procedures, it is necessary to consider both control of the glaucoma and the rate of complications.

A. Full-thickness Procedures

1. *Glaucoma control.* With regard to control of progressive glaucomatous damage, with or without additional anti-glaucoma medication, good results have been achieved with each of the standard full-thickness filtering procedures, *i.e.*, sclerectomy,[22–27, 119] trephination,[15, 32–34] and thermal sclerostomy.[36–40, 119, 126] The reported success rates for all of these operations generally range between 75 and 95%. One study, however, suggested that thermal sclerostomy, despite its simplicity in concept, may be more difficult for the novice surgeon to perform effectively, as compared to a posterior lip sclerectomy.[119] This may relate to the experience required to make an adequate fistula with cautery.

2. *Complications.* A more significant difference between full-thickness filtering procedures may be seen when analyzing the complication rates of the different techniques. As previously noted, filtering procedures with a large fistula, such as trephination, may be associated with a higher incidence of complications, including prolonged flat anterior chambers in the early postoperative period and bleb leakage with possible endophthalmitis in the late period after surgery.[113, 114] Nevertheless, when all aspects of glaucoma control and complication rates are considered together, it is not possible to demonstrate clear-cut superiority for any one full-thickness glaucoma filtering procedure.

B. Trabeculectomy vs Full-thickness Filtering Procedures

1. *Glaucoma control.* Numerous studies have been reported regarding experience with the various forms of trabeculectomy. In general, these studies all indicate successful glaucoma control in the range of that reported for full-thickness filtering procedures, but with a variable reduction in the incidence of complications.[44, 49, 54–69, 127–135] Studies which have specifically compared trabeculectomies and full-thickness operations have also shown comparable glaucoma control,[136, 137] although some surveys suggested slightly better intraocular pressure control with full-thickness procedures.[12, 138–141]

It is generally felt that glaucoma control among *black patients* is poorer than in white populations for most filtering procedures, although this has not been substantiated in all studies. With regard to trabeculectomies in blacks, the reported success rates have mostly been in the same range as those for whites,[142–145] although some series have had less than 75% success with standard trabeculectomies.[56, 146] Some surgeons have noted improved pressure control when the trabeculectomy technique is modified to enhance filtration around the scleral flap.[56, 147] Comparative studies of trabeculectomies and full-thickness filtering procedures within black populations have also been conflicting, with one series showing comparable glaucoma control,[148] while better control was achieved with a trabeculectomy in one study[149] and with a full-thickness procedure in another.[150]

It is reasonably well-established that children do worse with filtering procedures in general, and this appears to apply to trabeculectomies.[151] One study found no evidence that trabeculectomy is better than other procedures for advanced pediatric glaucomas.[152]

2. *Complications.* Virtually all studies agree that complication rates are lower with trabeculectomies as compared to full-thickness filtering procedures.[12, 44, 49, 54–69, 127–141, 153] This has led some surgeons to feel that selected cases can even be performed on an outpatient basis.[154] However, it is important to note that complications do occur with the trabeculectomy procedure as with other filtering operations. Some of the complications which have been reported following a trabeculectomy include flat anterior chambers,[155] significant postoperative hyphemas,[155] a 28% incidence of cataracts,[120] endophthalmitis,[114] and expulsive hemorrhage.[156]

References

1. Benedikt, O: The effect of filtering operations. Klin Monatsbl Augenheilkd 170:10, 1977.
2. Kronfeld, PC: The chemical demonstration of transconjunctival passage of aqueous after antiglaucomatous operations. Am J Ophthal 35:38, 1952.
3. Galin, MA, Baras, I, McLean, JM: How does a filtering bleb work? Trans Am Acad Ophthal Otol 69:1082, 1965.
4. Teng, CC, Chi, HH, Katzin, HM: Histology and mechanism of filtering . operations. Am J Ophthal 47:16, 1959.
5. Kornblueth, W, Tenenbaum, E: The inhibitory effect of aqueous humor on the growth of cells in tissue cultures. Am J Ophthal 42:70, 1956.
6. Herschler, J, Claflin, AJ, Fiorentino, G: The effect of aqueous humor on the growth of subconjunctival fibroblasts in tissue culture and its implications for glaucoma surgery. Am J Ophthal 89:245, 1980.
7. Radius, RL, Herschler, J, Claflin, A, Fiorentino, G: Aqueous humor changes after experimental filtering surgery. Am J Ophthal 89:250, 1980.
8. Albrink, WS, Wallace, AC: Aqueous humor as a tissue culture nutrient. Proc Soc Exp Biol Med 77:754, 1951.
9. Maumenee, AE: External filtering operations for glaucoma: the mechanism of function and failure. Trans Am Ophthal Soc 58:319, 1960.
10. Luntz, MH: Trabeculectomy using a fornix-based conjunctival flap and tightly sutured scleral flap. Ophthalmology 87:985, 1980.
11. Luntz, MH, Freedman, J: The fornix-based conjunctival flap in glaucoma filtration surgery. Ophthal Surg 11:516, 1980.
12. Shields, MB: Trabeculectomy vs full-thickness filtering operation for control of glaucoma. Ophthal Surg 11:498, 1980.
13. Kapetansky, FM: Trabeculectomy, or trabeculectomy plus tenectomy: a comparative study. Glaucoma 2:451, 1980.
14. Sugar, HS: Surgical anatomy of glaucoma. Surv Ophthal 13:143, 1968.
15. Sugar, HS: Further experience with limboscleral trephination. EENT Mthly 47:165, 1968.
16. Rainin, EA: Limbal-based conjunctival flap retractor. Ann Ophthal 7:599, 1975.
17. Freedman, J: Iridectomy technique in trabeculectomy. Ophthal Surg 9:45, 1978.
18. Pape, LG, Balazs, EA: The use of sodium hyaluronate (Healon) in human anterior segment surgery. Ophthalmology 87:699, 1980.

19. Wilensky, JT, Snyder, D, Gieser, D: Steroid-induced ocular hypertension in patients with filtering blebs. Ophthalmology 87:24, 1980.
20. LaGrange, F: Iridectomie et sclerectomie combinees dans le traitement du glaucome chronique. Arch d'Opht 26:481, 1906.
21. Holth, S: Sclerectomie avec la pince emporte-piec dans le glaucome, de preference apres incision a la pique. Ann d'Ocul 142:1, 1909.
22. Gass, JD: Anterior lip sclerectomy. A microsurgical technique for filtering operation for control of glaucoma. Ann Ophthal 2:355, 1970.
23. Potts, AM: Some rationalizations on chronic open-angle glaucoma. Am J Ophthal 86:743, 1978.
24. Berens, C: Iridocorneosclerectomy for glaucoma. Am J Ophthal 19:470, 1936.
25. McPherson, SD Jr, McCurdy, D: Anterior posterior lip sclerectomy. Proc Ann Staff Conf, McPherson Hosp 13:19, 1974.
26. Gershen, HF: Lateral lip sclerectomy. Arch Ophthal 86:534, 1971.
27. Iliff, CE, Haas, JS: Posterior lip sclerectomy. Am J Ophthal 54:688, 1962.
28. Regan, EF: Scleral cautery with iridectomy—an experimental study. Trans Am Ophthal Soc 61:219, 1963.
29. Elliot, RH: A preliminary note on a new operative procedure for the establishment of a filtering cicatrix in the treatment of glaucoma. Ophthalmoscope 7:804, 1909.
30. Fergus, F: Treatment of glaucoma by trephining. Br Med J 2:983, 1909.
31. Elliot, RH: Sclero-corneal Trephining in the Operative Treatment of Glaucoma. George Pulman and Sons, London, 1913.
32. Sugar, HS: Limboscleral trephination. Am J Ophthal 52:29, 1961.
33. Sugar, HS: Limboscleral trepanation eleven years' experience. Arch Ophthal 85:703, 1971.
34. Sugar, HS: Limbal trepanation: fourteen years' experience. Ann Ophthal 7:1399, 1975.
35. Preziosi, CL: The electro-cautery in the treatment of glaucoma. Br J Ophthal 8:414, 1924.
36. Scheie, HG: Retraction of scleral wound edges as a fistulizing procedure for glaucoma. Am J Ophthal 45:220, 1958.
37. Wadsworth, JAC: Corneoscleral cautery pathology and technique. Arch Ophthal 94:633, 1976.
38. Shaffer, RN, Hetherington, J Jr, Hoskins, HD Jr: Guarded thermal sclerostomy. Am J Ophthal 72:769, 1971.
39. Polychronakos, DJ: Modification of Scheie's fistulizing operation for glaucoma. Arch Ophthal 79:736, 1968.
40. Vinswanathan, B, Brown, IAR: Peripheral iridectomy with scleral cautery for glaucoma. Arch Ophthal 93:34, 1975.
41. King, JH, Wadsworth, JAC: An Atlas of Ophthalmic Surgery, 2nd Ed. JB Lippincot, Philadelphia, 1970.
42. Litwin, RL: Successful argon laser sclerostomy for glaucoma. Ophthal Surg 10:22, 1979.
43. Sugar, HS: Experimental trabeculectomy in glaucoma. Am J Ophthal 51:623, 1961.
44. Cairns, JE: Trabeculectomy. Preliminary report of a new method. Am J Ophthal 66:673, 1968.
45. Rich, AM, McPherson, SD: Trabeculectomy in the owl monkey. Ann Ophthal 5:1082, 1973.
46. Spencer, WH: Histologic evaluation of microsurgical glaucoma techniques. Trans Am Acad Ophthal Otol 76:389, 1972.
47. Schmitt, H: Histological examination on disks obtained by goniotraphining with scleral flap. Klin Monatsbl Augenheilkd 167:372, 1975.
48. Taylor, HR: A histologic survey of trabeculectomy. Am J Ophthal 82:733, 1976.
49. Cairns, JE: Trabeculectomy. Trans Am Acad Ophthal Otol 75:1395, 1971.
50. Shields, MB, Shelburne, JD, Bell, SW: The ultrastructure of human limbal collagen. Invest Ophthal Vis Sci 16:864, 1977.

51. Shields, MB, Bradbury, MJ, Shelburne, JD, Bell, SW: The permeability of the outer layers of limbus and anterior sclera. Invest Ophthal Vis Sci 16:866, 1977.
52. Benedikt, O: The mode of action of trabeculectomy. Klin Monatsbl Augenheilkd 167:679, 1975.
53. Benedikt, O: Demonstration of aqueous outflow patterns of normal and glaucomatous human eyes through the injection of fluorescein solution in the anterior chamber. Albrecht Graefes Arch Klin Exp Ophthal 199:45, 1976.
54. Krasnov, MM: A modified trabeculectomy. Ann Ophthal 6:178, 1974.
55. Dellaporta, A: Experiences with trepano-trabeculectomy. Trans Am Acad Ophthal Otol 79:362, 1975.
56. Welsh, NH: Trabeculectomy with fistula formation in the African. Br J Ophthal 56:32, 1972.
57. Watson, PG: In discussion of Marmion, VJ: Anterior sclerectomy, a controlled trial. Trans Ophthal Soc UK 89:523, 1969.
58. Watson, PG: Surgery of the glaucomas. Br J Ophthal 56:299, 1972.
59. Watson, PG, Barnett, F: Effectiveness of trabeculectomy in glaucoma. Am J Ophthal 79:831, 1975.
60. Hollwich, F, Fronimopoulos, J, Junemann, G, Christakis, C, Lambrou, N: Indication, technique and results of goniotrephining with scleral flap in primary chronic glaucoma. Klin Monatsbl Augenheilkd 163:513, 1973.
61. Jackson, AH: Lamellar limboscleral trephination in the surgical treatment of glaucoma. Ann Ophthal 5:1137, 1973.
62. Fronimopoulos, J, Christakis, C: Goniotrepanation (Gotrep) and further observations on this operation for chronic glaucoma. Albrecht Graefes Arch Klin Exp Ophthal 193:135, 1975.
63. Papst, W, Brunke, R: Goniotrepanation as a second fistulizing procedure. Klin Monatsbl Augenheilkd 176:915, 1980.
64. Smith, BF, Schuster, H, Seidenberg, B: Subscleral sclerectomy: A double-flap operation for glaucoma. Am J Ophthal 71:884, 1971.
65. Vasco-Posada, J: Glaucoma: esclerectomia subescleral. Arch Soc Am Oftal Optom 6:237, 1967.
66. Soll, DB: Intrascleral filtering procedure for glaucoma. Am J Ophthal 75:390, 1973.
67. Soll, DB: Further experiences with the intrascleral filtering procedure for glaucoma. Trans Am Acad Ophthal Otol 78:365, 1974.
68. Ganias, F: Thermotrabeculocanalotomy: preliminary report. Ann Ophthal 7:1107, 1975.
69. Schimek, RA, Williamson, WR: Trabeculectomy with cautery. Ophthal Surg 8:35, 1977.
70. Beckman, H, Fuller, TA: Carbon dioxide laser scleral dissection and filtering procedure for glaucoma. Am J Ophthal 88:73, 1979.
71. Beckman, H, Fuller, TA, Boyman, R, Mandell, G, Nathan, LE Jr: Carbon dioxide laser surgery of the eye and adnexa. Ophthalmology 87:990, 1980.
72. Kottow, MH: Trabeculectomy with scleral wick. Technique and early results. Ophthalmologica 179:99, 1979.
73. Lee, PF, Shihab, ZM, Fu, Y: Modified trabeculectomy: a new procedure for neovascular glaucoma. Ophthal Surg 11:181, 1980.
74. Herschler, J, Agness, D: A modified filtering operation for neovascular glaucoma. Arch Ophthal 97:2339, 1979.
75. Egerer, I, Freyler, H: Aqueous outflow following seton operations. Klin Monatsbl Augenheilkd 174:93, 1979.
76. Krejci, L: Hydrogel capillary drain for glaucoma: Nine years' clinical experience. Glaucoma 2:259, 1980.
77. Molteno, ACB: New implant for drainage in glaucoma. Clinical trial. Br J Ophthal 53:606, 1969.
78. Molteno, ACB, Van Rooyen, MMB, Bartholomew, RS: Implants for draining neovascular glaucoma. Br J Ophthal 61:120, 1977.
79. Ancker, E, Molteno, ACB: Surgical treatment of chronic aphakic glaucoma with

the Molteno Plastic implant. Klin Monatsbl Augenheilkd 177:365, 1980.

80. Krupin, T, Podos, SM, Becker, B, Newkirk, JB: Valve implants in filtering surgery. Am J Ophthal 81:232, 1976.

81. Krupin, T, Kaufman, P, Mandell, A, Ritch, R, Asseff, C, Podos, SM, Becker, B: Filtering valve implant surgery for eyes with neovascular glaucoma. Am J Ophthal 89:338, 1980.

82. Petursson, GJ, Fraunfelder, FT: Repair of an inadvertent buttonhole or leaking filtering bleb. Arch Ophthal 97:926, 1979.

83. Awan, KJ, Spaeth, PG: Use of isobutyl-2-cyanoacrylate tissue adhesive in the repair of conjunctival fistula in filtering procedures for glaucoma. Ann Ophthal 6:851, 1974.

84. Ferry, AP: Hemorrhage into the lens as a complication of glaucoma surgery. Am J Ophthal 81:351, 1976.

85. Bellows, AR, Chylack, LT, Jr, Epstein, DL, Hutchinson, BT: Choroidal effusion during glaucoma surgery in patients with prominent episcleral vessels. Arch Ophthal 97:493, 1979.

86. Sugar, HS: Treatment of hypotony following filtering surgery for glaucoma. Am J Ophthal 71:1023, 1971.

87. Hutchinson, BT: Choroidal detachment and flat anterior chamber after filtering surgery in open-angle glaucoma. In Controversy in Ophthalmology, Brockhurst, RJ, Boruchoff, SA, Hutchinson, BT, Lessell, S, eds. WB Saunders Co, Philadelphia, 1977, p. 248.

88. Chylack, LT Jr, Bellows, AR: Molecular sieving in suprachoroidal fluid formation in man. Invest Ophthal Vis Sci 17:420, 1978.

89. Simmons, RJ, Kimbrough, RL: Shell tamponade in filtering surgery for glaucoma. Ophthal Surg 10:17, 1979.

90. Cashwell, LF Jr, Simmons, RJ: Adjunctive techniques to glaucoma filtering surgery. Pers Ophthal 4:115, 1980.

91. Stewart, RH, Kimbrough, RL: A method of managing flat anterior chamber following trabeculectomy. Ophthal Surg 11:382, 1980.

92. Hawkins, ME, Kanarek, IE, Ackerman, J: Use of the ophthalmodynamometer in salvaging failing filtering blebs. Ann Ophthal 11:1090, 1979.

93. Galin, MA, Baras, I, Cavero, R: Stimulation of a filtering bleb. Arch Ophthal 74:777, 1965.

94. Harris, LS, Kahanowicz, Y: Unsuccessful eccentric perilimbal suction after filtering surgery. Am J Ophthal 79:112, 1975.

95. Galin, MA, Hung, PT: Further observations on eccentric perilimbal suction cup application. Ann Ophthal 9:69, 1977.

96. Prialnic, M, Savir, H: Transient ocular hypertension following trabeculectomy. Br J Ophthal 63:233, 1979.

97. O'Connell, EJ, Karseras, AG: Intraocular surgery in advanced glaucoma. Br J Ophthal 60:124, 1976.

98. Lawrence, GA: Surgical treatment of patients with advanced glaucomatous field defects. Arch Ophthal 81:804, 1979.

99. Lichter, PR, Ravin, JG: Risks of sudden visual loss after glaucoma surgery. Am J Ophthal 78:1009, 1974.

100. Cohen, JS, Shaffer, RN, Hetherington, J Jr, Hoskins, D: Revision of filtration surgery. Arch Ophthal 95:1612, 1977.

101. Swan, KC: Reopening of nonfunctioning filters—simplified surgical techniques. Trans Am Acad Ophthal Otol 79:342, 1975.

102. Yanoff, M, Scheie, HG, Allman, MI: Endothelialization of filtering bleb in iris nevus syndrome. Arch Ophthal 94:1933, 1976.

103. Ticho, U, Ivry, M: Reopening of occluded filtering blebs by argon laser photocoagulation. Am J Ophthal 84:413, 1977.

104. Sinnreich, Z, Barishak, R, Stein, R: Leaking filtering blebs. Am J Ophthal 86:345, 1978.

105. Scheie, HG, Guehl, JJ III: Surgical management of overhanging blebs after filtering procedures. Arch Ophthal 97:325, 1979.

106. Kanski, JJ: Treatment of late endophthalmitis associated with filtering blebs. Arch Ophthal 91:339, 1974.
107. Abel, R Jr, Binder, PS, Bellows, R: Postoperative bacterial endophthalmitis. Section I. Ann Ophthal 8:731, 1976.
108. Binder, PS, Abel, R Jr, Bellows, R: Postoperative bacterial endophthalmitis. Section II. Ann Ophthal 8:1129, 1976.
109. Abel, R Jr, Binder, PS, Bellows, R: Postoperative bacterial endophthalmitis: Section III. Ann Ophthal 8:1253, 1976.
110. Forster, RK: Etiology and diagnosis of bacterial postoperative endophthalmitis. Ophthalmology 85:320, 1978.
111. Baum, JL: The treatment of bacterial endophthalmitis. Ophthalmology 85:350, 1978.
112. Hattenhauer, JM, Lipsich, MP: Late endophthalmitis after filtering surgery. Am J Ophthal 72:1097, 1971.
113. Tabbara, KF: Late infections following filtering procedures. Ann Ophthal 8:1228, 1976.
114. Freedman, J, Gupta, M, Bunke, A: Endophthalmitis after trabeculectomy. Arch Ophthal 96:1017, 1978.
115. Shammas, HF, Zubyk, NA, Stanfield, TF: Sympathetic uveitis following glaucoma surgery. Arch Ophthal 95:638, 1977.
116. Pasticier-Tetreau, M: Etude des opacifications cristalliniennes dans les suites lointaines des operations antiglaucomateuses. Ann Oculist 206:733, 1973.
117. Haas, J: Surgical treatment of open-angle glaucoma. In Symposium on Glaucoma, New Orleans Ophthalmologic Society. St Louis, CV Mosby Co, 1967, p 183.
118. Sugar, HS: Cataract and filtering surgery. Am J Ophthal 69:740, 1970.
119. Marion, JR, Shields, MB: Thermal sclerostomy and posterior lip sclerectomy: a comparative study. Ophthal Surg 9:67, 1978.
120. Chauvaud, D, Clay-Fressinet, C, Pouliquen, Y, Offret, G: Opacification of the lens after trabeculectomy. Arch Ophthal (Paris) 36:379, 1976.
121. Cotlier, E, Baskin, M, Kim, JO, Lueck, K: Lysophosphatidyl choline and cataracts in uveitis. Arch Ophthal 94:1159, 1976.
122. Harris, LS, Galin, MA: Delayed spontaneous hyphema following successful sclerotomy with cautery in three patients. Am J Ophthal 72:458, 1971.
123. Michels, RG, Rice, TA: Bimanual bipolar diathermy for treatment of bleeding from the anterior chamber angle. Am J Ophthal 84:873, 1977.
124. Spaeth, GL, Rodrigues, MM: Staphyloma as a late complication of trabeculectomy. Ophthal Surg 8:81, 1977.
125. Putterman, AM, Urist, MJ: Upper eyelid retraction after glaucoma filtering procedures. Ann Ophthal 7:263, 1975.
126. Sofranko, JE: Statistical results of Scheie procedures. Proc Ann Staff Meet McPherson Hosp 9:76, 1971.
127. McPherson, SD, Cline, JW, McCurdy, D: Recent advances in glaucoma surgery, trabeculotomy and trabeculectomy. Ann Ophthal 9:91, 1978.
128. Jerndal, T, Lundstrom, M: 330 trabeculectomies—a follow-up study through ½-3 years. Acta Ophthal 55:52, 1977.
129. Loewenthal, LM: Trabeculectomy as treatment for glaucoma: a preliminary report. Ann Ophthal 9:1179, 1977.
130. Wilson, P: Trabeculectomy: Long-term follow-up. Br J Ophthal 61:535, 1977.
131. Schwartz, AL, Anderson, DR: Trabecular surgery. Arch Ophthal 92:134, 1974.
132. D'Ermo, F, Bonomi, L, Doro, D: A critical analysis of the long-term results of trabeculectomy. Am J Ophthal 88:829, 1979.
133. Zaidi, AA: Trabeculectomy: a review and 4-year follow-up. Br J Ophthal 64:436, 1980.
134. Jay, JL, Murray, SB: Characteristics of reduction of intraocular pressure after trabeculectomy. Br J Ophthal 64:432, 1980.
135. Watson, PG, Grierson, I: The place of trabeculectomy in the treatment of glaucoma. Ophthalmology 88:175, 1981.

136. Drance, SM, Vargas, E: Trabeculectomy and thermosclerectomy: A comparison of two procedures. Can J Ophthal 8:413, 1973.

137. Schwartz, PL, Ackerman, J, Beards, J, Wesseley, Z, Goodstein, S, Ballen, PH: Further experience with trabeculectomy. Ann Ophthal 8:207, 1976.

138. Spaeth, GL, Joseph, NH, Fernandes, E: Trabeculectomy: A re-evaluation after three years and a comparison with Scheie's procedure. Trans Am Acad Ophthal Otol 79:349, 1975.

139. Spaeth, GL: A prospective, controlled study to compare the Scheie procedure with Watson's trabeculectomy. Ophthal Surg 11:688, 1980.

140. Watkins, PH Jr, Brubaker, RF: Comparison of partial-thickness and full-thickness filtration procedures in open-angle glaucoma. Am J Ophthal 86:756, 1978.

141. Blondeau, P, Phelps, CD: Trabeculectomy vs thermosclerostomy. A randomized prospective clinical trial. Arch Ophthal 99:810, 1981.

142. Freedman, J, Shen, E, Ahrens, M: Trabeculectomy in a Black American glaucoma population. Br J Ophthal 60:573, 1976.

143. Ferguson, JG Jr, Macdonald, R Jr: Trabeculectomy in blacks: A two-year follow-up. Ophthal Surg 8:41, 1977.

144. David, R, Friedman, J, Luntz, MH: Comparative study of Watson's and Cairn's trabeculectomies in a Black population with open angle glaucoma. Br J Ophthal 61:117, 1977.

145. BenEzra, D, Chirambo, MC: Trabeculectomy. Ann Ophthal 10:1101, 1978.

146. Miller, RD, Barber, JC: Trabeculectomy in black patients. Ophthal Surg 12:46, 1981.

147. Thommy, CP, Bhar, IS: Trabeculectomy in Nigerian patients with open-angle glaucoma. Br J Ophthal 63:636, 1979.

148. Sandford-Smith, JH: The surgical treatment of open-angle glaucoma in Nigerians. Br J Ophthal 62:283, 1978.

149. Bakker, NJA, Manku, SI: Trabeculectomy versus Scheie's operation: a comparative retrospective study in open-angle glaucoma in Kenyans. Br J Ophthal 63:643, 1979.

150. Kietzman, B: Glaucoma surgery in Nigerian eyes: a five-year study. Ophthal Surg 7:52, 1976.

151. Stewart, RH, Kimbrough, RL, Bachh, H, Allbright, M: Trabeculectomy and modifications of trabeculectomy. Ophthal Surg 10:76, 1979.

152. Beauchamp, GR, Parks, MM: Filtering surgery in children: barriers to success. Ophthalmology 86:170, 1979.

153. McPherson, SD Jr: The present status of filtering operations for glaucoma. Pers Ophthal 4:107, 1980.

154. Kimbrough, RL, Stewart, RH: Outpatient trabeculectomy. Ophthal Surg 11:379, 1980.

155. Layden, WE: Complications of trabeculectomy. Pers Ophthal 1:182, 1977.

156. Tarakji, MS, Matta, CS: Expulsive hemorrhage: report of five cases. Ann Ophthal 10:1269, 1978.

Chapter 32

IRIDECTOMIES

IRIDECTOMIES

The iridectomy is one of the oldest surgical procedures for glaucoma, having been introduced by von Graefe[1] in 1857. However, it did not obtain its current popularity until 1920, when Curran[2] explained its mechanism in the relief of angle-closure glaucoma due to relative pupillary block. Today, some form of iridectomy is the preferred treatment for most cases of angle-closure glaucoma.

I. MECHANISM OF ACTION

The concept of relative pupillary block as the most common cause of primary angle-closure glaucoma was considered in Chapter 8. An opening in the iris bypasses the increased resistance to aqueous humor flow between the lens and pupillary portion of the iris by creating a new communication from the posterior to anterior chamber (Fig. 32.1). This relieves the relatively higher pressure in the posterior chamber and allows the peripheral iris to fall away from the trabecular meshwork.[2-6] Contrary to an earlier impression,[5] an iridectomy does not cause a deepening of the axial depth of the anterior chamber.[7]

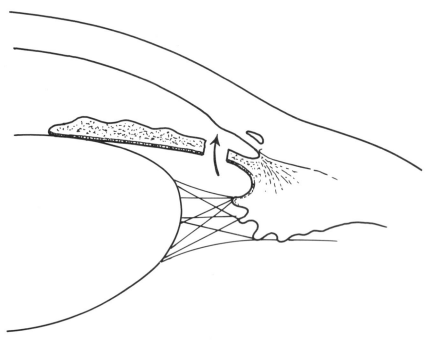

Figure 32.1. Mechanism of iridectomy. Communication between anterior and posterior chambers **(arrow)** bypasses the pupillary block, which relieves the relatively higher pressure in the posterior chamber, allowing peripheral iris to fall away from the trabecular meshwork.

Although the traditional surgical approach is to make the iridectomy in peripheral iris,[8, 9] experience with laser iridectomies suggests that success of the procedure is not related to placement of the iridectomy, as long as it is peripheral to the collarette and not in an area of posterior synechiae.[7] Furthermore, the effect of an iridectomy appears to be independent of the size of the opening in the iris.[7]

II. SURGICAL IRIDECTOMIES

A. Basic Technique

The most commonly used surgical approach is the *peripheral iridectomy* as described by Chandler[9] (Fig. 32.2).

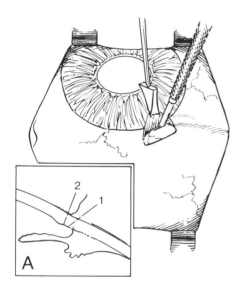

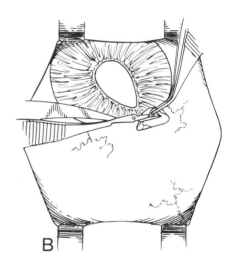

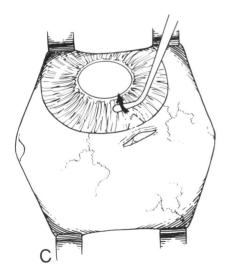

Figure 32.2.   Peripheral iridectomy. **A:** incision into anterior chamber may be placed **(1)** behind the corneolimbal junction or **(2)** in peripheral cornea (note the slant of each incision); **B:** peripheral iris is grasped with smooth forceps and excised with iris scissors; **C:** remaining iris is reposited by a gentle stroking action across the cornea **(arrow)**.

1. In one of the superior quadrants, a small conjunctival flap is prepared with either a fornix or limbus base.

2. A 3 to 4 mm incision is made into the anterior chamber, beginning approximately 1 to 1.5 mm behind the corneolimbal junction.

3. If the iris prolapses, it is lifted up with iris forceps and a small section is excised using iris scissors that are held parallel to the limbus. If the iris does not spontaneously come through the limbal opening, a slight pressure on the posterior margin of the incision may cause the prolapse. Factors that may prevent prolapse of the iris are considered later in this chapter under "Prevention and Management of Complications." When iris prolapse cannot be achieved, the iris is grasped with smooth forceps, and brought up through the incision to make the iridectomy. The iris is then reposited by a gentle stroking action across the cornea in a direction away from the incision, using a blunt instrument such as a muscle hook.

4. In closing the wound, a single suture may be placed through both the limbal wound and conjunctiva if a fornix-based flap was used. With a limbus-based flap, closure of the conjunctiva alone may be sufficient, if the limbal incision was beveled slightly to achieve spontaneous apposition.

B. Modifications

1. *Corneal incision.* Some surgeons prefer to make the incision into the anterior chamber through clear cornea adjacent to the corneolimbal junction.[10-12] The main advantage is that the undamaged conjunctiva remains available for future filtering surgery if required. The incision is usually placed perpendicular to the limbus in order to reach peripheral iris (Fig. 32.2), and suture closure is generally necessary. However, some surgeons feel suturing is not essential,[10] especially if the incision is beveled posteriorly.[12]

2. *Transfixation* is a technique in which the anterior chamber is entered at the limbus with a narrow cataract knife. Several incisions in the iris are then made as the blade is passed across the anterior segment of the eye (Fig. 32.3).[13] This approach has been favored by some surgeons for the management of iris bombe' in an inflamed eye, in the hope that it would reduce the danger of hemorrhage. However, one study showed that a peripheral iridectomy does not have a greater incidence of bleeding, and the author preferred the latter procedure in this clinical situation.[14]

3. *Sector iridectomy.* Some surgeons feel that there are times when a sector iridectomy has advantages over a peripheral iridectomy. Such situations might include 1) the need for the larger optical opening, 2) to facilitate future cataract extraction, 3) when a retinal detachment is suspected, or 4) in the treatment of pupillary block glaucoma in aphakia.[13] In the technique described by King and Wadsworth,[13] a larger limbal incision is required so that the iris can be grasped within 1 to 2 mm of the pupillary margin and brought well out through the

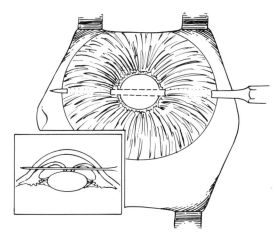

Figure 32.3.   Transfixation. Multiple iridotomies are created as a narrow cataract knife is passed across the anterior segment.

wound. A radial cut is then made across the iris at one side of the exposed portion, the iris is torn at its root, and a second incision is made across the other side of the exposed tissue. This creates a truly basal iridectomy. An alternative approach is to grasp mid-peripheral iris, withdraw it until the pupillary margin is exposed, and excise the tissue with a single cut.

C. Prevention and Management of Complications

1. *Operative complications*
 a. *Failure of spontaneous iris prolapse.* Factors that may prevent the peripheral iris from spontaneously prolapsing through the limbal incision include 1) inaccurate placement of the incision, 2) a hypotonous eye, 3) peripheral anterior synechiae, 4) a hole in the iris elsewhere, and 5) ciliary-iridial processes. Alternative surgical approaches in this situation were considered earlier in the chapter under "Basic Techniques."
 b. *Hemorrhage.* Cut edges of the iris normally do not bleed. However, hemorrhage may occur if inflammation or neovascularization is present. To minimize bleeding in these situations, the use of bipolar microcauterization of the iris surface before cutting the iridectomy has been suggested.[15, 16] In addition, iris scissors have been described with insulation and an electric current, which allows simultaneous cutting and cauterization of the iris.[17] Brisk bleeding may also occur if the ciliary body is inadvertently cut. The bleeding can usually be stopped by placing a large air bubble in the anterior chamber for several minutes.
 c. *Incomplete iridectomy.* It is not uncommon to cut only the stroma of the iris, leaving intact pigment epithelium, which prevents a successful operation. This complication should be avoided at the time of surgery by checking the iridectomy specimen for the presence

of the dark pigment epithelium and by transillumination through the iridectomy if there is any doubt as to its patency. If the complication is discovered postoperatively, the epithelial layer must either be penetrated with laser therapy or with a second surgical procedure.

d. *Injury to the lens* or disruption of the lens zonules with possible dislocation of the lens and vitreous loss should be avoided by gentle surgical manipulation. Intralenticular hemorrhage has also been reported as a rare complication of iridectomy.[18]

2. *Postoperative complications*

a. *Elevated intraocular pressure.* If the anterior chamber is flat, malignant (ciliary block) glaucoma or an incomplete iridectomy should be considered. These situations were discussed in Chapter 19. A formed anterior chamber suggests that permanent obstruction of the trabecular meshwork may be present. This should initially be managed with anti-glaucoma medications, although a filtering procedure may later be required if medical therapy is inadequate.

b. *Hyphemas* should be handled conservatively with elevation of the head and limited activity.

c. *Cataracts.* The frequency with which peripheral iridectomies lead to cataract formation is somewhat controversial. However, several studies indicate that some degree of lenticular opacity occurs in up to half of the cases with an acute angle-closure glaucoma attack and in one-third of the eyes treated prophylactically.[19-22] The mechanism of this complication is uncertain, although the frequency increases with age.

III. LASER IRIDECTOMIES

Laser Iridectomies (or iridotomies). Although the complications noted above for surgical iridectomies are uncommon and usually not serious, with the exception of cataracts, they do represent an important consideration. Furthermore, the hospitalization and operating room costs create an ever increasing disadvantage with any surgical procedure. Preliminary experience with laser iridectomies suggests a potential for significant advantage in these areas.

A. Techniques

The procedure may be performed on an outpatient basis, with the only anesthesia being a drop of topical anesthetic. Some surgeons prefer to place a diagnostic contact lens on the cornea, although this is not essential. A *continuous wave argon laser* appears to give the best results,[23-32] although success has also been reported with pulsed argon,[27, 28, 33, 34] pulsed ruby,[35, 36] neodynium,[35, 36] Q-switched ruby,[37] or dye lasers.[38] Settings with the argon laser are generally a 50 to 100 μ spot size with energy levels of 500 to 2000 mw and a duration of 0.1 to 0.2 sec.[27, 28, 32] The iridectomy is normally made in a superior quadrant in mid to peripheral iris. The basic technique is to begin with a low-energy setting and increase the power as required. Some surgeons have suggested first stretching the iris or creating a hump with the low-energy burns,[23, 24, 29, 31] although this does not appear to be necessary.[32] The required number of laser applications varies considerably, but averaged 60 to 87 for a single sitting in one series.[29] Penetration of the pigment epithelium is usually indicated by a cloud of pigment entering the anterior chamber from the laser therapy site, and patency of the iridectomy should be confirmed by observing transillumination through the opening. Dilating the pupil after completion of a laser iridectomy is suggested as a means of confirming that an effective iridectomy has been achieved.[32]

B. Results

In most series, a successful laser iridectomy was possible in approximately 95% of the cases, although some patients required one or more additional treatment sessions. Best results were obtained in eyes with medium pigmentation of the iris, while both light blue and dark brown irides were the most difficult to penetrate.[27, 28, 32] As the surgeon's experience increases, the amount of treatment required to achieve an iridectomy decreases,[32] and a successful laser iridectomy should be possible in nearly all cases.

Ultrastructural studies of iris specimens with failed pulsed argon laser iridectomies revealed severe edema, coagulation necrosis, focal vascular occlusion, and hemorrhage in the first few hours following laser treatment. After several days, cell debris and collapsed cell processes were seen. The iris was thin and irregular at 42 days, had a dense matted appearance at 8 months, and showed a depression, with pigment dispersion, irregular stroma, and disruption of the dilator muscle at 2 years.[33, 34]

C. Complications[27, 28, 32, 39]

Corneal endothelial and epithelial burns at the site of treatment are common and occasionally prevent completion of the iridectomy at the same session. However, the corneal clouding clears within days and leaves no sequelae. Lens opacification usually occurs behind the iridectomy, but does not appear to spread centrally. Retinal burns may occur when the iris pigment epithelium is penetrated, and the laser beam, therefore, should be directed well away from the posterior pole of the fundus. Transient anterior uveitis is common and is minimized by the use of topical steroids for the first several days. A transient pressure elevation may occur, presumably due to the dispersion of iris pigment and debris into the trabecular meshwork, although this rarely causes permanent outflow obstruction. In a small number of cases, pigment gradually closes the iridectomy during the first few weeks, but this can be easily dislodged with low-energy laser applications.

D. Indications

As experience with laser iridectomy grows, the technique is being used with increasing frequency in place of surgical iridectomy for the treatment of eyes with angle-closure glaucoma as well as for prophylaxis of the fellow eye. Specific situations in which laser iridectomy has a particular advantage include 1) pupillary block glaucoma in aphakia[25, 32] or pseudophakia, 2) pupillary block associated with a dislocated lens,[27, 28] 3) chronic angle-closure glaucoma,[32] 4) as a diagnostic measure in combined-mechanism or malignant (ciliary block) glaucomas,[27, 28] and 5) to penetrate an incomplete surgical iridectomy.[40, 41]

References

1. von Graefe, A: Uber die Iridectomie bie Glaucom und uber den glaucomatosed process. Arch Ophthal 3:456, 1857.
2. Curran, EJ: A new operation for glaucoma involving a new principle in the aetiology and treatment of chronic primary glaucoma. Arch Ophthal 49:131, 1920.
3. Banziger, T: The mechanism of acute glaucoma and the explanation for the effectiveness of iridectomy for the same. Ber Deutsch Ophthal Ges 43:43, 1922.
4. Chandler, PA: Narrow-angle glaucoma. Arch Ophthal 47:695, 1952.
5. Barkan, O: Narrow-angle glaucoma. Pupillary block and the narrow-angle mechanism. Am J Ophthal 37:332, 1954.
6. Barkan, O: Iridectomy in narrow-angle glaucoma. Am J Ophthal 37:504, 1954.
7. Jacobs, IH, Krohn, DL: Central anterior chamber depth after laser iridectomy. Am J Ophthal 89:865, 1980.
8. Barkan, O: Peripheral iridectomy. Technique, mechanism and the cause of hemorrhage. Am J Ophthal 37:889, 1954.
9. Chandler, PA: Peripheral iridectomy. Arch Ophthal 72:804, 1964.
10. Weene, LE: Self-sealing incision for peripheral iridectomy. Ophthal Surg 9:64, 1978.
11. Freeman, LB, Ridgway, AEA: Peripheral iridectomy via a corneal section: a follow-up study. Ophthal Surg 10:53, 1979.
12. Ahmad, N: Transcorneal peripheral iridectomy. Ophthal Surg 11:124, 1980.
13. King, JH, Wadsworth, JAC: An Atlas of Ophthalmic Surgery, 2nd ed. JB Lippincott Co, Philadelphia, 1970, p 416.
14. Curran, RE: Surgical management of iris bombe'. Arch Ophthal 90:464, 1973.
15. Kass, MA, Hersh, SB, Albert, DM: Experimental iridectomy with bipolar microcautery. Am J Ophthal 81:451, 1976.
16. Hersh, SB, Kass, MA: Iridectomy in rubeosis iridis. Ophthal Surg 7:19, 1976.
17. Hashmi, MS, McCarthy, JP: Cauterising iris scissors. Br J Ophthal 63:754, 1979.
18. Feibel, RM, Bigger, JF, Smith, ME: Intralenticular hemorrhage following iridectomy. Arch Ophthal 87:36, 1972.
19. Sugar, HS: Cataract formation and refractive changes after surgery for angle-closure glaucoma. Am J Ophthal 69:747, 1970.
20. Floman, N, Berson, D, Landau, L: Peripheral iridectomy in closed angle glaucoma—late complications. Br J Ophthal 61:101, 1977.
21. Godel, V, Regenbogen, L: Cataractogenic factors in patients with primary angle-closure glaucoma after peripheral iridectomy. Am J Ophthal 83:180, 1977.
22. Krupin, T, Mitchell, KB, Johnson, MF, Becker, B: The long-term effects of iridectomy for primary acute angle-closure glaucoma. Am J Ophthal 86:506, 1978.
23. L'Esperance, FA Jr, James, WA Jr: Argon laser photocoagulation of iris abnormalities. Trans Am Acad Ophthal Otol 79:321, 1975.
24. Abraham, RK, Miller, GL: Outpatient argon laser iridectomy for angle closure glaucoma: a two-year study. Trans Am Acad Ophthal Otol 79:529, 1975.
25. Anderson, DR, Forster, RK, Lewis, ML: Laser iridotomy for aphakic pupillary block. Arch Ophthal 93:343, 1975.
26. Pollack, IP, Patz, A: Argon laser iridotomy: an experimental and clinical study. Ophthal Surg 7:22, 1976.

27. Pollack, IP: Use of argon laser energy to produce iridotomies. Tr Am Ophthal Soc 77:674, 1979.

28. Pollack, IP: Use of argon laser energy to produce iridotomies. Ophthal Surg 11:506, 1980.

29. Podos, SM, Kels, BD, Moss, AP, Ritch, R, Anders, MD: Continuous wave argon laser iridectomy in agle-closure glaucoma. Am J Ophthal 88:836, 1979.

30. Yassur, Y, Melamed, S, Cohen, S, Ben-Sira, I: Laser iridotomy in closed-angle glaucoma. Arch Ophthal 97:1920, 1979.

31. Ritch, R, Podos, SM: Argon laser treatment of angle-closure glaucoma. Pers Ophthal 4:129, 1980.

32. Quigley, HA: Long-term follow-up of laser iridotomy. Ophthalmology 88:218, 1981.

33. Schwartz, LW, Rodrigues, MM, Spaeth, GL, Streeten, B, Douglas, C: Argon laser iridotomy in the treatment of patients with primary angle-closure or pupillary block glaucoma: a clinicopathologic study. Ophthalmology 85:294, 1978.

34. Rodriques, MM, Streeten, B, Spaeth, GL, Schwartz, LW: Argon laser iridotomy on primary angle closure or pupillary block glaucoma. Arch Ophthal 96:2222, 1978.

35. Beckman, H, Sugar, HS: Laser iridectomy therapy of glaucoma. Arch Ophthal 90:453, 1973.

36. Beckman, H, Barraco, R, Sugar, HS, Gaynes, E, Blau, R: Laser iridectomies. Am J Ophthal 72:393, 1971.

37. Bonney, CH, Gaasterland, DE: Low-energy, Q-switched ruby laser iridotomies in Macaca mulatta. Invest Ophthal Vis Sci 18:278, 1979.

38. Bass, MS, Cleary, CV, Perkins, ES, Wheeler, CB: Single treatment laser iridotomy. Br J Ophthal 63:29, 1970.

39. Ritch, R: The treatment of angle-closure glaucoma. Ann Ophthal 11:1373, 1979.

40. Snyder, WB, Vaiser, A, Hutton, WL: Laser iridectomy. Trans Am Acad Ophthal Otol 79:381, 1975.

41. Tessler, HH, Peyman, GA, Huamonte, F, Menachof, I: Argon laser iridotomy in incomplete peripheral iridectomy. Am J Ophthal 79:1051, 1975.

Chapter 33

SURGERY FOR CHILDHOOD GLAUCOMAS

SURGERY FOR CHILDHOOD GLAUCOMAS

The operative techniques considered in this chapter are used mainly for the treatment of primary congenital glaucoma and certain developmental glaucomas with associated anomalies. However, limited success has also been reported with some forms of adult-onset glaucoma.

I. MECHANISM OF ACTION

The mechanism of these operations differs from that of filtering procedures in that an abnormal tissue in the anterior chamber angle is incised, which allows aqueous to flow into the normal outflow system. This can be accomplished in two fundamental ways: an *ab interno* (goniotomy) or *ab externo* (trabeculotomy) approach.

II. GONIOTOMY

A. Basic Technique (Fig. 33.1)

A technique for goniotomy was described by Barkan[1] in 1938, and is still preferred by many pediatric glaucoma surgeons. The procedure can be performed with a binocular head loupe,[1] although the operating microscope provides better visualization.[2]

1. The patient's head is rotated away from the side of the surgery and the operative eye is slightly abducted. A surgical goniolens is then placed over the nasal cornea, leaving 2 to 3 mm of temporal cornea exposed for the knife entry. Fixation of the globe is essential, and this can be accomplished with locking forceps which are held by an assistant.

2. The goniotomy knife is made to penetrate the cornea 1 mm anterior to the limbus at 10 o'clock in the right eye or 4 o'clock in the left eye. The blade is passed across the anterior chamber to a point in the anterior chamber angle 180° from the entry site. The shaft of the knife is tapered to maintain a water tight seal. Numerous modifications of Barkan's goniotomy knife have been described, including attached fiber-optics for intraocular illumination.[3]

3. Using the tip of the goniotomy blade, the angle tissue is incised posterior to Schwalbe's line for approximately one-third of the angle circumference. The intent is to incise only the abnormal layer of tissue in front of the trabecular meshwork, and this is best judged by observing a white line develop as the cut edge of tissue retracts posteriorly and sclera is seen through intact trabecular meshwork.

4. The knife is then withdrawn with caution not to injure adjacent ocular structures, and the anterior chamber is deepened with air or a balanced salt solution. If bilateral surgery is needed, it has been suggested that both procedures can be done at the same operation,[4]

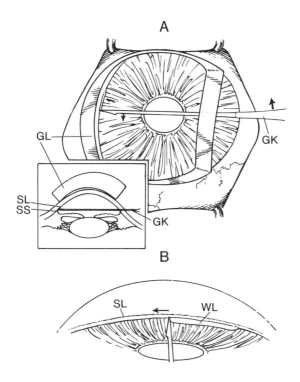

Figure 33.1. Goniotomy. **A:** with a surgical goniolens (GL) positioned on the cornea, a goniotomy knife **(GK)** is inserted through peripheral cornea and passed across the anterior chamber to the angle in the opposite quadrant; **B:** under direct gonioscopic visualization, angle tissue is excised between Schwalbe's line **(SL)** and scleral spur **(SS)** for approximately one-third of the chamber angle circumference. This creates a white line **(WL)** as the cut edge of tissue retracts from the incision. **Arrows** indicate the direction of knife movement during incision of angle tissue.

although these should be done with different sets of instruments. Postoperative management consists of topical antibiotics, a miotic, and topical steroids.

B. Variations

1. *Goniopuncture.* Scheie[5, 6] described a form of filtering surgery which utilized the goniotomy technique and was designed primarily for children in whom standard goniotomies had failed. In this procedure, saline is first injected beneath Tenon's capsule near the inferior limbus to create a bleb. A Scheie needle-knife is then made to penetrate the peripheral cornea just below the horizontal plane and the blade is passed across the anterior chamber diagonally to the inferior angle. The trabecular meshwork and limbal tissue are penetrated with the tip of the blade until it is visible in the sub-Tenon's bleb. The knife is then removed and the anterior chamber is deepened with saline.

2. *Goniodiathermy.*[7] A disadvantage of goniopuncture is that the limbal incision tends to scar closed. To avoid this, a technique was developed in which an intraocular diathermy probe is introduced into the goniopuncture tract to cause a gaping of the wound edges. Preliminary experience in rabbits was felt to be encouraging.

3. *Direct goniotomy.* When corneal clouding prevents visualization for standard goniotomy, it has been suggested that the goniotomy might be performed directly through a 60° limbal incision.[8] However, most surgeons prefer a trabeculotomy in these cases.

4. *Trabeculodialysis.* In this modified goniotomy, the trabecular meshwork is scraped from the scleral sulcus with the flat side of a goniotomy blade.[9] This technique is especially useful in *glaucoma associated with inflammation*, presumably because the trabecular tissue is friable and easily scraped away in these cases.[9-11] A histologic study has confirmed that this operation works by establishing a communication between the anterior chamber and Schlemm's canal.[11]

C. Complications

1. *Operative complications*

a. Placement of the incision is critical in performing a goniotomy. If the incision is too posterior, bleeding from the ciliary body may occur, while an incision that is too anterior will have no effect. Iridodialysis or cyclodialysis may also be inadvertently created during a goniotomy procedure.[4]

b. Loss of the anterior chamber during the operation prevents adequate visualization of the angle structures and increases the risk of damage to ocular structures. If this occurs, the knife should be withdrawn and the chamber should be deepened with balanced salt solution through the entry site.

c. As with any operation under general anesthesia, the risks of the anesthesia must also be considered. In a series of 401 goniotomies under general anesthesia, the most serious complication was cardio-pulmonary arrest, which occurred in 1.8%.[4]

2. *Postoperative complications*

a. A moderate hyphema is common after goniotomy, but rarely leads to serious sequelae. In the series of 401 goniotomies, postoperative bleeding was reported in 0.6%, but useful vision was lost in only one case.[4] Postoperative infection is rare.

b. Permanent visual impairment following surgery for glaucoma in children may be on an anatomical basis, but is more often due to amblyopia and large refractive errors.[12] An important aspect of the postoperative management is to anticipate these causes of reduced vision and treat them appropriately.

III. TRABECULOTOMY

In 1960, Burian[13] and Smith[14] independently described techniques for incising the trabecular meshwork from an *ab externo* approach. The procedure was modified by Harms and Dannheim,[15-17] who reported success in adults as well as children, although the primary interest has been as an alternative to goniotomy. It should be noted, however, that this operation differs from goniotomy not only by the external approach, but also in the fact that the full-thickness of trabecular meshwork is incised.

A. Basic Technique

The *basic technique*, as described by McPherson,[18] encompasses aspects of the procedures developed by Allen and Burian,[13, 19] and Harms and Dannheim[15-17] (Fig. 33.2).

1. A conjunctival flap is prepared in the manner described for filtering surgery, and a 2 × 4 mm limbus-based, partial-thickness scleral flap is dissected.

2. A radial incision is made across the sclerolimbal junction until Schlemm's canal is cut. To confirm the identity of the canal, a nylon suture may be threaded into one of the cut ends and observed gonioscopically to insure that the suture is in the canal.

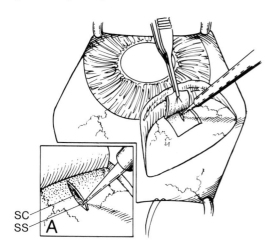

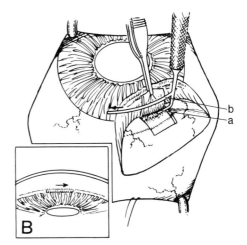

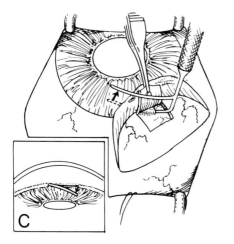

Figure 33.2. Trabeculotomy. **A:** beneath a partial-thickness scleral flap, a radial incision is made across the sclerolimbal junction until Schlemm's canal **(SC)** is identified just anterior to the circumferential fibers of scleral spur **(SS)**; **B:** the internal arm **(a)** of a trabeculotome is threaded into Schlemm's canal, using the external, parallel arm **(b)** as a guide; inset shows the gonioscopic appearance of the internal arm as it moves through the canal **(arrow)**; **C:** the trabeculotome is rotated **(arrows)** causing the internal arm to tear through the trabecular meshwork into the anterior chamber.

3. One arm of a McPherson trabeculotome is threaded into Schlemm's canal, using the other, parallel arm as a guide. The trabeculotome is then rotated so that the arm within the canal tears through trabecular meshwork into the anterior chamber. The same procedure is then performed on the other side of the radial incision.

4. The scleral and conjunctival flaps are closed in the manner described for filtering procedures. Postoperative care includes the use of topical miotics, antibiotics, and steroids.

B. Variations

1. *Combined trabeculotomy-trabeculectomy.* If Schlemm's canal cannot be located with certainty, which is not uncommon in highly buphthalmic eyes, it is possible to convert the procedure to a trabeculectomy by removing a block of deep limbal tissue beneath the scleral flap. In addition, the two procedures can be combined by first performing the trabeculotomy and then creating the fistula beneath the scleral flap. In some situations, such as the Sturge-Weber syndrome in which the exact mechanism of the glaucoma is uncertain (see Chapter 10), the combined procedure may offer the best chance of success.[20] A similar combined technique has been suggested for late onset congenital glaucoma in which a 2 × 2 mm block of tissue beneath the scleral flap is excised, but without penetrating the trabecular meshwork.[21] This procedure was reported to be successful in all of seven eyes, five of which had diffuse filtering blebs.[21]

2. *Electrocautery* has been utilized in modified trabeculotomies by insulating all sides of the probe except that exposed to the trabecular meshwork.[22-24] By burning an opening in the meshwork, it is felt that fibrotic closure of the severed edges is avoided. Success has been reported with this technique in patients with primary open-angle glaucoma, as well as congenital glaucoma.[24] A similar approach has also been described in which electrical discharges are used to create holes in the trabecular meshwork.[25]

3. *Laser* applications have also been used to create holes in the trabecular meshwork,[26-32] and success has been reported with the continuous wave[26-30] or pulsed argon laser,[29, 30] as well as the Q-switched ruby laser.[31, 32] The procedure basically consists of making a series of high energy burns in approximately two clock hours of the trabecular meshwork.[30] It is presumed that the mechanism of pressure reduction is the creation of holes in the meshwork, although studies in primates suggest that the lesions remain patent for the first week or two and then begin to close.[28] An alternative possibility is that the laser energy produces a radial or circumferential "tightening" of the meshwork, which improves outflow.[30] This concept will be discussed further in Chapter 35.

4. Other experimental types of trabeculotomy utilize *aqueous veins* to localize Schlemm's canal by threading a probe through a large vein and into the canal[33] or by forcing air into a vein, which causes multiple ruptures in the meshwork.[34]

C. Complications[35]

1. If Schlemm's canal is not properly identified, a false passage may be created either into the interior chamber or the suprachoroidal space. The latter may result in the creation of a cyclodialysis and possible hyphema. As previously noted, if Schlemm's canal cannot be identified, the procedure can be converted to a trabeculectomy. When the probe is rotated into the anterior chamber, it may strip Descemet's membrane if it is too far anterior, or damage the iris or lens if it is too far posterior.

2. As with all intraocular glaucoma procedures, postoperative bleeding and infection are potential complications.

IV. COMPARISON OF PROCEDURES

Opinions differ regarding the procedure of choice for the management of congenital glaucoma. Many pediatric glaucoma surgeons prefer the time-honored *goniotomy*, utilizing trabeculotomy only in cases with marked corneal clouding or after repeated goniotomy failures. Early reports indicated that only one-third[36] to one-half[37] of the cases were successfully controlled after the initial procedure. With one or more goniotomies, however, the reported success rate increases to a range of 77 to 88%.[37-39]

Other surgeons prefer *trabeculotomy* as the initial procedure for most cases of primary congenital glaucoma. Reports of experience with trabeculotomies for the treatment of congenital glaucoma describe success rates ranging from 62 to 95%.[38, 40-46] Success is less with older children[40, 46] and in cases of secondary glaucoma,[44, 46] primary open-angle glaucoma,[41, 42] and angle-closure glaucoma.[42] However, one surgeon reported success in all of 12 eyes with the exfoliation syndrome.[47] Continued study is needed to more clearly define the relative benefits of goniotomy versus trabeculotomy in the management of primary congenital glaucoma, and to further evaluate the value of these procedures in the other forms of glaucoma.

References

1. Barkan, O: Technic of goniotomy. Arch Ophthal 19:217, 1938.
2. Draeger, J: New microsurgical techniques to improve chamber angle surgery. Glaucoma 2:403, 1980.
3. Amoils, SP, Simmons, RJ: Goniotomy with intraocular illumination. A preliminary report. Arch Ophthal 80:488, 1968.
4. Litinsky, SM, Shaffer, RN, Hetherington, J, Hoskins, HD: Operative complications of goniotomy. Trans Am Acad Ophthal Otol 83:78, 1977.
5. Scheie, HG: Goniopuncture—a new filtering operation for glaucoma. Arch Ophthal 44:761, 1950.
6. Scheie, HG: Goniopuncture: an evaluation after eleven years. Arch Ophthal 65:38, 1961.
7. Kozart, DM, Cameron, JD: Goniodiathermy: experimental studies on *ab interno* filtration. Ann Ophthal 10:1597, 1978.
8. Fernandez, JL, Galin, MA: Technique of direct goniotomy. Arch Ophthal 90:305, 1973.

9. Haas, J: Goniotomy in aphakia. *In* The Second Report on Cataract Surgery, Welsh, R, ed. Miami Educational Press, Miami, 1971, p 551.
10. Hoskins, HD, Hetherington, J Jr, Shaffer, RN: Surgical management of the inflammatory glaucomas. Pers Ophthal 1:173, 1977.
11. Herschler, J, Davis, B: Modified goniotomy for inflammatory glaucoma. Histologic evidence for the mechanism of pressure reduction. Arch Ophthal 98:684, 1980.
12. Biglan, AW, Hiles, DA: The visual results following infantile glaucoma surgery. J Ped Ophthal Strab 16:377, 1979.
13. Burian, HM: A case of Marfan's syndrome with bilateral glaucoma. With description of a new type of operation for developmental glaucoma (trabeculotomy *ab externo*). Am J Ophthal 50:1187, 1960.
14. Smith, R: A new technique for opening the canal of Schlemm. Preliminary report. Br J Ophthal 44:370, 1960.
15. Harms, H: Glaukom-Operationen am Schlemm's chen Kanal. Sitzungsber. der 114. Versammlung des Vereins Rhein-Westf, Augenarzta, 1966.
16. Harms, H, Dannheim, R: Trabeculotomy results and problems. *In* Microsurgery in Glaucoma, MacKensen, C, ed, Karger, Basel, 1970, p 121.
17. Dannheim, R: Trabeculotomy. Trans Am Acad Ophthal Otol 76:375, 1972.
18. McPherson, SD Jr: Results of external trabeculotomy. Am J Ophthal 76:918, 1973.
19. Allen, L, Burian, HM: Trabeculotomy ab externo. Am J Ophthal 53:19, 1962.
20. Board, RJ, Shields, MB: Combined trabeculotomy-trabeculectomy for the management of glaucoma associated with Sturge-Weber syndrome. Ophthal Surg 12:813, 1981.
21. Rothkoff, L, Blumenthal, M, Biedner, B: Trabeculotomy in late onset congenital glaucoma. Br J Ophthal 63:38, 1979.
22. Moses, RA: Electrocautery puncture of the trabecular meshwork in enucleated human eyes. Am J Ophthal 72:1094, 1971.
23. Maselli, E, Sirellini, M, Pruneri, F, Galantino, G: Diathermo-trabeculotomy ab externo. A new technique for opening the canal of Schlemm. Br J Ophthal 59:516, 1975.
24. Maselli, E, Galantino, G, Pruneri, F, Sirellini, M: Diathermo-trabeculotomy *ab externo*: indications and long-term results. Br J Ophthal 61:675, 1977.
25. Hager, H, Hauck, W, Heppke, G, Hoffmann, R, Resewitz, EP: Experimental principles of trabecular-electro-puncture (TEP). Albrecht Graefes Arch Klin Exp Ophthal 185:95, 1972.
26. Hager, H: Special microsurgery interventions. Part 2. First experiences with the Argon Laser Apparatus 800. Klin Monatsbl Augenheilkd 162:437, 1973.
27. Ticho, U: Laser Application to the angle structures in animals and in human glaucomatous eyes. Adv Ophthal 34:201, 1977.
28. Ticho, U, Cadet, JC, Mahler, J, Sekeles, E, Bruchim, A: Argon laser trabeculotomies in primates: evaluation by histological and perfusion studies. Invest Ophthal Vis Sci 17:667, 1978.
29. Worthen, DM, Wickham, MG: Argon laser trabeculotomy. Trans Am Acad Ophthal Otol 78:371, 1974.
30. Wickham, MG, Worthen, DM: Argon laser trabeculotomy: long-term follow-up. Ophthalmology 86:495, 1979.
31. Krasnov, MM: Laseropuncture of anterior chamber angle in glaucoma. Am J Ophthal 75:674, 1973.
32. Krasnov, MM: Q-switched laser goniopuncture. Arch Ophthal 92:37, 1974.
33. Bonnet, M, Schiffer, HP: On trabeculotomy ab externo. Localisation of the canal of Schlemm by passing a catheter through an aqueous vein. Klin Monatsbl Augenheilkd 161:563, 1972.
34. Jocson, VL: Air trabeculotomy. Am J Ophthal 79:107, 1975.
35. McPherson, SD Jr, Cline, JW, McCurdy, D: Recent advances in glaucoma surgery, trabeculotomy and trabeculectomy. Ann Ophthal 9:91, 1977.
36. Kiffney, GT, Meyer, GW, McPherson, SD Jr: The surgical management of congenital glaucoma. So Med J 53:989, 1960.

37. Haas, J: End results of treatment. Trans Am Acad Ophthal Otol 59:333, 1953.
38. Promesberger, H, Busse, H, Mewe, L: Befunde und operative Therapie beim Buphthalmus. Klin Monatsbl Augenheilkd 176:186, 1980.
39. Broughton, WL, Parks, MM: An analysis of treatment of congenital glaucoma by goniotomy. Am J Ophthal 91:566, 1981.
40. McPherson, SD Jr, McFarland, D: External trabeculotomy for developmental glaucoma. Ophthalmology 87:302, 1980.
41. Luntz, MH, Livingston, DG: Trabeculotomy ab externo and trabeculectomy in congenital and adult-onset glaucoma. Am J Ophthal 83:174, 1977.
42. Urrets-Zavalia, A Jr: Indications et resultats de la trabeculotomie. Ann d'Oculist 205:647, 1972.
43. Gregersen, E, Kessing, SV: Congenital glaucoma before and after the introduction of microsurgery. Results of "macrosurgery" 1943–1963 and of microsurgery (trabeculotomy/ectomy) 1970–1974. Acta Ophthal 55:422, 1977.
44. Luntz, MH: Congenital, infantile, and juvenile glaucoma. Ophthalmology 86:793, 1979.
45. Blumenthal, M: Surgical approach to the trabeculum. Glaucoma 3:525, 1980.
46. Dannheim, R, Haas, H: Visual acuity and intraocular pressure after surgery in congenital glaucoma. Klin Monatsbl Augenheilkd 177:296, 1980.
47. Gillies, WE: Trabeculotomy in pseudoexfoliation of the lens capsule. Br J Ophthal 61:297, 1977.

Chapter 34

CYCLODESTRUCTIVE PROCEDURES

CYCLODESTRUCTIVE PROCEDURES

All of the operations discussed in the preceding chapters lower the intraocular pressure by improving the rate of aqueous outflow. An alternative approach is *to reduce the rate of aqueous production*, which can be accomplished by destroying a portion of the ciliary processes. These techniques are not often the first operation of choice, because the results are hard to predict and damage to ocular structures or inflammation often leads to complications. However, the cyclo-destructive procedures constitute a valuable adjunct in our surgical armamentarium for cases in which other operations have repeatedly failed or are felt to be contraindicated.

I. CYCLOCRYOTHERAPY

The most commonly used cyclodestructive technique involves *freezing* the ciliary body. This approach was suggested by Bietti[1] in 1950.

A. Mechanism of action

1. *Physical principles of cryosurgery.*[2] The ability of a freezing source, or cryogen, to freeze tissue depends on its ability to remove heat, which is a function of the boiling point of the source. For example, liquid nitrogen boils at −195.6°C and is an excellent cryogen. When the freezing source is applied to a tissue, a hemispherical iceball will develop, composed of different thermogradients, or temperature zones. The temperature at any point within the iceball depends upon: 1) the distance from the cryogen, with gradually increasing temperatures at progressively greater distances due to a resupplying of heat by blood vessels; and 2) the rate of freezing, with a rapid freeze producing colder temperatures near the edge of the growing iceball.

2. *Biological principles of cryosurgery.*[2] There are two phases of cryoinjury-induced *in vivo* cell death.

a. Initially, freezing of extracellular fluid concentrates the remaining solutes, which leads to cellular dehydration and is the probable mechanism of cell death associated with a slow freeze. When the rate of cooling is rapid, intracellular ice crystals develop. Although these crystals are not always lethal to the cell, a slow thaw leads to the formation of larger crystals, which are highly destructive to the cell by an uncertain mechanism. Maximum cell death is achieved with a *rapid freeze* and a *slow thaw*.

b. Later, superimposed hemorrhagic infarction results from obliteration of the microcirculation within the frozen tissue. *Ischemic necrosis* is the histologic hallmark of cryoinjured tissue.

3. *Cyclocryotherapy* presumably destroys the ability of ciliary

processes to produce aqueous humor by the biphasic mechanism of cell death outlined above. Animal studies have revealed significant differences between the temperature of the cryoprobe and the temperature within the treated tissues.[3, 4] In living eyes, a temperature of −60 to −80°C over the sclerolimbal area produced a temperatue of approximately −10°C at the tips of the ciliary processes after a lag of 20 to 30 sec.[4] The latter temperature is near the minimum thermogradient at which cryoinjury normally occurs.[2] Ciliary body blood flow in rabbits is reduced 50 to 60% when treated with −80°C cryoapplications for 60 sec.[5] Histologic studies of eyes treated with cyclocryotherapy show destruction of vascular, stromal, and epithelial elements of the ciliary processes with replacement by fibrous tissue.[4, 6–8] Ciliary epithelium has been observed to regenerate in monkey, but not in human eyes.[8]

In addition to lowering the intraocular pressure, cyclocryotherapy may provide relief of pain by the destruction of corneal nerves. Wallerian degeneration of corneal nerve fibers was observed in rabbits following cyclocryotherapy, although regeneration began within 9 to 16 days.[9]

B. Techniques

1. *Cryoinstruments.* Either nitrous oxide or carbon dioxide gas cryosurgical units may be used. The standard "glaucoma" probe has a tip diameter of 4 mm.[10] A modified cryoprobe with a curved 3 × 6 mm tip has been developed to reduce the number of applications required.[11] An automatic timer to monitor the duration of each application has also been described.[12]

2. *Cryoprobe placement.* With the 4-mm tip, the nearest edge of the probe is placed 2.5 mm from the corneolimbal junction to concentrate the maximum freezing effect over the ciliary processes (Fig. 34.1).[13] It has also been suggested that transillumination may be helpful by delineating the pars plicata.[13, 14] Most surgeons treat two to three quadrants, with three to four cryoapplications per quadrant. The number of cryolesions may be influenced to a degree by preoperative parameters, such as the type of glaucoma, the intraocular pressure level, and the number of previous cyclocryotherapy procedures. However, there are no precise guidelines by which an individual patient's response to therapy can be predicted, and it is best to err on the side of under-treatment rather than to run the risk of phthisis. One recommended approach is to limit each treatment session to six applications or less over 180° of the globe.[13]

3. *Freezing technique.* A study of human eyes with direct visualization of the ciliary body during cyclocryotherapy revealed that a freeze of −75°C for 30 sec produced visible ice crystals only in the valleys between ciliary processes, while a 1-min freeze resulted in an iceball at the tips of the processes.[15] Most surgeons prefer −60 to −80°C applications for 60 sec.[10, 13–15] As previously noted, a rapid freeze and slow, unassisted thaw produce the maximum cell death.[2]

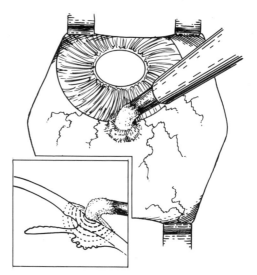

Figure 34.1.   Cyclocryotherapy technique, showing placement of probe and shape of iceball (inset).

Opinions differ as to the value of repeating the freeze in the same site. In the cryosurgical management of tumors, multiple freeze/thaw cycles have been shown to produce increasingly greater tissue destruction.[2] However, this does not necessarily imply optimum treatment, and further study is needed with regard to cyclocryotherapy. If the initial procedure does not adequately lower the intraocular pressure after 1 month, cyclocryotherapy may be repeated one or more times as required. In one series of 61 eyes, 14 required two or more procedures.[10]

4. *Postoperative management.* For approximately the first 24 hr, the patient may experience intense pain, and strong analgesics are often required. It has also been noted that subconjunctival steroids seem to minimize the postoperative pain.[13] In addition, frequent topical corticosteroids, antibiotics, and a cycloplegic-mydriatic should be used routinely starting on the day of surgery. Since the intraocular pressure may remain elevated for a day or more after the treatment, it is advisable to keep the patient on his pre-operative anti-glaucoma medications until a pressure reduction is observed.

C. Complications

1. *Uveitis* occurs in all cases and is usually intense, with the frequent formation of a fibrin clot. One study suggests that the inflammation is prostaglandin-induced and might be minimized by pretreatment with aspirin.[16] In addition, a chronic aqueous flare may persist due to permanent disruption of the blood-aqueous barrier, but this does not require treatment.

2. *Hyphema* is a common complication, especially in eyes with neovascular glaucoma, and usually clears with conservative management.

3. *Hypotony.* A major disadvantage of all cyclodestructive proce-

dures is that nothing can be done to reverse the hypotony or phthisis, if this should occur. Although this complication is less common with cyclocryotherapy than with other cyclodestructive operations,[10] it does occur and is best avoided by treating a limited area each time. It is far better to repeat the treatment several times than to produce phthisis by over-treatment.

4. Other complications associated with cyclocryotherapy include choroidal detachment with a flat anterior chamber,[17] papilledema in monkeys due to reduced intraocular pressure,[18] intravitreal neovascularization from the ciliary body,[19] anterior segment ischemia in neovascular glaucoma following 360° of cryotherapy,[20] and proliferation of retinal glial cells and pigmented epithelial cells in monkeys.[21] Ocular rigidity in rabbit studies was found to be low initially, but then rose significantly after approximately 2 weeks, which is important to consider if indentation tonometry is being used.[22]

D. Indications

As previously noted, cyclocryotherapy is usually reserved for situations in which other glaucoma operations have repeatedly failed or in which the surgeon wishes to avoid intraocular surgery. Two conditions in which this procedure is reported to have particular value are glaucoma after a penetrating keratoplasty[23, 24] and chronic open-angle glaucoma in aphakia.[25] Cyclocryotherapy has also been advocated for the management of neovascular glaucoma,[26, 27] although the main benefit in this disease appears to be relief of pain,[28, 29] since visual results have been poor despite reasonable pressure control.

II. OTHER CYCLODESTRUCTIVE PROCEDURES

A. Penetrating Cyclodiathermy

This technique was introduced by Vogt[30] in 1940. The sclera is penetrated 2.5 to 5 mm from the corneolimbal junction by a 1.0 to 1.5 mm electrode, and a diathermy current of 40 to 45 ma is applied for 10 to 20 sec.[30–32] This may be done with or without preparation of a conjunctival flap. One or two rows of diathermy lesions are generally placed several millimeters apart for approximately 180°. The mechanism of permanent intraocular pressure reduction is probably cell death within the ciliary body, as in the case of cyclocryotherapy.[6] In addition, it has been felt that the more posteriorly placed lesions may create a draining fistula in the region of the pars plana.[32]

Early reports of experience with cyclodiathermy were encouraging.[33, 34] However, subsequent study revealed a low success rate and a significant incidence of hypotony. In a review of 100 cases, 5% had lasting, useful reduction in intraocular pressure, while about the same number developed phthisis.[32] These results undoubtedly vary to some degree according to the specific technique that is used.

B. Cycloelectrolysis

Berens and co-workers,[35] in 1949, described a technique which employs the use of low frequency galvanic current to create a chemical reaction within the ciliary body. This leads to the formation of sodium hydroxide, which is caustic to the tissue of the ciliary body. The resulting structural changes seen in studies with rabbit eyes were tissue destruction with hemorrhage and vasodilation, especially in the anterior ciliary processes.[36]

C. Cyclophotocoagulation

The laser has also been used to create cell death within the ciliary body for reduction of intraocular pressure. It has been reported that ciliary body photocoagulation through the conjunctiva and sclera can be achieved with ruby or neodynium laser.[37, 38] However, the transpupillary route in aphakic eyes offers a more direct approach to the ciliary processes, and a contact lens with attached scleral depressor has been developed for this purpose.[39] Successful transpupillary photocoagulation of individual ciliary processes with the argon laser in rabbits[40] and man[41] has been reported, although one study indicated that a limiting factor was adequate access to a sufficient number of ciliary processes.[42]

References

1. Bietti, G: Surgical intervention on the ciliary body. New trends for the relief of glaucoma. JAMA 142:889, 1950.
2. Wilkes, TD, Fraunfelder, FT: Principles of cryosurgery. Ophthal Surg 10:21, 1979.
3. de Roetth, A, Jr: Ciliary body temperatures in cryosurgery. Arch Ophthal 85:204, 1971.
4. Quigley, HA: Histological and physiological studies of cyclocryotherapy in primate and human eyes. Am J Ophthal 82:722, 1976.
5. Green, K, Hull, DS, Bowman, K: Cyclocryotherapy and ocular blood flow. Glaucoma 1:141, 1979.
6. Edmonds, C, de Roetth, A Jr, Howard, GM: Histopathologic changes following cryosurgery and diathermy of the rabbit ciliary body. Am J Ophthal 69:65, 1970.
7. Ferry, AP: Histopathologic observations on human eyes following cyclocryotherapy for glaucoma. Trans Am Acad Ophthal Otol 83:90, 1977.
8. Smith, RS, Boyle, E, Rudt, LA: Cyclocryotherapy. A light and electron microscopic study. Arch Ophthal 95:284, 1977.
9. Wener, RG, Pinkerton, RMH, Robertson, DM: Cryosurgical induced changes in corneal nerves. Can J Ophthal 8:548, 1973.
10. Bellows, AR, Grant, WM: Cyclocryotherapy in advanced inadequately controlled glaucoma. Am J Ophthal 75:679, 1973.
11. Machemer, R: Modified cryoprobe for retinal detachment surgery and cyclocryotherapy. Am J Ophthal 83:123, 1977.
12. Machemer, R, Lashley, R: Automatic timer for cryotherapy. Am J Ophthal 83:125, 1977.
13. Bellows, AR: Cyclocryotherapy: its role in the treatment of glaucoma. Pers Ophthal 4:139, 1980.
14. Wesley, RE, Kielar, RA: Cyclocryotherapy in treatment of glaucoma. Glaucoma 3:533, 1980.
15. Burton, TC: Cyclocryotherapy. In Current Concepts of Ophthalmology, vol 4, Blodi, FC, ed. CV Mosby Co, St Louis, 1974.
16. Chavis, RM, Vygantas, CM, Vygantas, A: Experimental inhibition of prostaglandin-like inflammatory response after cryotherapy. Am J Ophthal 82:310, 1976.
17. Kaiden, JS, Serniuk, RA, Bader, BF: Choroidal detachment with flat anterior chamber after cyclocryotherapy. Ann Ophthal 11:1111, 1979.

18. Minckler, DS, Tso, MOM: Experimental papilledema produced by cyclocryotherapy. Am J Ophthal 82:577, 1976.
19. Goldberg, MF, Ericson, ES: Intravitreal ciliary body neovascularization. Ophthal Surg 8:62, 1977.
20. Krupin, T, Johnson, MF, Becker, B: Anterior segment ischemia after cyclocryotherapy. Am J Ophthal 84:426, 1977.
21. Yamishita, H, Sears, ML: Complications of cyclocryosurgery. Glaucoma 2:273, 1980.
22. Paterson, CA, Paterson, EF, Briggs, SA: Experimental cryosurgery. Effect upon ocular rigidity and intraocular pressure. Arch Ophthal 86:425, 1971.
23. West, CE, Wood, TO, Kaufman, HE: Cyclocryotherapy for glaucoma pre- or postpenetrating keratoplasty. Am J Ophthal 76:485, 1973.
24. Binder, PS, Abel, R Jr, Kaufman, HE: Cyclocryotherapy for glaucoma after penetrating keratoplasty. Am J Ophthal 79:489, 1975.
25. Bellows, AR, Grant, WM: Cyclocryotherapy of chronic open-angle glaucoma in aphakic eyes. Am J Ophthal 85:615, 1978.
26. Feibel, RM, Bigger, JF: Rubeosis iridis and neovascular glaucoma. Evaluation of cyclocryotherapy. Am J Ophthal 74:862, 1972.
27. Faulborn, J, Hoster, K: Results of cyclocryotherapy in case of hemorrhagic glaucoma. Klin Monatsbl Augenheilkd 162:513, 1973.
28. Faulborn, J, Birnbaum, F: Cyclocryotherapy of haemorrhagic glaucoma: clinical long time and histopathologic results. Klin Monatsbl Augenheilkd 170:651, 1977.
29. Krupin, T, Mitchell, KB, Becker, B: Cyclocryotherapy in neovascular glaucoma. Am J Ophthal 86:24, 1978.
30. Vogt, A: Cyclodiathermypuncture in cases of glaucoma. Br J Ophthal 24:288, 1940.
31. King, JH, Wadsworth, JAC: An Atlas of Ophthalmic Surgery, 2nd ed. JB Lippincott Co, Philadelphia, 1970, p 448.
32. Walton, DS, Grant, WM: Penetrating cyclodiathermy for filtration. Arch Ophthal 83:47, 1970.
33. Albaugh, CH, Dunphy, EB: Cyclodiathermy. Arch Ophthal 27:543, 1942.
34. Stocker, FW: Response of chronic simple glaucoma to treatment with cyclodiathermy puncture. Arch Ophthal 34:181, 1945.
35. Berens, C, Sheppard, LB, Duel, AB Jr: Cycloelectrolysis for glaucoma. Trans Am Ophthal Soc 47:364, 1949.
36. Sheppard, LB: Retrociliary cyclodiathermy versus retrociliary cycloelectrolysis. Effects on the normal rabbit eye. Am J Ophthal 46:27, 1958.
37. Beckman, H, et al: Transscleral ruby laser irradiation of the ciliary body in the treatment of intractable glaucoma. Trans Am Acad Ophthal Otol 76:423, 1972.
38. Beckman, H, Sugar, HS: Neodymium laser cyclocoagulation. Arch Ophthal 90:27, 1973.
39. Slezak, H: Results of depression biomicroscopy of the posterior chamber. Am J Ophthal 72:1073, 1971.
40. Lee, PF, Pomerantzeff, O: Transpupillary cyclophotocoagulation of rabbit eyes. An experimental approach to glaucoma surgery. Am J Ophthal 71:911, 1971.
41. Lee, PF: Argon laser photocoagulation of the ciliary processes in cases of aphakic glaucoma. Arch Ophthal 97:2135, 1979.
42. Merritt, JC: Transpupillary photocoagulation of the ciliary processes. Ann Ophthal 8:325, 1976.

Chapter 35

CYCLODIALYSIS, COMBINED PROCEDURES, AND MISCELLANEOUS GLAUCOMA OPERATIONS

CYCLODIALYSIS, COMBINED PROCEDURES, AND MISCELLANEOUS GLAUCOMA OPERATIONS

I. CYCLODIALYSIS

Cyclodialysis, as an operation for glaucoma, was described by Heine[1] in 1905. The procedure has been employed as an alternative to filtering surgery, although it is no longer in common use, primarily due to the unpredictable results. One situation in which it may offer specific advantages, however, is in combination with cataract surgery, which will be considered later in this chapter.

A. Theories of Mechanism

Cyclodialysis is a separation of the ciliary body from the scleral spur, which creates a direct communication between the anterior chamber and the suprachoroidal space. One theory holds that this lowers the intraocular pressure by increasing extracanalicular (or uveoscleral) outflow.[2-4] Another hypothesis proposes reduced aqueous production, due to altered ciliary body anatomy, as the main cause of pressure lowering.[5, 6] It may be that both mechanisms are involved in a successful cyclodialysis procedure. This was suggested by an intraocular manometric study of a glaucoma patient before and after cyclodialysis, which revealed both improved outflow and reduced aqueous production.[7]

B. Basic Technique (Fig. 35.1)[1, 8]

1. An incision is made through conjunctiva and Tenon's capsule approximately 8 mm from the corneolimbal junction, usually in a superior quadrant between the insertions of two rectus muscles. A 3 to 4 mm full-thickness scleral incision, 4 to 6 mm from the anatomical limbus, is then made parallel to the limbus.

2. A cyclodialysis spatula is inserted through the scleral incision and into the suprachoroidal space. Staying close to the inner scleral surface, the spatula is advanced until the tip enters the anterior chamber. Lateral movements of the spatula tip are then made to either side of the entry point to separate about one-third of the ciliary body from the scleral spur.

An alternative technique is to create the cyclodialysis with multiple forward thrusts of the spatula, by which up to one-half of the ciliary body can be disinserted.[9] Air injection into the anterior chamber has been advocated as a means of holding the cleft open during the early postoperative period,[10, 11] and a cannulated cyclodialysis spatula is available for this purpose.[12] Other modifications of the cyclodialysis spatula include a rounded, shorter handle, to facilitate use under the

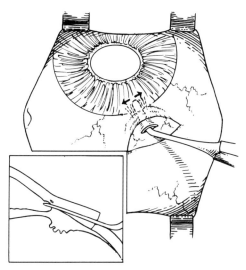

Figure 35.1. Cyclodialysis. A cyclodialysis spatula is passed through a full-thickness scleral incision and the suprachoroidal space until it enters the anterior chamber. With lateral movements of the spatula tip (*arrows*), approximately one-third of the ciliary body is separated from the scleral spur.

operating microscope,[13] a shorter blade with a blunt tip, for increased safety,[13] and a fiber-optic tip, to facilitate visualization within the suprachoroidal space and anterior chamber.[14]

3. A peripheral iridectomy is normally not used with a cyclodialysis, although such a combination has been described and reported to give good results.[15] After withdrawal of the spatula, only the conjunctiva is closed.

4. Postoperative management includes topical antibiotics and corticosteroids. In addition, the use of a miotic has been recommended to keep the cyclodialysis cleft open through traction on the longitudinal ciliary muscle.[2, 16]

C. Variations

1. *Implants* (setons) of various material have been inserted into the cyclodialysis cleft to keep it open,[7, 17-20] although no evidence of lasting success has been provided for any of these techniques.

2. *Iridocyclo-retraction.* Krasnov[21] described a technique for the treatment of chronic angle-closure glaucoma in which two or three scleral pedicles are folded forward into a cyclodialysis cleft to keep the angle open. A modification of this technique, using a single scleral pedicle, was designed to maintain a patent cyclodialysis cleft in aphakic eyes.[22] Reports concerning the usefulness of this procedure for the treatment of chronic glaucoma in aphakia are conflicting.[22, 23]

3. Another attempt to utilize cyclodialysis in aphakic eyes has been described in which a block of sclera beneath a partial-thickness scleral flap is removed at the incision site for the cyclodialysis spatula to

establish external filtration through the suprachoroidal space and around the scleral flap.[24]

D. Complications[8, 9]

1. *Intraoperative hemorrhage* is a frequent complication of cyclodialysis. The risk may be minimized by making a more anterior scleral incision, avoiding anterior ciliary arteries, and keeping the cyclodialysis spatula close to the sclera to avoid perforating the ciliary body. When brisk bleeding does occur, it can usually be stopped by placing a large air bubble in the anterior chamber for several minutes.

2. *An improper spatula position* can cause several complications. If the cyclodialysis spatula is too far anterior as it enters the anterior chamber, it may strip Descemet's membrane or otherwise damage the cornea. A position that is too posterior may tear the ciliary body or iris, injure the lens, or rupture the hyaloid face and possibly cause vitreous loss.

3. *Hypotony* is a common postoperative complication of cyclodialysis. Penetrating cyclodiathermy or cyclocryotherapy to "wall off" the cleft may correct the problem, but the results are highly unpredictable.[16] Techniques for surgical closure of the cyclodialysis cleft have also been described.[25, 26]

4. *Failure to control the intraocular pressure* is usually associated with closure of the cyclodialysis cleft, which may result from hemorrhage, excessive inflammation, or an inadequate initial cleft. As previously noted, the risk of this complication can be reduced by the use of miotics, which presumably keep the cyclodialysis cleft open by traction of the ciliary musculature.[2, 16] A complication of cyclodialysis that may occur at any time after surgery, is a sudden, marked rise in the intraocular pressure. This is felt to be associated with closure of the cleft, and can be reversed, in some cases, with the use of miotics.

II. COMBINED CATARACT EXTRACTION AND GLAUCOMA SURGERY

A. Indications

Lens extraction combined with glaucoma surgery has a slightly greater risk of complications than a cataract operation alone as well as a lower chance of glaucoma control than with filtering surgery alone. For this reason, in managing a patient with cataracts and chronic glaucoma, the surgeon should consider each of the following surgical options and select the approach that seems to be most appropriate for each patient.

1. *Cataract extraction alone.* When the intraocular pressure is well controlled on a relatively low and well-tolerated medical regimen and optic nerve head damage is not advanced, most surgeons prefer a cataract extraction alone.[27–31] It has been reported that medical control

of the glaucoma is often easier after routine cataract surgery.[27-30] However, the long-term benefit of cataract surgery on glaucoma has not been clearly established, and it is generally agreed that this benefit is proportionally less with increasing severity of the glaucoma. Furthermore, with newer suturing techniques and tighter wound closure, a transient intraocular pressure rise in the early postoperative period is common, and this may pose a serious threat to the patient with advanced glaucomatous optic atrophy.

When a cataract extraction is performed on an eye with chronic glaucoma, especially if miosis is marked, it is often advisable to make a sector iridectomy or multiple sphincterotomies and a peripheral iridectomy.[32] This facilitates delivery of the lens, and also improves postoperative visualization of the fundus.

2. *Filtering surgery alone.* When the glaucoma is uncontrolled medically and poses an immediate threat to the patient's vision, the surgical procedure of choice is the one which has the greatest chance of controlling the intraocular pressure. In the hands of most surgeons, this is a filtering procedure performed alone. In some cases, the vision may be improved after filtering surgery by eliminating the need for a miotic, thereby postponing the need for cataract surgery.

When extraction of the cataract ultimately becomes necessary in an eye with a functioning filtering bleb, surgeons generally prefer to make the cataract incision away from the bleb, either inferiorly[33] or through clear cornea superiorly.[34, 35] One study revealed better results when the previous glaucoma procedure had been performed at the 6 o'clock position,[36] although this is technically more difficult and may reduce the chances of success with the filtering operation. Poor results have been reported in attempts to combine intraocular lens implantation in eyes with pre-existing filtering blebs.[37]

3. *Combined cataract extraction and glaucoma surgery.* Despite the problems associated with combining the cataract extraction and glaucoma procedure in a single operation, there are times when this approach may be in the patient's best interest. Such situations include cases in which 1) the glaucoma is under borderline medical control, especially when epinephrine is required or the patient has significant drug-induced side effects, 2) the glaucomatous optic atrophy is advanced, 3) there is an urgent need to restore vision as well as a need for glaucoma surgery, or 4) two operations are not feasible.

B. Techniques

The main problem with combining most glaucoma filtering techniques with a cataract extraction is the transient *shallow or flat anterior chamber*, which leads to significantly more complications in the inflamed, aphakic eye. For this reason, the preferred combined operations employ a glaucoma procedure that is less likely to cause loss of the anterior chamber.

1. *Cyclodialysis and cataract extraction* has been used as a com-

bined procedure for many years, with reports of good results.[38-42] However, in one large series, an analysis of the postoperative course suggested that the intraocular pressure reduction in many cases was due to the effect of the cataract surgery, rather than the cyclodialysis.[41] Since this effect may be lost with the newer techniques of wound closure, and considering the unpredictable nature of cyclodialysis, many surgeons have turned to alternative combined procedures.

2. *Trabeculectomy and cataract extraction* (Fig. 35.2). The protective scleral flap over a limbal fistula, which reduces the chances of an early postoperative flat anterior chamber, makes the guarded filtering procedure particularly desirable for combined procedures.[30, 31, 43-51] Reported techniques vary considerably, but the basic approach involves preparation of the partial-thickness scleral flap and limbal fistula in the usual manner, followed by extension of the corneoscleral incision from either side of the fistula. After removal of the lens, both scleral flap and corneoscleral incision are closed with multiple sutures. The conjunctival flap is closed in the manner described for glaucoma filtering procedures.

A simplified technique for creating a guarded fistula in conjunction with cataract surgery is to prepare a very beveled corneoscleral incision and remove one or more bites from the posterior lip of the incision with a scleral punch (Fig. 35.3).[52] A technique of combining a trabeculectomy and cyclodialysis with lens removal has also been described.[53]

3. *Trabeculotomy and cataract extraction* (Fig. 35.4). McPherson[54] has reported a technique in which a trabeculotomy is performed through a radial incision at 12 o'clock adjacent to a partial-thickness

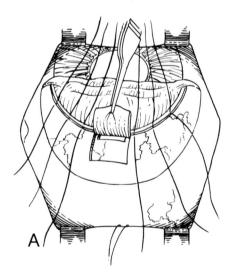
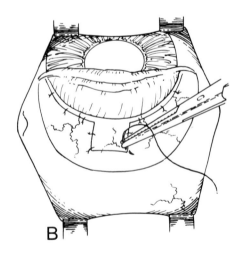

Figure 35.2. Trabeculectomy and cataract extraction. **A:** partial-thickness scleral flap and deep limbal fistula are prepared and the cataract incision is extended from either side; **B:** following lens extraction, the cataract incision and scleral flap are approximated with multiple sutures.

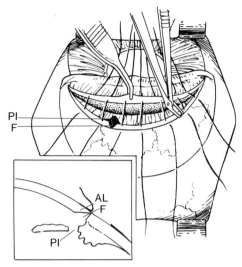

Figure 35.3. Simplified guarded filtering procedure and cataract extraction.[52] A sclerectomy punch is used to excise one or more blocks of tissue from the posterior lip of a beveled cataract incision. The original procedure has been modified by placing a peripheral iridectomy **(PI)** beneath each fistula **(F)**. When the cataract incision is closed, the anterior lip **(AL)** provides a protective partial-thickness flap over each fistula **(inset)**.

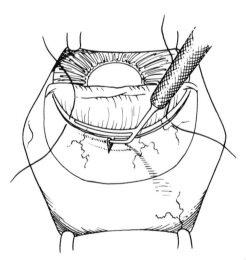

Figure 35.4. Trabeculotomy and cataract extraction.[54] A trabeculotomy is first performed posterior to a partial-thickness cataract incision. The cataract extraction is then completed in a standard manner.

corneoscleral incision. The cataract wound is then extended full-thickness, and an intracapsular cataract extraction is completed in a standard manner. Good results have been obtained with the preliminary experience.

III. MISCELLANEOUS GLAUCOMA OPERATIONS

A. Sinusotomy

Based on the theory that some cases of primary open-angle glaucoma result from increased resistance to aqueous outflow in the intrascleral outlet channels, Krasnov[55] developed an operation in which a 1.5-mm strip of sclera is excised to expose one-fourth to one-third of Schlemm's canal. However, it is not clear as to whether the benefit of this procedure comes from eliminating the abnormal outlet channels or from relieving the collapse of Schlemm's canal.[56, 57] Studies suggest that the latter is more likely.[56, 57]

B. Goniospasis

As noted in the discussion of miotic drugs, a centripetal pull on the scleral spur usually improves aqueous outflow, presumably by altering the anatomy of the trabecular meshwork and/or Schlemm's canal. Cairns[58] sought to apply this principle to a surgical procedure in which a portion of peripheral iris is displaced centrally by a taut suture anchored at two points in the limbus. Although the preliminary experience was said to be encouraging, the usefulness of this procedure has yet to be confirmed.

C. Vitrectomy Techniques in the Treatment of Glaucoma

The ever-expanding role of vitreous surgery in the management of ocular disease has grown to encompass many forms of secondary glaucoma. These were discussed in Section Two, and the following is a review of the more significant situations in which vitrectomy may be useful.[59, 60]

1. *Pupillary block glaucoma in aphakia* (Chapter 19). When surgical intervention is required, an iridectomy is usually effective. In recalcitrant cases, however, removal of the anterior vitreous by pars plana vitrectomy may be necessary.

2. *Malignant (ciliary block) glaucoma* (Chapter 19). This condition has been reported to respond well to vitrectomy in either the aphakic or phakic eye.

3. *Lens-induced glaucomas* (Chapter 14). When lens-induced uveitis and secondary glaucoma result from a posteriorly dislocated, hypermature cataract or from lens particles in the vitreous following surgery or trauma, removal of the offending material with vitrectomy instruments usually offers the safest, most effective treatment.

4. *Blood-induced glaucomas* (Chapter 17). In cases of traumatic hyphema in which surgical evacuation of the clot is indicated, the use of a vitrectomy instrument through a limbal incision is one effective surgical approach.[61-63] When the glaucoma is due to blood in the vitreous, which is coming forward to cause ghost cell or hemolytic glaucoma, it may be necessary to perform a complete pars plana vitrectomy to eliminate the source of the offending cells.[64]

5. *Epithelial ingrowth* (Chapter 19). A pars plana vitrectomy has

been successfully used to remove the involved iris and vitreous in these difficult cases.[65]

6. *Vitreo-retinal abnormalities of the newborn* (Chapter 15). *Persistent hyperplastic primary vitreous* or the retrocorneal mass in *retrolental fibroplasia*, both of which can cause angle-closure glaucoma by a forward displacement of the lens-iris diaphragm, may be removed by vitrectomy techniques.

D. Laser Techniques in the Treatment of Glaucoma

The benefits of laser technology have also been applied to many aspects of glaucoma therapy. The following list includes a summary of the techniques that have been considered in previous chapters and one additional laser procedure that has not yet been discussed.

1. *Filtering procedures* (Chapter 31). Preliminary experience has been reported with the use of laser energy to create a full-thickness glaucoma fistula,[66] or a fistula beneath a scleral flap.[67]

2. *Iridectomy* (Chapter 32). The laser has well-established value in the creation of full-thickness iridectomies and in the penetration of incomplete surgical iridectomies.

3. *Photomydriasis* (Chapter 19). Photocoagulation of the iris can also be used to treat pupillary block glaucoma in aphakia or pseudophakia, by applying a series of low energy burns near the pupillary margin.[68-70] This produces mydriasis, which may break the pupillary block.

4. *Cyclophotocoagulation* (Chapter 34). Preliminary experience has been reported with attempts to reduce aqueous production by destroying ciliary processes with transscleral or transpupillary laser applications.

5. *Goniophotocoagulation* (Chapter 15). As noted in the discussion of neovascular glaucoma, new vessels crossing the scleral spur may be obliterated with laser application. Preliminary experience suggests that goniophotocoagulation may be a useful adjunct for the treatment of this disorder.[71, 72]

6. *Trabeculotomy* (Chapter 33). Several studies have indicated that holes can be created in the trabecular meshwork with laser energy, but the long-term benefit of this is controlling the intraocular pressure has yet to be established.

7. *Laser trabecular therapy*. Wise and Witter[73] described the use of evenly spaced argon laser applications to the full circumference of the trabecular meshwork in patients with primary open-angle glaucoma. They postulated that traction on the tissue between the burns shortens the total circumference of the meshwork, thereby causing it to be displaced centrally, which opens the intertrabecular spaces[73] (a widening of Schlemm's canal might also be postulated). The basic technique consists of making 100 to 120 laser burns with settings of 800 to 1200 mw, 50 μ in diameter, and 0.1 sec duration, evenly spaced for 360° on the trabecular meshwork.[74] Although the mechanism of action has not been proven, preliminary clinical experience by several independent investigative teams suggests that this may become an

important therapeutic modality in the management of open-angle glaucoma.[74-76]

References

1. Heine, L: Die Cyklodialyse, eine neue Glaucomoperation. Deutsche Med Wehnschr 31:825, 1905.
2. Barkan, O: Cyclodialysis: its mode of action. Histologic observations in a case of glaucoma in which both eyes were successfully treated by cyclodialysis. Arch Ophthal 43:793, 1950.
3. Bill, A: The routes for bulk drainage of aqueous humour in rabbits with and without cyclodialysis. Doc Ophthal 20:157, 1966.
4. Pederson, JE, Gaasterland, DE, MacLellan, HM: Experimental ciliochoroidal detachment. Effect on intraocular pressure and aqueous humor flow. Arch Ophthal 97:536, 1979.
5. Auricchio, G: Considerations on mechanism of action of cyclodialysis. Boll Ocul 35:401, 1956.
6. Chandler, PA, Maumenee, AE: A major cause of hypotony. Trans Am Acad Ophthal Otol 52:563, 1961.
7. Gills, JP Jr, Paterson, CA, Paterson, ME: Action of cyclodialysis utilizing an implant studied by manometry in a human eye. Exp Eye Res 6:75, 1967.
8. Ascher, KW: Some details of the technique of cyclodialysis. Am J Ophthal 50:1207, 1960.
9. O'Brien, CS, Weih, J: Cyclodialysis. Arch Ophthal 42:606, 1949.
10. Haisten, MW, Guyton, JS: Cyclodialysis with air injection: technique and results in ninety-four consecutive operations. Arch Ophthal 59:507, 1958.
11. Miller, RD, Nisbet, RM: Cyclodialysis with air injection in black patients. Ophthal Surg 12:92, 1981.
12. Randolph, ME: A new cyclodialysis instrument. Am J Ophthal 30:1063, 1947.
13. Simmons, RJ, Kimbrough, RL: A modified cyclodialysis spatula. Ophthal Surg 10:67, 1979.
14. Cohen, SW, Banko, W, Nath, S: A fiber-optics cyclodialysis spatula. Ophthal Surg 10:74, 1979.
15. Romem, M, Pasco, M: Peripheral iridectomy and cyclodialysis as simultaneous operation in glaucoma surgery. Acta Ophthal 50:26, 1972.
16. Chandler, PA, Grant, WM: Glaucoma, 2nd ed. Lea & Febiger, Philadelphia, 1979, p 307.
17. Gills, JP: Cyclodialysis implants in human eyes. Am J Ophthal 61:841, 1966.
18. Streeten, BW, Belkowitz, M: Experimental hypotony with silastic. Arch Ophthal 78:503, 1967.
19. Richards, RD: Long-term results of gonioplasty. Am J Ophthal 70:715, 1970.
20. Portney, GL: Silicone elastomer implantation cyclodialysis. A negative report. Arch Ophthal 89:10, 1973.
21. Krasnov, MM: Iridocyclo-retraction in narrow-angle glaucoma. Br J Ophthal 55:389, 1971.
22. Aviner, Z: Modified Krasnov's iridocycloretraction for aphakic glaucoma. Ann Ophthal 7:859, 1975.
23. Sugar, HS: Experiences with some modifications of cyclodialysis for aphakic glaucoma. Ann Ophthal 9:1045, 1977.
24. Ackerman, J, Kanarek, I, Shamah, M, Rand, WJ: A new approach to aphakic glaucoma: a subscleral filtering cyclodialysis. Glaucoma 1:176, 1979.
25. Best, W, Hartwig, H: Traumatic cyclodialysis and its treatment. Klin Monatsbl Augenheilkd 170:917, 1977.
26. Tate, GW Jr, Lynn, JR: A new technique for the surgical repair of cyclodialysis induced hypotony. Ann Ophthal 10:1261, 1978.
27. Bigger, JF, Becker, B: Cataracts and primary open-angle glaucoma: the effect of uncomplicated cataract extraction on glaucoma control. Trans Am Acad Ophthal Otol 75:260, 1971.

28. Randolph, ME, Maumenee, AE, Iliff, CE: Cataract extraction in glaucomatous eyes. Am J Ophthal 71:328, 1971.
29. Kornzweig, AL, Schneider, J: Cataract extraction in glaucoma cases: a retrospective study of 94 cases. Ann Ophthal 6:959, 1974.
30. Palimeris, G, Chimonidou, E, Magouritsas, N, Velissaropoulos, P: Cataract extraction in chronic simple glaucoma. Ophthal Surg 5:62, 1974.
31. Spaeth, GL: The management of patients with conjoint cataract and glaucoma. Ophthal Surg 11:780, 1980.
32. Kolker, AE, Stewart, RH, LeBlanc, RP: Cataract extraction in glaucomatous patients. Arch Ophthal 84:63, 1970.
33. Baloglou, P, Matta, C, Asdourian, K: Cataract extraction after filtering operations. Arch Ophthal 88:12, 1972.
34. Riise, P: Influence of cataract operation on the pressure in glaucoma eyes operated with iridencleisis. Acta Ophthal 50:436, 1972.
35. Kondo, T: Cataract extraction after filtering operation. Glaucoma 1:165, 1979.
36. Polychronakos, DJ, Chryssafis, B: Cataract extraction after Scheie's operation. Klin Monatsbl Augenheilkd 165:234, 1974.
37. Alpar, JJ: Cataract extraction and lens implantation in eyes with pre-existing filtering bleb. Am Intra-ocular Implant Soc J 5:33, 1979.
38. Kopaeva, VG: Results of cataract extraction in glaucomatous patients. Vestn Oftalmol 4:43, 1968.
39. Galin, MA, Baras, I, Sambursky, J: Glaucoma and cataract. A study of cyclodialysis-lens extraction. Am J Ophthal 67:522, 1969.
40. Shmeleva, VV, Mukhina, EA: Combined cataract extraction and cyclodialysis. Vestn Oftalmol 85:30, 1972.
41. Shields, MB, Simmons, RJ: Combined cyclodialysis and cataract extraction. Trans Am Acad Ophthal Otol 81:286, 1976.
42. Montgomery, D, Gills, JP: Extracapsular cataract extraction, lens implantation and cyclodialysis. Ophthal Surg 11:343, 1980.
43. Rich, W: Cataract extraction with trabeculectomy. Trans Ophthal Soc UK 94:458, 1974.
44. Bregeat, P: Cataract surgery and trabeculectomy at the same time. Klin Monatsbl Augenheilkd 167:505, 1975.
45. Jerndal, T, Lundstrom, M: Trabeculectomy combined with cataract extraction. Am J Ophthal 81:227, 1976.
46. Stewart, RH, Loftis, MD: Combined cataract extraction and thermal sclerostomy versus combined cataract extraction and trabeculectomy. Ophthal Surg 7:93, 1976.
47. Johns, GE, Layden, WE: Combined trabeculectomy and cataract extraction. Am J Ophthal 88:973, 1979.
48. Ganias, F: Combined thermotrabeculocanalotomy cataract extraction. Ann Ophthal 11:674, 1979.
49. Edwards, RS: Trabeculectomy combined with cataract extraction: a follow-up study. Br J Ophthal 64:720, 1980.
50. Klemen, UM: Uniphasic glaucoma—cataract surgery: anterior sclerectomy versus goniotrephining. Glaucoma 2:437, 1980.
51. Freedman, J: Combined cataract and glaucoma surgery. Glaucoma 3:51, 1981.
52. Spaeth, GL, Sivalingam, E: The partial-punch: A new combined cataract-glaucoma operation. Ophthal Surg 7:53, 1976.
53. Galin, MA, Hung, PT, Obstbaum, SA: Cataract extraction in glaucoma. Am J Ophthal 87:124, 1979.
54. McPherson, SD Jr: Combined trabeculotomy and cataract extraction as a single operation. Tr Am Ophthal Soc 74:251, 1976.
55. Krasnov, MM: Sinusotomy. Foundations, results, prospects. Trans Am Acad Ophthal Otol 76:368, 1972.
56. Nesterov, AP: Role of the blockade of Schlemm's canal in pathogenesis of primary open-angle glaucoma. Am J Ophthal 70:691, 1970.
57. Ellingsen, BA, Grant, WM: Trabeculotomy and sinusotomy in enucleated human

eyes. Invest Ophthal 11:21, 1972.

58. Cairns, JE: Goniospasis: A method designed to relieve canalicular blockade in primary open-angle glaucoma. Ann Ophthal 8:1417, 1976.
59. McCuen, BW II: The treatment of secondary glaucoma with vitrectomy techniques and instrumentation. Pers Ophthal 4:155, 1980.
60. Taylor, HR, Michels, RG, Stark, WJ: Vitrectomy methods in anterior segment surgery. Ophthal Surg 10:25, 1979.
61. Diddie, KR, Ernest, JT: Rotoextractor evacuation of total hyphema. Ophthal Surg 7:49, 1976.
62. Stern, WH, Mondal, KM: Vitrectomy instrumentation for surgical evacuation of total anterior chamber hyphema and control of recurrent anterior chamber hemorrhage. Ophthal Surg 10:34, 1979.
63. McCuen, BW, Fung, WE: The role of vitrectomy instrumentation in the treatment of severe traumatic hyphema. Am J Ophthal 88:930, 1979.
64. Brucker, AJ, Michels, RG, Green, WR: Pars plana vitrectomy in the management of blood-induced glaucoma with vitreous hemorrhage. Ann Ophthal 10:1427, 1978.
65. Stark, WJ, Michels, RG, Maumenee, AE, Cupples, H: Surgical management of epithelial ingrowth. Am J Ophthal 85:772, 1978.
66. Litwin, RL: Successful argon laser sclerostomy for glaucoma. Ophthal Surg 10:22, 1979.
67. Beckman, H, Fuller, TA: Carbon dioxide laser scleral dissection and filtering procedure for glaucoma. Am J Ophthal 88:73, 1979.
68. Patti, JC, Cinotti, AA: Iris photocoagulation therapy of aphakic pupillary block. Arch Ophthal 93:347, 1975.
69. Theodossiadis, G: A new argon-laser-approach for the management of aphakic pupillary block. Klin Monatsbl Augenheilkd 169:153, 1976.
70. Obstbaum, SA, Galin, MA, Barasch, KR, Baras, I: Laser photomydriasis in pseudophakic pupillary block. Am Intra-ocular Implant Soc J 7:28, 1981.
71. Simmons, RJ, Dueker, DK, Kimbrough, RL, Aiello, LM: Goniophotocoagulation for neovascular glaucoma. Trans Am Acad Ophthal Otol 83:80, 1977.
72. Simmons, RJ, Depperman, SR, Deuker, DK: The role of gonio-photocoagulation in neovascularization of the anterior chamber angle. Ophthalmology 87:79, 1980.
73. Wise, JB, Witter, SL: Argon laser therapy for open-angle glaucoma. A pilot study. Arch Ophthal 97:319, 1979.
74. Wise, JB: Long-term control of adult open angle glaucoma by argon laser treatment. Ophthalmology 88:197, 1981.
75. Schwartz, AL, Whitten, ME, Bleiman, B, Martin, D: Argon laser trabecular surgery in uncontrolled phakic open angle glaucoma. Ophthalmology 88:203, 1981.
76. Wilensky, JT, Jampol, LM: Laser therapy for open angle glaucoma. Ophthalmology 88:213, 1981.

AUTHOR INDEX

Frenkel, M, 319
Freyler, H, 473
Fridman, AH, 292
Fried, K, 208
Friedberg, DN, 319
Friedburg, D, 291
Friedenwald, JS, 42, 73, 74, 433
Friedland, BR, 434
Friedman, A, 129
Friedman, AH, 227, 236, 319, 355, 375
Friedman, AI, 402
Friedman, BZ, 193
Friedman, J, 476
Friedman, L, 167
Friedman, Z, 195
Friedmann, AI, 129
Frisen, L, 107
Fritch, CD, 319
Fronimopoulos, J, 473
Fu, Y, 473
Fuchs, E, 101, 250, 308
Fuerry, DP, III, 419
Fujimoto, F, 308
Fujino, T, 100
Fuller, IB, 73
Fuller, TA, 473, 516
Fung, WE, 516
Furg, WE, 320
Furman, M, 403, 404

G

Gaasterland, DE, 38, 39, 103, 371, 375, 400, 447, 485, 514
Gaffney, HP, 162
Gafner, VF, 101
Gage, J, 329
Gal, A, 401
Galantino, G, 494
Galin, MA, 71, 102, 163, 193, 194, 195, 320, 352, 353, 355, 383, 400, 402, 417, 420, 421, 422, 423, 424, 439, 471, 474, 475, 493, 515, 516
Gallin-Cohen, PF, 72
Galloway, NR, 400, 401
Gandhi, N, 161
Gandiglio, G, 227
Gangitano, JL, 434
Ganias, F, 195, 473, 515
Ganley, JP, 160, 162
Garg, LC, 423, 433
Garlikov, RS, 403
Garner, A, 422
Garner, LL, 416, 417
Garrison, RJ, 104, 165
Gartner, J, 70
Gartner, S, 236, 290, 292

Gasparini, J, 166
Gass, JD, 472
Gass, JDM, 235, 353
Gasset, AR, 382, 401
Gay, AJ, 290, 416
Gaylow, JR, 355
Gaynes, E, 485
Geeraets, WJ, 419
Geijer, C, 100
Gelart, SS, 447
Gelatt, KN, 76, 374, 375
Gelber, EC, 132
George, TW, 106, 107, 132, 162
Gerhard, JP, 131
Gershen, HF, 472
Getson, AJ, 422
Ghartey, KN, 357
Ghosh, M, 273
Gibbs, D, 356
Gideoni, O, 164
Gieser, D, 365, 472
Gifford, H, 274
Gilbert, HD, 320
Giles, CL, 319
Gillies, WE, 273, 495
Gills, JP, Jr, 195, 514, 515
Gillspie, JE, 423
Gilman, BG, 75
Gipson, CC, 36, 433
Gipson, IK, 39
Gipstein, RM, 440
Girard, LJ, 161
Gitter, KA, 102, 236
Glaser, B, 320
Glaser, BM, 291
Glaser, JS, 106, 131
Glass, JL, 434
Gleser, DK, 193
Gloster, J, 106, 107, 132, 193, 418
Gnad, HD, 356, 365
Goar, E, 250
Godel, V, 366, 484
Goder, G, 101
Godfrey, WA, 307
Goes, F, 402, 403
Goffmann, R, 494
Golberg, DB, 226, 356
Golberg, L, 382
Goldberg, B, 236
Goldberg, I, 401, 419, 423
Goldberg, LS, 307
Goldberg, MF, 273, 274, 290, 292, 293, 294, 319, 320, 357, 503
Goldberg, RE, 106
Goldman, MH, 74
Goldmann, H, 42, 73, 101, 128,

129, 164, 167
Goldthwaite, D, 132
Goldwyn, R, 161
Golman, VH, 74
Gombos, GM, 353
Goodart, R, 292, 382
Goodstein, S, 476
Goodwin, T, 447
Gordon, GG, 365
Gordon, JM, 356
Gordon, L, 401
Gordon, M, 167
Gore, SM, 425
Goren, SB, 433
Gorin, G, 192
Gorn, RA, 319
Gottinger, W, 272
Gould, AL, 422
Grabie, MT, 440
Gragoudas, ES, 106, 291, 420
Graham, PA, 160
Gramer, E, 226
Grant, WM, 38, 40, 41, 42, 43, 71, 72, 73, 74, 105, 107, 131, 160, 162, 164, 192, 193, 194, 195, 227, 235, 237, 256, 257, 273, 274, 290, 291, 292, 293, 307, 309, 320, 351, 352, 353, 371, 399, 402, 404, 421, 433, 434, 502, 503, 514, 515
Graue, EL, 226
Graves, SA, 72
Grayson, M, 250
Greco, JJ, 403
Green, K, 39, 71, 72, 401, 417, 446, 447, 502
Green, WR, 101, 105, 226, 236, 307, 320, 354, 355, 419, 516
Greene, ME, 75
Gregersen, E, 495
Gregg, JM, 447
Gregor, Z, 225
Gregory, DS, 423
Greve, EL, 129
Grey, RHB, 357
Grierson, I, 39, 40, 41, 42, 400, 475
Grieten, J, 365
Grodzki, WF Jr, 38, 42, 74, 76, 165, 356, 399
Grolman, B, 75
Grote, P, 72, 208, 209
Grudsky, A, 365
Guehl, JJ, III, 474
Guilbault, N, 162, 250
Gum, GG, 76, 375
Gunn, PM, 425
Gupta, AK, 375

Gupta, M, 475
Gupta, S, 418
Gustin, J, 416
Gutman, FA, 292
Guy, J, 103
Guyton, JS, 514
Gwin, RM, 76, 375

H

Haas, H, 495
Haas, JS, 161, 291, 354, 472, 475, 494, 495
Hadden, OB, 235
Haegerstrom-Portnoy, G, 447
Hager, H, 494
Hagler, WS, 73
Hahn, KA, 165
Haik, GM, 43
Haimann, MH, 353, 424
Hajek, S, 163
Halasa, AH, 195, 293, 421
Halberg, GP, 75, 107
Hall, GA, 195
Hallett, JW, 235
Halpern, BL, 319
Halpin, JA, 366
Hamasaki, D, 100, 104, 194, 353
Hamilton, AG, 72
Hamilton, PB, 38
Hammer, M, 319
Hamming, N, 227
Handrup, B, 70
Haney, WP, 226
Hanible, JE, 129
Hanna, C, 250, 401
Hanna, R, 382
Hanno, R, 227
Hanselmayer, H, 250
Hanson, JW, 225, 226
Hansson, HA, 208
Hara, J, 308
Hara, K, 36
Hara, S, 273
Harbin, R, 422
Harbin, TS, Jr, 73, 160, 310, 401, 419
Hardberger, R, 382
Harding, C, 272
Hargett, NA, 419, 422, 434
Harms, C, 249
Harms, H, 129, 132, 209, 494
Harnoncourt, K, 433
Harrenhauer, J, 273
Harrington, DO, 106, 128, 129, 131, 352
Harris, GJ, 291, 371
Harris, JA, 291
Harris, LS, 163, 193, 353, 383,

400, 402, 403, 404, 417, 474, 475
Harris, WA, 446
Harrison, R, 404, 419, 420
Harstein, J, 401
Hart, FD, 307
Hart, W, Jr, 420
Hart, WM, Jr, 130, 132, 160, 167
Hartwig, H, 514
Harvey, J, 418
Hashimoto, JM, 42, 309, 352
Hass, I, 422
Hatem, G, 446
Hatt, MU, 421
Hattenhauer, JM, 475
Hauck, W, 494
Havener, WH, 382, 402, 433, 440
Hawkins, ME, 474
Hayasaka, S, 41, 417
Hayes, TL, 38
Hayreh, SS, 100, 101, 102, 104, 130, 160, 291, 310, 352, 355, 357
Haywood, JR, 434
Hecht, G, 382
Heckbert, S, 417
Heckenlively, J, 226
Heijl, A, 130
Heilmann, K, 132
Hein, HF, 274
Heine, L, 514
Heintz-DeBree, C, 165
Heinze, J, 320
Helfgott, MA, 161
Hellman, L, 71
Henderson, JW, 106, 320, 371
Hendrickson, AE, 103, 104
Henkind, P, 70, 71, 102, 104, 226, 290, 291, 355
Henley, W, 164, 166
Henville, JD, 72
Hepler, RS, 446, 447
Hepner, GW, 440
Heppke, G, 494
Herbst, RW, 273
Herbst, SF, 401, 402
Hermannspann, U, 71
Hernandez, MR, 365
Herschler, J, 106, 249, 293, 329, 352, 354, 355, 366, 471, 473, 494
Hersh, EM, 309
Hersh, SB, 484
Hetheringon, J Jr, 102
Hetherington, J, 493
Hetherington, J, Jr, 107, 167,

192, 208, 209, 250, 309, 371, 424, 472, 474, 494
Hetherington, J Jr, 42, 105
Hetland-Eriksen, J, 42, 73
Heydenreich, A, 356
Hiatt, RL, 73, 165
Hickey, TE, 421
Hidayat, A, 237
Higgins, RG, 37, 70, 417
Hiles, DA, 162
Hill, K, 320
Hiller, R, 161
Hillman, JS, 193
Hillmas, JS, 192
Hils, DA, 494
Hilton, GF, 290
Hinman, F, Jr, 440
Hippel, E, 226
Hirose, T, 227
Hirschhorn, K, 70
Hirst, LW, 225, 249
Hitchings, RA, 102, 104, 105, 106, 132, 162, 225, 227, 291, 309, 354
Hittner, HM, 226, 294
Hocker, LO, 275
Hodapp, E, 365
Hodes, C, 71
Hoepner, J, 226, 294
Hoffmann, F, 38
Hogan, MJ, 100, 101, 274, 308, 329
Holland, MG, 36, 274, 417, 418, 433
Hollenhorst, RW, 292
Hollows, FC, 105, 160
Hollwich, F, 163, 307, 473
Holly, FJ, 382
Holm, O, 37
Holm, OC, 105
Holmberg, A, 36, 39, 404
Holmberg, AS, 352
Holmes, JH, 404
Holmin, C, 130, 132
Holter, O, 70
Holth, S, 472
Holtmann, HW, 441
Holtz, SJ, 74
Hood, CI, 354
Hoover, GS, 41
Hoover, RE, 130, 355
Hopkins, JL, 129, 329
Hopkins, RE, 236
Horie, T, 70, 160, 418
Horlington, M, 400
Horsmanheimo, A, 273
Horven, I, 74, 320
Hoskins, HD, Jr, 132, 164, 290,

SUBJECT INDEX

A

Aceclidine, 397
Acetazolamide, 314, 428, 431
  test, 151
Acetohexamide, 431
Acetylcholine, 386, 388
Acetylcholinesterase, 386, 397
Acid burns, 328
Acid mucopolysaccharides, 23
Actin filaments, 20, 21
Acute angle-closure glaucoma, 125
Adenosine triphosphate, 387
Adenovirus, 301
Adenyl cyclase, 156, 387, 389, 446
Adrenergic drugs, 181, 406
Adrenergic nervous system, 386
Adrenergic potentiators, 389
Adrenergic supersensitivity, 408
Adrenochrome pigmentation, 409
Agranulocytosis, 431
Alcohol, 50, 439
Alkali burns, 328
Allen separator, 99
Alpha-adrenergic agonists, 389
Alpha-adrenergic antagonists, 389
Alpha-adrenergic receptors, 386
Alpha-methyl-para-tyrosine, 408
Amino acids, aqueous humor and, 15
Aminocarproic acid, 314
Amphetamines, 51
Amphotheric drugs, 380
Amyloidosis, primary familial, 262, 263
Anesthesia, 490
  filtering procedures, 455
Angiogenesis factors, 280
Angioscotomata, 121
Angle recession, 325
Aniridia, 216, 219, 266
Ankylosing spondylitis, 298
Antazoline, 446
Anterior chamber, angle, 7
Anterior chamber cleavage syndrome, 212
Anterior ciliary arteries, 9
Anterior ischemic optic neuropathy, 88, 98, 143
Anticholinergics, 51, 181
Anticonvulsants, 51
Antifibrinolytic agents, 314
Anti-nuclear antibodies reactions, 157
Aphakia
  glaucoma in, 339, 415, 465, 501, 507
  visual field and, 118
Aplastic anemia, 431
Apparent limbus, 449
Applanometer, 63
Aqueous humor, 6, 454
  active transfer, 12
  amino acids, 12

  ascorbate, 15
  ascorbic acid, 12
  bicarbonate, 12
  carbonic anhydrase, 12
  chloride, 12
  diffusion, 12
  paracentesis, 15
  plasmoid aqueous, 15
  potassium, 12
  production, 12
  sodium, 12
  ultrafiltration, 12
  uveitis, 15
Aqueous veins of Ascher, 18
Arachidonic acid, 445
Argon laser, 284, 461
Artery occlusion
  carotid, 124
  ophthalmic, 124
Arthritis, 297
Aspirin, 303, 430
Astigmatism, visual field and, 118
Astroglial supportive tissue, 83
Astrogliocytes, 78, 81
Atenolol, 416
Atropine, 388, 396
Autonomic nervous system, 385
Axenfeld's anomaly, 213
Axoplasmic flow, 83, 86
Azathioprine, 303

B

Band keratopathy, 396
Barbiturates, 50
Baring of the circumlinear vessel, 95
Barkan focal illuminator, 27
Barkan's membrane, 204, 206
Barraquer tonometer, 63
Basset hounds, spontaneous glaucoma, 373
Bayoneting at the disc edge, 93
Beagles, spontaneous glaucoma, 373
Bean-pot cupping, 97
Behcet's disease, 304
Benzalkonium chloride, 381, 397
Beta-adrenergic agonists, 389
Beta-adrenergic antagonists, 389
Beta-adrenergic receptors, 386
Betamethasone, 363
Bicarbonate
  aqueous humor and, 15
  depletion, 430
Bishydroxycoumarin, 446
Bjerrum's rhomboid, 127
Bjerrum's scotoma, 122
Black cornea, 410
Blepharospasm, 201
Blind spot, 111

DATE DUE

NO 12 '9			